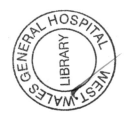
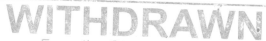

Maternal–Fetal Evidence Based Guidelines

SERIES IN MATERNAL-FETAL MEDICINE

Available

Vincenzo Berghella, *Obstetric Evidence Based Guidelines*
ISBN 9780415701884

Howard Carp, *Recurrent Pregnancy Loss: Causes, Controversies and Treatment*
ISBN 9780415421300

Of related interest

Joseph J Apuzzio, Anthony M Vintzelos, Leslie Iffy, *Operative Obstetrics*
ISBN 9781842142844

Isaac Blickstein, Louis G Keith, *Prenatal Assessment of Multiple Pregnancy*
ISBN 9780415384247

Tom Bourne, George Condous, *Handbook of Early Pregnancy Care*
ISBN 9781842143230

Gian Carlo Di Renzo, Umberto Simeoni, *The Prenate and Neonate: The Transition to Extrauterine Life*
ISBN 9781842140444

Asim Kurjak, Guillermo Azumendi, *The Fetus in Three Dimensions: Imaging, Embryology and Fetoscopy*
ISBN 9780415375238

Asim Kurjak, Frank A Chervenak, *Textbook of Perinatal Medicine*, second edition
ISBN 9781842143339

Catherine Nelson-Piercy, *Handbook of Obstetric Medicine*, third edition
ISBN 9781841845807

Dario Paladini, Paolo Volpe, *Ultrasound of Congenital Fetal Anomalies*
ISBN 9780415414449

Donald M Peebles, Leslie Myatt, *Inflammation and Pregnancy*
ISBN 9781842142721

Felice Petraglia, Jerome F Strauss, Gerson Weiss, Steven G Gabbe, *Preterm Birth: Mechanisms, Mediators, Prediction, Prevention and Interventions*
ISBN 9780415392273

Ruben A Quintero, *Twin-Twin Transfusion Syndrome*
ISBN 9781842142981

Baskaran Thilaganathan, Shanthi Sairam, Aris T Papageorghiou, Amor Bhide, *Problem Based Obstetric Ultrasound*
ISBN 9780415407281

Maternal–Fetal Evidence Based Guidelines

Edited By

Vincenzo Berghella MD FACOG
Director, Division of Maternal–Fetal Medicine
Professor, Department of Obstetrics and Gynecology
Jefferson Medical College of Thomas Jefferson University
Philadelphia, PA
USA

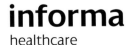

© 2007 Informa UK Ltd

First published in the United Kingdom in 2007 by Informa Healthcare, Telephone House, 69-77 Paul Street, London EC2A 4LQ. Informa Healthcare is a trading division of Informa UK Ltd. Registered Office: 37/41 Mortimer Street, London W1T 3JH. Registered in England and Wales number 1072954.

Tel: +44 (0)20 7017 6000
Fax: +44 (0)20 7017 6699
Email: info.medicine@tandf.co.uk
Website: www.informahealthcare.com

Although every effort has been made to ensure that all owners of copyright material have been acknowledged in this publication, we would be glad to acknowledge in subsequent reprints or editions any omissions brought to our attention.

Although every effort has been made to ensure that drug doses and other information are presented accurately in this publication, the ultimate responsibility rests with the prescribing physician. Neither the publishers nor the authors can be held responsible for errors or for any consequences arising from the use of information contained herein. For detailed prescribing information or instructions on the use of any product or procedure discussed herein, please consult the prescribing information or instructional material issued by the manufacturer.

A CIP record for this book is available from the British Library.

Library of Congress Cataloging-in-Publication Data

Data available on application

ISBN-10: 0 415 43281 2
ISBN-13: 978 0 415 43281 8

Distributed in North and South America by
Taylor & Francis
6000 Broken Sound Parkway, NW, (Suite 300)
Boca Raton, FL 33487, USA
Within Continental USA
Tel: 1 (800) 272 7737; Fax: 1 (800) 374 3401
Outside Continental USA
Tel: (561) 994 0555; Fax: (561) 361 6018
Email: orders@crcpress.com

Distributed in the rest of the world by
Thomson Publishing Services
Cheriton House
North Way
Andover, Hampshire SP10 5BE, UK
Tel: +44 (0)1264 332424
Email: tps.tandfsalesorder@thomson.com

Composition by C&M Digitals (P) Ltd, Chennai, India
Printed and bound in India by Replika Press Pvt. Ltd
Cover image: Leonardo da Vinci, The babe in the Womb ©2007 The Royal Collection, Her Majesty Queen Elizabeth II

Contents

List of contributors   vii
Acknowledgments   xi
Dedication   xiii
List of abbreviations   xv
Introduction   xix
How to 'read' this book   xxi

Part I
Maternal medical complications   1

1. Hypertensive disorders   3
    Jason K Baxter

2. Cardiac disease   23
    Shailen Shah

3. Dermatoses of pregnancy   31
    Dana Correale and Jason B Lee

4. Pregestational and gestational diabetes   43
    Patrice ML Trauffer

5. Hypothyroidism   56
    Alisa B Modena

6. Hyperthyroidism   63
    Alisa B Modena

7. Prolactinoma   68
    Vincenzo Berghella

8. Nausea/vomiting of pregnancy and
    hyperemesis gravidarum   73
    Vincenzo Berghella

9. Intrahepatic cholestasis of pregnancy   78
    Vincenzo Berghella

10. Pregnancy after liver transplantation   81
    *Fabrizio di Francesco, Cataldo Doria, and Ignazio
    R Marino*

11. Maternal anemia   86
    Karen Feisullin

12. Sickle cell disease   91
    Jolene Seibel-Seamon

13. von Willebrand disease   97
    Vincenzo Berghella

14. Care of the Jehovah's Witness
    pregnant woman   101
    Regina L Arvon

15. Renal disease   103
    Alisa B Modena

16. Seizures   113
    Meriem K Bensalem Owen and Franca Cambi

17. Headache   118
    Tarvez Tucker

18. Spinal cord injury   123
    Leonardo Pereira

19. Cancer   127
    Elyce Cardonick

20. Smoking   137
    Julie Takeuchi Crawford and Jorge E Tolosa

21. Depression   144
    David J Lynn and Elisabeth JS Kunkel

22. Respiratory disease   155
    Lauren A Plante

23. Antiphospholipid syndrome   175
    James Airoldi

24. Systemic lupus erythematosus   179
    Vincenzo Berghella

25. Trauma   183
    Lauren A Plante

26. Venous thromboembolism and anticoagulation   192
    James Airoldi

27. Inherited thrombophilia   205
    James Airoldi

28. Hepatitis A   213
    James Airoldi

29. Hepatitis B   215
    James Airoldi

30. Hepatitis C   219
    James Airoldi

31. HIV   223
    Amanda M Cotter and A Marie O'Neill

32. Gonorrhea   234
    A Marie O'Neill

33. Chlamydia   239
    A Marie O'Neill

34. Syphilis   245
    A Marie O'Neill

35. Trichomonas   253
    A Marie O'Neill

36. Group B streptococcus   256
    Marianne Vendola

37. Vaccination   264
    A Marie O'Neill

Part II
Fetus   271

38. Multiple gestations   273
    Edward J Hayes

39. Fetal growth restriction   286
    Juan Carlos Sabogal and Stuart Weiner

40. Fetal macrosomia   294
    Suneet P Chauhan and Everett F Magann

41. CMV   297
    Marianne Vendola

42. Toxoplasmosis   302
    Marianne Vendola

43. Parvovirus   306
    Marianne Vendola

44. Herpes   310
    Marianne Vendola

45. Varicella   315
    Marianne Vendola

46. Fetal death   320
    Irina D Burd

47. Hemolytic disease of the fetus/neonate   327
    *Giancarlo Mari, Farhan Hanif,
    and Kathryin Drennan*

48. Neonatal alloimmune thrombocytopenia   337
    Jason K Baxter

49. Non-immune hydrops fetalis   344
    Arianna Bonato and Dennis C Wood Jr

50. Sonographic assessment of amniotic fluid:
    oligohydramnios and polyhydramnios   352
    Everett F Magann and Suneet P Chauhan

51. Antepartum testing   360
    *Christopher R Harman, Michelle L Kush,
    and Ahmet A Baschat*

52. Fetal lung maturity   383
    Sarah Poggi

Index   389

Contributors

James Airoldi MD
Division of Maternal-Fetal Medicine
Department of Obstetrics and Gynecology
Jefferson Medical College of Thomas Jefferson University
Philadelphia, PA
USA

Regina L Arvon MD
Associate Director
Prenatal Diagnosis Program
California Pacific Medical Center
San Francisco, CA
USA

Ahmet A Baschat MD MB BCH
Associate Professor
Department of Obstetrics, Gynecology,
    and Reproductive Sciences
University of Maryland
Baltimore, MD
USA

Jason K Baxter MD MSCP
Assistant Professor
Division of Maternal-Fetal Medicine
Department of Obstetrics and Gynecology
Jefferson Medical College of Thomas Jefferson University
Philadelphia, PA
USA

Meriem K Bensalem Owen MD
Assistant Professor
Department of Neurology
University of Kentucky
Lexington, KY
USA

Vincenzo Berghella MD
Director, Division of Maternal-Fetal Medicine
Professor, Department of Obstetrics and Gynecology
Jefferson Medical College of Thomas Jefferson University
Philadelphia, PA
USA

Arianna Bonato MD
Migjorn Homebirth
Barcelona
Spain

Irina D Burd MD PHD
Division of Maternal-Fetal Medicine
University of Pennsylvania
Philadelphia, PA
USA

Franca Cambi MD PHD
Associate Professor
Department of Neurology
University of Kentucky
Lexington, KY
USA

Elyce Cardonick MD
Associate Professor
Division of Maternal-Fetal Medicine
Department of Obstetrics and Gynecology
Cooper University Hospital
Camden, NJ
USA

Suneet P Chauhan MD
Director, Division of Maternal-Fetal Medicine
Aurora Health Care
West Allis, WI
USA

Amanda M Cotter MD MSPH
Associate Professor
Director of the Perinatal HIV Service
Division of Maternal-Fetal Medicine
Department of Obstetrics and Gynecology
Miller School of Medicine, University of Miami
Miami, FL
USA

Dana Correale MD
Department of Dermatology and Cutaneous Biology
Jefferson Medical College of Thomas Jefferson University
Philadelphia, PA
USA

Julie Takeuchi Crawford MD
Chief Resident Physician
Department of Obstetrics and Gynecology
Oregon Health and Science University
Portland, OR
USA

Fabrizio di Francesco MD
Division of Transplantation
Department of Surgery
Jefferson Medical College of Thomas Jefferson University
Philadelphia, PA
USA

Cataldo Doria MD PHD
Interim Director,
    Division of Transplantation
Associate Professor, Department of Surgery
Jefferson Medical College of Thomas Jefferson University
Philadelphia, PA
USA

Kathryin Drennan MD
Division of Maternal-Fetal Medicine
Department of Obstetrics and Gynecology
Wayne State University
Detroit, MI
USA

Karen Feisullin MD
Director, Women's Health
Community Health Services
Clinical Assistant Staff
Department of Obstetrics and Gynecology
Hartford, CT
USA

Farhan Hanif MD
Divison of Maternal-Fetal Medicine
Department of Obstetrics and Gynecology
Wayne State University
Detroit, MI
USA

Christopher R Harman MD
Department of Obstetrics, Gynecology
    and Reproductive Sciences
University of Maryland Medical Center
Baltimore, MD
USA

Edward J Hayes MD MSCP
Division of Maternal-Fetal Medicine
Department of Obstetrics and Gynecology
Jefferson Medical College of Thomas Jefferson University
Philadelphia, PA
USA

Elisabeth JS Kunkel MD FAPM
Vice Chairman
Department of Psychiatry and Human Behavior
Jefferson Medical College of Thomas Jefferson University
Philadelphia, PA
USA

Michelle L Kush MD
Department of Obstetrics, Gynecology,
    and Reproductive Sciences
University of Maryland Medical Center
Baltimore, MD
USA

Jason B Lee MD
Director of Dermatopathology and Residency Program
Associate Professor and Clinical Vice-Chairman
Jefferson Dermatology Associates
Department of Dermatology and Cutaneous Biology
Jefferson Medical College of Thomas Jefferson University
Philadelphia, PA
USA

David J Lynn MD
Chief, Department of Psychiatry
Hines Veterans Administration Hospital
Professor of Psychiatry
Loyola University Stritch School of Medicine
Chicago, IL
USA

Everett F Magann MD
Chairman
Department of Obstetrics and Gynecology
Naval Medical Center - Portsmouth
Portsmouth, VA
USA

Giancarlo Mari MD
Director of Fetal Therapy
Division of Maternal-Fetal Medicine
Professor, Department of Obstetrics and Gynecology
Wayne State University
Detroit, MI
USA

Ignazio R Marino MD FACS
Division of Transplantation
Professor, Department of Surgery
Jefferson Medical College of Thomas Jefferson University
Philadelphia, PA
USA

Alisa B Modena MD
Division of Maternal-Fetal Medicine
Virtua Health System
Voorhes, NJ
USA

A Marie O'Neill, MD
Division of Maternal-Fetal Medicine
Department of Obstetrics and Gynecology
Jefferson Medical College of Thomas Jefferson University
Philadelphia, PA
USA

Leonardo Pereira MD
Assistant Professor
Division of Maternal-Fetal Medicine
Department of Obstetrics and Gynecology
Oregon Health and Science University
Portland, OR
USA

Lauren A Plante MD MPH
Associate Professor
Division of Maternal-Fetal Medicine
Department of Obstetrics and Gynecology
Jefferson Medical College of Thomas Jefferson University
Philadelphia, PA
USA

Sarah Poggi MD
Perinatal Diagnostic Center
Inova Alexandria Hospital
Clinical Assistant Professor
Division of Maternal-Fetal Medicine
Department of Obstetrics and Gynecology
Georgetown University
Alexandria, VA, and Washington DC
USA

Juan Carlos Sabogal MD
Department of Obstetrics and Gynecology
Jefferson Medical College of Thomas Jefferson University
Philadelphia, PA
USA

Jolene Seibel-Seamon MD
Division of Maternal-Fetal Medicine
Department of Obstetrics and Gynecology
Jefferson Medical College of Thomas Jefferson University
Philadelphia, PA
USA

Shailen Shah MD
Division of Maternal-Fetal Medicine
Virtua Health System
Assistant Professor
Department of Obstetrics and Gynecology
Jefferson Medical College of Thomas Jefferson University
Voorhes, NJ, and Philadelphia, PA
USA

Jorge E Tolosa MD MSCE
Associate Professor
Division of Maternal-Fetal Medicine
Department of Obstetrics and Gynecology
Oregon Health and Science University
Portland, OR
USA

Patrice ML Trauffer MD
Capital Health Systems
Mercer Perinatal Group
Trenton, NJ
USA

Tarvez Tucker MD
American Migraine Center
Moreland Hills, OH
USA

Marianne Vendola MD
Department of Obstetrics and Gynecology
University of Rome "La Sapienza"
Rome
Italy

Stuart Weiner MD
Director, Reproductive Imaging
Division of Maternal-Fetal Medicine
Department of Obstetrics and Gynecology
Jefferson Medical College of Thomas Jefferson University
Philadelphia, PA
USA

Dennis C Wood Jr BA RDMS RDCS RCPT
Director, Fetal Cardiology
Division of Maternal-Fetal Medicine
Department of Obstetrics and Gynecology
Jefferson Medical College of Thomas Jefferson University
Philadelphia, PA
USA

Acknowledgments

Drs Jorge Tolosa, Suneet Chauhan, Jason Baxter, Lauren Plante, Bud Weiner, Leo Pereira, Regina Arvon, Alisa Modena, Amen Ness, Marie O'Neill, Jim Airoldi, Ted Hayes, John Visintine for reviewing and improving many of these guidelines.

My 'bosses' and mentors, for having given me a chance to practice the job I love, and showing me how to be an obstetrician: my father Andrea Berghella, Stanley Zinberg, Ron Wapner, Richard Depp, Ronald Bolognese, and Louis Weinstein. Finally, but perhaps most importantly, Lynn Stierle, for having been my trusted and patient assistant all these years.

Dedication

To Paola, Andrea, Pietro, mamma and papà, for giving me the serenity,
love, and strength at home now, then, and in the
future to fulfill my dreams and spend my talents as best as I could.

Abbreviations

Ab	antibody
AC	abdominal circumference
ACA	anticardiolipin antibody
ACE	angiotensin-converting enzyme
ACOG	American College of Obstetricians and Gynecologists
ACS	acute chest syndrome
ADR	autonomic dysreflexia
AF	amniotic fluid
AFI	amniotic fluid index
AFP	alpha fetoprotein
AFV	amniotic fluid volume
Ag	antigen
AIDS	acquired immunodeficiency syndrome
ALT	alanine aminotransferase
ANA	antinuclear antibodies
APAs	antiphospholipid antibodies
APS	antiphospholipid syndrome
aPT	activated prothrombin time
aPTT	activated partial thromboplastin time
AROM	artificial rupture of membranes
ART	assisted reproductive technologies
ARV	antiretroviral therapy
ASA	aspirin
ASD	atrial septal defect
AST	aspartate aminotransferase
AT III	antithrombin III
AZT	ziduvudine
bid	'bis in die', i.e. twice per day
BPD	biparietal diameter
BPD	bronchopulmonary dysplasia
BPP	biophysical profile
BMI	body mass index
BP	blood pressure
CAFS	conotruncal anomaly face syndrome
CAP	community-acquired pneumonia
CBC	complete blood count
CD	cesarean delivery
CDC	Center for Disease Control
CF	cystic fibrosis
CHD	congenital heart defect
CL	cervical length
CMV	cytomegalovirus
CNS	central nervous system
CRL	crown–rump length
CSE	combined spinal epidural
CSF	cerebrospinal fluid
CT	computed tomography
CVS	chorionic villus sampling
DES	diethylstilbestrol
DIC	disseminated intravascular coagulation
DM	diabetes mellitus
DNA	deoxyribonucleic acid
DRVVT	dilute Russell's viper venom time
DV	ductus venosus
DVP	deepest vertical pocket
DVT	deep vein thrombosis
ECV	external cephalic version
EDC	estimated date of confinement
EDD	estimated date of delivery (synonym of EDC)
EF	ejection fraction
EKG	electrocardiogram
ERCD	elective repeat cesarean delivery
FBS	fetal blood sampling
FDA	Food and Drug Administration
FFN	fetal fibronectin
FGR	fetal growth restriction
FHR	fetal heart rate
FISH	fluorescent in-situ hybridization
FLM	fetal lung maturity
FOB	father of baby
FPO	fetal pulse oximetry
FPR	false-positive rate
FTS	first trimester screening
FVL	factor V Leiden
g	grams
GA	gestational age
GBS	group B streptococcus
GDM	gestational diabetes mellitus
GI	gastrointestinal
HAART	highly active antiretroviral therapy
HAV	hepatitis A virus
HBsAg	hepatitis B surface antigen
HBV	hepatitis B virus
HCG	human chorionic gonadotropin
Hct	hematocrit
HCV	hepatitis C virus

HG	hyperemesis gravidarum		PC	protein C
Hgb	hemoglobin		PCEA	patient-controlled epidural analgesia
HIE	hypoxic-ischemic encephalopathy		PCI	placental cord insertion
HIV	human immunodeficiency virus		PCR	polymerase chain reaction
HR	heart rate		PE	pulmonary embolus
HSG	hysterosalpinogram		PFTs	pulmonary function tests
HSV	herpes simplex virus		PGM	prothrombin gene mutation
HTN	hypertension		PID	pelvic inflammatory disease
IAI	intra-amniotic infection		PIH	pregnancy-induced hypertension
ICU	intensive care unit		PL	pregnancy loss
IM	intramuscular		PNC	prenatal care
IND	investigational new drug		po	'per os', i.e. by mouth
ITP	idiopathic thrombocytopenic purpura		PPH	postpartum hemorrhage
IUGR	intrauterine growth restriction (synonym of FGR)		PPHN	persistent pulmonary hypertension of the newborn
IUPC	intrauterine pressure catheter		PPROM	preterm premature rupture of membranes
IV	intravenous		PRBC	packed red blood cells
IVH	intraventricular hemorrhage		PROM	preterm rupture of membranes
IVIG	intravenous immune globulin		PS	protein S
L&D	Labor and Delivery (unit)		PSV	peak systolic velocity
LA	lupus anticoagulant		PT	prothrombin time
Lab	laboratory		PTB	preterm birth
LBW	low birth weight (infants)		PTL	preterm labor
LFTs	liver function tests		PTT	partial thromboplastin time
LMP	last menstrual period		PTU	propylthiouracil
LMW	low molecular weight		PUBS	percutaneous umbilical blood sampling
LMWH	low molecular weight heparin		qd	once a day
LPD	luteal phase defect		qid	four times per day
LR	likelihood ratio		qhs	before bedtime
LR	lactated Ringer's solution		QS	quadruple screen
MAS	meconium aspiration syndrome		RBC	red blood cell
MCA	middle cerebral artery		RCT	randomized controlled trial
MCV	mean corpuscular volume		RDS	respiratory distress syndrome
MoM	multiple of the median		REPL	recurrent early pregnancy loss
MRI	magnetic resonance imaging		RNA	ribonucleic acid
MTHFR	methylenetetrahydrofolate reductase		ROM	rupture of membranes
MVP	maximum vertical pocket		RPL	recurrent pregnancy loss
NA	not available		RPR	rapid plasma reagin
NAIT	neonatal alloimmune thrombocytopenia		RR	respiratory rate
NEC	necrotizing enterocolitis		Rx	treatment
NICU	neonatal intensive care unit		SAB	spontaneous abortion
NIH	National Institute of Health		SC	subcutaneous
NIH	non-immune hydrops		SCI	spinal cord injury
NRFHR	non-reassuring fetal heart rate		SDP	single deepest pocket
NRFHT	non-reassuring fetal heart testing		SIDS	sudden infant death syndrome
NRFS	non-reassuring fetal status		SLE	systemic lupus erythematosus
NS	normal saline		SPTB	spontaneous preterm birth
NSAIDs	non-steroidal anti-inflammatory drugs		STD	sexually transmitted diseases (synonym of STI)
NST	non-stress test			
NT	nuchal translucency		STI	sexually transmitted infection
NTDs	neural tube defects		STS	second trimester screening
n/v	nausea and/or vomiting		TB	tuberculosis
OR	operating room		TG	*Toxoplasma gondii*
PAPP-A	pregnancy-associated plasma protein-A		tid	three times per day

TOL	trial of labor	U/S (or u/s)	ultrasound
TRAP	twin reversal arterial perfusion	VAS	visual analogue scale
TSH	thyroid-stimulating hormone	VBAC	vaginal birth after cesarean
TSI	thyroid-stimulating immunoglobulins	VDRL	venereal disease research laboratory
TTTS	twin–twin transfusion syndrome	VSD	ventricular septal defect
TVU	transvaginal ultrasound	VTE	venous thromboembolism
UA	umbilical artery	WHO	World Health Organization
UFH	unfractionated heparin		

Introduction

To me, pregnancy has always been the most fascinating and exciting area of interest, as care involves not one, but at least two persons – the mother and the fetus – and leads to the miracle of a new life. I was a third-year medical student, when, during a lecture, a resident said: 'I went into obstetrics because this is the easiest medical field. Pregnancy is a physiology process, and there isn't much to know. It's simple'. I knew from my 'classic' background that 'obstetrics' means to 'stand by, stay near', and that indeed pregnancy used to receive no medical support at all.

After almost 20 years practicing obstetrics, I know now that while physiologic and at times simple, obstetrics and maternal–fetal medicine can be the **most complex of the medical fields**: pregnancy is based on a different physiology than for non-pregnant women, can include any medical disease, requires surgery, etc. It is not so simple. In fact, ignorance can kill, in this case with the health of the woman and her baby both at risk. Too often I have gone to a lecture, journal club, rounds, or other didactic event to hear presented only one or a few articles regarding the subject, without the presenter reviewing the pertinent best literature and data. It is increasingly difficult to read and acquire all the knowledge that is published, certainly in obstetrics, with over 20 journals publishing on this subject. Some residents or even authorities would state at times that 'there is no evidence' on a topic. Indeed, we used to be the field with the worst use of randomized trials.[1] As the best way to find something is to look for it, my co-authors and I searched for the best evidence. On careful investigation, we found data on almost everything we do in obstetrics, especially on our interventions. Indeed, **our field is now the pioneer for a number of meta-analyses and extension of work for evidence based reviews.**[2] Obstetricians are now blessed with lots of data, and should make the best use of it.

The **aims** of this book are to **summarize the best evidence available in the obstetrics and maternal–fetal medicine literature,** and make the results of randomized trials and meta-analyses **easily accessible to guide clinical care.** The intent is to bridge the gap between knowledge (the evidence) and its easy application. To reach these goals, we reviewed all trials on effectiveness of interventions in obstetrics. **Millions of pregnant women have participated in thousands of properly conducted randomized controlled trials (RCTs).** The efforts and sacrifice of mothers and their fetuses for science should be recognized at least by

Table 1	*Obstetric evidence*
> 600 current Cochrane reviews	
Hundreds of other current meta-analyses	
Thousands of RCTs	
Millions of pregnant women randomized	

the physician's awareness and understanding of these studies. Some of the trials have been summarized in over 600 Cochrane reviews, with hundreds of other meta-analyses also published in obstetric topics (Table 1). All of the Cochrane Reviews, other meta-analyses and trials in obstetrics and maternal–fetal medicine were reviewed and referenced. The material presented in single trials or meta-analyses is too detailed to be readily translated to advice for the busy clinician who needs to make dozens of clinical decisions a day. Even the Cochrane Library, the undiscussed leader for evidence based medicine efforts, has been criticized for its lack of flexibility and relevance in failing to be more easily understandable and clinically readily usable.[3] It was the gap between research and clinicians that needed to be filled, making sure that proven **interventions** are clearly highlighted, and are included in today's care. All pilots fly planes under similar rules to maximize safety; by analogy, all obstetricians should manage all aspects of pregnancy with similar, evidence based rules. Indeed, **only interventions that have been proven to provide benefit should be used routinely.** On the other hand, *primum non nocere*: interventions that have clearly been shown to be not helpful or indeed harmful to mother and/or baby should be avoided. Another aim of the book is to make sure the pregnant woman and her unborn child are not penalized by the medical community. In most circumstances, medical disorders of pregnant women can be treated as in non-pregnant adults. Moreover, there are several effective interventions for preventing or treating specific pregnancy disorders.

Evidence based medicine is the concept of treating patients according to the best available evidence. While George Bernard Shaw said: 'I have my own opinion, do not confuse me with the facts', this can be a deadly approach, especially in medicine, and may compromise two or more lives at the same time in obstetrics and maternal–fetal medicine. What should be the basis for our interventions in medicine? Meta-analyses allow summarizing of the best research

Table 2	*Why did we write this book?*

Many aims:

- Improve the health of women and their children
- 'Make it easy to do it right'
- Clinical best care
- Research ideas
- Education
- Develop lectures
- Decrease disease, use of detrimental interventions, therefore costs
- Reduce medico-legal risks

Table 3	*Who is this book for?*

- Generalists
- Residents
- Nurses
- Medical students
- MFM attendings
- MFM fellows
- Other consultants on pregnancy
- Even lay public who wants to know 'the evidence'
- Politicians responsible for health care

data available. As such, they provide the best guidance for 'effective' clinical care.[4] It is unscientific and unethical to practice medicine or to teach or conduct research without first knowing all that has already been proven.[4] In the absence of trials or meta-analyses, lower-level evidence is reviewed. This book aims at providing a current systematic review of the evidence, **so that current practice and education, as well as future research, can be based on the full story from the best-conducted research, not just the latest data or someone's opinion** (Table 2). These evidence based guidelines cannot be used as a 'cookbook', or a document dictating the best care. The knowledge from the best evidence presented in the guidelines needs to be integrated with other knowledge gained from clinical judgment, individual patient circumstances, and patient preferences, to lead to best medical practice. These are guidelines, not rules. Even the best scientific studies are not always perfectly related to any given individual, and clinical judgment must still be applied to allow the best 'particularizations' of the best knowledge for the individual, unique patient. Evidence based medicine informs clinical judgment, but does not substitute it. However, it is important to understand that greater clinical experience by the physician actually correlates with inferior quality of care, if not integrated with knowledge of the best evidence.[5] The appropriate treatment is given in only 50% of visits to general physicians.[5] At times, limitations in resources may also limit the physicians' knowledge. Guidelines and clinical pathways based on evidence not only point to the right management but also can decrease medico-legal risk.[6]

We aimed for brevity and clarity. Suggested management of the healthy or sick mother and child is stated as straightforwardly as possible, **for everyone to easily understand and implement** (Table 3). If you find the Cochrane Reviews, scientific manuscripts and books difficult to 'translate' into care of your patients, this book is for you. We wanted to prevent information overload. On the other hand, as stated by Albert Einstein, 'everything should be made as simple as possible, but not simpler'. Key management points are highlighted at the beginning of each guideline, and in bold in the text. The chapters are divided in two volumes: one of obstetrics and one on maternal–fetal medicine. Please contact vincenzo.berghella@jefferson.edu or www.jefferson.edu/mfm for any comments, criticisms, corrections, missing evidence, etc.

I have the most fun discovering the best ways to alleviate discomfort and disease. The search for the best evidence for these guidelines has been a wonderful, stimulating journey. Keeping up with evidence-based medicine is exciting. The most rewarding part, as a teacher, is the dissemination of knowledge. I hope, truly, that this effort will be helpful to you, too.

References

1. Cochrane AL. 1931–1971: a critical review, with particular reference to the medical profession. In: Medicines for the Year 2000. London: Office to Health Economics; 1979: 1–11. [review]
2. Dickersin K, Manheimer E. The Cochrane Collaborations: evaluation of health care services using systematic reviews of the results of randomized controlled trials. Clin Obstet Gynecol 1998: 41: 315–31. [review]
3. Summerskill W. Cochrane Collaborations and the evolution of evidence. Lancet 2005; 366: 1760. [review]
4. Chalmers I. Academia's failure to support systematic reviews. Lancet 2005; 365: 469. [III]
5. Arky RA. The family business – to educate. N Engl J Med 2006; 354: 1922–6. [review]
6. Ransom SB, Studdert DM, Dombrowski MP, Mello MM. Brennan TA. Reduced medico-legal risk by compliance with obstetric clinical pathways: a case-control study. Obstet Gynecol 2003; 101: 751–5. [II-2]

How to 'read' this book

The knowledge from all currently available randomized controlled trials (RCTs) and meta-analyses in obstetrics is summarized and easily available for clinical implementation. Key management points are highlighted at the beginning of each guideline, and in bold in the text. Relative risks and 95% confidence intervals from studies are generally not quoted, unless trends were evident, to avoid crowding the text. Instead, the straight recommendation for care is made if one intervention is superior to the other, with the percent improvement often quoted to assess degree of benefit. If there is insufficient evidence to compare interventions or managements, this is clearly stated.

An evidence based book must be based on adequate references, so to let "res ipsa loquitur" ('things speak for themselves'). Cochrane Reviews with 0 RCT are not referenced, and, instead of referencing a meta-analysis with only one RCT, the actual RCT is referenced. If a meta-analysis includes >10 RCTs, not all RCTs are referenced, for brevity and because they can be easily accessed by reviewing the meta-analysis. If new RCTs are not included in meta-analysis, they are obviously referenced. Each reference was reviewed and evaluated for quality according to a modified method as outlined by the US Preventive Services Task Force (www.ahrq.gov):

I	Evidence obtained from at least one properly designed randomized controlled trial.
II-1	Evidence obtained from well-designed controlled trials without randomization.
II-2	Evidence obtained from well-designed cohort or case-control analytic studies, preferably from more than one center or research group.
II-3	Evidence obtained from multiple time series with or without the intervention. Dramatic results in uncontrolled experiments could also be regarded as this type of evidence.
III (review)	Opinions of respected authorities, based on clinical experience, descriptive studies, or reports of expert committees.

These levels were quoted after each reference. For RCTs and meta-analyses, the number of subjects studied was stated, and, sometimes, more details were provided to aid the reader to understand the study better.

Part I

Maternal medical complications

A. Cardiology

1. Hypertensive disorders
2. Cardiac disease

B. Dermatology

3. Dermatoses of pregnancy

C. Endocrinology

4. Pregestational and gestational diabetes
5. Hypothyroidism
6. Hyperthyroidism
7. Prolactinoma

D. Gastroenterology

8. Nausea/vomiting of pregnancy and hyperemesis gravidarum
9. Intrahepatic cholestasis of pregnancy
10. Pregnancy after liver transplantation

E. Hematology

11. Maternal anemia
12. Sickle cell disease
13. Von Willebrand disease
14. Care of the Jehovah's Witness pregnant woman

F. Nephrology

15. Renal disease

G. Neurology

16. Seizures
17. Headache
18. Spinal cord injury

H. Oncology

19. Cancer

I. Psychiatry and Abuse

20. Smoking
21. Depression

J. Pulmonology

22. Respiratory disease

K. Rheumatology

23. Antiphospholipid syndrome
24. Systemic lupus erythematosus

L. **Trauma**

25. Trauma

M. **Thromboembolic Disease**

26. Venous thromboembolism and anticoagulation
27. Inherited thrombophilia

N. **Infectious Diseases**

28. Hepatitis A
29. Hepatitis B
30. Hepatitis C
31. HIV
32. Gonorrhea
33. Chlamydia
34. Syphilis
35. Trichomonas
36. Group B streptococcus
37. Vaccination

1

Hypertensive disorders*

Jason K Baxter

CHRONIC HYPERTENSION

KEY POINTS

- Chronic hypertension (HTN) in **pregnancy** is defined as either (a) a **history of hypertension preceding the pregnancy** or (b) a **blood pressure ≥ 140/90 mmHg prior to 20 weeks' gestation**.
- Severe HTN has been defined as systolic blood pressure (SBP) ≥ 160/180 mmHg or diastolic blood pressure (DBP) ≥ 110 mmHg. **High-risk HTN has been defined in pregnancy as that associated with secondary hypertension, target organ damage (left ventricular dysfunction, retinopathy, dyslipidemia, maternal age > 40 years old, microvascular disease, prior stroke), previous loss, SBP ≥ 180 mmHg or DBP ≥ 110 mmHg.**
- **Complications** of chronic HTN include (maternal) worsening HTN; superimposed pre-eclampsia; severe pre-eclampsia; eclampsia, HELLP syndrome; cesarean delivery, and (uncommonly) **pulmonary edema, hypertensive encephalopathy, retinopathy, cerebral hemorrhage, and acute renal failure**, and (fetal) **growth restriction; oligohydramnios; placental abruption; preterm birth; and perinatal death**.
- **Prevention** (mostly pre-pregnancy) consists of **exercise, weight reduction, proper diet**, and **restriction of sodium intake**.
- **Initial evaluation** may include, in addition to **history** and **physical examination, liver function tests (LFTs); platelets; creatinine; urine analysis; and 24-hour urine for total protein (and creatinine clearance)**. Women with high-risk, severe, or long-standing HTN may need an electrocardiogram (EKG) and echocardiogram, as well. If hypertension is newly diagnosed and has not been evaluated previously, a medical consult may be indicated to assess for possible etiological factors (renal artery stenosis, pheochromocytoma, hyperaldosteronism, etc.).
- There is **insufficient evidence** to assess **bed rest** for managing HTN in pregnancy.
- Blood pressure (BP) decreases physiologically in the first and second trimester in pregnancy, especially in women with HTN. **As blood pressure is usually < 140/90 mmHg at the first visit for hypertensive women, often antihypertensive drugs not only do not need to be increased but also can be stopped.** Often BP will increase again in the third trimester, leading to work-up for pre-eclampsia, and, if pre-eclampsia is absent, restarting of antihypertensive drugs. So antihypertensive medications should probably **be started (or increased, modified) in pregnancy only when SBP ≥ 160 mmHg or DBP ≥ 100 mmHg on two occasions. The goal is to maintain a BP of around 140–150/90–100 mmHg. With end-organ damage (high-risk HTN), e.g. renal disease, diabetes with vascular disease, or left ventricular dysfunction, these thresholds should probably be lowered to < 140/90 mmHg.**
- **Labetalol is considered the current antihypertensive drug of choice** by many experts, based on limited trial data. Dosing can start at 100 mg twice a day, with maximum dose of 1200 mg twice a day. **Nifedipine** is a reasonable alternative, started at 10 mg twice a day, with maximum dose of 120 mg/day. **Angiotensin-converting enzyme (ACE) inhibitors are contraindicated** in pregnancy.

---

*Hypertensive disorders of pregnancy include chronic hypertension, gestational hypertension, pre-eclampsia, HELLP syndrome, and eclampsia.

Diagnosis/definition

Chronic hypertension in pregnancy is defined as either a history of hypertension preceding the pregnancy or a blood pressure ≥ 140/90 mmHg prior to 20 weeks' gestation. Though controversial, the 5th Korotkoff sound is used for the diastolic reading. Blood pressure (BP) measurements can be obtained using a manual or an automated cuff with the patient in the sitting position. Severe hypertension is defined as systolic blood pressure (SBP) ≥ 160 mmHg or diastolic blood pressure (DBP) ≥ 110 mmHg. In **non-pregnant** adults: BP < 120/80 mmHg is normal; BP 120–139/80–89 mmHg is prehypertension; BP 140–159/ 90–99 mmHg is stage 1 hypertension; and BP ≥ 160/100 mmHg is stage 2 hypertension.

Epidemiology/incidence

Hypertension (HTN) occurs in about **1–5%** of pregnant women. Hypertension in pregnancy is the second leading cause of maternal mortality in the USA, accounting for about 15% of such deaths. Hypertensive disorders such as hypertension, gestational hypertension, pre-eclampsia, or HELLP syndrome occur in 12–22% of pregnancies.

Etiology/basic pathophysiology

Hypertension mostly develops as a complex quantitative trait affected by both genetic and environmental factors.

Classification

Severe HTN has been defined as SBP ≥ 160–180 mmHg and DBP ≥ 110 .[1] **High-risk** HTN has been defined in pregnancy as that associated with **secondary hypertension, target organ damage (left ventricular dysfunction, retinopathy, dyslipidemia, maternal age > 40 years old, microvascular disease, prior stroke), previous loss, SBP ≥ 180 mmHg or DBP ≥ 110 mmHg.** For gestational HTN, see below.

Risk factors/associations

Renal disease; collagen vascular disease; antiphospholipid syndrome; diabetes; other endocrine disorders such as thyrotoxicosis, Cushing's disease, hyperaldosteronism, pheochromocytoma, or coartation of the aorta.

Complications[2]
Maternal

Worsening HTN, superimposed pre-eclampsia (20%), severe pre-eclampsia, eclampsia, HELLP, and cesarean delivery. Pulmonary edema, hypertensive encephalopathy, retinopathy, cerebral hemorrhage, and acute renal failure are uncommon, but are more common with severe HTN.

Fetal

Growth restriction (8–15%); oligohydramnios, placental abruption (0.7–1.5%, about a two-fold increase), preterm birth (PTB; 12–34%), and perinatal death (2–4-fold increase).

All these complications have higher incidences with severe or high-risk hypertension.

Management
Principles

Pregnancy is characterized by increased blood volume, decreased colloid oncotic pressure (see also Chapter 2 of *Obstetric Evidence Based Guidelines*). Physiological BP decrease in first and second trimester may mask chronic HTN.

Initial evaluation/work-up
History

Antihypertensive drugs; prior work-up; end-organ damage; and prior obstetric history.

Physical examination

Blood pressure; edema.

Laboratory tests

Baseline values must be known in order to be able to compare in cases of possible later pre-eclampsia. **Liver function tests (LFTs); platelets; creatinine; urine analysis; 24-hour urine for total protein (and creatinine clearance); antinuclear antibodies (ANA); anticardiolipin antibody (ACA) and lupus anticoagulant (LA)** (see also Chapter 23). An early glucose challenge test may be indicated. Coagulation studies (especially fibrinogen) are usually not indicated, except in specific severe cases. Creatinine clearance (ml/min) is calculated as:

(Urine creatinine (mg/dl) × Total urine volume (ml)/ (serum creatinine (mg/dl) × 1440 minutes)

Other tests

Maternal electrocardiogram (EKG), echocardiogram **and ophthalmological examination** are suggested, especially in women with high-risk or severe hypertension.

Work-up

It is important to identify cardiovascular risk factors, any reversible cause of hypertension, and assess for target organ damage or cardiovascular disease. Reversible causes include chronic kidney disease, coartation of the aorta, Cushing's syndrome, drug-induced/related causes, **pheochromocytoma, hyperaldosteronism, renovascular hypertension** (renal artery stenosis), thyroid/parathyroid disease, and sleep apnea. **If hypertension is newly diagnosed and has not been evaluated previously, a medical consult** may be indicated to assess for any of these factors. Secondary hypertension, target organ damage (left ventricular dysfunction, retinopathy, dyslipidemia, maternal age >40 years old, microvascular disease, prior stroke), previous loss, SBP ≥ 180 mmHg or DBP ≥ 110 mmHg are associated with higher risks in pregnancy.

Prevention

Thirty minutes of **exercise** three times per week in women with mild hypertension, gestational hypertensive disorders, or a family history of hypertensive disorders may decrease DBP, as per a very small trial.[3] **Weight reduction** preconception is recommended if overweight. A **proper diet** should be rich in fruits, vegetables, low-fat dairy foods, with reduced saturated and total fats. **Restriction of sodium intake** to the same < 2.4 g sodium daily intake recommended for essential hypertension is beneficial in non-pregnant adults. Strongly discourage the use of alcohol and tobacco.

Screening/diagnosis

Initial BP evaluation may help to identify women with chronic hypertension, while third trimester BP readings aid in pre-eclampsia screening. **A BP of ≥ 120/80 mmHg in the first or second trimester is not normal,** and is associated with later risks of pre-eclampsia. **Blood pressure should be taken properly.** Appropriate measurement of BP includes using Korotkoff phase V, appropriate cuff size (length 1.5 × upper arm circumference, or a cuff with a bladder that encircles ≥ 80% of the arm), and position so that the woman's arm is at the level of the heart (sitting up), at rest.

Preconception counseling

There are significant risks associated with hypertension and pre-eclampsia in pregnancy. All women should be counseled appropriately regarding the possible complications and preventive and management strategies for hypertensive disorders in pregnancy. Angiotensin-converting enzyme (ACE) inhibitors and angiotensin type II (AII) receptor antagonists should be discontinued. A complete evaluation and work-up, as described above, should be done, especially if there is a several-year history of hypertension and/or hypertension never fully evaluated. Baseline tests can also be obtained for later comparison. Abnormalities should be addressed and managed appropriately (see specific chapters). If, for example, serum creatinine (Cr) is > 1.4 mg/dl, the woman should be aware of increased risks in pregnancy (pregnancy/fetal loss, reduced birthweight, preterm delivery, and accelerated deterioration of maternal renal disease). Even mild renal disease (Cr = 1.1 − 1.4 mg/dl) with uncontrolled HTN is associated with 10× higher risk of fetal loss.

Prenatal care

Often BP monitoring at home is suggested in pregnancies with HTN. There is no randomized controlled trial (RCT) evidence to support the use of ambulatory BP monitoring during pregnancy.

Therapy
Lifestyle changes

There are no trials to assess lifestyle changes other than bed rest in pregnancy. Weight reduction in pregnancy is not recommended. The diet should be rich in fruits, vegetables, and low-fat dairy foods, with reduced saturated and total fats, and with sodium intake restricted to < 2.4 g of sodium daily.

Bed rest
There is **insufficient evidence** to demonstrate any differences between bed rest (in or out of the hospital) for reported outcomes overall. Compared with routine activity at home, some bed rest in hospital for **non-proteinuric hypertension** is associated with a 42% reduced risk of severe hypertension and a borderline 47% reduction in risk of preterm birth in one trial.[4] The trials do not address possible adverse effects of bed rest. Three times more women in the bed rest group opt not to have the same management in future pregnancies, if the choice is given. There are no significant differences for any other outcomes.[4]

Antihypertensive drugs

Common types
Methyldopa (Aldomet). This drug was the preferred first-line treatment historically, since it is associated with stable uteroplacental blood flow and fetal hemodynamics, and no long-term adverse effects seen in exposed children (up

to 7.5 years old; best documentation of fetal safety of any antihypertensive drug). Liver disease is a contraindication. The initial dose is usually 250 mg two or three times a day, with highest dose 500 mg four times a day (2 g/day). Side effects include dry mouth and drowsiness/somnolence.

Labetalol (alpha- and beta-blocker). Labetalol is the **current drug of choice** of many experts, based on limited trial data (see below).[1] Dosing can start at 100 mg twice a day, with a maximum dose of 1200 mg twice a day. As with other drugs, generally a different agent should not be added until the maximum doses of the first drug are achieved.

Beta-blockers. Atenolol has been associated with fetal growth restriction (FGR) in pregnancy compared with placebo, and with higher mortality in non-pregnant adults compared to other agents, and should probably be avoided. There is insufficient evidence to assess if other drugs in this class (or even other classes) are associated with the same effect (see below).

Calcium channel blockers (especially nifedipine). There is no known association with birth defects, with reassuring long-term follow-up of babies up to 1.5 years. Nifedipine can be started at 10 mg twice a day, with a maximum dose of 120 mg/day. Long-acting nifedipine XL can be started at 30 mg, with 120 mg as maximum dose. Very rare cases of neuromuscular blockade have been reported when nifedipine is used simultaneously with magnesium sulfate. This blockade is reversible with a 10% solution of calcium gluconate.

Diuretics. Women who use diuretics from early in pregnancy do not have the physiological increase in plasma volume, which poses a theoretical concern since pre-eclampsia is associated with reduced plasma volume. Nonetheless, the reduction in plasma volume associated with diuretics has not been associated with adverse effects on outcomes. Diuretics are not contraindicated in pregnancy, except in settings where uteroplacental perfusion is already reduced (i.e. pre-eclampsia and FGR). This is usually the drug of first choice for some non-pregnant adults. The initial dose is usually 12.5 mg twice a day, with a maximum dose of 50 mg/day.

Angiotensin-converting enzyme (ACE) inhibitors (or AII receptor antagonists). These drugs are contraindicated in the first trimester because they might be associated with a two-fold increase in malformations, and later because they are associated with FGR, oligohydramnios, neonatal renal failure, and neonatal death.

Effectiveness
Mild to moderate HTN. This is usually defined in the trials as a SBP of 140–169 mmHg or a DBP of 90–109 mmHg. In pregnant women with **mild to moderate hypertension**, antihypertensive drugs are associated with a **48% reduction of the risk of developing severe hypertension,** which is expected given their effects in non-pregnant adults. There is **no difference in pre-eclampsia, preterm birth, small for gestational age, perinatal death** (non-significant 29% reduction), **or any other outcomes.**[5] Improvement in control of maternal BP with use of drugs would be worthwhile only if it were reflected in substantive benefits for the mother and/or baby, and none have been clearly demonstrated.

Compared to placebo/no beta-blocker, oral beta-blockers decrease by 63% the risk of severe hypertension and by 56% the need for additional antihypertensives. Maternal hospital admission may be decreased, neonatal bradycardia increased, and respiratory distress syndrome decreased, but these outcomes are reported in only a small proportion of trials.[6] There are insufficient data for conclusions about the effect on perinatal mortality or preterm birth.[6] Compared with controls not taking antihypertensives, women receiving **beta-blockers** had a 36–56% increase in small for gestational age (SGA) birthweight and a three-fold **increase in birthweight < 5% percentile.**[5,6] **The woman's natural BP may be necessary for adequate placental perfusion, so that artificial lowering of the BP may then impair fetal growth.** There is insufficient evidence to assess if beta-blockers are more detrimental in this respect than other antihypertensive regimens. Compared with methyldopa, beta-blockers appear to be no more effective and probably equally as safe. Single small trials have compared beta-blockers with hydralazine, nicardipine, or isradipine. It is unusual for women to change drugs due to side effects.[6] Other antihypertensive agents seem better than methyldopa for reducing (by 51%) the risk of fetal death.[5] Other outcomes are only reported by a small proportion of studies, and there are no clear differences.

As BP is usually < 140/90 mmHg at the first visit for hypertensive women, often antihypertensive drugs not only do not need to be increased but also can be stopped. Often BP will increase again in the third trimester, leading to work-up for pre-eclampsia, and, if pre-eclampsia is absent, restarting of antihypertensive drugs. So **antihypertensive medications should probably be started (or increased, modified) in pregnancy only when SBP ≥ 160 mmHg, or DBP ≥ 100 mmHg on two occasions.** This is to decrease the risk of cerebrovascular accidents and cardiovascular (e.g. congestive heart failure) and renal complications. **The goal is to maintain BP at around 140–150/90–100 mmHg. With end-organ damage (high-risk HTN) – e.g. renal disease, diabetes with vascular disease, or left ventricular dysfunction – these thresholds should probably be lowered to < 140/90 mmHg.**

Severe HTN   (This is usually defined in the trials as SBP ≥ 160 mmHg or diastolic DBP ≥ 110 mmHg.) There is insufficient evidence to assess benefits and risks of different antihypertensive drugs for severe HTN. Hydralazine is the most common drug evaluated in trials. **Diazoxide** and **ketanserin** should probably be **avoided**.[7] Diazoxide, given as 75 mg bolus injections, appears to be associated with maternal hypotension requiring treatment. Ketanserin is less effective than hydralazine at reducing BP. There is no other clear evidence that any one of the other antihypertensive agents is better than another for women with severe hypertension during pregnancy.[7] Therefore, the choice of antihypertensive should depend on the experience and familiarity of an individual clinician with a particular drug, and on what is known about adverse maternal and fetal side effects. Exceptions are diazoxide and ketanserin, which are probably not good choices (see also below under severe pre-eclampsia).

Antepartum testing

Increased perinatal morbidity and mortality is mainly attributed to superimposed pre-eclampsia and/or FGR; therefore, look to detect these early.

Initial **dating ultrasound**, preferably in the first trimester (FTS at 11–14 weeks), **anatomy ultrasound** at around 18–20 weeks, and **ultrasound for growth** at 28–32 weeks are suggested (see also Chapter 3 of *Obstetric Evidence Based Guidelines*).

Antenatal testing (usually with weekly non-stress tests [NSTs]) is suggested starting around 32 weeks, especially if poorly controlled or severe HTN, FGR, or pre-eclampsia. Umbilical artery Doppler is recommended in cases of FGR (see Chapter 39). For uterine artery Doppler, see under pre-eclampsia.

Delivery

Often preterm birth (either spontaneous or iatrogenic) occurs because of complications. In the uncomplicated pregnancy with hypertension, the pregnancy should probably be delivered by the estimated date of confinement (EDC).

Anesthesia

See below under pre-eclampsia, and also Chapter 10 of *Obstetric Evidence Based Guidelines*.

Post-partum/breastfeeding

Methyldopa, labetalol, beta-blockers, calcium channel blockers, and most other agents are safe with breastfeeding, with the possible exception of ACE inhibitors, because low concentrations in breast milk could affect neonatal renal function.

GESTATIONAL HYPERTENSION
Definition

Sustained (on at least two occasions, 6 hours apart) BP ≥ 140/90 mmHg after 20 weeks, without proteinuria, other signs or symptoms of pre-eclampsia, or a prior history of HTN. Formerly known as pregnancy induced hypertension (PIH). Severe gestational HTN is defined similarly, except that the cut-offs are ≥ 160/110 mmHg.

Incidence

About 6–17% in healthy nulliparous women.

Complications and management

This condition is usually associated with good outcomes, similar to low-risk pregnant women,[8] so that **close surveillance for development of pre-eclampsia** but no other interventions are usually needed. Severe gestational HTN is associated with higher morbidities than mild pre-eclampsia, with incidences of abruption, PTB, and SGA similar to severe pre-eclampsia. If gestational HTN develops before 30 weeks or is severe, there is a high (50%) rate of progression to pre-eclampsia.

PRE-ECLAMPSIA
KEY POINTS

- **Pre-eclampsia** is defined as sustained (at least twice, 6 hours but not > 7 days apart) **BP ≥ 140/90 mmHg** (in the absence of chronic HTN), and proteinuria (**≥ 300 mg in 24 hours in a woman without prior proteinuria**).
- **Superimposed pre-eclampsia** is defined as proteinuria (≥ 300 mg in 24 hours in a woman without prior proteinuria) after 20 weeks in a woman with chronic HTN.
- **Severe pre-eclampsia** is defined as pre-eclampsia with any of: BP ≥ 160/110 mmHg, proteinuria ≥ 5 g in 24 hours, platelets < 100 000/mm³, aspartate aminotransferase (AST) and/or ALT ≥ 70 U/L, persistent headache or other cerebral or visual disturbances

(including grand mal seizures), persistent epigastric (or right upper quadrant) pain, pulmonary edema, or oliguria (< 500 ml urine in 24 hours).

- **HELLP syndrome** is defined as **hemolysis, AST or ALT ≥ 70 U/L, platelets < 100 000/mm³**.
- **Eclampsia** is defined as seizures in the presence of pre-eclampsia and/or HELLP syndrome.
- **Complications** of pre-eclampsia include (maternal) HELLP syndrome, disseminated intravascular coagulation (DIC), pulmonary edema, abruptio placentae, renal failure, seizures (eclampsia), cerebral hemorrhage, liver hemorrhage, and (fetal/neonatal) PTB, FGR, perinatal death, and hypoxemia-neurological injury.
- **Low-dose aspirin** (at least **81 mg/day starting preferably around 12 weeks and before 20 weeks**) given to women with **risk factors for pre-eclampsia** is associated with a **19% reduction** in the risk of **pre-eclampsia**, a small (8%) reduction in the risk of PTB < 37 weeks, an 8% reduction in SGA babies, and a 16% reduction in perinatal deaths.
- **Low-dose aspirin** in women with **abnormal uterine Doppler** at 14–24 weeks is associated with a **22% reduction** in pre-eclampsia, with insufficient data to assess other important outcomes.
- While **calcium supplementation** is associated with a 42% reduction in the incidence of high blood pressure and a 65% reduction in the risk of pre-eclampsia, especially in women at high risk of hypertension and those with low baseline calcium intake, the **largest trial** reported **no reduction** in the rate, severity, or timing of onset of pre-eclampsia.
- **Vitamin C** 1000 mg/day and **vitamin E** 400 mg/day starting in the early second trimester are associated with an 18% reduction in risk of pre-eclampsia, an 8% trend for reduction in **PTB**, and no effect on SGA or fetal or neonatal death. Given the fact that the two largest most recent trials do not show any maternal or fetal benefit, not even a reduction in pre-eclampsia, and that in one of them the intervention is associated with pre-eclampsia appearing 8 days earlier and more frequent gestational hypertension, antioxidant therapy should **not be recommended for prevention of pre-eclampsia**.
- Work-up for pre-eclampsia should include, apart from history and physical examination (BP), AST and ALT, platelets, creatinine, and 24-hour urine for total protein (and creatinine clearance). It is **important to know the baseline values**; hence, these tests should be obtained at the first prenatal visit in women with risk factors.
- **Magnesium is the drug of choice for prevention of eclampsia**, as it is associated with a 59% **reduction in the risk of eclampsia**, a 36% reduction in **abruption**, and a non-statistically significant but clinically important 46% reduction in **maternal death**. The reduction is similar, regardless of severity of pre-eclampsia, with

about 400 women needing to be treated to prevent eclampsia for mild pre-eclampsia, 71 for severe pre-eclampsia, and 36 for pre-eclampsia with central nervous system (CNS) symptoms. The **intravenous** route at **1 g/h is preferable, usually given at least in active labor and for 12–24 hours postpartum**, but for a shorter or longer period depending on the severity of pre-eclampsia, without mandatory serum monitoring.

- **Antihypertensive drugs** for the treatment of **severe HTN** with pre-eclampsia are usually **labetalol, nifedipine, or hydralazine**.
- **Severe pre-eclampsia at ≥ 32–34 weeks** warrants **expedited delivery**, possibly after steroids for fetal maturity between 32 and 33 6/7 weeks. Expedited delivery even at **< 32 weeks** is suggested for **uncontrollable BP** in spite of continuing increase in antihypertensive drugs, **persistent headache and/or visual/CNS symptoms, epigastric pain, vaginal bleeding, persistent oliguria, preterm labor, preterm premature rupture of membranes (PPROM), platelets < 100 000/mm³, and non-reassuring fetal heart rate testing**.
- There is **insufficient evidence to recommend the use of dexamethasone** or other steroids for therapy specific for HELLP syndrome.
- In **about 15% of cases, hypertension or proteinuria** may be **absent before eclampsia**. A **high index of suspicion for eclampsia** should be maintained in **all cases of hypertensive disorders in pregnancy**, in particular those with CNS (e.g. headache, visual) disturbances.
- In eclampsia, the first priorities are **airway, breathing, and circulation**.
- **Magnesium sulfate is certainly the drug of choice for preventing recurrence of eclampsia**, as it is also associated with maternal and fetal/neonatal benefits.
- Women with **prior pre-eclampsia or its complications** are not only at **increased risk of recurrence** but also at **increased risk of cardiovascular disease in the future**.

Diagnoses/definitions
Pre-eclampsia

Sustained (at least twice, 6 hours but not > 7 days apart) BP ≥ 140/90 mmHg (in the absence of chronic HTN) and **proteinuria (300 mg in 24 hours in a woman without prior proteinuria)**.[9,10] BP should be measured with adequate cuff size, position of the heart at arm level, and with calibrated equipment. The accuracy of dipstick urinalysis with a 1 + (0.1 g/L) threshold as well as random protein-to-creatinine ratios in the prediction of significant proteinuria by 24-hour urine is poor.[11] **Mild pre-eclampsia** is usually defined as pre-eclampsia not meeting severe criteria (see below). 'Toxemia' is a lay term. The '30–15 rule' and edema have been eliminated as criteria for pre-eclampsia.

Superimposed pre-eclampsia

Proteinuria (≥ 300 mg in 24 hours in a woman without prior proteinuria) after 20 weeks in a woman with chronic HTN.

Severe pre-eclampsia

Pre-eclampsia, with any one of the following criteria:

- BP ≥ 160/110 mmHg (two occasions, ≥ 6 hours apart)
- proteinuria ≥ 5 g in 24 hours. Some propose 2 g in 24 hours, instead
- platelets < 100 000/mm³ (and/or evidence of microangiopathic hemolytic anemia)
- increased hepatic transaminases (AST and/or ALT ≥ 70 U/L)
- persistent headache or other cerebral or visual disturbances (including grand mal seizures)
- persistent epigastric (or right upper quadrant) pain
- pulmonary edema
- oliguria (< 500 ml urine in 24 hours).

FGR, an increased serum creatinine >1.2 mg/dl, or other conditions are associated with worse outcomes with pre-eclampsia, but are not always considered criteria for severe pre-eclampsia.

HELLP (**H**emolysis, **E**levated **L**iver enzymes and **L**ow **P**latelet count) syndrome

Hemolysis (microangiopathic hemolytic anemia, with at least two of the following: schistocytes, Burr cells in peripheral smear; serum bilirubin ≥ 1.2 mg/dl; low serum haptoglobin), **AST or ALT** (liver enzymes) at least twice the level of normal, or ≥ 70 U/L, **platelets** < 100 000/mm³.

Eclampsia

Seizures in the presence of pre-eclampsia and/or HELLP syndrome.

Symptoms

Persistent headache or other cerebral or visual disturbances (including grand mal seizures) and persistent epigastric (or right upper quadrant) pain are criteria for severe pre-eclampsia. Edema, especially central, should prompt evaluation of pre-eclampsia.

Epidemiology/incidence

In healthy nulliparous women, about 7% (most at term and mild).

Etiology/basic pathophysiology

Pre-eclampsia is a **systemic** disease of unknown etiology. It is associated with **endothelial disease** and with **vasospasm** and **sympathetic overactivity**. Trophoblastic invasion by the placenta into the spiral arteries of the uterus is **incomplete**, resulting in **reduced perfusion**. Hypoxia, free radicals, oxidative stress, and activation of endothelium are characteristics. Thromboxane (which is associated with vasoconstriction, platelet aggregation, and decreased uteroplacental blood flow) is increased, while prostacyclin (which has opposite effects) is decreased. FGR is also theorized to develop as a result of defective placentation and the imbalance between prostacyclin and thromboxane.

- Alterations of the immune response.
- *Vascular*: vasospasm and subsequent hemoconcentration are associated with contraction of intravascular space; **capillary leak** and decreased colloid oncotic pressure may predispose to pulmonary edema.
- *Cardiac*: usually reduced cardiac output, decreased plasma volume, and increased systemic vascular resistance.
- *Hematological*: thrombocytopenia and hemolysis with HELLP syndrome (also elevated lactate dehydrogenase [LDH]).
- *Hepatic*: elevated AST, ALT; subcapsular hematoma.
- *CNS*: eclampsia, intracranial hemorrhage, headache, blurred vision, scotomata, hyperreflexia, and temporary blindness.
- *Renal*: vasospasm, hemoconcentration, and decreased renal blood flow, resulting in oliguria (rarely leading to acute tubular necrosis, possibly leading to acute renal failure).
- *Fetal*: impaired uteroplacental blood flow (FGR, oligohydramnios, abruption, and non-reassuring fetal heart rate testing [NRFHT]).

Classification

See 'mild' vs severe, above.

Risk factors/associations

Nulliparity, limited sperm exposure, primipaternity, 'dangerous father' (for pre-eclampsia), donor eggs and/or sperm, multifetal gestation, prior pre-eclampsia, chronic HTN, diabetes, vascular and connective tissue disease, nephropathy, antiphospholipid syndrome (APS), obesity, insulin resistance, young maternal age (YMA) or advanced maternal age (AMA), African-American race, family history of pre-eclampsia, maternal low birth weight, low socioeconomic status, increased soluble fms-like tyrosine kinase 1 (sFlt-1), reduced placental growth factor (PlGF), and higher fetal cells in maternal circulation. A change in partner is usually associated with a protective effect if prior pregnancy had pre-eclampsia. Previous pregnancy with same partner seems to be protective, albeit for a short (1–3 years) time. While case reports have associated pre-eclampsia with some thrombophilias, only hyperhomocysteinemia is associated with pre-eclampsia in prospective studies, with no studies to assess interventions for this association (see also Chapter 27). Smoking is associated with decreased incidence of pre-eclampsia. There are no sensitive prediction tests. Abnormal **uterine Doppler** findings in the second trimester have a sensitivity of 20–60%, and a positive predictive value of 6–40%, depending on prevalence of pre-eclampsia.

Complications

Complications depend on gestational age at time of diagnosis, severity of disease, presence of other medical conditions, and, of course, management. Most cases of mild pre-eclampsia at term do not convey significant risks. Rates of complications **for severe preeclampsia** are in parentheses.[12]

Maternal

HELLP syndrome (20%); **DIC** (10%); **pulmonary edema** (2–5%); **abruptio placentae** (1–4%); **renal failure** (1–2%); **seizures** (eclampsia) (< 1%); **cerebral hemorrhage** (< 1%); **liver hemorrhage** (< 1%); and death (rare).

Fetal/neonatal

PTB (15–60%); **FGR** (10–25%); **perinatal death** (1–2%); **hypoxemia-neurological injury** (< 1%); and long-term cardiovascular morbidity (rate unknown – fetal origin of adult disease).

Management (Figures 1.1–1.3)[12,13]

Principles

Pre-eclampsia is one of the most common, and perhaps most typical, obstetric complications. It is important to understand that pre-eclampsia's **only cure is delivery**. As such, pre-eclampsia is a temporary disease, which resolves usually 24–48 hours after delivery. Remember that there are two patients: delivery is always good for the mother, but not always for the baby, especially if very premature. In general, most patients with pre-eclampsia are otherwise healthy.

Prevention

Aspirin

General prevention.   Aspirin acts to inhibit thromboxane synthesis, which could theoretically improve uteroplacental blood flow and fetal growth.

Compared with placebo or no treatment, antiplatelet agents such as **low-dose aspirin** given to women with risk factors for pre-eclampsia are associated with a **19% reduction** in the risk of **pre-eclampsia**.[14,15] This reduction occurs regardless of risk status at trial entry or whether a placebo is used, and irrespective of the dose of aspirin or gestation at randomization. Low-dose aspirin is also associated with a small **(8%) reduction** in the risk of **PTB < 37 weeks**, an 8% reduction in **SGA** babies, and a **16% reduction in perinatal deaths**.[14,15] There are no significant differences between treatment and control groups in any other measures of outcome.

When studied in women at risk for FGR or pre-eclampsia (prior preeclampsia/gestational hypertension, prior FGR, HTN, etc.), aspirin prophylaxis (50 or 81 mg/day) is associated with a significant reduction in the risk of SGA babies. Data suggest that the **preventive effect of aspirin may be greater at doses between 100 and 150 mg/day** and in women prophylaxed earlier (< 20 weeks). Women with history of severe pre-eclampsia requiring delivery prior to 32 weeks or FGR (any gestational age) should receive aspirin prophylaxis **at least 81 mg/day, starting preferably around 12 weeks and before 20 weeks.** Aspirin prophylaxis should be discontinued before delivery, by 37–38 weeks. Aspirin use has been shown to be safe for the fetus, even in the first trimester.[16]

Prevention in women with abnormal uterine Doppler ultrasound.   Abnormal uterine artery Doppler ultrasound in the second trimester has been associated with an increased risk of pre-eclampsia. My meta-analysis of the 7 RCTs ($n = 1277$) comparing **low-dose** (50–150 mg/day) **aspirin** with placebo or no treatment in women with abnormal uterine Doppler ultrasound at 14–24 weeks reveals that **pre-eclampsia is decreased by 22%** (relative risk [RR] 0.78, 95% confidence interval [CI] 0.62–0.97).[17–23] There are **insufficient data to assess other important outcomes**, as SGA, abruption, and perinatal death. The largest trial[24] trying to assess this intervention had a different study design from the others, and cannot be included in this meta-analysis. Women with abnormal uterine artery Doppler ultrasound were randomized to having the Doppler ultrasound done and always getting aspirin if abnormal, or not receiving

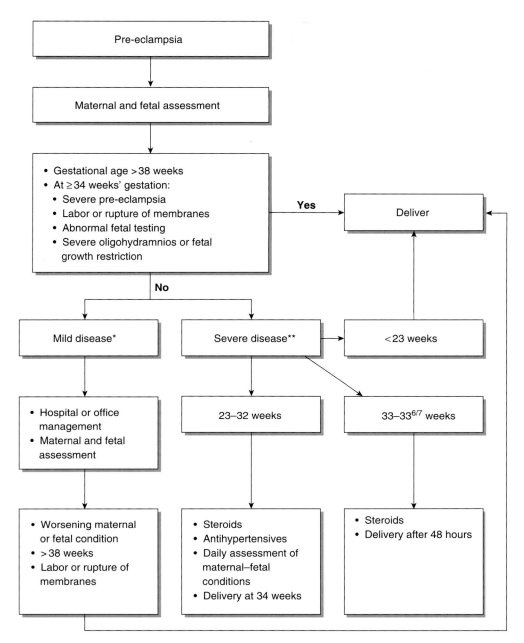

Figure 1.1
Management of pre-eclampsia. (Adapted from Sibai et al.[12])
* See Figure 1.2 for details
**See Figure 1.3 for details

the Doppler ultrasound screening. There were no differences in these two groups in any of the outcomes.[24] **Therefore, it is still unclear if aspirin improves outcomes in pregnant high-risk women with abnormal uterine Doppler results.**

Calcium

Compared with placebo or no treatment, calcium supplementation is associated with a 42% **reduction in the** **incidence of high blood pressure.**[25] The effect is greater among women at high risk of developing hypertension (53%), and those with low baseline dietary calcium (62%). Calcium supplementation is also associated with a 65% **reduction in the risk of pre-eclampsia.** The effect was greatest in women at high risk of hypertension (78%), and those with low baseline calcium intake (71%). There is no overall effect on the risk of PTB, although there is a 55% reduction in risk amongst women at high risk of developing

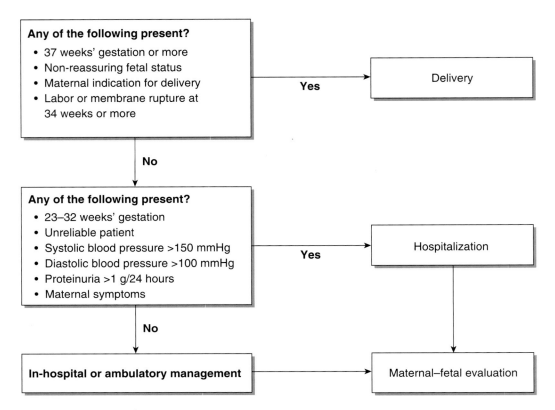

Figure 1.2
Management of mild pre-eclampsia in healthy women. (Adapted from Sibai.[13])

hypertension.[25] There is no evidence of any effect of calcium supplementation on fetal death or death before discharge from hospital. Calcium supplementation is associated with a 55% reduction in babies with low birth weight (< 2500 g) in women at high risk of hypertension. In one study, childhood SBP > 95th percentile was reduced by 41%.[25] The **largest trial**, though, reported **no reduction** in the rate or severity of pre-eclampsia or the timing of onset.[26] Optimum dosage and the effect on some substantive outcomes require further investigation.

Antioxidant therapy

Pre-eclampsia has been associated in some studies (but not in others) with oxidative stress. Antioxidative therapy (e.g. vitamins C and E) has been tested as a preventive intervention. In my own meta-analysis of the 9 trials published so far, compared with placebo, **vitamin C** 1000 mg/day and **vitamin E** 400 mg/day given usually starting in the early second trimester are associated with an **18% reduction** in risk of **pre-eclampsia** (RR=0.82, 95% CI 0.72–0.93), an 8% trend for reduction in **PTB** (RR=0.92, 95% CI 0.83–1.02), and no effect on **SGA or fetal or neonatal**

death.[27–29] Given that the two largest most recent trials[28,29] do not show any maternal or fetal benefit, not even a reduction in pre-eclampsia, and that in one of them[29] the intervention is associated with pre-eclampsia appearing 8 days earlier and more frequent gestational hypertension, antioxidant therapy should **not be recommended for prevention of pre-eclampsia.**

Magnesium

There is insufficient evidence to assess magnesium as a preventive intervention for pre-eclampsia.

Fish oil supplementation

There is insufficient evidence to assess omega-3 fatty acids as a preventive intervention for pre-eclampsia.

Salt intake

Compared with advice to continue a normal diet, advice to reduce dietary salt intake is associated with similar outcomes, including the incidence of pre-eclampsia.[30] In the

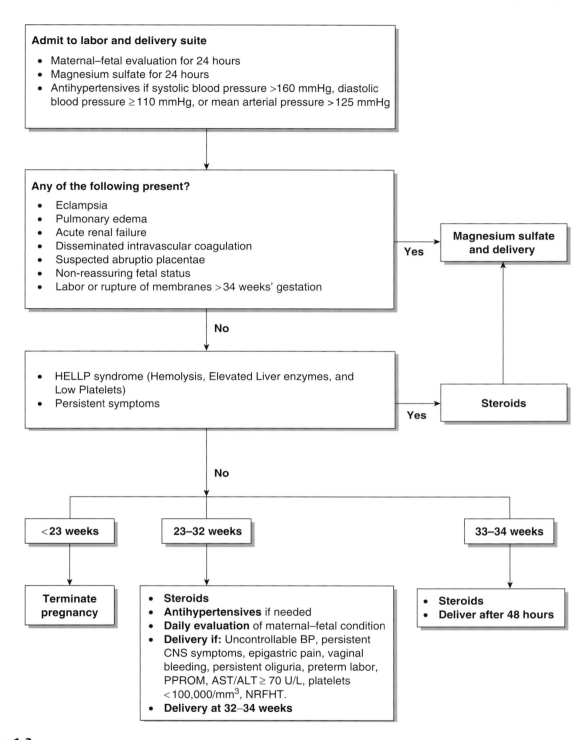

Figure 1.3
Management of severe preeclampsia < 34 weeks. (Adapted from Sibai.[13])

absence of evidence that advice to alter salt intake during pregnancy has any beneficial effect for prevention of pre-eclampsia or any other outcome, either reliance on the non-pregnancy data on beneficial salt restricted diet or personal preference can guide salt intake.

Preconception counseling

Preventive measures are as per chronic hypertension, as described above, plus avoidance of risk factors, if feasible.

Diagnosis

Diagnosis is described above.

History

Headache; blurry vision, 'spots in front of eyes'; and abdominal pain.

Physical examination

BP; edema (especially of hands, face; excessive quick weight gain); increased reflexes. Period when hypertension is first documented (before or after 20 weeks) is important.

Work-up

Laboratory tests: AST and ALT; platelets; creatinine; and 24-hour urine for total protein (and creatinine clearance). It is important to know the baseline values of these tests in the woman when either not pregnant or at least in the beginning of the pregnancy to be able to compare in women being evaluated for pre-eclampsia or its complications. Therefore, these tests should be obtained at the first prenatal visit in women with significant risk factors (e.g. chronic hypertension, diabetes, collagen disorders, APS, prior pre-eclampsia, and HELLP). Coagulations studies (especially fibrinogen) can be obtained only in severe cases. Uric acid is neither sensitive nor specific, and has not been shown to be helpful in management. Repeat laboratory tests can be performed as clinically indicated.

Evaluate for symptoms and laboratory tests to distinguish pre-eclampsia from chronic HTN, and to assess disease progression and severity.

Counseling

Delivery (the only definite treatment) is always appropriate for the mother, but may not be so for the fetus. The woman should be instructed on the signs and symptoms of pre-eclampsia and severe pre-eclampsia. The management plan should always consider gestational age, maternal and fetal status, and the presence of labor or preterm premature rupture of membranes (PPROM). Expectant management aims to palliate the maternal condition to allow for fetal maturation and cervical ripening. Consider corticosteroid administration to accelerate fetal lung maturity between 24 and 33 6/7 weeks. BP (several times/day), urine for protein, fluid input and output, weight, laboratory tests (as above), and fetal status should be closely monitored.

Activity

There is insufficient evidence to assess the effect of activity restriction in women with pre-eclampsia, as no trials have evaluated this intervention as inpatient or outpatient.

Admission

Management of proteinuric and non-proteinuric hypertension in day care units has similar clinical outcomes and costs but greater maternal satisfaction compared with hospital admission.[31–33] Hospitalization may be indicated in cases in which the woman is unreliable, ≥2 SBPs > 150 mmHg or DBP >100 mmHg, proteinuria ≥1 g in 24 hours, or persistent maternal symptoms.

Magnesium prophylaxis

Magnesium is the drug of choice for prevention of eclampsia. Compared with placebo or no anticonvulsant, magnesium sulfate is associated with a 59% reduction in the risk of eclampsia, a 36% reduction in abruption, and a non-statistically significant but clinically important 46% reduction in maternal death.[34] The reduction of the risk of eclampsia is consistent across the subgroups. In particular, the reduction is similar regardless of severity of pre-eclampsia. As eclampsia is more common among women with severe pre-eclampsia than among those with mild pre-eclampsia, the number of women who would need to be treated to prevent one case of eclampsia is greater for non-severe (mild) pre-eclampsia (i.e. 400 for mild pre-eclampsia, 71 for severe pre-eclampsia, and 36 for those with CNS symptoms).[35] In women with mild pre-eclampsia, the incidence of eclampsia may be only < 1/200, and magnesium has not been shown to affect perinatal outcome, possibly because too few ($n = 357$) women with mild pre-eclampsia have been enrolled in the two specific trials.[35] In women with severe pre-eclampsia, the incidence of eclampsia decreases 61%, from 2% in the placebo group to 0.6% in the magnesium group (4 trials).[34,35] Magnesium is also associated with a trend for a 33% decrease in abruption in women with severe pre-eclampsia. Women allocated to magnesium sulfate have a small increase (5%) in the risk of cesarean section. There is no overall difference in the risk of fetal or neonatal death. Side effects, in particular flushing, occur in 24% of women on magnesium, compared with 5% of controls. Almost all the data on side effects and safety come from studies that used either the intramuscular (IM) regimen for maintenance therapy, or the intravenous (IV) route with 1 g/h, and for around 24 hours. Intravenous administration is preferable, where there are appropriate resources, as side effects and injection site problems are lower. Magnesium is usually given at least in active labor and for 12–24 hours postpartum, but can be given for a shorter or longer period depending on the

Table 1.1 *Maternal serum magnesium concentrations associated with toxicity*

	Serum magnesium concentration		
	mmol/L	mEq/L	mg/dl
Loss of patellar reflexes	3.5–5	7–10	8.5–12
Respiratory depression	5–6.5	10–13	12–16
Altered cardiac conduction	>7.5	>15	>18
Cardiac arrest	>12.5	>25	>30

severity of pre-eclampsia (monitored for this purpose in particular with maternal urine output). Most trials managed magnesium **without serum monitoring,** but with clinical monitoring of respiration, tendon reflexes, and urine output. If serum levels are used, Table 1.1 shows the correlations with side effects. Monitoring of patellar reflexes can be used to avoid toxicity. The use of higher doses and longer duration cannot be supported by trial data. Magnesium sulfate for pre-eclampsia prophylaxis does not significantly affect labor but is associated with higher use of oxytocin.[36]

Compared with phenytoin, magnesium sulfate is associated with a **95% better reduction in the risk of eclampsia,** and with a 21% increased risk of cesarean section.[34]

Compared with **nimodipine,** magnesium sulfate is associated with a **67% better reduction in the risk of eclampsia.** There is insufficient evidence on other agents, such as diazepam or methydopa.[34]

Plasma volume expansion

Blood plasma volume increases gradually in women during pregnancy. The increase is usually greater for women with multiple pregnancies and less for those with small babies. Plasma volume is reduced in women with pre-eclampsia. There are **insufficient data** to assess any effect of plasma volume for outcomes in women with pre-eclampsia. The three small trials compared a colloid solution with no plasma volume expansion. For every outcome reported, the confidence intervals are very wide and cross the no-effect line.[37]

Antihypertensive therapy

Patients with SBP consistently ≥ 160 mmHg and/or DBP ≥ 100 (severe HTN) should be placed on antihypertensive medication; this includes those women with pre-eclampsia or its complications (HELLP, etc.). As stated above, it is appropriate to initiate therapy at lower blood pressures in patients with evidence of end-organ damage (renal, cardiovascular, etc.) and diabetes. ACE inhibitors are contraindi-

cated in pregnancy. Any patient requiring antihypertensive agents may be placed on home BP monitoring if managed as an outpatient. There are no trials on this intervention in pre-eclampsia. Types of medications include:

- **Labetalol:** 20 mg IV bolus, then 40 mg, 80 mg, 80 mg as needed, every 10 minutes (maximum 220 mg total dose).
- **Nifedipine:** 10–20 mg orally, may repeat in 30 minutes (caution with magnesium sulfate). This drug is associated with diuresis when used postpartum.
- **Hydralazine:** 5–10 mg IV (or IM) every 20 minutes. Change to another drug if no success by 30 mg (maximum dose). Hydralazine may be associated with more maternal side effects and NRFHT than IV labetalol or oral nifedipine.[38]
- **Sodium nitroprusside** (rarely needed): start at 0.25 μg/kg/min to a maximum of 5 μg/kg/min.

Antiplatelet agents

Five trials compared antiplatelet agents with placebo or no antiplatelet agent for the treatment of pre-eclampsia.[14] There are insufficient data for any firm conclusions about the possible effects of these agents when used for treatment of pre-eclampsia.

Antepartum testing

Antenatal testing (usually with NSTs) at diagnosis and repeated weekly; twice weekly for FGR or oligohydramnios. Umbilical artery Doppler ultrasound is recommended at least weekly if FGR is present. Ultrasound for fetal growth and amniotic fluid assessment should be performed at diagnosis and every 3 weeks if still pregnant.

Anesthesia

(See also Chapter 10 of *Obstetric Evidence Based Guidelines.*) Regional anesthesia is preferred, but contraindicated with coagulopathy or platelets < 85 000/mm³. Patients with hypertension may benefit from epidural analgesia, as it may improve uterine perfusion through several pathways (localized neuraxial vasodilatory effect, reduced catecholamine release). **Epidural analgesia is the analgesia of choice in hypertensive pregnant women.** Patients with hypertension, pre-eclampsia, and eclampsia are at increased risk for hemodynamic instability during both labor and surgical anesthesia. Some, but not all studies, have found a higher incidence of hypotension in parturients receiving a spinal vs epidural. Methods to prevent hypotension should be employed. The prevention, rather than treatment, of hypotension has been associated with better outcomes for the fetus. In women with severe pre-eclampsia, a careful approach is necessary for either regional or general anesthesia. Provided this is followed, they are associated with similar, good outcomes in a small trial.[39] Women with severe pre-eclampsia who must undergo **general anesthesia are at risk for an extremely exaggerated hypertensive response to intubation** and often benefit from pretreatment with an antihypertensive such as labetalol immediately prior to induction. Prophylaxis with magnesium sulfate for pre-eclampsia/eclampsia can potentiate neuromuscular blockade in patients receiving general anesthesia, so care must be taken in using intermediate- to long-acting non-depolarizing muscle relaxants.

Delivery (see Figures 1.1–1.3)

Invasive hemodynamic monitoring in pre-eclamptic women, even with severe cardiac disease, renal disease, refractory HTN, pulmonary edema, or unexplained oliguria, is **usually unnecessary**, especially since Swan–Ganz catheters have been associated with complications and no improvements in outcomes in non-pregnant critically ill adults. There are no trials on this intervention in pregnancy.

Timing
There are **insufficient data** to assess when the best time to deliver is in the presence of pre-eclampsia. In the absence of severe criteria, or preterm labor, and the presence of reassuring fetal testing, most clinicians suggest expectant management, with delivery for development of any severe criteria. Some clinicians suggest delivery even with 'mild' pre-eclampsia at ≥ 37–38 weeks.

Mode
Vaginal delivery is preferred, with induction of labor reasonable if severe. With severe pre-eclampsia, especially < 30 weeks in a nullipara, the chances of a successful induction are about 30–40%. If the woman is stable, and accepts this low incidence of success, induction may be reasonable, especially in a woman desiring a large family, if management includes a clear endpoint for delivery (e.g. within 24 hours).

PRE-ECLAMPSIA COMPLICATIONS
Superimposed pre-eclampsia
Prognosis may be much worse for mother and fetus than either diagnosis (chronic hypertension and pre-eclampsia) alone. Complications are similar to pre-eclampsia, but more common and severe (e.g. PTB 50–60%, FGR 5%, abruption 2–5%, perinatal death 1–5%). There are no specific trials to guide management, which should follow management as per pre-eclampsia (see Figures 1.1–1.3), with even more caution given the higher morbidity and mortality.

Severe pre-eclampsia
See above for pre-eclampsia.

Management (see Figure 1.3)
Magnesium sulfate
See above for pre-eclampsia.

Plasma volume expansion
The addition of **plasma volume expansion** as a temporazing treatment does not improve maternal or fetal outcome in women with early preterm severe pre-eclampsia.[40]

Timing of delivery (see Figure 1.3)
In the presence of severe pre-eclampsia at **≥ 32–34 weeks, expedited delivery,** possibly after steroids for fetal maturity between 32 and 33 6/7 weeks if safe, is recommended, given the high maternal incidence of complications with expectant management. Timing the delivery of a very premature infant < 32–34 weeks in the presence of severe pre-eclampsia is a difficult clinical decision. When the mother's life is in danger, there is no doubt that delivery is the only correct course of action. This situation is rare. More usually, the risks of maternal morbidity if the pregnancy is continued have to be constantly balanced against the hazards of prematurity to the fetus if it is delivered too early. The options are expeditious delivery or expectant management, but there are only two small trials comparing these approaches at 28 weeks to 32–34 weeks. In general, an interventionist approach with **expedited delivery** is suggested **for uncontrollable BP** in spite of continuing increase in antihypertensive drugs, **persistent headache and/or visual/CNS symptoms, epigastric pain, vaginal bleeding, persistent oliguria, preterm labor, PPROM, AST/ALT ≥ 70 U/L, platelets < 100 000/mm³, NRFHT.**[41] Women with renal disease, systemic lupus erythematosus (SLE), insulin-dependent diabetes, or multiple gestations require very careful management if expectantly managed. Massive proteinuria, even > 10 g in 24 hours, is not associated per se with worse maternal or neonatal outcomes compared with proteinuria of < 10 g or even < 5 g, and so should probably not be a criterion for delivery by itself. The presence of FGR requires even closer monitoring, is associated with worse outcomes, and is seldom associated with delay of delivery > 48 hours (enough to allow steroids for fetal maturation). There are insufficient data for reliable conclusions comparing these two policies for outcome for the mother. For the baby, there is insufficient evidence for reliable conclusions about the effects on fetal or neonatal death. Babies whose mothers are allocated to the **immediate delivery** group have 2.3-fold **more hyaline membrane disease,** 5.5-fold **more necrotizing**

Table 1.2 *Signs and symptoms of HELLP syndrome*	
Condition	Frequency (%)
Hypertension	85
Proteinuria	87
Right upper quadrant, or epigastric pain	40–90
Nausea or vomiting	29–84
Headaches	33–60
Visual changes	10–20
Mucosal bleeding	10
Jaundice	5

HELLP, Hemolysis, Elevated Liver enzymes, and a Low Platelet count.
Adapted from Sibai.[43]

Table 1.3 *Complications of HELLP*	
Complication	Frequency (%)
Maternal death	1
Adult respiratory distress syndrome (ARDS)	1
Laryngeal edema	1–2
Liver failure or hemorrhage	1–2
Acute renal failure	3
Pulmonary edema	6–8
Pleural effusions	10–15
Abruptio placentae	10–15
Disseminated intravascular coagulation	10–15
Marked ascites	10–15
Perinatal death	7–20
PTB	70

HELLP, Hemolysis, Elevated Liver enzymes, and a Low Platelet count;
PTB, preterm birth.
Adapted from Sibai.[43]

enterocolitis, and are 32% more likely to need admission to a neonatal intensive care unit (NICU) than those allocated an expectant policy.[41] Nevertheless, babies allocated to the interventionist policy are 64% less likely to be SGA. There were no statistically significant differences between the two strategies for any other outcomes. **Expectant management of severe pre-eclampsia remote from term warrants hospitalization at a tertiary facility, daily antenatal testing, and laboratory studies at frequent intervals, with the decision to prolong pregnancy determined day to day.**

HELLP

Epidemiology

Approximately 72% of cases are diagnosed antepartum, and 28% postpartum (of which 80% < 48 hours, and 20% ≥ 48 hours postpartum). Of the antepartum cases, about 70% occur 28–36 weeks, 20% > 37 weeks (few postpartum), and about 10% < 28 weeks.

Diagnosis

See above. If only one or two criteria are present, some use the term 'partial HELLP syndrome'.

Signs and symptoms

It is important to note that 15% have no hypertension, and 13% no proteinuria (Table 1.2).[42]

Complications

Complications (Table 1.3) of HELLP syndrome are somewhat similar in incidence and severity to those of severe pre-eclampsia, once gestational age is controlled.[42] If profound hypovolemic shock occurs, suspect liver hematoma. If confirmed, liver hematoma is best managed conservatively.

Management

See Figure 1.4 for management.[43]

Work up

Laboratory tests as for severe pre-eclampsia, plus peripheral smear evaluation.

Specific therapy

Corticosteroids. Five small trials have assessed dexamethasone vs placebo/no treatment and are summarized in a meta-analysis,[44–49] with one more recent trial.[50] The dose of dexamethasone was usually 10 mg IV every 6–12 hours for 2–3 doses, followed by 5–6 mg IV 6–12 hours later for 2–3 more doses. Compared with placebo/no treatment, **dexamethasone is not associated with any significant differences in maternal mortality** and morbidity due to placental abruption, pulmonary edema, and liver hematoma or rupture. Dexamethasone is associated with a tendency to a greater platelet count increase over 48 hours in the meta-analysis (but this is not confirmed in the largest trial),[50] about 2–4 less mean number of hospital stay days, and longer (41 vs 15 hours) mean interval to delivery.[49] There are **no**

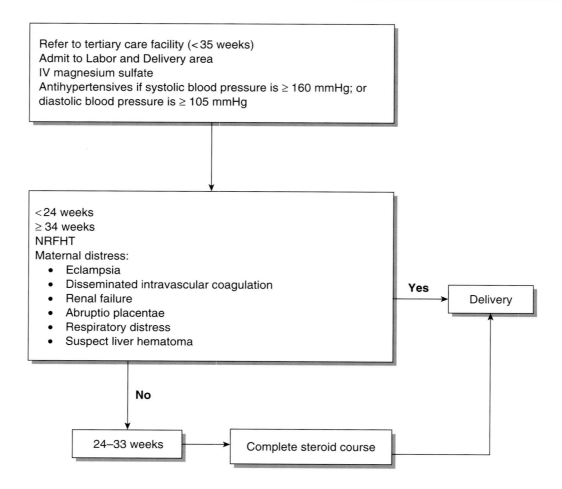

Figure 1.4
Management of HELLP syndrome. HELLP, Hemolysis, Elevated Liver enzyme levels, and Low Platelet count.
(Adapted from Sibai.[43])

significant differences in perinatal mortality or morbidity due to respiratory distress syndrome, need for ventilatory support, intracerebral hemorrhage, necrotizing enterocolitis, and a 5-minute Apgar < 7. The mean birth weight is significantly greater by 247 g in the group allocated to dexamethasone. The largest and only placebo-controlled trial[50] failed to show any significant differences between dexamethasone and placebo, with a shorter platelet recovery and hospitalization in the subgroup with platelets < 50,000/mm³.

Compared with betamethasone, dexamethasone is not associated with significant differences in maternal and perinatal morbidity or mortality, except for significantly better oliguria, mean arterial pressure, mean increase in platelet count, mean increase in urinary output, and liver enzyme elevations, in one small trial.[45]

Given no significant improvements in important maternal and fetal outcomes, there is still **insufficient evidence to recommend the use of dexamethasone or other steroids for therapy specific for HELLP** syndrome, and this approach should be considered experimental.

Anesthesia

Regional anesthesia is usually allowed by anesthesiologists in cases with platelet counts ≥ 75 000/mm³. General anesthesia may be safer in cases with lower platelet counts.

Delivery

Timing (see Figure 1.4)   Prompt delivery is indicated if HELLP is diagnosed at ≥ 34 weeks, or even earlier if multiorgan dysfunction, DIC, liver failure or hemorrhage, renal failure, possible abruption, or NRFHT are present. Delivery can only be delayed for a maximum of 48 hours when at 24–33 6/7 weeks to give steroids for fetal maturity, but this management is not tested in trials. Although some women may have improvement in laboratory values in these 48 hours, delivery is still indicated in most cases.

Mode   Mode of delivery should generally follow obstetric indications, with HELLP syndrome not being an indication for cesarean per se. Counseling and managements should include the information that the incidence of cesarean delivery in trial of labor of nulliparous women or those with Bishop score < 5 with HELLP < 30 weeks is high.

With platelet count < 100 000/mm³, a drain may be indicated under and/or over the fascia in cases of cesarean delivery.

Eclampsia

Incidence

1 in 2000–3400 deliveries in Europe and other developed countries, and from 1 in 100 to 1 in 11 700 deliveries in developing countries. The onset may be antepartum (40–50%), intrapartum (20–35%), or postpartum (10–40%). Late postpartum eclampsia (> 48 hours but < 4 weeks after delivery) is rare, but can occur.

Definition

Eclampsia is the occurrence of ≥ 1 seizure(s) in association with pre-eclampsia.

Complications

The risk of **maternal death** is around **1–2%** in the developed world and up to **10%** in developing countries. An estimated 50 000 women die each year worldwide having had an eclamptic convulsion. **Perinatal mortality** is 6–12% in the developed world and up to 25% in developing countries. Other complications are similar and possibly more severe than severe pre-eclampsia cases (maternal – abruption 7–10%, DIC 7–11%, HELLP 10–15%, pulmonary edema 3–5%, renal failure 5–9%, aspiration pneumonia 2–3%, cardiopulmonary arrest 2–5%; perinatal: PTB 50%).[51]

Management
Principles

In about 15% of cases, hypertension or proteinuria may be absent before eclampsia. A high index of suspicion for eclampsia should be maintained in all cases of hypertensive disorders in pregnancy, in particular those with CNS symptoms (e.g. headache, visual disturbances). Up to 50% or more of cases of eclampsia, by occurring in women with no diagnosis of pre-eclampsia, or only mild disease, preterm or before hospitalization, may not be preventable.

The first priorities are **airway, breathing, and circulation (ABCs)**. Multidisciplinary care is essential, as several people are needed for immediate stabilization. Interventions include airway assessment, and placing the patient in the lateral decubitus position (to avoid aspiration). Maintain oxygenation with supplemental oxygen via an 8–10 L/min mask.

Obtain vital signs, and assess pulse oximetry. Supportive care includes a tongue blade inserted between the teeth (avoid inducing a gag reflex), and preventing maternal injury.

Work-up

Cerebral imaging is usually not necessary for the diagnosis and management of most women with eclampsia. It might be helpful in cases complicated by neurological deficits, coma, refractory to magnesium, or occuring > 48 hours after delivery.

Therapy

Magnesium sulfate is certainly the drug of choice for preventing recurrence of eclampsia, as it is associated with maternal and fetal/neonatal benefits compared with all interventions against which it has been tested.

Magnesium vs diazepam. Compared with diazepam, magnesium sulfate is associated with **reductions** in **maternal death** by 41%, in **further convulsions** from eclampsia by 56%, in **Apgar scores** < 7 at 5 minutes by 28%, and in **length of stay in a special care baby unit > 7 days** by 34%.[52]

Magnesium vs phenytoin. Compared with phenytoin, magnesium sulfate is associated with **reductions** of maternal complications, such as the **recurrence of convulsions** by 69%, **maternal death** by 50% (non-significant due to small numbers: RR=0.50, 95% CI 0.24–1.05), **pneumonia** by 56%, and **admission to the intensive care unit** by 33%. For the baby, magnesium sulfate is associated with 27% **fewer admissions to a special care baby unit** and 23% **fewer babies who died or were in a special care baby unit for > 7 days.**[53]

Magnesium vs lytic cocktail. Lytic cocktail is usually a mixture of Thorazine (chlorpromazine), Phenergan (promethazine), and Demerol (meperidine). Compared to a lytic cocktail, magnesium sulfate is associated with a **91% reduction in subsequent convulsions**, and with **88% less respiratory depression.** Magnesium sulfate is also associated with **75% fewer maternal deaths** than lytic cocktail, but the difference was not statistically significant due to small numbers.[54]

About 10% of women will have a **second seizure** even after a bolus of 6 g and maintenance of 2 g/h of magnesium sulfate. Another bolus of 2 g of magnesium sulfate can then be given IV over 3–5 minutes, and, rarely, if another convulsion occurs, sodium amorbital 250 mg IV over 3–5 minutes is necessary.[51]

Blood pressure should be maintained about 140–159/90–109 mmHg by antihypertensive agents, as described for pre-eclampsia.

Antepartum testing

NRFHT occurs in many cases of eclampsia, but usually resolves spontaneously in 3–10 minutes by **fetal in-utero resuscitation** with maternal support. Therefore, **NRFHT is not an indication for immediate cesarean delivery in case of eclampsia,** unless it continues > 10–15 minutes despite normal maternal oxygenation.

Delivery

Delivery should occur expeditiously, but only **when the mother is stable.** This requires a **multidisciplinary,** efficient, timely effort.

Postpartum management of pre-eclampsia

Eclampsia prophylaxis
Magnesium should be continued for at least 12 hours, and often for about 24 hours or at least until improvement in maternal urinary output (e.g. > 100 ml/h). In some cases of severe pre-eclampsia, eclampsia, HELLP, or continuing oliguria or other complications, magnesium may need to be continued for > 24 hours. Pre-eclampsia can worsen postpartum. Edema always worsens, and the woman should be aware of this. Eclampsia can still occur, especially in the first 48 hours post-delivery, but even up to ≥ 14 days postpartum.

Postpartum management of hypertension

There are no reliable data to guide management of women who are hypertensive postpartum or at increased risk of becoming so. Women should be informed that they will require long-term surveillance (and possible therapy) for hypertension at their postpartum visit.

For prevention in women who had antenatal pre-eclampsia, there are **insufficient data** to assess outcomes comparing furosemide or nifedipine with placebo/no therapy.[55] Compared with therapy, postpartum **furosemide 20 mg** orally for 5 days does not affect any outcomes in women with mild or superimposed pre-eclampsia.[56] In women with severe pre-eclampsia, this intervention normalizes blood pressure more rapidly and reduces the need for antihypertensive therapy, but does not affect the incidence of delayed complications or the length of hospitalization.[56] **L-arginine** therapy hastens recovery in postpartum pre-eclampsia.[57] Therefore, for women with antenatal hypertension, even that of pre-eclampsia, it is unclear whether or not they should routinely receive postpartum antihypertensive therapy. Although BP peaks on days 3–6 postpartum, whether or not routine postpartum treatment can prevent transient severe maternal hypertension and/or prolongation of maternal hospital stay has not been established.[55]

For treatment, there are insufficient data to assess the antihypertensives studied: these are oral timolol or hydralazine compared with oral methyldopa for treatment of mild to moderate postpartum hypertension, and oral hydralazine plus sublingual nifedipine compared with sublingual nifedipine.[55] Oral **nifedipine** (10 mg every 8 hours short-acting or 30 mg daily long-acting; maximum dose 120 mg/day) is a resonable choice, with **ACE inhibitors for women with diabetes or nephropathy.** If a clinician feels that hypertension is severe enough to treat, the agent used should be based on his/her familiarity with the drug.

Long-term counseling

Long-term counseling should involve review of recurrence, and preventive measures (see above). The risk of complications in the subsequent pregnancy depends on how early in gestation and severe the complications were, other underlying medical conditions, age of the woman at future pregnancy, same vs different partner, and many other variables (see risk factors above). In general, the **recurrence risk** of pre-eclampsia is about 20–30%. The recurrent risk of HELLP syndrome is about 5%, but pregnancies following one with HELLP syndrome have a 25–30% incidence of pre-eclampsia, 30–40% of PTB, 25% of SGA, and up to 5–10% of perinatal death.[58] Women with eclampsia have a risk or recurrence in the subsequent pregnancy of about 2%, with a risk of pre-eclampsia of about 25%. Moreover, **women with prior pre-eclampsia are at increased risk of cardiovascular disease in the future,** even premenopause if the pre-eclampsia occurred early in pregnancy or as a multipara, or in menopause if it happened at term in a primipara.

REFERENCES

1. Sibai BM. Chronic hypertension in pregnancy. Obstet Gynecol 2002; 100: 369–77. [review]
2. Chronic hypertension in pregnancy. ACOG Practice Bulletin No. 29, July 2001. [review]
3. Yeo SY, Steele NM, Chang M-C, et al. Effect of exercise on blood pressure in pregnant women with a high risk of gestational hypertensive disorders. J Reprod Med 2000; 45: 293–8. [RCT, $n = 16$]
4. Meher S, Abalos E, Carroli, G. Bed rest with or without hospitalization for hypertension during pregnancy. Cochrane Database Syst Rev 2007; 1. [meta-analysis: 4 RCTs, $n = 449$]
5. Abalos E, Duley L, Steyn DW, Henderson-Smart DJ. Antihypertensive drug therapy for mild to moderate hypertension during pregnancy. Cochrane Database of Syst Rev 2007; 1. [meta-analysis: 40 RCTs, $n = 3797$; 24 of which compared an antihypertensive drug with placebo/no antihypertensive drug, $n = 2815$]
6. Magee LA, Duley L. Oral beta-blockers for mild to moderate hypertension during pregnancy. Cochrane Database Syst Rev 2007;1. [meta-analysis: 29 RCTs, $n = 2500$]
7. Duley L, Henderson-Smart DJ. Drugs for treatment of very high blood pressure during pregnancy. Cochrane Database Syst Rev 2007; 1. [meta-analysis: 20 RCTs, $n = 1637$]

8. Sibai BM. Diagnosis and management of gestational hypertension and preeclampsia. Obstet Gynecol 2003; 102: 181–92. [review]

9. Diagnosis and management of preeclampsia and eclampsia. ACOG Practice Bulletin No. 33, January 2002. [review]

10. National High Blood Pressure Education Program Working Group Report on High Blood Pressure in Pregnancy. AJOG 2000; 183: S1–S22. [guideline]

11. Waugh JJ, Clark TJ, Divakaran TG, Khan KS, Kilby MD. Accuracy of urinalysis dipstick techniques in predicting significant proteinuria in pregnancy. Obstet Gynecol 2004; 103: 769–77. [review]

12. Sibai BM, Dekker G, Kupferminc M. Pre-eclampsia. Lancet 2005; 365: 785–99. [review]

13. Sibai BM. Expectant management of preeclampsia. OBG Management 2005; 3: 18–36. [review]

14. Knight M, Duley L. Henderson-Smart DJ, King JF. Antiplatelet agents for preventing and treating pre-eclampsia. Cochrane Database Syst Rev 2007; 1. [meta-analysis: 40 RCTs, $n = > 32\,000$. Prevention trials: 30 RCTs, $n = 30\,563$. Treatment trials: 5 RCTs]

15. Duley L, Henderson-Smart DJ, Knight M, King JF. Antiplatelet agents for preventing pre-eclampsia and its complications. Cochrane Database Syst Rev 2007; 1. [meta-analysis: 51 RCTs, $n = 36\,500$]

16. Kozer E, Nikfan S, Costei A, et al. Aspirin consumption during the first trimester of pregnancy and congenital anomalies: a meta-analysis. Am J Obstet Gynecol 2002; 187: 1623–30. [meta-analysis]

17. McParland P, Pearch JM, Chamberlain GV. Doppler ultrasound and aspirin in recognition and prevention of pregnancy-incuded hypertension. Lancet 1990; 335: 1552–5. [RCT, $n = 100$]

18. Bower SJ, Harrington KF, Schuchter K, McGirr C, Campbell S. Prediction of pre-eclampsia by abnormal uterine Doppler ultrasound and modification by aspirin. Br J Obstet Gynaecol 1996; 103: 625–9. [RCT, $n = 60$]

19. Morris JM, Fay RA, Ellwood DA, Cook CM, Devonald KJ. A randomized controlled trial of aspirin in patients with abnormal uterine artery blood flow. Obstet Gynecol 1996; 87: 74–8. [RCT, $n = 102$]

20. Harrington K, Kurdi W, Aquilina J, England P, Campbell S. A prospective management study of slow-release aspirin in the palliation of uteroplacental insufficiency predicted by uterine artery Doppler at 20 weeks. Ultrasound Obstet Gynecol 2000; 15: 13–8. [RCT, $n = 210$]

21. Vainio M, Kujansuu E, Iso-Mustajarvi M, Maenpaa J. Low dose acetylsalicylic acid in prevention of pregnancy-induced hypertension and intrauterine growth retardation in women with bilateral uterine artery notches. Br J Obstet Gynaecol 2002; 109: 161–7. [RCT, $n = 86$]

22. Yu CKH, Papageorghiou AT, Parra M, Palma Dias R, Nicolaides KH. Randomized controlled trial using low-dose aspirin in the prevention of pre-eclampsia in women with abnormal uterine artery Doppler at 23 weeks' gestation. Ultrasound Obstet Gynecol 2003; 22: 233–9. [RCT, $n = 554$]

23. Ebrashy A, Ibrahim M, Marzook A, Yousef D. Usefulness of aspirin therapy in high-risk pregnant women with abnormal uterine artery Doppler ultrasound at 14–16 weeks pregnancy: randomized controlled clinical trial. Croatian Med J 2005; 46(5): 826–31. [RCT, $n = 139$]

24. Subtil D, Goeusse P, Houfflin-Debarge V, et al. Randomized comparison of uterine artery Doppler and aspirin (100 mg) with placebo in nulliparous women: the Essai Regional Aspirine Mere-Enfant study (Part 2). BJOG 2003; 110: 485–91. [RCT, $n = 1\,860$]

25. Atallah AN, Hofmeyr GJ, Duley L. Calcium supplementation during pregnancy for preventing hypertensive disorders and related problems. Cochrane Database Syst Rev 2007; 1. [meta-analysis: 11 RCTs, $n = 6\,894$]

26. Levine RJ, Hauth JC, Curet LB, et al. Trial of calcium to prevent preeclampsia. NEngl J Med 1997; 337: 69–76. [RCT, $n = 4\,589$]

27. Rumbold A, Duley L, Crowther C, Haslam R. Antioxidants for preventing pre-eclampsia. Cochrane Database Syst Rev 2007; 1. [meta-analysis: 7 RCTs, $n = 6\,082$]

28. Rumbold AR, Crowther CA, Haslam RR, Dekker GA, Robinson JS. Vitamins C and E and the risks of preeclampsia and perinatal complications. N Engl J Med 2006; 354: 1796–806. [RCT, $n = 1\,877$]

29. Poston L, Briley AL, Seed PT, Kelly FJ, Shennan AH. Vitamin C and vitamin E in pregnant women at risk for pre-eclampsia (VIP trial): randomised placebo-controlled trial. Lancet 2006; 367: 1145–54. [RCT, $n = 2\,410$]

30. Duley L, Henderson-Smart D, Meher S. Altered dietary salt for preventing pre-eclampsia, and its complications. Cochrane Database Syst Rev 2007; 1. [meta-analysis: 2 RCTs, $n = 603$]

31. Kroner C, Turnbull D, Wilkinson C. Antenatal day care units versus hospital admission for women with complicated pregnancy. Cochrane Database Syst Rev 2007; 1. [meta-analysis: only Tuffnell – ref. 32 – included]

32. Tuffnell DJ, Lilford RJ, Buchan PC, et al. Randomised controlled trial of day care for hypertension in pregnancy. Lancet 1992; 339: 224–7. [RCT, included in Cochrane by Kroner]

33. Turnbull DA, Wilkinson C, Gerard C, et al. Clinical, psychological and economic effects of antenatal day care for three medical complications of pregnancy: a randomized controlled trial of 395 women. Lancet 2004; 363: 1104–9. [RCT, $n = 395$, not included in Cochrane by Kroner]

34. Duley L, Gulmezoglu AM, Henderson-Smart DJ. Magnesium sulphate and other anticonvulsants for women with pre-eclampsia. Cochrane Database Syst Rev 2007; 1. [meta-analysis: 6 RCTs, $n = 11\,444$]

35. Sibai BM. Magnesium sulfate prophylaxis in preeclampsia: lessons learned from recent trials. Am J Obstet Gynecol 2004; 190: 1520–6. [review]

36. Witlin AG, Friedman SA, Sibai BM. The effect of magnesium sulfate therapy on the duration of labor in women with mild preeclampsia at term: a randomized, double-blind, placebo-controlled trial. Am J Obstet Gynecol 1997; 176: 623–7. [RCT, $n = 135$]

37. Duley L, Williams J, Henderson-Smart DJ. Plasma volume expansion for treatment of pre-eclampsia. Cochrane Database Syst Rev 2007; 1. [meta-analysis: 3 RCTs, $n = 61$]

38. Magee LA, Cham C, Waterman EJ, Ohlsson A, von Dadelszen P. Hydralazine for treatment of severe hypertension in pregnancy: a meta-analysis. BMJ 2003; 327: 1–10. [meta-analysis]

39. Wallace D, Leveno KJ, Cunningham FG, et al. Randomized comparison of general and regional anesthesia for cesarean delivery in pregnancies complicated by severe preeclampsia. Obstet Gynecol 1995; 86: 193–9. [RCT, $n = 80$]

40. Ganzevoort W, Rep A, Bonsel GJ, et al. A randomised controlled trial comparing two temporising management strategies, one with and one without plasma volume expansion, for severe and early onset (24–34 weeks) pre-eclampsia. BJOG 2005; 112: 1358–68. [RCT, $n = 216$]

41. Churchill D, Duley L. Interventionist versus expectant care for severe pre-eclampsia before term. Cochrane Database Syst Rev 2007; 1. [meta-analysis: 2 RCTs, $n = 133$]

42. Sibai BM. A practical plan to detect and manage HELLP syndrome. OBG Management 2005; 4: 52–69. [review]

43. Sibai BM. Diagnosis, controversies, and management of the syndrome of hemolysis, elevated liver enzymes, and low platelet count. Obstet Gynecol 2004; 103: 981–91. [review]

44. Matchaba P, Moodley J. Corticosteroids for HELLP syndrome in pregnancy. Cochrane Database Syst Rev 2007; 1. [meta-analysis: 5 RCTs, $n = 170$]

45. Isler CM, Barrilleaux PS, Magann EF, Bass JD, Martin JN. A prospective, randomized trial comparing the efficacy of dexamethasone and betamethasone for the treatment of antepartum HELLP (hemolysis, elevated liver enzymes, and low platelet count) syndrome. Am J Obstet Gynecol 2001; 184(7): 1332–7. [RCT, $n = 41$. Dexamethasone vs betamethasone]

46. Magann EF, Perry KG, Meydrech EF, et al. Postpartum corticosteroids: accelerated recovery from the syndrome of hemolysis, elevated liver enzymes, and low platelets (HELLP). Am J Obstet Gynecol 1994; 171(4): 1154–8. [RCT, $n = 40$ (but only 25 with follow-up). Postpartum]

47. Magann EF, Bass D, Chauhan SP, et al. Antepartum corticosteroids: disease stabilization in patients with the syndrome of hemolysis, elevated liver enzymes, and low platelets (HELLP). Am J Obstet Gynecol 1994; 171: 1148–53. [RCT, $n = 25$. Antepartum]

48. Vigil-De Gracia P, Garcia-Caceres E. Dexamethasone in the post-partum treatment of HELLP syndrome. Int Gynecol Obstet 1997; 59: 217–21. [RCT, *n* = 34]

49. Yalcin OT, Sener T, Hassa H, Ozalp S, Okur A. Effects of postpartum corticosteroids in patients with HELLP syndrome. Int J Gynecol Obstet 1998; 61: 141–8. [RCT, *n* = 30]

50. Fonseca JE, Mendez F, Catano C, Arias F. Dexamethasone treatment does not improve the outcome of women with HELLP syndrome: a double-blind, placebo-controlled, randomized clinical trial. Am J Obstet Gynecol 2005; 193: 1591–8. [RCT, *n* = 132]

51. Sibai BM. Diagnosis, prevention and management of eclampsia. Obstet Gynecol 2005; 105: 402–10. [review]

52. Duley L, Henderson-Smart D. Magnesium sulphate versus diazepam for eclampsia. Cochrane Database Syst Rev 2007; 1. [meta-analysis: 7 RCTs, *n* = 1441]

53. Duley L, Henderson-Smart D. Magnesium sulphate versus phenytoin for eclampsia. Cochrane Database Syst Rev 2007; 1. [meta-analysis: 6 RCTs, *n* = 897]

54. Duley L, Gulmezoglu AM. Magnesium sulphate versus lytic cocktail for eclampsia. Cochrane Database Syst Rev 2007; 1. [meta-analysis: 2 RCTs, *n* = 199]

55. Magee L, Sadeghi S. Prevention and treatment of postpartum hypertension. Cochrane Database Syst Rev 2007; 1. [meta-analysis: 6 RCTs; 3 RCTs on prevention, *n* = 315; 3 RCTs on treatment, *n* = 144]

56. Ascarelli M, Johnson V, McCreary H, et al. Postpartum preeclampsia management with furosemide: a randomized clinical trial. Obstet Gynecol 2005; 105: 29–33. [RCT, *n* = 264]

57. Hladunewich MA, Derby GC, Lafayette RA, et al. Effect of L-arginine therapy on the glomerular injury of preeclampsia. Obstet Gynecol 2006; 107: 886–95. [RCT, *n* = 45]

58. Chames MC, Haddad B, Barton JR, Livingston JC, Sibai BM. Subsequent pregnancy outcome in women with a history of HELLP syndrome at ≤ 28 weeks of gestation. Am J Obstet Gynecol 2003; 188: 1504–8. [II-2]

2

Cardiac disease

Shailen Shah

KEY POINTS

- Normal pregnancy physiology – particularly increased intravascular volume, hypercoagulability, and decreased systemic vascular resistance – can severely exacerbate cardiac disease during pregnancy.
- **Relative hypervolemia,** rather than fluid restriction, and **avoidance of hypotension, constitute the key intrapartum management principle for many cardiac diseases.** Mitral stenosis is the main exception to this principle.
- Women with congenital heart disease should have a **fetal echocardiogram** at around 22 weeks.
- **Most cardiac diseases in pregnancy do *not* benefit from cesarean delivery,** and this can be reserved for usual obstetric indications.
- Pulmonary hypertension, Marfan syndrome with aortic root > 4 cm, and severe cardiomyopathy are associated with high maternal mortality, and patients should be counseled pre-pregnancy of this risk and provided alternatives to their own pregnancy.

BACKGROUND

For 'cardiac disease in pregnancy', this chapter reviews *maternal* cardiac disease. Concern for cardiac decompensation occurs when the heart, either from acquired or congenital, physiological or structural defects, is unable to accommodate pregnancy physiology or dynamics of parturition. There are no trials of intervention for cardiac disease in pregnancy.

SYMPTOMS/SIGNS

Symptoms and signs can include fatigue, limitation of physical activity, palpitations, tachycardia, shortness of breath, chest pain, dyspnea on exertion, and cyanosis. These symptoms and signs of cardiac disease can often be confused with common pregnancy complaints.

EPIDEMIOLOGY/INCIDENCE

Cardiac disease complicates 1–4% of pregnancies, but accounts for 10–25% of maternal mortality.[1–3] In the USA, congenital heart disease is more common than rheumatic heart disease as a result of medical care and surgical advances. Despite significant medical and surgical advances over the past two decades, cardiac disease remains a significant cause of maternal mortality.

GENETICS

When the mother has a congenital heart defect, the fetus is at increased risk for a congenital heart defect (generally 3–5%, but ranges from 1 to 15%). Therefore, **fetal echocardiography** (best if done at around 22 weeks) is recommended. DiGeorge syndrome (chromosomal deletion in 22q11), Marfan syndrome, and hypertrophic obstructive cardiomyopathy are all autosomal dominant conditions.

ETIOLOGY/BASIC PATHOPHYSIOLOGY/ PREGNANCY CONSIDERATIONS

The main function of the heart is to provide oxygen (and other nutrients), and remove carbon dioxide (and other wastes) to and from all end organs of the body, which include the uterus and fetus during pregnancy. The chief determinants of oxygen delivery include the amount carried by the blood (determined by the amount of hemoglobin and degree of saturation) and the delivery of that blood: primarily, cardiac output (determined by pre-load, afterload, cardiac contractility, and heart rate). Any disease process or pregnancy physiology that interferes with this main function of the heart can result in maternal and fetal morbidity and mortality.

Five principal physiological changes of pregnancy can complicate cardiac disease during pregnancy:[4]

1. *Decreased systemic vascular resistance.* Large ventricular septal defects (VSDs), for example, result in the shunting of blood from the left ventricle to the right ventricle because the systemic blood pressure is greater than the pulmonary blood pressure. Over time, this can result in pulmonary hypertension that can approach systemic blood pressures. Pregnancy, with its associated 20% decrease in systemic vascular resistance, can allow pulmonary pressures to equal or exceed systemic pressures, resulting in a reversal, or right to left shunting of blood. This would result in deoxygenated right ventricular blood entering the left ventricle, leading to decreased oxygen delivery to the body, and even cyanosis and death.[5]

2. *Increase in intravascular volume.* This volume increase occurs throughout pregnancy (50% increase), and is maximal by 32 weeks' gestation. Women with severe myocardial dysfunction, such as cardiomyopathy, may not be able to accommodate this physiological demand and experience congestive heart failure and pulmonary edema.

3. *Postpartum increase in intravascular volume from 'auto-transfusion' of blood from the contracted uterus and mobilization of third space fluid.* Women with mitral stenosis have restricted left ventricular filling. This postpartum vascular load could result in pulmonary edema.[6]

4. *Hypercoagulability.* This well-characterized pregnancy adaptation can dramatically heighten the chance of thromboembolism in at-risk patients. Pregnant women with artificial mechanical heart valves, for example, can develop fatal thromboses despite adequate heparin anticoagulation as a result of this physiology.[7,8]

5. *Marked increase in cardiac output during parturition.*[9] This increase occurs during pregnancy, and is both necessary for and partly 'worsened' by labor and delivery and the postpartum volume shift described above. In women whose cardiac output is fixed and very dependent on preload, like aortic stenosis, a negative volume shift from postpartum hemorrhage can result in a precipitous drop in cardiac output and lead to inadequate coronary and cerebral perfusion.[10]

Understanding these pathophysiological interactions forms the basis for understanding, anticipating, and managing patients with cardiac disease during pregnancy.

Table 2.1   *New York Heart Association classification of heart disease*

Class I
No symptoms or limitations
  Ordinary physical activity does not cause undue fatigue, dyspnea, palpitations, or angina

Class II
Slight limitation of physical activity
  Comfortable at rest
  Ordinary physical activity (e.g. carrying heavy packages) may result in fatigue, palpitations, or angina

Class III
Marked limitation of physical activity
  Comfortable at rest
  Less than ordinary physical activity (e.g. getting dressed) leads to symptoms

Class IV
Severe limitation of physical activity
  Symptoms of heart failure or angina are present *at rest* and worsen with any activity

CLASSIFICATION

Classification of women with heart disease by their clinical functional class (New York Heart Association [NYHA] system) is helpful, in particular preconception. Up to 40% of women who develop congestive heart failure during gestation begin their pregnancy without symptoms (class I)[11] (Table 2.1) and 15–55% of pregnant women with heart disease show deterioration by this system. Contemporary classification categorizes women according to an estimate of risk for mortality due to pregnancy and cardiac disease (Table 2.2).[12]

RISK FACTORS

Predictors of maternal complications include prior cardiac events, NYHA class III or IV (see Table 2.1), lesion classified as group II or, especially, III (see Table 2.2), left heart obstruction (mitral stenosis [MS], aortic stenosis [AS]), and significant left ventricular systolic dysfunction with ejection fraction [EF] ≤ 40%.

COMPLICATIONS

Today, with proper modern management, maternal mortality is predominantly restricted to patients with pulmonary hypertension (PHTN), coronary artery disease (CAD), cardiomyopathy, endocarditis, and sudden arrhythmia.[2,13]

Table 2.2 *Maternal risk associated with pregnancy*
Group I: minimal risk of mortality (< 1%) Atrial septal defect Ventricular septal defect (VSD) Pulmonic or tricuspid valvular disease Corrected tetralogy of Fallot Bioprosthetic heart valve Mitral stenosis, NYHA classes I and II Marfan syndrome, normal aorta Aortic or mitral insufficiency Hypertrophic cardiomyopathy
Group II: moderate risk of mortality (5–15%) Mitral stenosis, NYHA classes III and IV Artificial mechanical heart valve, if anticoagulation with heparin Aortic stenosis Coarctation of the aorta, uncomplicated Uncorrected tetralogy of Fallot (TOF) Myocardial infarction
Group III: major risk of mortality (> 25%) Pulmonary hypertension (PHTN) Coarctation of aorta, complicated Marfan syndrome, with aortic root > 4 cm Severe dilated cardiomyopathy

NYHA, New York Heart Association.

These groups can be used to determine general treatment principles. Neonatal complications mostly derive from preterm birth, miscarriage, and growth restriction.

MANAGEMENT
Preconception counseling

Women with **cardiac diseases that can be ameliorated** (invasively or non-invasively) **should be advised to do so before pregnancy** to decrease their pregnancy-related morbidity and mortality. These include significant mitral, aortic, or pulmonic stenosis, uncorrected tetralogy of Fallot (TOF), CAD, coarctation of the aorta, atrial septal defect (ASD) and VSD with mild or moderate PHTN.[14] Coexisting disorders such as anemia, thyroid disease, or hypertension should be treated and controlled before pregnancy.

Counseling should include diet and activity modifications, infection prevention and control, and review of prognosis, possible complications, and management in a future pregnancy.

Patients with group III lesions or significant dilated cardiomyopathy (including persistent peripartum cardiomyopathy) should be advised *not* to conceive because they have an unacceptable risk of mortality. Contraception and sterilization counseling should be offered. If such patients present postconceptually, pregnancy termination should be offered.[14]

Prenatal care/antepartum testing

The patient should be questioned and examined during frequent prenatal visits for cardiac failure. **A maternal echocardiogram** allows assessment of heart function. Pulmonary hypertension, which can be often overestimated by this modality, may need to be confirmed by cardiac catheterization. An electrocardiogram (EKG) shows physiological changes such as QRS axis shift to left (because of elevated diaphragm), and minor ST- and T-wave changes in lead III. Fetal growth ultrasounds should be performed every 4 weeks when there is concern for developing intrauterine growth restriction. This can be coupled with serial antenatal testing at 34 weeks.[15] Postdatism is often best avoided. Finally, future contraceptive plans, including sterilization, should be reviewed.[12,16]

General management

Certain general principles apply to most women with cardiac disease:

1. *Antepartum activity modification.* This can be used to minimize maternal exertion and oxygen demand in the pregnant patient with limited cardiac output or cyanotic heart disease.[12] Strict bed rest should be avoided to prevent thromboembolism.
2. *Treat coexisting medical conditions.* The morbidity of cardiac disease can be compounded by medical conditions such as anemia, hypertension, or thyroid disease. Therefore, these conditions should be optimized to minimize their comorbidity.[14]
3. *Collaborative care by multiple specialists.* Pregnant patients with cardiac disease are very complex, and should be **managed by a multidisciplinary team of specialists from a variety of areas,** including obstetrics, maternal–fetal medicine, cardiology, and anesthesiology.[17]
4. *Labor in the lateral decubitus position.* This maximizes blood return to the heart by decreasing vena caval compression by the gravid uterus, and therefore, maximizes cardiac output.[18,19] This preload preservation can be critical to the woman with cardiac compromise.[12,16]
5. *Epidural anesthesia.* This minimizes pain, sympathetic stress, oxygen utilization, and fluctuations in cardiac output. Sometimes 'just' a narcotic epidural should be used, avoiding the sympathetic blockade (and consequent hypotension) of local anesthetics. Spinal anesthesia should be avoided, and an epidural should be dosed

slowly with adequate prehydration (intravenous [IV] fluids) to minimize the risk of hypotension and its consequent drop in preload, leading to decreased cardiac output.[12,20–22]

6. *Oxygen, particularly during labor and delivery, as necessary.* Keeping maternal $PaO_2 \geq 70$ mmHg allows for adequate maternal and fetal hemoglobin oxygen saturation.[16,22]

7. *Bacterial endocarditis prophylaxis.* While antibiotic prophylaxis is not necessary for most obstetric procedures, it can be considered for uncomplicated vaginal delivery in high-risk patients (**prosthetic cardiac valve, prior endocarditis, complex congenital heart disease, and surgically constructed systemic pulmonary shunts or conduits**), and should be given to high-risk or moderate-risk (other congenital cardiac malformations, rheumatic heart disease, hypertrophic cardiomyopathy, and mitral valve prolapse with leaflet thickening and/or regurgitation) women undergoing complicated vaginal delivery (vaginal or rectal lacerations, manual exploration of the uterus).[23] Antibiotic prophylaxis at cesarean delivery (even without maternal cardiac disease) is associated with decrease in operative infection. The recommended antibiotic regimen for cardiac prophylaxis is ampicillin 2.0 g and gentamicin 1.5 mg/kg (maximum 120 mg) IV preprocedure, followed by ampicillin 1.0 g orally 6 hours later. This should be started in the active phase of labor 1–2 hours before delivery is anticipated. Vancomycin 1.0 g can be substituted in the penicillin-allergic patient.[23]

8. *Cesarean delivery is usually reserved for obstetric indications.* Operative delivery is associated with greater blood loss, increased pain, and prolonged bed rest compared with vaginal delivery, and therefore can complicate the gravida with heart disease. While labor induction and/or assisted second stage may be necessary for certain maternal or fetal indications, **cesarean delivery should be used for the usual obstetric reasons.**[15,16,21]

9. *Invasive hemodynamic monitoring with a pulmonary artery catheter (PAC).* Although the safety and utility of PACs in critically ill non-pregnant patients have been recently questioned,[24–26] they may be helpful in managing certain high-risk conditions that are preload dependent, such as critical AS or PHTN.[12,16]

10. *Most patients benefit from avoiding hypotension during labor and delivery.* Although not true for all patients, most patients with group 2 and 3 cardiac lesions will benefit from avoiding hypotension or hypovolemia. **To avoid hypotension, keep the woman on the 'wet' side, avoid hemorrhage, replenish blood loss adequately, avoid spinal anesthesia, hydrate at least 1L of IV fluids before 'slow' epidural, and avoid supine hypotension.**

Pregnancy management of specific diseases

Palpitations

Work-up should include thyroid function, and ruling out drugs, alcohol, caffeine, or smoking, as well as an EKG and echocardiogram. A woman can be counseled that premature atrial and ventricular contractions are increased in pregnancy, and are usually benign.

Ventricular septal defect

Pregnancy outcome is usually good. Rule out PHTN, especially in large, long-standing cases. In the absence of PHTN, mortality is unlikely.[27] Intrapartum, avoid fluid overload.[27]

Eisenmenger's syndrome/pulmonary hypertension

It is important to avoid a false-positive diagnosis of PHTN by echocardiogram, as up to 30% of women with this diagnosis (pulmonary artery systolic pressure > 30–40 mmHg) by echocardiography have normal pulmonary pressures by pulmonary artery catheterization. Whereas not all patients require pulmonary catheterization confirmation, it is a useful test when the diagnosis is in doubt or mild, and can be done either antepartum or just before induction (the latter timing allows the catheter to remain in place for labor management). Over time, in women with unrepaired VSD, ASD, or patent ductus arteriosus (PDA), the left to right shunt leads to PHTN, right to left shunt, and consequently decreased pulmonary perfusion, and hypoxemia. Even with modern management, a high risk of maternal death remains.[28] Some of this mortality is secondary to thromboembolic events.[29] Delayed postpartum death can be seen 4–6 weeks after delivery, possibly secondary to loss of pregnancy-associated hormones and increased pulmonary vascular resistance (PVR).[12,29] As **hypotension** can fatally precipitate decreased pulmonary perfusion and oxygenation (and reverse the left to right cardiac shunt; see pathophysiology above), leading to sudden death, it **must be avoided**. As such, patients are better managed on the 'wet' side, even at the expense of mild pulmonary edema. This allows a margin of safety against unexpected hemorrhage or drug-induced hypotension.[29] PAC may be useful in this regard.[12] Avoid increase in PVR and myocardial depressants. Anticoagulant prophylaxis may be useful in preventing thromboembolic risk, and IV prostacyclin (or its analogues), endothelin-receptor antagonist (Bosentan) (contra-indicated in pregnancy), or inhaled nitric oxide may be helpful in reducing PVR while sparing the systemic vascular resistance (SVR).[30,31]

Coarctation of the aorta

If surgically corrected, maternal outcome is good. There is an increased risk for maternal mortality when associated with aneurysmal dilation or associated cardiac lesions (VSD, PDA).[32] Avoid hypotension, myocardial depression, and bradycardia.[33]

Tetralogy of Fallot

TOF consists of VSD, pulmonary stenosis, hypertrophy of right ventricle, and overriding aorta. Corrected lesions do well, but uncorrected ones are still associated with high maternal mortality.[34] Because of the VSD-associated shunting in uncorrected cases, **hypotension,** myocardial depressants, and bradycardia **should be avoided.**[12]

Mitral stenosis

Women with >1.5 cm^2 mitral valve area usually have good outcomes. When significant (valve area < 1.5 cm^2) mitral stenosis is present, left ventricular filling is limited, which leads to fixed cardiac output. If the pregnant patient is unable to accommodate the volume shifts that occur during gestation and puerperium, pulmonary edema can result (see pathophysiology above). Antenatally, percutaneous balloon valvuloplasty may be relatively safely performed in certain patients.[35] As cardiac output is dependent on adequate diastolic filling time, **tachycardia** can result in hemodynamic decompensation (hypotension and fall in cardiac output) and should be **avoided.** Intrapartum, therefore, short-acting beta-blockers should be considered when the pulse rate exceeds 90–100 beats/min.[12,36] Whereas inadequate preload will decrease cardiac output, too much will result in pulmonary edema, particularly postpartum when pulmonary capillary wedge pressure (PCWP) can rise up to 16 mmHg.[6] As frank pulmonary edema is unusual with PCWP < 28–30 mmHg,[37] PAC and cautious, individualized intrapartum diuresis to a predelivery target of 14 mmHg (while normal is 6–9 mmHg, mitral stenosis patients often need elevated wedge pressures to maintain left ventricular filling) is desirable in some patients.[12,37] Patients with moderate stenosis with only mild fluid overload can often be managed with just fluid restriction to complement their insensible loss during labor.[12] Avoid decrease in SVR, and increase in PVR.

Aortic stenosis

The major issue is fixed and limited cardiac output through a restricted valve area. Mortality is related to degree of stenosis, with > 100 mmHg of shunt gradient associated with 15–20% mortality. Congestive heart failure (CHF), syncope, and previous cardiac arrest are other contraindications to pregnancy.

Hypotension and decreased preload can lead to a precipitous drop in cardiac output. Consequently, **hypotension should be avoided.**[38] PAC monitoring may be helpful to increase the PCWP to the 15–17 mmHg range to maintain a margin of safety against unexpected blood loss or hypotension (although the data are insufficient for an evidence-based recommendation).[12,16] This range of PCWP minimizes risk of frank pulmonary edema even with normal postpartum fluid shifts, and furthermore, hypovolemia is potentially more dangerous in these patients than pulmonary edema. Avoid decrease in venous return, and tachycardia.

Mitral and aortic insufficiency

These lesions are usually well tolerated in pregnancy. Avoid arrhythmia, bradycardia, increase in SVR, and myocardial depressants.

Mechanical heart valves

Women who anticipate ultimately needing valve replacement surgery should be encouraged to complete childbearing before valve replacement. For women with mechanical heart valves, optimal anticoagulation during pregnancy is controversial. The highest risk is with first-generation mechanical valves (Starr–Edwards, Bjork–Shiley) in the mitral position, followed by second-generation valves (St Jude) in the aortic position. These women need to be **therapeutically anticoagulated throughout pregnancy and postpartum, with blood levels frequently (usually weekly) checked to ensure therapeutic levels of anticoagulation.** With unfractionated heparin, mid-interval activated partial thromboplastin time (PTT) should be maintained at about 60–80 seconds. With warfarin the international normalized ratio (INR) should be maintained at 2.0–3.0. With low molecular weight heparin, peak anti Xa level should be about 0.8–1.2 and trough 0.6–0.7. Warfarin throughout pregnancy and postpartum is probably the regimen associated with the least maternal risks of thromboembolism, but in the first trimester warfarin is associated with a 10–15% teratogenic risk (nasal hypoplasia, optic atrophy, digital anomalies, mental impairment). On the other hand, **heparin throughout pregnancy can be ineffective.**[7,8] A common option utilizes unfractionated **heparin during the first trimester to minimize teratogenesis, warfarin for the majority of pregnancy (12–36 weeks), and unfractionated heparin again in the last month to prepare for delivery and allow for epidural anesthesia.**[39,40] While this management may be efficacious, fetal risk is not completely eliminated.[41] Low molecular weight heparin in this setting has been associated with reports of valve thrombosis, with an FDA (Food and Drug Administration) warning against its use in this setting (although this decision was criticized).[42,43] Regarding delivery, therapeutic anticoagulation should be stopped during active labor and for delivery, with therapeutic heparin restarted about 6–12 hours after delivery, and warfarin restarted in an overlapping fashion (to avoid paradoxical thrombosis) 24–36 hours after delivery (the night after delivery). Extensive counseling on all these options and risks is required.

Marfan syndrome

Marfan syndrome is an autosomal dominant generalized connective tissue disorder, with 80% of affected women having a family history of this condition. Its main risk in pregnancy is aortic aneurysm, leading to rupture and dissection. Women with a personal or family history of Marfan syndrome should have an **echocardiogram,** possibly a slit lamp examination to look for ectopia lentis, and **genetic counseling.** Prognosis is reasonable when there is no aortic root involvement (<5% mortality), although mortality can still occur. There is a risk of aortic rupture, dissection, and mortality (up to 50%) in pregnancy w**hen the aortic root is dilated beyond 4 cm,** such that pregnancy is contraindicated in these women before repair. This may result from the 'shearing force' of normal pregnancy increase in blood volume and cardiac output.[44–46] Prenatally, serial maternal echocardiograms to follow the cardiac root should be performed.[45] **Hypertension should be avoided,** and **beta-blockade therapy** should be considered. Whereas pregnancy data are limited for this last recommendation, long-term use in non-pregnant patients has been shown to slow the progression of aortic root dilation.[47] Avoid positive inotropic drugs, and plan epidural (watch for dural ectasia, present in about 90% of patients with Marfan syndrome) to reduce cardiovascular stress. If cesarean delivery is required, retention sutures should be considered because of generalized connective tissue weakness.[12]

Hypertrophic cardiomyopathy

Previously called idiopathic hypertrophic subaortic stenosis, hypertrophic cardiomyopathy can be inherited as autosomal dominant, with variable penetrance. It can result in left ventricular hypertrophy, leading to obstruction of the left ventricular outflow. The decrease in SVR of pregnancy can worsen outflow obstruction. Also, tachycardia decreases diastolic filling time, compromising cardiac output. Peripartum management focuses on avoiding tachycardia (treatment with beta-blockade) and hypotension.[48,49]

Dilated cardiomypathy

The left ventricle is hypokinetic, cardiac output falls, and can be associated with arrhythmia and possible CHF. Etiology includes autoimmune, alcohol, infection, and genetic factors. When severe dilated cardiomyopathy is present, a possible option is prepregnancy transplantation.

Peripartum cardiomyopathy

This condition is defined as cardiomyopathy (with EF <45%) occurring during the last 4 weeks of pregnancy or within 5 months postpartum (peaks at 2 months postpartum), without other cause. The incidence is 1/3000–4000 live births. Risk factors are older maternal age, multiparity, African-American race, multiple gestation, and hypertensive disorders of pregnancy. Serial echocardiography, medical management (**digoxin, diuretics,** and afterload reduction – **hydralazine** and/or **beta-blockers** during pregnancy; angiotensin-converting enzyme [ACE] inhibitors postpartum), anticoagulation if EF is <35%, and possible intrapartum PAC in severe patients are useful for management.[12,50–53]

Regarding future pregnancies after a diagnosis of peripartum cardiomyopathy, persistent dilated cardiomyopathy with abnormal EF predicts a high risk of mortality with subsequent gestation, and should be discouraged. Even women with "normal" echocardiograms (EF ≥ 45–50%) after recovering from peripartum cardiomyopathy can have persistent 'subclinical' low contractile reserve,[51] with up to 21% risk of developing symptoms of CHF in a future pregnancy, but a < 5% risk of maternal death.[54]

Coronary artery disease

Underlying risks factors, such as diabetes, obesity, hypercholesterolemia, smoking, hypertension, and stress, should be individually addressed and treated, ideally before conception. Stable angina can be treated with nitrates, calcium channel blockers, and/or beta-blockers in pregnancy. With unstable angina, the woman should be counseled regarding severe risks, and offered termination if early enough in pregnancy. Myocardial infarction (MI) is rare in reproductive-age women, with a 1:10 000 incidence in the pregnancy. When MI occurs in the third trimester or within 2 weeks of labor, there is a high (20%) maternal mortality risk.[54] Women with prior MI with recovered heart function and optimally controlled CAD can anticipate a successful pregnancy.[55] Management of MI during pregnancy is similar to management in non-pregnant patients, including coronary angioplasty (or stent), although thrombolytic therapy is a relative contraindication.[16,54,56] Heparin and beta-blockers are recommended. If labor occurs within 4 days of an MI, cesarean delivery is often advocated.[57] Women with a prior MI should wait at least 1 year after the MI, and ensure normal cardiac function before pregnancy. In such circumstances, a future pregnancy is associated with low risk of maternal or fetal morbidity or mortality.

CONCLUSION

With medical and surgical advances, and advancing maternal age, heart disease complicating pregnancy is increasingly common. Understanding the physiological changes of pregnancy and their effect on specific cardiac conditions forms the basis for management during pregnancy. Optimizing cardiac function and decreasing the risk of cardiac decompensation by proper management and close prenatal surveillance will allow most pregnant women with heart disease to enjoy a favorable maternal and fetal outcome.

REFERENCES

1. Koonin LM, Atrash HK, Lawson HW, et al. Maternal mortality surveillance, United States 1979–1986. MMWR CDC Surveill Summ 1991; 40: 1–13. [II-3]
2. DeSweit M. Maternal mortality from heart disease in pregnancy. Br Heart J 1993; 69: 524. [II-3]
3. Berg CJ, Atrash HK, Koonin LM, et al. Pregnancy-related mortality in the United States, 1987–1990. Obstet Gynecol 1996; 88: 161–7. [II-3]
4. American College of Obstetricians and Gynecologists. Cardiac disease in pregnancy. Technical Bulletin No. 168, June 1992. [III]
5. Sinnenberg RJ. Pulmonary hypertension in pregnancy. South Med J 1980; 73: 1529–31. [III]
6. Clark SL, Phelan JP, Greenspoon J, et al. Labor and delivery in the presence of mitral stenosis: central hemodynamic observations. Am J Obstet Gynecol 1985; 152: 984–8. [II-3]
7. Oakley CM, Doherty P. Pregnancy in patients after heart valve replacement. Br Heart J 1976; 38: 1140–8. [II-3]
8. Golby AJ, Bush EC, DeRook FA, et al. Failure of high-dose heparin to prevent recurrent cardioembolic strokes in a pregnancy patient with a mechanical heart valve. Neurology 1992; 42: 2204–6. [III]
9. van Oppen ACC, Stigter RH, Bruinse HW. Cardiac output in normal pregnancy: a critical review. Obstet Gynecol 1996; 87: 310–18. [III]
10. Arias F, Pineda J. Aortic stenosis and pregnancy. J Reprod Med 1978; 20: 229–32. [II-3]
11. Sciscione AC, Callen NA. Pregnancy and contraception: congenital heart disease in adolescents and adults. Cardiol Clin 1993; 11: 701–9. [III]
12. Foley MR. Cardiac disease. In: Dildy GA, Belfont MA, Suade G, et al., eds. Critical Case Obstestrics, 4th edn. Molden, MA: Blackwell Publishing Company; 2004. [II-3]
13. Jacob S, Bloebaum L, Shah G, et al. Maternal mortality in Utah. Obstet Gynecol 1998; 91: 187–91. [II-3]
14. Blanchard DG, Shabetai R. Cardiac diseases. In: Creasy RK, Resnik R, Iams JD, eds. Maternal Fetal Medicine Principles and Practice, 5th edn. Philadelphia, PA: WB Saunders; 2004. [III]
15. McFaul PB, Dornan JC, Lamki H, et al. Pregnancy complicated by maternal heart disease: a review of 519 women. BJOG 1988; 95: 861–7. [III]
16. Tomlinson, MW. Cardiac disease. In: James DK, Steer PJ, Weiner CP, Gonik B, eds. High-Risk Pregnancy Management Options, 3rd edn. Philadelphia, PA: WB Saunders; 2006. [III]
17. Surgue D, Blake S, MacDonald D. Pregnancy complicated by maternal heart disease at the National Maternity Hospital, Dublin, Ireland, 1969–1978. Am J Obstet Gynecol 1981; 139: 1–6. [III]
18. Ueland K, Novy MJ, Peterson EN, et al. Maternal cardiovascular dynamics IV. The influence of gestational age on maternal cardiovascular response to posture and exercise. Am J Obstet Gynecol 1969; 104: 856. [II-3]
19. Clark SL, Cotton DB, Pivarnik JM, et al. Position change and hemodynamic profiling during normal third-trimester pregnancy and postpartum. Am J Obstet Gynecol 1991; 164: 883. [II-3]
20. Vadhera RB. Anesthesia for the critically ill parturient with cardiac disease and pregnancy induced hypertension. In: Dildy G, Belfort M, Suade G, et al, eds. Critical Care Obstetrics, 4th edn. Malden, MA: Blackwell Publishing; 2004. [III]
21. Siu S, Sermer M, Colman J, et al. Prospective multicenter study of pregnancy outcome in women with heart disease. Circulation 2001; 104: 515–21. [II-3]
22. Sobrevilla LA, Cassinella MT, Carcelen A, et al. Human fetal and maternal oxygen tension and acid–base status during delivery at high altitude. Am J Obstet Gynecol 1971; 111: 1111–18. [III]
23. Dajani AS, Taubert KA, Wilson W, et al. Prevention of bacterial endocarditis: recommendations of the American Heart Association. JAMA 1997; 277: 1794–801. [III]
24. Bernard G, Sopko G, Cerra F, et al. Pulmonary artery catheterization and clinical outcomes: National Heart, Lung, and Blood Institute and Food and Drug Administration Workshop Report. JAMA 2000; 283: 2568–72. [III]
25. Sandham JD, Hull RD, Brant RF, et al. A randomized, controlled trial of the use of pulmonary artery-catheters in high-risk surgical patients. N Engl J Med 2003; 348: 5–14. [I]
26. Parsons PE. Progress in research on pulmonary-artery catheters. N Engl J Med 2003; 348: 66–8. [III]
27. Schaefer G, Arditi LI, Solomon HA, et al. Congenital heart disease and pregnancy. Clin Obstet Gynecol 1968; 11: 1048–63. [III]
28. Avila WS, Grinberg M, Snitcowsky R, et al. Maternal and fetal outcome in pregnant women with Eisenmenger's syndrome. Eur Heart J 1995; 16: 460–4. [III]
29. Weiss BM, Zemp L, Seifert B, et al. Outcome of pulmonary vascular disease in pregnancy: a systematic overview from 1978–1996. J Am Coll Cardiol 1998; 31: 1650–7. [III]
30. Stewart R, Tuazon D, Olson G, et al. Pregnancy and primary pulmonary hypertension. Chest 2001; 119: 973–5. [III]
31. Lam GK, Stafford RE, Thorp J, Moise KJ Jr, Cairns BA. Inhaled nitric oxide for primary pulmonary hypertension in pregnancy. Obstet Gynecol 2001; 98: 895–8. [II-3]
32. Deal K, Wooley CF. Coarctation of the aorta and pregnancy. Ann Intern Med 1973; 78: 706–10. [III]
33. Koszalka MF. Cardiac disease in pregnancy. In: Foley MR Jr, Strong TH, Garite TJ, eds. Obstetric Intensive Care: A Practical Manual. Philadelphia, PA: WB Saunders; 1997. [III]
34. Shime J, Mocarski EJ, Hastings D, Webb GD, MCLaughlin PR. Congenital heart disease in pregnancy: short- and long-term implications. Am J Obstet Gynecol 1987; 156: 313–22. [III]
35. Iung B, Cormier B, Elias J, et al. Usefulness of percutaneous balloon commissurotomy for mitral stenosis during pregnancy. Am J Cardiol 1994; 73: 398–400. [III]
36. Al Kasab SM, Sabag T, Al Zailbag M, et al. β-adrenergic receptor blockade in the management of pregnant women with mitral stenosis. Am J Obstet Gynecol 1990; 163: 37–40. [III]
37. Forrester JS, Swan HJC. Acute myocardial infarction: a physiological basis for therapy. Crit Care Med 1974; 2: 283–92. [II-3]
38. Lao TT, Stemmer M, Magee L, et al. Congenital aortic stenosis and pregnancy: a reappraisal. Am J Obstet Gynecol 1993; 169: 540–5. [III]
39. Vongpatanasin W, Hillis LD, Lange RA. Prosthetic heart valves. N Engl J Med 1996; 335: 407–16. [III]
40. Ad hoc committee of the Working Group on Valvular Heart Disease, European Society of Cardiology: guidelines for prevention of thromboembolic events in valvular heart disease. J Heart Valve Dis 1993; 2: 398–410. [III]

41. Briggs GG, Freeman RK, Yaffe SJ, eds. Drugs in Pregnancy and Lactation. Baltimore, MD: Lippincott, Williams and Wilkins; 1994.

42. Ginsberg JS, Chan WS, Bates SM, et al. Anticoagulation of pregnant women with mechanical heart valves. Arch Intern Med 2003; 163: 694–8. [III]

43. Anticoagulation and enoxaparin use in patients with prosthetic heart valves and/or pregnancy. Fetal Matern Med Consensus Rep 2002; 3: 1–20. [III]

44. Pyeritz RE. Maternal and fetal complications of pregnancy in the Marfan syndrome. Am J Med 1981; 71: 784–90. [III]

45. Rossiter JP, Repke JT, Morales AJ, et al. A prospective longitudinal evaluation of pregnancy in the Marfan syndrome. Am J Obstet Gynecol 1995; 173: 1599–606. [III]

46. Lipscomb KJ, Smith JC, Clarke B, et al. Outcome of pregnancy in women with Marfan's syndrome. BJOG 1997; 104: 201–6. [II–3]

47. Shores J, Berger KR, Murphy EA, et al. Progression of aortic dilatation and the benefit of long term β-adrenergic blockade in Marfan's syndrome. N Engl J Med 1994; 330: 1335–41. [II–3]

48. Maron BJ. Hypertrophic cardiomyopathy: a systematic review. JAMA 2002; 287: 1308–20. [III]

49. Fairley CJ, Clarke JT. Use of esmolol in a parturient with hypertrophic obstructive cardiomyopathy. Br J Anaesth 1995; 74: 801–4. [II–3]

50. Demakis JG, Rahimtoola SH, Sutton GC, et al. Natural course of peripartum cardiomyopathy. Circulation 1971; 44: 1053–61. [III]

51. Lampert MB, Weinert L, Hibbard J, et al. Contractile reserve in patients with peripartum cardiomyopathy and recovered left ventricular function. Am J Obstet Gynecol 1997; 176: 189–95. [II-3]

52. Witlin AG, Mabie WC, Sibai BM. Peripartum cardiomyopathy: an ominous diagnosis. Am J Obstet Gynecol 1997; 176: 182–8. [III]

53. Elkayam U, Tummala PP, Rao K, et al. Maternal and fetal outcomes of subsequent pregnancies in women with peripartum cardiomyopathy. N Engl J Med 2001; 344: 1567–71. [II-3]

54. Roth A, Elkayam RA. Acute myocardial infarction associated with pregnancy. Ann Intern Med 1996; 125: 751–62. [III]

55. Vinatier D, Virelizier S, Depret-Mosser S, et al. Pregnancy after myocardial infarction. Eur J Obstet Gynecol Reprod Biol 1994; 56: 89–93. [III]

56. Garry D, Leikin E, Fleisher AG, et al. Acute myocardial infarction in pregnancy with subsequent medical and surgical management. Obstet Gynecol 1996; 87: 802–4. [III]

57. Mabie WC, Anderson GD, Addington MB, et al. The benefit of cesarean section in acute myocardial infarction complicated by premature labor. Obstet Gynecol 1988; 71: 503–6. [III]

3

Dermatoses of pregnancy

Dana Correale and Jason B Lee

BACKGROUND

Stretch marks are the only pregnancy-related dermatological condition for which there are trials for interventions. Pregnancy-specific dermatoses (PSD), as well as melanoma in pregnancy, are not well studied, with no specific trials regarding treatment. Most evidence regarding pathogenesis and etiology, as well as typical disease presentation, is based on case reports and case series. PSD have been plagued by synonyms and eponyms in the past. However, more recent efforts have established a more unified nomenclature, which has improved communication among physicians regarding some of the rarer and more recently described entities. Table 3.1 provides a summary of the pregnancy-specific dermatoses. Multidisciplinary management involving a dermatologist expert in dermatological conditions in pregnancy is of paramount importance.

STRIAE GRAVIDARUM

KEY POINTS

- The **exact cause** of striae gravidarum (SG) is **unknown**, but the strongest associated risk factors for their development are the presence of pre-existing breast and thigh striae and a family history.
- **There is no widely available product that has been shown to prevent the formation of SG.** Massage with either **Trofolastin cream** or **Verum ointment** is associated with a **decrease in the development of SG**.
- **Topical tretinoin and various types of laser therapy have been shown to be helpful in the treatment of SG.**

Table 3.1 *A summary of the pregnancy-specific dermatoses*				
Dermatosis	Course	Skin findings	Fetal risks	Treatment
PUPPP	Third trimester. Resolution postpartum	Urticarial lesions on the abdomen, often within striae with sparing of the periumbilical area. Extension to upper thighs and buttocks	None	High potency topical steroids
PFP	Second or third trimester. Resolution within 1–2 months postpartum	Follicular papules and pustules	None	Mid to high potency topical corticosteroids
PP	Second or third trimester. Resolution postpartum	Excoriated papules over extremities and occasionally abdomen	None	Mid to high potency topical steroids
IH	Third trimester. Persists after delivery if untreated	Symmetric, erythematous patches with peripheral superficial sterile pustules on flexural skin	Placental insufficiency and fetal loss	Systemic corticosteroids

PUPPP, pruritic urticarial papules and plaques of pregnancy; PFP, pruritic folliculitis of pregnancy; PP, prurigo of pregnancy; IH, impetigo herpetiformis.

Diagnosis/definition

Striae distensae (SD), or stretch marks, do not represent a disease, but rather they are a cosmetic problem for many people. They often occur for the first time during pregnancy and are referred to as striae gravidarum (SG). SD initially appear as linear patches that are red to purple in color and lack noticeable surface change (striae rubra). With time, their color fades to lighter than normal skin tone. They become atrophic or depressed with a fine, wrinkled surface (striae alba).

Symptoms

SD are largely asymptomatic. They may be slightly pruritic in their early stages.

Epidemiology/incidence

The prevalence of SG ranges from 50 to 90%.[1] The mean gestational age for the onset of SG is 25 weeks.[1]

Genetics

There is no known clear genetic cause of SG; however, there may be a familial tendency to develop them.[1]

Etiology/basic pathology

Many theories exist regarding the etiology of SG. Rapid weight gain, baseline weight, hormonal changes, and greater change in abdominal and hip girth during pregnancy have been associated in the past with SG.[1,2] None of these theories has been supported by any recent studies. It is known, however, that elastin and fibrillin fibers, components of the dermal extracellular matrix, are reduced in SD.[3]

Risk factors/associations

The factors most strongly associated with the development of SG are the **presence of breast or thigh striae**, having a **mother with SG**, having **additional family members with SG**, and non-white race. In contrast, pre-pregnancy body mass index (BMI), mean weight gain during pregnancy, mean percent weight gain, and mean change in BMI seem not to be associated with the development of SG.[1]

Management

Prevention

Massage with Trofolastin cream containing *Centella asiatica* extract, alpha-tocopherol, and collagen–elastin hydrolysates applied daily is associated with a 59% **decrease in the development of SG** compared with massage with placebo.[4] Overall, 56% of the placebo group developed SG compared with 34% of the Trofolastin group. **Massage with Verum ointment** containing tocopherol, essential fatty acids, panthenol, hyaluronic acid, elastin, and menthol is also associated with a 74% **decrease in the development of SG** compared with no treatment, so it is unclear in this study if the massage or the Verum ointment or the combination of the two was beneficial.[4] In women with stretch marks from a previous pregnancy, there is no benefit. It should be noted that neither of these compounds is widely available, nor is it known what their active ingredient, if any, might be. There is the suggestion from the second study that bland emollients and massage alone may be of benefit in preventing the formation of SG.

Therapy

Once SG have formed, there are treatment options. Topical tretinoin 0.1% cream has been shown to reduce the appearance of SG/SD when used on early lesions (striae rubra).[5] It is important to note that once striae have become white and atrophic, topical tretinoin was shown to have no benefit in a double-blind, placebo-controlled study.[6] Topical tretinoin (Retin A) works by binding to cytoplasmic proteins and nuclear receptors of keratinocytes and altering downstream gene transcription. Their end biological effect is to regulate the growth and differentiation of keratinocytes.[7] In addition to regulating keratinocyte proliferation, topical retinoids have been shown to decrease fine wrinkling, increase dermal collagen, and repair elastin fiber formation.[8] Improvement in the appearance of SD/SG is probably the result of this particular biological effect. Tretinoin is pregnancy category C. Its use is contraindicated during breastfeeding, which makes it difficult to use during the early stages of SG. The side effects of tretinoin therapy are erythema, desquamation, and photosensitivity limited to the application site.

In addition to tretinoin therapy, improvement in the appearance of SD/SG can be achieved with laser therapy. **Laser therapy** is a rapidly evolving field, with new lasers and applications emerging on a regular basis. Two large, blinded studies using an objective grading system evaluating the treatment of SD using a 585-nm pulsed dye laser have shown improvement in their appearance.[9] Both increases and decreases in collagen production have been shown post-treatment, depending on the wavelength and energy density of the laser used. An increase in dermal elastin content has also been shown in biopsies obtained after laser therapy.[9] Again, newer, more erythematous striae respond more favorably to pulsed dye laser treatment. This may be a more reasonable treatment option during the postpartum period, as laser therapy is believed to be safe in breastfeeding women. A more recent study evaluating the effects of an XeCl excimer ultraviolet B (UVB) laser and a ultraviolet UVB light device showed repigmentation of striae alba.[2]

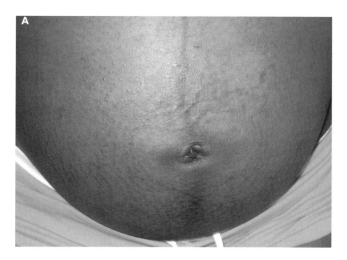
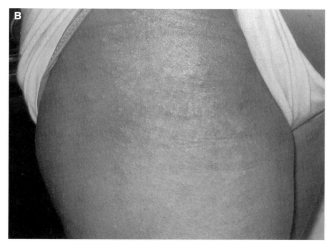

Figure 3.1
Pruritic urticarial papules and plaques of pregnancy (PUPPP). A 28-year-old primigravida with abrupt onset of extremely pruritic urticarial papules on the abdomen (A) and thighs (B) during her 39th week of pregnancy. Note the predilection for the abdominal striae with periumbilical sparing.

Repigmentation was associated with an increase in melanin content, hypertrophy of melanocytes, and an increase in the number of melanocytes 6 months after treatment.

PRURITIC URTICARIAL PAPULES AND PLAQUES OF PREGNANCY

KEY POINTS

- Pruritic urticarial papules and plaques of pregnancy (PUPPP) is an extremely pruritic urticarial eruption occurring during the third trimester of pregnancy.
- There is no associated fetal morbidity or mortality.
- The mainstay of **treatment** is **topical steroids.**

Historic notes

This entity was originally described by Lawley and collegues in 1979 in a series of seven patients.[10]

Diagnosis/definition

Pruritic urticarial papules and plaques of pregnancy (PUPPP) is characterized by urticarial lesions that **begin on the abdomen**, often within abdominal striae, and spare the periumbilical area (Figure 3.1). Lesions frequently spread to the **upper thighs and buttocks and occasionally may affect the arms.** The face, palms, and soles are usually spared. Despite the severe pruritus, there is notable lack of excoriation. As its name implies, PUPPP is polymorphous. Clinical lesions may appear vesicular, targetoid, or purpuric. This eruption is seen mostly in primigravidas with onset in the third trimester of pregnancy. It resolves shortly after delivery, but there have been a few cases reported in which onset of the disease has occurred in the post partum period.[11–13] The diagnosis is primarily clinical. Histopathological examination of affected skin most often yields non-specific findings.

Symptoms

The eruption is accompanied by extreme pruritus. The itching is often so severe that it may interfere with sleep.

Epidemiology/incidence

PUPPP is one of the most common dermatoses of pregnancy. It occurs in approximately 0.5% of pregnancies.[14]

Genetics

There are no known genetic factors in PUPPP. In fact, some studies have looked for, but failed to document an HLA (human leukocyte antigen) association.[15,16]

Etiology/basic pathology

To date, there are no widely accepted theories to explain the etiology of this disease. Associated factors include increased abdominal distention secondary to excessive maternal weight gain and fetal birth weight,[12,16,17] increased incidence of multiple pregnancy,[11,14,16,18] not autoimmune mechanisms,[19] but decreased serum cortisol levels,[20,21] and fetal DNA migration in PUPPP skin lesions.[22]

Complications

There have been no consistent maternal or fetal complications associated with PUPPP, with newborns not affected with any related skin disease.[13,16,20]

Work-up

The most important disease to exclude when diagnosing PUPPP is herpes gestationis (HG), which can present with urticarial lesions in the absence of more prototypical blisters. HG is usually a widespread eruption which begins on the abdomen but does not show a predilection for striae nor spares the periumbilical area. HG represents an expression of the autoimmune blistering disease bullous pemphigoid during pregnancy. HG is rare, but it is associated with significant maternal morbidity and fetal morbidity and mortality.[20,23] Exclusion of HG relies on the clinical presentation, but direct immunofluorescence (DIF) of affected skin may be required in equivocal cases. There are no consistent DIF findings in PUPPP.[12,13,16,20,24] When positive DIF findings have been reported in PUPPP, they have been considered non-diagnostic for any particular disease.[13,24] In contrast, HG is associated with very consistent and reliable DIF findings.[23]

Management

Preconception counseling

The vast majority of cases of PUPPP do not recur with subsequent pregnancies[10,16,20] or oral contraceptive use.[10,16] A few women affected by PUPPP have been reported to have episodes of transient hives while breastfeeding after the initial eruption resolved.[10]

Therapy

The majority of cases of PUPPP can be effectively managed with **high-potency topical steroids**.[10,16,20] This class of medication does not cause any known fetal complications when used properly. In rare cases of prolonged and widespread use, significant systemic absorption could occur. In severe and widespread cases, short courses of oral corticosteroids have been used effectively.[10,16,20] The reader is referred to later in this chapter for the guideline for impetigo

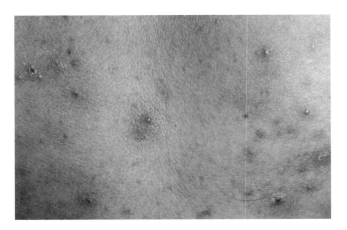

Figure 3.2
Pruritic folliculitis of pregnancy. A 28-year-old woman with erythematous, follicular papules on the abdomen.

herpetiformis (IH) for a more detailed information on the use and safety of steroids in pregnancy. There is one reported case of severe PUPPP that required delivery by cesarean section at 35 weeks' gestation for intractable pruritus uncontrolled by topical and oral corticosteroids.[25] In this case, the patient's symptoms were significantly improved within 12 hours of delivery.

PRURITIC FOLLICULITIS OF PREGNANCY

KEY POINTS

- Pruritic folliculitis of pregnancy (PFP) is a **benign** eruption presenting in the second or third trimester.
- There is no underlying infectious etiology.
- There are no adverse maternal or fetal outcomes.
- The mainstay of **therapy** is **topical corticosteroids**.

Historic notes

PFP was originally described by Zoberman and Farmer in 1981 in a series of 6 pregnant patients.[26]

Diagnosis/definition

PFP is characterized by pruritic, follicular papules with some discrete pustules in a primarily truncal distribution (Figure 3.2). The eruption occurs anywhere from the 4th to 9th month of gestation and resolves by 1–2 months postpartum. The rash may recur with subsequent pregnancies. Histopathological examination of affected skin shows a sterile folliculitis.[26] Immunoreactive deposit is not detected in DIF in PFP.[26–28]

Symptoms

PFP is usually accompanied by mild to moderate pruritus.

Epidemiology/incidence

There are no formal data available that document the incidence of PFP. This entity may be under-reported because of frequent mistaken diagnoses of bacterial folliculitis.[27,29,30]

Etiology/basic pathology

The underlying etiology of PFP is unknown. One case report suggests that *Pityrosporum* yeast may be a causative agent.[31] The vast majority of case reports fail to reveal any causative organism by special staining during histopathological examination or by culture.[26,27,29,32,33] Some clinicians have proposed a hormone-related etiology based on the similarity of PFP to steroid acne,[34] but a recent controlled, prospective study did not show any change in androgen levels in patients with PFP.[28]

Pregnancy considerations

There is one case report of premature delivery secondary to placental abruption at 32 weeks.[33] There is a reported increase in the male to female birth ratio.[28] Otherwise, there are no reports of adverse maternal or fetal outcomes in PFP.

Work-up

The diagnosis of PFP relies mostly on its clinical features. We advocate performing a routine Gram stain and culture on a primary pustule to rule out routine bacterial folliculitis. Skin biopsy for histopathology may be necessary for equivocal cases.

Management

Therapy

The mainstay of therapy is **mid- to high-potency topical corticosteroids**.[26,28,29] The reader is referred to the guideline for PUPPP (above) for a discussion on the use of topical corticosteroids during pregnancy. A recently reported alternative treatment in recalcitrant cases of PFP is narrowband UVB phototherapy.[33] The mechanism of action of UVB is not entirely defined, but it is believed that UV radiation can depress certain components of the cell-mediated immune system and thereby exert beneficial effects in a wide variety of inflammatory skin diseases.[35] UVB treatment is considered safe during pregnancy.[35]

PRURIGO OF PREGNANCY
KEY POINTS

* Prurigo of pregnancy (PP) is an intensely pruritic eruption confined mostly to the extremities.
* The mainstay of **therapy** is **topical steroids**.
* There is no associated maternal or fetal morbidity or mortality.

Historic notes

Prurigo of pregnancy (PP) was first described by Nurse in 1968.[36] His case series of 31 patients is the largest group of women with PP to be described to date. A synonym for this skin disease is prurigo gestationis of Besnier.

Diagnosis/definition

PP is diagnosed by its clinical features. The eruption consists of pruritic papules occurring on the extensor surface of the extremities and occasionally the abdomen (Figure 3.3). Excoriation is often present. The lesions appear between the 25th and 30th weeks of gestation. In the original description of this disease, there was no tendency toward recurrence in subsequent pregnancies. However, others have found that this is not the case.[37] The eruption resolves in the postpartum period, but there have been a few patients in which lesions have persisted for as long as 3 months after delivery.[36] A skin biopsy shows non-specific histopathological changes.

Symptoms

The papules are intensely pruritic.

Epidemiology/incidence

In Nurse's original report, the incidence was calculated as 1 in 300 pregnancies. A more recent prospective analysis of pruritic eruptions during pregnancy yielded an incidence of PP of 1 in 450 pregnancies.[37]

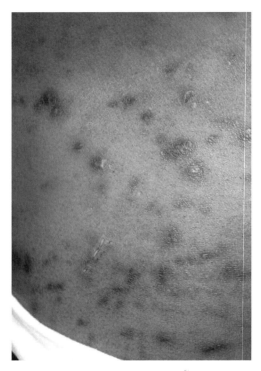

Figure 3.3
Prurigo of pregnancy. Grouped excoriated papules on the thigh of a 24-year-old primigravida with a prior history of asthma and seasonal allergies.

Etiology/basic pathology

There is no definitive evidence regarding the etiology of PP. One theory is that women who are affected have an underlying predisposition to atopy either by personal history or family history and that this predisposition is unmasked during pregnancy.[38] Evidence to support this theory is that some women with PP have elevated serum immunoglobulin E (IgE) levels.[38,39] Evidence for atopy by personal and/or family history has been present in some series[38,39] and absent in others.[37] There have not been any significant changes detected in levels of β-human chorionic gonadotropin (β-HCG), estradiol, or cortisol in women with PP vs controls.[37,39]

Risk factors/associations

There may be an association between PP and a personal or family history of an atopic diathesis (atopic dermatitis, allergic rhinitis, asthma).[38,39]

Complications

There are no large-scale epidemiological studies investigating maternal or fetal morbidity. No case series has ever reported any associated fetal or maternal complications[36,38,39] except for one patient who exhibited intrauterine growth restriction.[37]

Work-up

The diagnosis of PP rests on the clinical features of the eruption. In all cases, DIF has been negative[37–39] and therefore is not indicated.

Management

Therapy

The mainstay of therapy for PP is **mid- to high-potency topical steroids**.[36–40] This class of medication does not cause any known fetal complications when used properly. In rare cases of prolonged and widespread use, significant systemic absorption could occur.

IMPETIGO HERPETIFORMIS
KEY POINTS

- Impetigo herpetiformis (IH) represents **pustular psoriasis** that occurs during pregnancy.
- Most patients have no prior history of psoriasis.
- There is an **increased risk of placental insufficiency and fetal loss.**
- Patients are at risk for recurrence of disease with subsequent pregnancies.
- The mainstay of **therapy** is **oral corticosteroids.**

Historic notes

This disease was first described in 1872 by Von Hebra in a series of 5 pregnant women, 40 years before the first description of generalized pustular psoriasis.[41]

Diagnosis/definition

Impetigo herpetiformis (IH) is characterized by symmetric, erythematous patches with peripheral superficial sterile pustules (Figure 3.4). There is **no underlying infectious etiology** despite the name this disorder was given. The

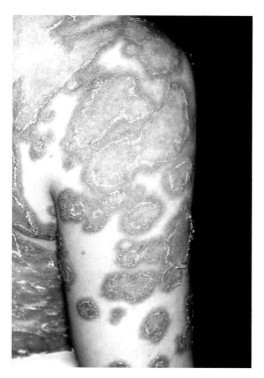

Figure 3.4
Impetigo herpetiformis. A 26-year-old pregnant woman with erythematous plaques bordered by tiny pustules on the trunk and extremities. There was no prior history of psoriasis. (Reprinted with permission from Imai et al.[46] Archives of Dermatology, January 2002, Volume 138, p. 129. Copyright © (2002), American Medical Association. All rights reserved.)

eruption begins over the intertriginous and flexural skin and expands outward. Older lesions may become crusted or secondarily infected.

Symptoms

Patients may report very mild itching or burning at the sites of the lesions; however, most are asymptomatic. There may be accompanying fever, malaise, diarrhea, and vomiting.

Epidemiology/incidence

There are no formal epidemiological data. IH is very rare, with only about 100 cases being reported in the literature. The eruption most often occurs in the third trimester, but can occur as early as the first trimester. Most women do not have a prior history of psoriasis.

Genetics

Generalized pustular psoriasis is associated with HLA types B17 and Cw6.[42]

Etiology/basic pathology

IH is probably a **variant of pustular psoriasis** that occurs during pregnancy.[42–44] The basic underlying etiology is unknown. Many theories exist, including hormonal dysregulation and electrolyte imbalance, but these are based on a few case reports. Histopathology of the skin shows a characteristic sterile pustule containing polymorphonuclear neutrophils in the epidermis referred to as a spongiform pustule of Kogoj, which is indistinguishable from findings that are seen in pustular psoriasis. There may also be elongation of the rete ridges and overlying parakeratosis.

Risk factors/associations

Patients usually do not have a prior history of psoriasis and there is no evidence that having such a history increases the risk of IH in pregnancy.[43]

Complications

The most important complication is **placental insufficiency and fetal death,** the etiology of which is unknown.[42,43] There may be hypocalcemia or decreased vitamin D levels as a result of hypoparathyroidism or hypoalbuminemia.[42,43,45] If severe, these changes may lead to tetany or seizure.

Pregnancy management

Patients must be monitored closely with fetal ultrasound and fetal testing because of the risk of placental insufficiency.[41]

Principles

Pregnancy is speculated to be a trigger for IH.[43] The effect of the disease on the pregnancy is discussed above.

Work-up

Work-up includes **skin biopsy** for routine histopathology as well as a second specimen for DIF in order to rule out other pregnancy-specific dermatoses such as herpes gestationis. When the presentation is accompanied by systemic symptoms, systemic infection must be ruled out with blood cultures as well as bacterial and viral cultures of one or more pustules. Serum calcium, vitamin D, and hypoparathyroid levels should be monitored. The patient should be questioned regarding the history of skin eruptions during any previous pregnancies.

Prevention

None.

Preconception counseling

Any patient with a history of IH should be counseled that it may recur with subsequent pregnancies.

Therapy

The mainstay of therapy of IH is **systemic corticosteroids**, usually in the form of prednisone at a dose of 15–30 mg/day. Doses as high as 60–80 mg/day may be required.[43] Evidence for varying levels of effectiveness is based on case reports.[41,42,44,46] Once the disease is under control, steroids may be tapered very slowly. Disease rebound is common with rapid tapering. The mechanism of action of corticosteroids is broad suppression of the immune system. They exert inhibitory effects on cell trafficking, as well as the humoral and cytotoxic portions of the immune system. Corticosteroids have well-documented side effects in humans, including hypothalamic–pituitary axis (HPA) suppression, hyperglycemia, hyperlipidemia, cushingoid changes, osteoporosis, peptic ulcer disease, cataracts, and opportunistic infections. Fetal HPA suppression must be considered when corticosteroids are given near the time of delivery.[47] Oral corticosteroids should be used with caution during lactation. They are excreted into human breast milk but do not have any known adverse reaction or potential in infants.

When IH is insufficiently controlled with corticosteroids alone, the next therapeutic option is cyclosporin A (CsA). Doses of 3–10 mg/kg/day have been reported in the treatment of IH.[46,48,49] Again, medication should be tapered to the lowest possible dose that results in control of the disease. The mechanism of action is inhibition of calcineurin with resultant decrease in interleukin-2 production by CD4+ T cells. CsA also inhibits interferon-γ production by T cells. CsA is pregnancy category C. The most serious adverse effects are renal dysfunction and hypertension.[47] Renal function and blood pressure should be monitored during therapy. In a study of transplant recipients treated with CsA during pregnancy, there was no evidence of teratogenicity.[50] However, 44.5% of infants were born at less than 37 weeks' gestation and 44.3% weighed less than 2500 g at birth.[50] CsA is excreted in human breast milk and breastfeeding should be avoided during therapy.

CUTANEOUS MELANOMA
KEY POINTS

- **Pregnancy** at the time of diagnosis or subsequent to the diagnosis of melanoma has **no impact on overall survival, tumor thickness, or disease-free survival.**
- **Pregnant women who are diagnosed with melanoma should not be counseled or managed any differently from a non-pregnant woman with a similar stage of disease.**

Diagnosis/definition

Cutaneous melanoma is a malignant neoplasm of melanocytes that arises in the skin. Melanomas often display irregularities in color, border, and symmetry, although these observations are neither sensitive nor specific (Figure 3.5). Even the most experienced dermatologist may have difficulty differentiating a benign pigmented lesion from a malignant one. The gold standard for the **diagnosis** of melanoma is **excisional biopsy of the entire lesion** for tissue pathology. Biopsy specimens of all clinically pigmented lesions should be evaluated by an experienced dermatopathologist.

Symptoms

Melanomas are usually asymptomatic. They may rarely itch or bleed spontaneously.

Epidemiology/incidence

The lifetime risk of melanoma for a caucasian person born in the USA in 2001 is 1 in 7.[51] The estimated incidence of melanoma during pregnancy is between 2.8 and 5 in 100 000.[52]

Genetics

A rare group of patients with a family history of melanoma and many moles may carry inherited mutations in *CDKN2A* and *CDK4*. An individual who carries one of these mutations has a 60–90% lifetime risk of melanoma.[53]

Classification

There are four main clinical types of melanoma: superficial spreading, acral lentiginous, lentigo maligna, and nodular melanoma. The clinical type bears no significance to the

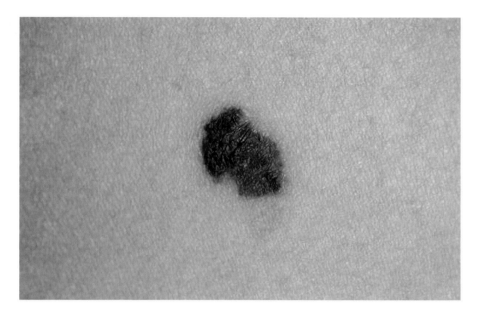

Figure 3.5
Melanoma. A 25-year-old with a new, irregularly pigmented, asymmetric lesion in her back that had been gradually expanding over the past several months. Note the irregular borders.

prognosis of melanoma; rather, the **Breslow depth, which is a measure of tumor thickness, and ulceration** are the two major factors that have been shown to **impact prognosis.**[54]

Risk factors

The major risk factors are fair skin, blue or green eyes, blond or red hair, inability to tan, intense intermittent sun exposure (especially during childhood), use of tanning beds, and inherited mutations in *CDKN2A* or *CDK4.*[51,53]

Complications

Melanoma is a malignant neoplasm that can metastasize to regional lymph nodes as well as viscera. In general, the thicker the primary cutaneous melanoma, the higher the likelihood for metastasis at the time of diagnosis.

Pregnancy considerations

For many years it was believed that pregnancy had an adverse impact on survival in patients diagnosed with malignant melanoma. This belief was based on case reports and uncontrolled series in which confounding variables were not accounted for: namely, tumor thickness at the time of diagnosis.[52,55] Several large, retrospective, controlled cohort studies of women who were diagnosed with

melanoma during their pregnancy have confirmed that this is *not* the case.[52,56,57] In fact, these recent large cohort studies have shown that there is **no difference in overall survival or tumor thickness between pregnant and non-pregnant age- and disease stage-matched patients.**[52,56,57] The **disease-free survival rate** is the same in pregnant and non-pregnant women.[57] **Pregnancy in women who have been previously diagnosed with melanoma does not affect overall survival.**[52] An important point related to pregnancy and melanoma is the concept that benign nevi may darken and change during pregnancy. There has been debate in recent years regarding this belief. In fact, there has been no study to date that has documented a significant change in size or color of benign nevi during pregnancy in normal, healthy women. The clinical lesions that are reported by patients to darken or change during pregnancy are usually non-pigmented lesions, such as dermatofibromas or skin tags.[58] Photographic documentation and blinded comparison by physicians do not show any change in size of nevi between the first and third trimester of pregnancy.[59] Women with the *dysplastic nevus syndrome (DNS)* may have an increased rate of change in clinically dysplastic nevi with pregnancy,[60] but women with DNS represent only a very small portion of the population. Histopathological study of nevi removed during pregnancy fails to detect a statistically significant difference in criteria for atypia.[58] So, **any nevus that changes during pregnancy should be considered suspect and be carefully considered for excisional biopsy,** not observation. The belief that nevi may normally darken and change during pregnancy may lead to a false sense of security and a delay in the diagnosis of melanoma.[55,58,59]

Pregnancy specific management

There is no difference in pregnancy outcomes, including cesarean delivery, length of stay, risk of low birth weight, prematurity, or neonatal death.[55] Pregnant women who are diagnosed with melanoma **should not be counseled any differently than non-pregnant women** with a similar stage of disease with respect to both pregnancy outcomes and their overall prognosis.[55] There are approximately 22 cases of placental metastases of melanoma reported in the literature. Indeed, of all malignancies that tend to metastasize to the placenta, melanoma is the most common.[55] However, metastasis to the fetus and/or placenta is an extremely rare event and has occurred exclusively in the setting of hematogenous dissemination of metastatic disease in the mother.[61–63] **Placental involvement** implies a fatal prognosis for the mother and an approximately 22% risk of metastasis to the fetus.[63]

Work-up

The extensiveness of the work-up of primary cutaneous melanoma is primarily based on tumor thickness at the time of diagnosis. Initial diagnosis is made by tissue pathology. It is strongly recommended that all suspicious lesions be removed by **excisional biopsy with narrow margins** for diagnostic purposes.[64] Once the diagnosis of melanoma is made, all patients should have a thorough review of systems and a physical examination, with special attention given to the lymph nodes. There is no evidence that routine laboratory tests and imaging studies detect occult metastases in asymptomatic patients with tumors < 4.0 mm in thickness.[53,64] Therefore, **chest X-ray, serum lactate dehydrogenase, and hemoglobin are reserved for patients who are symptomatic or have tumors that are thicker than 4.0 mm at the time of initial diagnosis.** Patients should be taught to give themselves monthly self-examinations and should be seen 1–4 times per year for the first 2 years after the initial diagnosis and then 1–2 times yearly thereafter.[64] The goal of follow-up is to detect recurrence or a new primary lesion. Screening tests should be ordered based on symptomatology and physical examination findings during follow-up care. **Sentinel lymph node biopsy** in melanoma is still a relatively controversial procedure at this date. It is used to detect occult nodal metastases at the time of diagnosis and is generally reserved for patients **with tumors that are ≥1.0 mm in thickness.**[53] Sentinel lymph node biopsy should be performed at the time of definitive excision. This procedure is

considered safe to perform during pregnancy.[55] For patients with microscopic or clinically apparent nodal disease, a full metastatic work-up is indicated,[53] including bloodwork and computed tomography (CT) or magnetic resonance imaging (MRI) of the chest, abdomen, and pelvis. MRI is preferable in pregnant patients because it is the safer alternative.[55]

Management
Prevention

General preventive measures include the use of sun protection via sunscreens and protective clothing, especially during childhood and adolescence. Regular skin examination by a physician is recommended. Melanomas that are detected by a physician are diagnosed at an earlier stage than those detected by patients; however, a direct reduction in mortality has not been documented.[54]

Preconception counseling

Since melanomas tend to recur within the first 2 years after diagnosis, women should be counseled to wait this length of time before conceiving.[51,55] Again, there is no evidence that pregnancy results in a higher rate of recurrence, but it seems unwise to conceive if there is *any* risk for recurrence of a potentially fatal disease.

Therapy

The treatment of melanoma is primarily surgical. After the initial diagnostic biopsy, **excision of the primary lesion with 0.5–2 cm margins,** depending on tumor thickness, is recommended.[53,64] Patients with evidence of metastasis can be considered for surgical debulking and/or adjuvant therapy.[53]

References

1. Chang ALS, Agredano YZ, Kimball AB. Risk factors associated with striae gravidarum. J Am Acad Dermatol 2004; 51: 881–5. [III]
2. Goldberg DJ, Marmur ES, Schmults C, et al. Histologic and ultrastructural analysis of ultraviolet B laser and light source treatment of leukoderma in striae distensae. Dermatol Surg 2005; 31: 385–7. [II-3]
3. Watson REB, Parry EJ, Humphries JD, et al. Fibrillin microfibrils are reduced in skin exhibiting striae distensae. Br J Dermatol 1998; 138: 931–7. [II-3]
4. Young GL, Jewell D. Creams for preventing stretch marks in pregnancy. Cochrane Database Syst Rev 2007; 1. [meta-analysis: 2 RCTs, n=130]

5. Kang S, Kim KJ, Griffiths CEM, et al. Topical tretinoin (retinoic acid) improves early stretch marks. Arch Dermatol 1996; 132: 519–26. [I]
6. Pribanich S, Simpson FG, Held B, et al. Low-dose tretinoin does not improve striae distensae: a double-blind, placebo-controlled study. Cutis 1994; 54: 121–4. [I]
7. Wolverton SE. Comprehensive Dermatologic Drug Therapy. Philadelphia: WB Saunders, 2001: 578–94. [III]
8. Kligman AM, Grove GL, Hirose R, et al. Topical tretinoin for photo-damaged skin. J Am Acad Dermatol 1986; 15: 836–59. [II-1]
9. McDaniel DH. Laser therapy of stretch marks. Dermatol Clin 2002; 20: 67–76. [III]
10. Lawley TJ, Hertz KC, Wade TR, et al. Pruritic urticarial papules and plaques of pregnancy. JAMA 1979; 241: 1696–9. [III]
11. Roger D, Vaillant L, Lorette G. Pruritic urticarial papules and plaques of pregnancy are not related to maternal or fetal weight gain. Arch Dermatol 1990; 126: 1517. [III]
12. Cohen LM, Capeless EL, Krusinski PA, et al. Pruritic urticarial papules and plaques of pregnancy and its relationship to maternal–fetal weight gain and twin pregnancy. Arch Dermatol 1989; 125: 1534–6. [III]
13. Aronson IK, Bond S, Fiedler VC, et al. Pruritic urticarial papules and plaques of pregnancy: clinical and immunopathologic observations in 57 patients. J Am Acad Dermatol 1998; 39: 933–9. [II-3]
14. Powell FC. Pruritic urticarial papules and plaques of pregnancy and multiple pregnancies. J Am Acad Dermatol 2000; 43: 730–1. [II-3]
15. Weiss R, Hull P. Familial occurrence of pruritic urticarial papules and plaques of pregnancy. J Am Acad Dermatol 1992; 26: 715–17. [III]
16. Yancey KB, Hall RP, Lawley TJ. Pruritic urticarial papules and plaques of pregnancy. J Am Acad Dermatol 1984; 10: 473–80. [II-3]
17. Beckett MA, Goldberg NS. Pruritic urticarial papules and plaques of pregnancy and skin distension. Arch Dermatol 1991; 127: 125–6. [III]
18. Kroumpouzos G, Cohen LM. Specific dermatoses of pregnancy: an evidence-based systematic review. Am J Obstet Gynecol 2003; 188: 1083-92. [meta-analysis, n = 282]
19. Alcalay J, Ingber A, Kafri B, et al. Hormonal evaluation and autoimmune background in pruritic urticarial papules and plaques of pregnancy. Am J Obstet Gynecol 1988; 158: 417–20. [II-3]
20. Callen JP, Hanno R. Pruritic urticarial papules and plaques of pregnancy (PUPPP). J Am Acad Dermatol 1981; 5: 401–5. [II-3]
21. Vaughan Jones SA, Hern S, Nelson-Piercy C, et al. A prospective study of 200 women with dermatoses of pregnancy correlating clinical findings with hormonal and immunopathological profiles. Br J Dermatol 1999; 141: 71–81. [II-2; n = 44]
22. Aractingi S, Berkane P, LeGoue' C, et al. Fetal DNA in skin of polymorphic eruptions of pregnancy. Lancet 1998; 352: 1898–901. [II-2]
23. Kroumpouzos GK, Cohen LM. Dermatoses of pregnancy. J Am Acad Dermatol 2001; 45: 1–19. [III]
24. Alcalay J, Ingber A, David M, et al. Pruritic urticarial papules and plaques of pregnancy. J Reprod Med 1987; 32: 315–16. [II-3]
25. Beltrani VP, Beltrani VS. Pruritic urticarial papules and plaques of pregnancy: a severe case requiring early delivery for relief of symptoms. J Am Acad Dermatol 1991; 26: 266–7. [III]
26. Zoberman E, Farmer ER. Pruritic folliculitis of pregnancy. Arch Dermatol 1981; 117: 20–22. [III]
27. Kroumpouzos G, Cohen LM. Pruritic folliculitis of pregnancy. J Am Acad Dermatol 2000; 43: 132–4. [III]
28. Vaughan Jones SA, Hern S, Nelson-Piercy C, et al. A prospective study of 200 women with dermatoses of pregnancy correlating clinical findings with hormonal and immunopathological profiles. Br J Dermatol 1999; 141: 71–81. [II-2]
29. Fox GN. Pruritic folliculitis of pregnancy. Am Fam Physician 1989; 39: 189–93. [III]
30. Kroumpouzos G, Cohen LM. Specific dermatoses of pregnancy: an evidence-based review. Am J Obstet Gynecol 2003; 188: 1083–92. [III]
31. Parlak AH, Boran C, Topcuoglu MA. Pityrosporum folliculitis during pregnancy: a possible cause of pruritic folliculitis of pregnancy. J Am Acad Dermatol 2005; 52: 528–9. [III]
32. Wilkinson SM, Buckler H, Wilkinson N, et al. Androgen levels in pruritic folliculitis of pregnancy. Clin Exp Dermatol 1995; 20: 234–6. [III]
33. Reed J. Pruritic folliculitis of pregnancy treated with narrowband (TL-01) ultraviolet B phototherapy. Br J Dermatol 1999; 141: 177–9. [III]
34. Black MM. Prurigo of pregnancy, papular dermatitis of pregnancy, and pruritic folliculitis of pregnancy. Semin Dermatol 1989; 8: 23–5. [III]
35. British Photodermatology Group. An appraisal of narrowband (TL-01) UVB phototherapy. British Photodermatology Group workshop report. Br J Dermatol 1997; 137: 327–30. [III]
36. Nurse DS. Prurigo of pregnancy. Australas J Dermatol 1968; 9: 258–67. [III]
37. Roger D, Vaillant L, Fignon A, et al. Specific pruritic diseases of pregnancy. Arch Dermatol 1994; 130: 734–9. [II-2]
38. Holmes RC, Black MM. The specific dermatoses of pregnancy. J Am Acad Dermatol 1983; 3: 405–12. [II-3]
39. Vaughan Jones SA, Hern S, Nelson-Piercy C, et al. A prospective study of 200 women with dermatoses of pregnancy correlating clinical findings with hormonal and immunopathological profiles. Br J Dermatol 1999; 141: 71–81. [II-2]
40. Black MM. Prurigo of pregnancy, papular dermatitis of pregnancy, and pruritic folliculitis of pregnancy. Semin Dermatol 1989; 8: 23–5. [III]
41. Lotem M, Katzenelson V, Rotem A, et al. Impetigo herpetiformis: a variant of pustular psoriasis or a separate entity? J Am Acad Dermatol 1989; 20: 338–41. [III]
42. Breier-Maly J, Ortel B, Breier F, et al. Generalized pustular psoriasis of pregnancy (impetigo herpetiformis). Dermatology 1999; 198: 61–4. [III]
43. Kroumpouzos GK, Cohen LM. Dermatoses of pregnancy. J Am Acad Dermatol 2001; 45: 1–19. [III]
44. Chang SE. Impetigo herpetiformis followed by generalized pustular psoriasis: more evidence of the same disease entity. Inte J Soc Dermatol 2003; 42: 754–5. [III]
45. Ott F, Krakowski A, Tur E, et al. Impetigo herpetiformis with lowered serum level of vitamin D and its diminished intestinal absorption. Dermatologica 1982; 164: 360–5. [III]
46. Imai N, Watanabe R, Fujiwara H, et al. Successful treatment of impetigo herpetiformis with oral cyclosporine during pregnancy. Arch Dermatol 2002; 138: 128–9. [III]
47. Wolverton SE. Comprehensive Dermatologic Drug Therapy. Philadelphia: WB Saunders; 2001: 109–39, 205–22. [III]
48. Raddadi AA, Damanhoury ZB. Cyclosporin and pregnancy. Br J Dermatol 1999; 140: 1197–8. [III]
49. Finch TM, Tan CY. Pustular psoriasis exacerbated by pregnancy and controlled by cyclosporine A. Br J Dermatol 2000; 142: 582–4. [III]
50. Lamarque V, Leleu MF, Monka C, Krupp P. Analysis of 629 pregnancy outcomes in transplant recipients treated with Sandimmun. Transplant Proc 1997; 29: 2480. [II-3 n = 629]
51. Lang PE. Current concepts in the management of patients with melanoma. Am J Clin Dermatol 2002; 3: 401–26. [III]
52. Lens MB, Rosdahl I, Ahlbom A, et al. Effect of pregnancy on survival in women with cutaneous malignant melanoma. J Clin Oncol 2004; 22: 4369–75. [II-2]
53. Tsao H, Atkins MB, Sober AJ. Management of cutaneous melanoma. N Engl J Med 2004; 351: 998–1012. [III]
54. Thompson JA. The revised American Joint Committee on Cancer staging system for melanoma. Semin Oncol 2002; 29: 361–9. [III]
55. Katz VL, Farmer RM, Dotters D. From nevus to neoplasm: myths of melanoma in pregnancy. Obstet Gynecol Surv 2002; 57: 112–19. [III]
56. O'Meara AT, Cress R, Xing G, et al. Malignant melanoma in pregnancy. A population-based evaluation. Cancer 2005; 103: 1217–26. [II-2]
57. Daryanani D, Plukker JT, De Hullu JA, et al. Pregnancy and early-stage melanoma. Cancer 2003; 97: 2248–53. [II-2]

58. Foucar E, Bentley TJ, Laube DW, et al. A histopathologic evaluation of nevocellular nevi in pregnancy. Arch Dermatol 1985; 121: 350–4. [II-2]

59. Pennoyer JW, Grin CM, Driscoll MS, et al. Changes in size of melanocytic nevi during pregnancy. J Am Acad Dermatol 1997; 36: 378–82. [II-2]

60. Ellis DL. Pregnancy and sex steroid hormone effects on nevi of patients with the dysplastic nevus syndrome. J Am Acad Dermatol 1991; 25: 467–82. [II-3]

61. Borden EC. Melanoma and pregnancy. Semin Oncol 2000; 27: 654–6. [III]

62. Altman JF, Lowe L, Redman B, et al. Placental metastasis of maternal melanoma. J Am Acad Dermatol 2003; 49: 1150–4. [III]

63. Alexander A, Harris RM, Grossman D, et al. Vulvar melanoma: diffuse melanosis and metastasis to the placenta. J Am Acad Dermatol 2004; 50: 293–8. [III]

64. Sober AJ, Chuang T, Duvic M, et al. Guidelines of care for primary cutaneous melanoma. J Am Acad Dermatol 2001; 45: 579–86. [III]

4

Pregestational and gestational diabetes

Patrice ML Trauffer

KEY POINTS

- **Poorly controlled** diabetes mellitus (DM) in pregnancy is associated with **increased risks of** first trimester miscarriage; congenital malformations (especially cardiac defects and central nervous system [CNS] anomalies); fetal death; preterm birth; pre-eclampsia; ketoacidosis; polyhydramnios; macrosomia; operative (both vaginal and cesarean) delivery and birth injury (including brachial plexus); delayed lung maturity; respiratory distress syndrome (RDS); jaundice, hypoglycemia, hypocalcemia; perinatal mortality; and long-term obesity, type II DM, and lower IQ.
- Prevention of pregestational DM complications and prevention of gestational diabetes can often be achieved with weight loss and exercise before pregnancy.
- **Preconception counseling of pregestational DM should include weight loss, exercise, appropriate diet, and glucose testing with treatment of hyperglycemia** as appropriate. Normalization (**hemoglobin A_{1c} < 6%**) of glucose levels before and during pregnancy **prevents most if not all of the complications of DM during gestation.**
- In pregestational diabetes pregnancies, **fasting glucose < 95 mg/dl and 2-hour postprandial < 120 mg/dl** should be achieved and maintained at all times with diet, exercise, and insulin therapy as necessary.
- There is insufficient evidence to assess the safety and efficacy of all oral hypoglycemic agents in pregestational diabetes.
- **Diabetes ketoacidosis is treated with aggressive hydration and intravenous insulin.**
- In pregestational diabetes, timing of delivery is about 39 weeks, and cesarean delivery (CD) may be offered if estimated fetal weight is > 4500 g.
- **In gestational diabetes (GDM), diet and glucose monitoring with insulin if needed aimed at achieving fasting glucose < 95 mg/dl and 2-hour postprandial < 120 mg/dl** is associated with similar incidence of CD, **reduced macrosomia,** similar special care baby unit admission, but **reduced risk of shoulder dystocia, of neonatal**

hypoglycemia, **no birth trauma** (bone fracture, nerve palsy) (vs 1%), and **no perinatal death** (vs 1%) compared with no treatment or diet alone.

- Compared with insulin therapy, **glyburide is equally as efficacious in glucose control and results in similar pregnancy outcomes** (including incidences of macrosomia, CD, neonatal hypoglycemia, admission to NICU, and other neonatal outcomes) **for gestational diabetics** in the second and third trimester (starting at 11 weeks).
- In GDM, **exercise** is associated with a similar rate of macrosomia compared with insulin, improvement in glycemic control when done with diet compared with diet only, and improvement in cardiovascular fitness.
- Women with GDM should be screened for diabetes 6–8 weeks postpartum.

PREGESTATIONAL DIABETES
Diagnosis/definition

Diabetes is defined as a metabolic abnormality characterized by elevated circulating glucose. **The diagnoses of diabetes and impaired glucose tolerance outside of pregnancy are established based on formal laboratory criteria** (Table 4.1).[1,2] As different countries use either mmol/L or mg/dl for glucose values, a comparison is provided (Table 4.2). Women with impaired glucose tolerance are at an increased risk of developing diabetes in the future and/or in pregnancy. An acceptable diagnostic alternative for diabetes is a random glucose > 200 mg/dl associated with symptoms consistent with diabetes, such as polyuria.

Symptoms

Women are often asymptomatic, but classic symptoms of uncontrolled diabetes are polydypsia, polyuria, and polyphagia.

Table 4.1	*Criteria for the diagnosis of diabetes mellitus in the non-pregnant state*[a]	
Normal values	Impaired fasting glucose or impaired glucose tolerance	Diabetes mellitus
FPG: < 110 mg/dl	FPG: 110–125 mg/dl	FPG: ≥ 126 mg/dl
75 g, 2-hour OGTT: 2-hour PG < 140 mg/dl	75-g, 2-h OGTT: 2-hour PG 140–199 mg/dl	75- g, 2-hour OGTT: 2-hour PG ≥ 200 mg/dl
		Symptoms of diabetes and PG (without regard to time since last meal) ≥ 200 mg/dl

FPG, fasting plasma glucose; OGTT, oral glucose tolerance test; PG, plasma glucose. The diagnosis of diabetes mellitus should be confirmed on a separate day by any of these three tests.
[a]Data from Expert Committee on the Diagnosis and Classification of Diabetes Mellitus.[2]

Table 4.2	*Glucose equivalents*	
mmol/L	mg/dl	
5.9	105	
6.7	120	
7.77	140	
8.0	144	
11.0	198	

Epidemiology/incidence

Pregestational diabetes mellitus (DM) complicates approximately 1%[2–4] of all pregnancies.

Basic pathophysiology

The etiology of the disease varies and includes a primary insulin production defect, insulin receptor abnormalities, end-organ insulin resistance, and as a secondary effect of another disease process, such as cystic fibrosis. Type I diabetics are usually insulin deficient, related to a destruction of the pancreatic islet β-cells by an autoimmune process, possibly initiated by a viral infection. These individuals usually develop disease early in life, require insulin replacement, and become acutely symptomatic with ketoacidosis if no therapy is initiated. In contrast, Type II diabetics continue to produce insulin but do so at diminished levels. They are often hyperinsulinemic, at least in the early stages; relative hypoinsulinemia may (or may not) develop later. Insulin resistance is the cardinal feature. In addition, many exhibit insulin resistance at the level of the receptor on the end organs. The onset of disease for these individuals is usually later in life, gradual but progressive, and linked to obesity. This is rapidly changing: disease is now being seen at earlier and earlier ages, including childhood and adolescence. Both

groups can be further subclassified based on the presence of vascular complications, such as hypertension, renal disease, and retinopathy. The same physiological changes of pregnancy that cause gestational diabetes (see below) also complicate achieving optimal glucose control in the pregestational diabetic.

Classification

The classification of diabetes has undergone recent revisions to reflect the physiology and implications of the disease process to facilitate the management of these patients. Priscilla White's classification has no proven clinical benefit.[3]

Risk factors/associations

Obesity, hypertension, advanced maternal age, non-white race, family history (type II diabetes), metabolic syndrome, etc.

Complications

The incidence of complications is inversely proportional to glucose control, with minimal complications if optimal glucose control. In poorly controlled DM, increased glucose in the mother causes consequent abnormal metabolism, whereas in the fetus it causes hyperinsulinemia and its consequences. Poorly controlled DM is associated with increased risks of first trimester miscarriage; congenital malformations (glycosylated hemoglobin < 7, no increased risk; 7–8.9, 5–10%; 9–10.9, 10–20%; ≥ 11 > 20%) (most common malformations are cardiac defects and central nervous system [CNS] anomalies, especially neural tube defects; most pathognomonic are sacral agenesis/caudal regression); fetal death; preterm birth (both iatrogenic [hypertensive complications] and spontaneous); pre-eclampsia; ketoacidosis; polyhydramnios; macrosomia (fetal increased insulin acts as growth factor; the degree of macrosomia is correlated with postprandial blood glucose values outside of the suggested parameters); operative (both vaginal and cesarean) delivery and birth injury (including brachial plexus) (both related to macrosomia); delayed lung maturity; respiratory distress syndrome (RDS); jaundice (due to the induced polycythemia), hypoglycemia, hypocalcemia, and polycythemia in the neonate, all related to elevated glucose levels and consequent hyperinsulinemia antenatally; and perinatal mortality. Long-term follow-up has shown higher rates of obesity, Type II DM, and lower IQ with uncontrolled DM in pregnancy.

Pregnancy considerations

The implications of any maternal disease on pregnancy outcome are important to delineate. Likewise, the effect of pregnancy on the disease state needs to be considered prior to embarking on a pregnancy. Because pregestational diabetes is a disease which affects the micro- and macrovascular system, the implications of pregnancy on the end organs most frequently affected by the disease need to be discussed. Diabetic **retinopathy** is the leading cause of blindness in reproductive years. Background retinopathy is characterized by retinal microaneurysms and dot-blot hemorrhages, while proliferative retinopathy is characterized by neovascularization. Proliferative diabetic retinopathy does progress in pregnancy as tightened glycemic control is achieved, but background retinopathy does not. Diabetic **nephropathy** occurs in 5–10% of pregestational diabetics, and can progress to end-stage renal disease, especially in women with a pre-pregnancy creatinine level of ≥1.5 mg/dl, or a 24-hour proteinuria of ≥3 g. Proteinuria does increase in diabetic patients as they approach term, particularly in those who have baseline nephropathy. Progression of renal insufficiency is not clearly linked to the physiologically increased glomerular filtration rate of pregnancy, although those with nephrotic range proteinuria and moderate to severe renal insufficiency may progress to end-stage renal disease. Diabetic **neuropathy** is not worsened per se in pregnancy although decreased gastrointestinal (GI) motility related to progesterone and mechanical factors may exacerbate underlying gastroparesis. The presence of **hypertension** (in 5–10% of women with pregestational DM) increases even more the risks of pre-eclampsia, fetal growth restriction, and fetal death. Progression of **cardiovascular** disease in the diabetic pregnant patient has not been reported, but symptomatic coronary artery disease is a contraindication to pregnancy in these diabetic women.

Pregnancy management
Principles

Strict glycemic control.

Work-up

- Careful history (review of glucose control and therapy; history of end-organ disease)
- Laboratory tests (preconceptionally or first trimester if feasible):
  - HgbA$_{1c}$
  - metabolic profile (glucose, creatinine)
  - urine culture – repeat each trimester
  - 24-hour urine collection for protein and creatinine clearance
  - thyroid stimulating hormone (TSH).
- Consider electrocardiogram (EKG), especially if concomitant hypertension (HTN).
- Consider ophthalmological consult to assess for any retinopathy, especially if long-standing or poorly controlled DM.

Management of pregestational diabetes mellitus (Figure 4.1)
Prevention

Weight loss, exercise, glucose testing with treatment of hyperglycemia as appropriate, leading to strict glucose control, prevent most if not all of the complications of DM in pregnancy.

Preconception counseling

The care of the pregestational diabetic is best instituted in the preconception period. The objectives of prepregnancy care are shown in Table 4.3. The frequency of maternal hospitalizations, length of NICU (neonatal intensive care unit) admission, congenital malformations, and perinatal mortality are reduced in DM women seeking consultation in preparation for pregnancy, but unfortunately only about one-third of these women receives such consultation.[5] In addition to advocating the use of folic acid, at least 400 μg for 3 months prior to pregnancy, this consultation affords the opportunity to screen for vascular consequences of the diabetes. Ophthalmological evaluation, EKG, and renal evaluation via a 24-hour urine collection for total protein and creatinine clearance will ascertain end-organ damage and determine ancillary pregnancy risks. A TSH should be checked, as 40% of young women with Type I diabetes have

Preconception prevention
Weight loss
Exercise
Glucose testing
Treatment of hyperglycemia as appropriate
Strict glucose control

Preconception evaluation
Normalization of the hemoglobin A_{1C} to at least within 1% of normal (<7%), best if <6%
Evaluate the presence of vascular disease:
- ophthalmological examination with retinal evaluation
- 24-hour urine for protein and creatinine clearance
- electrocardiogram
Nutritional counseling:
- 30–35 kcal/kg/day if normal weight
Institute glucose testing to include fasting and 2-hour postprandial values
Incorporate exercise regimen
Start or refine insulin regimen

Antepartum management
Insulin therapy adjusted by weight and pregnancy trimester as guided by glucose monitoring:
- Usual insulin requirement:
     first trimester 0.7–0.8 units/kg/day
     second trimester 0.8–1.0 units/kg/day
     third trimester 1.0–1.2 units/kg/day
     insulin dose: divided two-thirds in the a.m., one third in the p.m.
     a.m. insulin: two-third long-acting, one-third short-acting
     p.m. insulin: half long-acting, half short-acting
- Glucose monitoring:
     target fasting blood sugars: 60–95 mg/dl
     target 2-hour postprandial blood sugars: ≤120 mg/dl
Fetal surveillance:
- viability/dating scan
- maternal alpha-fetoprotein screening at 16–20 weeks
- detailed anatomic survey at 18–20 weeks
- echocardiogram at 20–22 weeks
- serial ultrasounds for growth in the second and third trimester
- antenatal assessments with NST/BPP weekly from 32–36 weeks, then twice weekly until delivery

Intrapartum management
Vaginal delivery unless clinical or ultrasound estimated fetal weight >4500 g
Elective delivery at 39 weeks or with amniocentesis-documented pulmonary maturity (see also Chapter 52)
IV insulin therapy with 1 U/ml in a saline solution to maintain blood sugars between 70 and 120 mg/dl
IV dextrose solution if blood sugars fall <70 mg/dl or with development of urinary ketones
For scheduled cesarean section, long-acting insulin administered in a.m., withholding the a.m. short-acting insulin dose
Hourly blood glucose monitoring

Postpartum management
Reduce the antepartum insulin dosing by half and administer it with the resumption of oral intake,
or restart pre-pregnancy oral agents if they were effective
Supplement breastfeeding mothers with 500 extra kcal compared with non-pregnant levels

Figure 4.1
Management of the pregestational diabetic. NST, non-stress test; BPP, biophysical profile.

hypothyroidism. Proliferative retinopathy should be treated with laser before pregnancy. The evaluation should emphasize the importance of tight glycemic control, with **normalization of the HgbA$_{1C}$ (aim for normal, which is <6%)**. Decreased spontaneous miscarriage, congenital anomalies, and other complications have been demonstrated in multiple studies when this goal has been attained. Women compliant with insulin pumps may continue this regimen.

Prenatal care

The principal management is a combination of diet, exercise, glucose monitoring, and insulin therapy. Women with Type I DM and glucose levels of >200 mg/dl should check their urine ketones. A glass of milk is preferable to juice for hypoglycemia. Glucagon should be immediately available.

Table 4.3   *The objectives of diabetes mellitus prepregnancy care*

Patient education
Assessment of the patient's medical condition
Optimum glycemic control (hemoglobin $A_{1c} < 6\%$) *prior to conception*
Folic acid supplementation (at least 400 µg) *prior to conception*

Table 4.4   *Diabetic diet*

35 kcal/kg/day (usually 2000–2400 kcal/day)	
3 meals, 3 snacks	
Composition:	
Carbohydrate (complex)	45%
Protein	20%
Fat (< 10% saturated)	35%

Table 4.5   *Target venous plasma glucose levels*

Fasting	60–90 mg/dl
Preprandial	60–100 mg/dl
1-hour postprandial	≤ 140 mg/dl
2-hour postprandial	< 120 mg/dl
3 a.m.	60–90 mg/dl

Diet (Table 4.4)

Nutritional requirements are adjusted based on the maternal body mass index (BMI), with women of normal BMI requiring 35 kcal/kg/day. Individuals below their ideal BMI need to increase this by an additional 5 kcal/kg/day, while obese individuals should decrease this value by 20%. The content should be distributed as 45% complex, high-fiber carbohydrates, 20% protein, and 35% primarily unsaturated fats.[3,5] The calories are distributed over three meals and three snacks, with breakfast receiving the smallest allotment at 15%, and the other two receiving near equal distribution. Saccharin, aspartame, acesulfame-k, maltodextrin, and sucralose may be used safely in moderate amounts. Carbohydrate counting and the help of a registered dietitian may provide benefit, but these two interventions have been insufficiently studied in pregnancy.

Exercise

Moderate exercise decreases the need for insulin therapy in Type II diabetics by increasing the glucose uptake in skeletal muscle, and therefore should be strongly encouraged for any diabetic patient.

Glucose monitoring

Frequent home glucose monitoring, both pre and postprandially, has been associated with enhanced glucose control and shorter interval to achieve target blood sugars. Capillary blood glucose ('fingerstick') measurements using a glucometer should be obtained at least 4 times/day – fasting, and 2 hours postprandial. Target levels are in Table 4.5. Some women will require another assessment at 3 a.m. for prevention of hypoglycemic episodes. Some women may be

followed with preprandial values as well as postprandial values: if used, the preprandial level target is ≤ 100 mg/dl and the 1-hour postprandial target is ≤ 140 mg/dl. HgbA$_{1c}$ is normal when < 6%,[3] whereas HgbA$_{1c}$ of 8% reflects a mean glucose level of 180 mg/dl, with each 1% higher or lower equal to a change of 30 mg/dl.

Oral hypoglycemic agents

There is insufficient evidence to assess the safety of all oral hypoglycemic agents in pregestational diabetes. There is also insufficient evidence to assess their effectiveness in glucose control in these patients. Therefore, even in women on oral hypoglycemic control before pregnancy, insulin therapy is recommended for glucose control, also due to the limited range of glucose excursions allowed during pregnancy.

Insulin

Insulin therapy is the mainstay in the management of all pregestational diabetics. All insulin types, except glargine and newest insulins, have been approved during pregnancy, including insulin pumps. Women compliant with insulin pumps have increased satisfaction, decrease in severe hypoglycemia, and better control of hyperglycemia.[3] A review of the insulin types and their onset and duration of action is given in Table 4.6. Inhaled insulin has been recently tested in non-pregnant adults, but there are as yet insufficient data for pregnancy management. Women, particularly those new to insulin therapy, need to be counseled about the differences in the various insulins in order to use them to their greatest efficacy. Close monitoring with at least weekly contact with a provider is suggested to maximize insulin adjustment. The goal of therapy is as shown in Table 4.5. The postprandial blood sugar has been found to have the greatest correlation with fetal macrosomia. While it has not been associated with adverse fetal outcomes, hypoglycemia can cause significant maternal morbidities. Glucagon should be available for home use in emergency situations.

Satisfactory metabolic control can usually be achieved with two or three injections of insulin daily. A combination of intermediate-acting (e.g. NPH) and short-acting (e.g. lispro) insulin may be employed. Insulin lispro should be given immediately before eating. Glargine cannot be mixed in the

Table 4.6 *Types of insulin and their pharmacokinetics*			
Type	Onset	Peak	Duration
Lispro/Aspart	1–15 minutes	1–2 hours	4–5 hours
Regular	30–60 minutes	2–4 hours	6–8 hours
NPH	1–3 hours	5–7 hours	13–18 hours
Lente	1–3 hours	4–8 hours	13–20 hours
Ultralente	2–4 hours	8–14 hours	18–30 hours
Glargine	1 hour	None	24 hours

Table 4.7 *Insulin requirements*	
Trimester	Units/kg/day
1	0.7–0.8
2	0.8–1.0
3	1.0–1.2

Patients on steroids, beta-mimetics, and multiple gestations often require larger doses.

Insulin regimen
- Morning (2/3 total dose): 2/3 NPH; 1/3 regular.
- Evening (1/3 total dose): 1/2 NPH; 1/2 regular.

same syringe with other insulins, and has not been sufficiently studied in pregnancy to assess efficacy, but has great potential, as it mimics the pump for basal dosing, and it's the basal insulin of choice in non-pregnant adults. Subcutaneous insulin pump therapy may be continued in women already compliant with this mode of therapy. Carbohydrate counting and the use of an insulin-to-carbohydrate ratio of 1 unit of insulin for every 15 g of carbohydrate in early gestation can allow for greater flexibility in eating, but has not been studied in a trial. As pregnancy advances with its concomitant insulin resistance, an increased ratio is required, with 1 unit covering a lower amount of carbohydrates, e.g. 1 unit per 10 g of carbohydrate. In general, 10 grams of carbohydrate elevate blood glucose by 30 mg/dL; while 1 unit of short acting insulin lowers the blood glucose by 30 mg/dL.

Useful sample calculations for the total daily insulin requirement and insulin regimen are given in Table 4.7.

Very tight vs tight control

There is insufficient evidence (owing to paucity of data) to assess the effect of tight vs very tight glycemic control in pregestational diabetic women. Compared with tight control (either fasting and 2-hour postprandial 5.6–6.7 mmol/L or fasting < 5.6 mmol/L and 1.5-hour postprandial < 7.8 mmol/L), **very tight control** (either fasting and 2-hour postprandial < 5.6 mmol/L or fasting < 4.4 mmol/L and 1.5-hour postprandial < 6.7 mmol/L) is associated with similar incidence of pre-eclampsia and cesarean delivery (CD), but a **lower incidence of neonatal hypoglycemia**, trends for improvements in other neonatal metabolic outcomes, with **increased incidence of maternal hypoglycemia** based on limited trial numbers.[6] There is no difference detected in perinatal outcome between the groups. There are no data to assess the clinical value in terms of prevention of significant long-term neonatal morbidity.

Diabetic ketoacidosis

Diabetic ketoacidosis can occur in 5–10% of women with pregestational type I diabetes. It is defined by elevated glucose (usually > 250 mg/dl), and positive serum ketones plus acidosis. Risk factors include type I diabetes, new-onset diabetes, infections (e.g. urinary tract infections or respiratory viruses), poor compliance, insulin pump failure, or treatment with beta-mimetics or steroids.[3] Symptoms are abdominal pain, nausea and vomiting, and altered sensorium. Laboratory tests should include an arterial blood gas (pH < 7.3), electrolytes (serum bicarbonate < 15 mEq/L, elevated anion gap), and serum and urinary ketones (elevated). **Aggressive hydration and intravenous (IV) insulin are the most important necessary interventions**, with close electrolytes (especially glucose and potassium) monitoring (Table 4.8). Fetal mortality may be up to 10%, even with aggressive management.

Antepartum testing (Table 4.9)

Fetal surveillance is required to determine if congenital anomalies are present and to minimize perinatal mortality. The nature of this surveillance is by convention and expert consensus rather than supported by well-performed trials. Because of the increased risk of birth defects, particularly congenital heart and neural tube defects, patients should be offered maternal alpha-fetoprotein screening at 16–18

Table 4.8   *Management of diabetic ketoacidosis in pregnancy*

- One liter intravenous (IV) **fluids** (isotonic sodium chloride), then 500–1000 ml for 2–4 hours. Continue 250 ml/hour until at least about 4 L have been replaced

- IV lispro or regular **insulin**: load 0.2–0.4 U/kg; then 2–10 U/hour

- Laboratory tests: arterial blood gas; serum glucose, ketones, electrolytes every 1–2 hours until normal. When glucose < 250 mg/dl, start 5% dextrose in normal saline IV fluids. When potassium low, replenish adequately. If pH < 7.1, add bicarbonate one ampule (4 mEq) to IV fluids (half normal saline)

- Diagnose and treat any underlying infection

Table 4.9   *Antepartum testing*

(A) Assessment of viability and exact gestational age – first trimester ultrasound

(B) Detection of congenital malformations:
1. If Hgb A_{1C} is elevated, transvaginal ultrasound at 13 weeks to rule out structural defects and assess four-chamber view of heart
2. Maternal serum alpha-fetoprotein level at 16 weeks
3. Anatomy ultrasound at 18–20 weeks
4. Fetal echocardiogram at 20–22 weeks

(C) Assessment of fetal growth:
1. Growth ultrasound examination at around 32 weeks

(D) Assessment of fetal well-being:
1. Maternal assessment of fetal activity ('fetal kick counts')
2. Non-stress tests (NSTs) weekly at 32 weeks until 36 weeks; then twice weekly until delivery. Begin at 32 weeks if maternal glycemic control is satisfactory, fetal growth is appropriate, and there are no coexisting maternal medical or obstetric complications. Begin earlier and increase frequency if the above conditions are not met

---

weeks' gestation, targeted ultrasonography at 18–20 weeks, and fetal echocardiography at 20–22 weeks. Ultrasound in the third trimester to evaluate fetal growth and frequent prenatal visits to review glucose control are also advocated. The use of fetal surveillance by the non-stress test (NST) and/or biophysical profile (BPP) is recommended by expert opinion[5] but the frequency and nature of the testing cannot be determined, since there is no randomized trial to direct effective screening. Women in good control start antepartum testing usually with weekly NSTs at 32 weeks. More frequent testing in the form of NST or BPP occurs after 36 weeks, with twice-weekly testing usually employed. Elective delivery < 39 weeks mandates some assessment of fetal lung maturity, with phosphatidylglycerol ≥ 3% accepted by most authorities as the laboratory value indicating the least risk for respiratory insufficiency (see also Chapter 52).

Delivery

Timing
Timing of delivery is usually delayed to the 39th week, unless maternal or fetal factors dictate earlier intervention, but should be accomplished by the EDD (estimated date of delivery) as perinatal mortality increases after this gestational age (GA).

Mode
Mode of delivery is generally vaginal, although **cesarean for macrosomia > 4500 g** as estimated by ultrasound has been proposed (see Chapter 40). The diagnosis of macrosomia is inexact by ultrasound and clinical estimation, confounding the ability to make a clear recommendation. Induction for macrosomia may not reduce birth trauma, and increases CD.[7]

Intrapartum glucose management
Intrapartum glucose management (Table 4.10) is targeted to maintain maternal glucose levels between 70 and 120 mg/dl. Often the insulin requirement is decreased due to the energy requirement of labor. The usual subcutaneous (SQ) intermediate-acting insulin (e.g. NPH) is given at bedtime, while the usual SQ morning (a.m.) insulin is withheld. IV insulin, dextrose solution, frequent (usually every 1 hour) glucose monitoring, and evaluation of urinary

Table 4.10 *Low-dosage constant insulin infusion for the intrapartum period*[a]

Blood glucose (mg/dl)	Insulin dosage (units/hour)	Fluids (125 ml/hour)
< 100	0	Dextrose/lactated Ringer's injection
100–140	1.0	Dextrose/lactated Ringer's injection
141–180	1.5	Normal saline
181–220	2.0	Normal saline
> 220	2.5	Normal saline

[a]Dilution is 25 U of regular insulin in 250 ml of normal saline with 25 ml flushed through line administered intravenously. A fingerstick glucose test is performed every 1–2 hours. The insulin pump and intravenous solution are adjusted accordingly. Adapted from ACOG Practice Bulletin.[3]

ketones are required to prevent a catabolic state and the development of ketoacidosis. Once active labor begins or glucose is < 70 mg/dl, IV 5% dextrose at 125 ml/h can be started. Once the glucose level > 100 mg/dl, short-acting (e.g. lispro or regular) IV insulin should be started. IV 5% dextrose and insulin infusions should be separate, and often should occur at the same time, to prevent ketonuria. Adjustments to the basal infusion rates are based on hourly fingerstick blood sugars while in labor. The use of the insulin pump, maintaining the basal rate, rather than using an IV insulin infusion, is an accepted alternative.

With CD, use of a single injection of long-acting insulin, an IV insulin infusion, or SQ pump at a basal rate are equal alternatives, until oral intake is assured and more standard dosing can be reinstituted. Insulin requirements are diminished postpartum and are generally half of the antepartum requirement.

Anesthesia

No specific adjustments necessary.

Postpartum/breastfeeding

Usual diabetic food intake should be restarted after delivery, with one-half of the predelivery dose or the prepregnancy dose (if this achieves euglycemia) restarted. If food intake cannot be restarted soon, glucose levels of > 140 mg/dl should be treated with pro re nata (prn; as required) coverage. Breastfeeding has increased maternal caloric demands and an additional 500 kcal/day needs to be added to the diet

to avoid hypoglycemia. All forms of contraception are available to diabetics, providing they have no contraindications.

Future (new therapeutic approaches)

Pancreatic islet cell transplant; inhaled insulin; non-invasive monitoring and control of blood sugars.

GESTATIONAL DIABETES
Screening/diagnosis
General

The definition of gestational diabetes (GDM) is hyperglycemia diagnosed ≥ 20 weeks during a pregnancy. The diagnosis of GDM is controversial as the reliability of the testing process and the significance of an abnormal result has not been formally established. The relative efficacy of one testing schema vs another in terms of identifying individuals who are at risk for adverse outcomes has not been studied in a trial. The population who should be offered screening has also not been uniformly identified, with selective screening advocated by the American College of Obstetricians and Gynecologists (ACOG).[8] Low-risk individuals in whom screening may not be necessary include women aged < 25 years old; ethnic origin of low risk (not: Hispanic, African, Native American, South or East Asian, or Pacific Islander); BMI < 25; no previous personal or family history of abnormal glucose tolerance; and no previous history of adverse obstetric outcomes associated with GDM.[8] However, universal screening is most commonly adopted despite studies demonstrating the efficacy of a selective screening process. The best GA at screening is 24–28 weeks to balance sensitivity and specificity, aware that the incidence of GDM (related to placental mass and hormone production) increases with GA. Women with risk factors should be screened preconceptionally or at the first prenatal visit (Table 4.11). About 5–10% of women with these risk factors will have early GDM, and these represent 40% of all GDM diagnosed later at 24–28 weeks. If the early screen is negative, a repeat screen should be performed at 24–28 weeks' gestation.

Diagnosis

One step testing

In most countries, the World Health Organization (WHO) 75 g one-step screening process is employed in women with risk factors, using fasting < 7.8 mmol/L (140 mg/dl) and 2-hour 7.8–11.0 mmol/L (140–198 mg/dl) as criteria for diagnosis.[9] This approach diagnoses twice as many women as having gestational diabetes as the two-step process generally

Table 4.11 *Risk factors for gestational diabetes mellitus*

Prior unexplained stillbirth

Prior infant with congenital anomaly (if not screened in that pregnancy)

Prior macrosomic infant

History of gestational diabetes

Family history of diabetes

Obesity

Chronic use of steroids

Age > 35 years old

Glycosuria

employed in North America,[10] and is the approach most commonly used by the trials on interventions.[9,11–14]

Two step testing
The first (screening) step involves a 50 g 1-hour oral glucose load (glucose challenge test), applied in the non-fasting state,[15] with a venous glucose value obtained 1 hour after. Glucose polymer solutions should be preferred to monomeric solutions.[16] Jelly beans have not been sufficiently tested to be a valid alternative.[17] A positive result on the screening test is defined as 130, 135, or 140 mg/dl. The lower threshold identifies 90% of gestational diabetics but subjects 20–25% of those screened to the second diagnostic test. In contrast, the higher value has a lower sensitivity of 80%, but subjects fewer women (14–18%) to further testing. Any of these thresholds is acceptable.[8] Over 80% of women with values ≥ 200 mg/dl meet a diagnosis of GDM. A definitive diagnosis of GDM is then made based on the results of a 100 g 3-hour oral glucose tolerance test (OGTT), administered after an overnight fast (8–14 hours), ideally following 3 days of unrestricted diet and activity, while the patient remains seated and refrains from smoking. Unfortunately, the criteria to establish this diagnosis are not universally accepted. The two competing tests and their

diagnostic levels are listed in Table 4.12. Two or more abnormal values on these tests establishes the diagnosis of GDM. The relative efficacy of these tests for establishing the population at risk for adverse outcomes by employing either of these tests has not been established, although the Carpenter–Coustan criteria identify more gestational diabetics. ACOG acknowledges that there are no studies to guide the choice of any one test and indicates that either diagnostic test can be used to diagnose gestational diabetes.[8] The Carpenter–Coustan stricter criteria increase by about 50% the number of women with a diagnosis of GDM compared with the National Diabetes Data Group (NDDG) criteria, with no evidence of benefit from any trials, but these pregnancies have elevated incidences of macrosomia and neonatal insulinemia. If GDM is diagnosed < 20 weeks, counseling and management should be as for pregestational diabetes. The presence or absence of fasting hyperglycemia further subdivides this category. If one abnormal value in the 3-hour GTT is present, the patient is counseled to avoid excess glucose consumption, and fasting and 2-hour postprandial glucose samples or a repeat 3-hour GTT can be obtained 3–4 weeks later.

Incidence

The incidence of GDM is 3–5%, representing one of the most common medical complications facing obstetricians; 88% of DM in pregnancy is GDM.[4,8]

Basic pathophysiology

The pathophysiology of GDM is insulin resistance caused by circulating hormonal factors, coming from two sources:

- placental production of human placental lactogen, progesterone, growth hormone, cortisol, and prolactin
- increased maternal steroid production.

Increased body weight and caloric intake also contribute to the insulin resistance and may offset the normally increased

Table 4.12 *Criteria for standard 100 g glucose load to diagnose gestational diabetes*

	National Diabetes Data Group		Carpenter–Coustan criteria	
	mg/dl	mmol/L	mg/dl	mmol/L
Fasting	105	5.8	95	5.3
1-hour	190	10.6	180	10.0
2-hour	165	9.2	155	8.6
3-hour	145	8.0	140	7.8

Preconception prevention
Weight loss
Exercise

Antepartum management
Nutritional counseling for dietary control
Fingerstick blood sugar assessments as fasting and 2-hour postprandial with fasting values <105 mg/dl and 2-hour postprandial <120 mg/dl
Exercise program
Insulin or oral hypoglycemic agent if diet not sufficient to obtain target blood sugars
Fetal surveillance:
  • NSTs weekly from 40 to 42 weeks, if diet controlled
  • NSTs weekly from 32 to 36 weeks; twice weekly from 36 to 40 weeks, if medicated

Intrapartum management
Induction of labor:
  • 40 weeks if medicated
  • 42 weeks if diet controlled
Cesarean section if EFW > 4500 g
Frequent glucose assessment:
  • every 1 hour if required medication
  • every 4 hours if diet controlled
  • Target blood sugars 70–120 mg/dl
IV insulin therapy if blood sugars greater than target blood sugars or with ketonuria
IV saline infusion at 125 ml/h unless ketonuric; then add 5% dextrose solution at rate to keep blood sugar in target range

Postpartum management
Standard 75 g glucose challenge test at 6-week postpartum visit

Figure 4.2
Management of the gestational diabetic.

insulin production in the pregnant woman.[4] Women with GDM have been found to have lower basal islet cell function in addition to their insulin resistance when compared with a non-diabetic cohort. The combination of the two factors contributes to the development of GDM. This insulin resistance and decreased insulin production persist in the postpartum state and lead to the development of type II diabetes in this population.

Risk factors/associations

Obesity, hypertension, advanced maternal age (AMA), metabolic syndrome, family history of type II DM, non-white ethnicity, previous macrosomia, etc. Pregnancy itself is a risk factor.

Complications

The incidence of complications is inversely proportional to glucose control. In poorly controlled DM, increased glucose in the mother causes consequent abnormal metabolism, whereas in the fetus it causes hyperinsulinemia, and its consequences.

Other complications are hypertensive disorders and pre-eclampsia; macrosomia; operative delivery and birth injury (confounded by maternal obesity; both related to macrosomia).[9]

Apart from neonatal hypoglycemia, no other metabolic derangement has been reported in the infant of the GDM mother, and the hypoglycemia is transitional in nature. Long-term adult disorders, such as glucose intolerance and obesity, have been postulated to occur more frequently in these neonates as in pregestational diabetes, but have not been verified by observational studies. Approximately 50% of women identified as having gestational diabetes will develop frank diabetes within 10 years, if followed longitudinally.

Prenatal care

Management of gestational diabetes (Figure 4.2)

Treatment of GDM consists of diet, exercise, and glucose monitoring, with medication reserved for use when glycemic control is not achieved with these modalities.

Diet

Dietary therapy consists of approximately 30 kcal/kg/day divided between three meals and three snacks in a 45% carbohydrate, 20% protein, and 35% unsaturated fat distribution (see above for pre-gestational DM). Since about 30–40% of gestational diabetics fail to achieve glucose control with diet alone, other interventions may be necessary. If two glucose levels are fasting > 99 mg/dl, or 2-hour postprandial ≥ 126 mg/dl at ≤ 35 weeks or ≥ 144 mg/dl after 35 weeks, or even just one 2-hour postprandial is ever ≥ 162 mg/dl, despite diet and exercise, medical therapy should be considered.[9]

Exercise

In women with GDM, exercise, as defined by 30 minutes of non-weight-bearing activity at 50% of aerobic capacity, has been associated with **similar rate of macrosomia compared with insulin,**[18] **improvement in glycemic control when done with diet compared with diet only,**[19] **and improvement in cardiovascular fitness.**[20]

Glucose monitoring

With a glucometer, fasting and 2-hour postprandial glucose levels should be followed daily. Compared with preprandial monitoring, **postprandial monitoring is associated with better change in HgbA$_{1C}$, lower rate of CD for dystocia, lower birth weight, and lower rate of neonatal hypoglycemia.**[21] Since the risk of macrosomia appears to be linked with postprandial hyperglycemia, following these values appears to be reasonable, and is what trials have tested.[9,12–14] Target goals (euglycemia) are fasting glucose between 60 and 95 mg/dl and 2-hour postprandial glucose <120 mg/dl. Achieving euglycemia decreases neonatal complications. If all values are within normal limits for extended periods, less-frequent monitoring can be considered.

Oral hypoglycemic agents

Concerns regarding the safety of oral hypoglycemic agents in pregnancy initially precluded their use during pregnancy. The second-generation sulfonylurea agents have been demonstrated to have less transplacental passage in both in-vitro and in-vivo models, with glyburide not detected in cord blood.[22] Compared with insulin therapy, **glyburide (Micronase, Diabeta, etc.) is equally as efficacious in glucose control and results in similar pregnancy outcomes (including incidences of macrosomia, CD, neonatal hypoglycemia, admission to ICN, and other neonatal outcomes) for gestational diabetics in the second and third trimester (starting at 11 weeks).**[22] Glyburide is started at 2.5 mg orally in a.m., with maximum dose 20 mg daily. At least 10–20% of women on this regimen do not achieve euglycemia, especially women with BMI > 30. Metformin (Glucophage) is currently being used in women with polycystic ovarian disease to treat the infertility related to anovulation. The incidences of miscarriage and gestational diabetes are decreased in women who are continued on this therapy throughout pregnancy. No attributable birth defects or adverse outcomes in this patient population have been reported. Although the literature is limited for these agents, the use of these two medications, in particular glyburide, can be supported during pregnancy, in view of their safety, efficacy, and decreased discomfort with absence of injections compared with insulin. However, this is not true for the other oral medications.

Insulin

As in pregestational DM, NPH and lispro can be used for glucose control. Doses are as calculated above, or starting with empiric regimens such as NPH 20 units and lispro 10 units at breakfast and dinner time, with adjustments as needed to achieve the above goals. No insulin regimen has been found to be superior to any other, so therapy is directed by the results of the glucose testing.

In women with GDM as defined by either one-step[9,12,13] or two-step[14] (using NDDG criteria) criteria, compared with no treatment or diet only, **diet and glucose monitoring with insulin** if needed is associated with similar incidence of CD, **reduced macrosomia, reduced risk of shoulder dystocia,** similar special care baby unit admission and neonatal hypoglycemia, **no birth trauma** (bone fracture, nerve palsy) (vs 1%), and **no perinatal death** (vs 1%).[9,11] **Mood and quality of life are improved,** while incidence of **depression decreases** with the above interventions.[9]

Antepartum testing

Antepartum fetal testing and ultrasound evaluations have not been standardly applied to the management of gestational diabetics, since there is no clear literature to provide direction:

- Euglycemia with diet only: no special testing necessary. Consider weekly NSTs starting at 40 weeks.
- Hyperglycemia or medication necessary: consider management similar to pregestational diabetics.

Ultrasound assessment of fetal weight is commonly employed but, owing to the inherent inaccuracy of predicting macrosomia, has not been supported by any studies.

Delivery

Timing, mode, and lung maturity
There is insufficient evidence to assess the timing and mode of delivery in gestational diabetics, as there is only one small trial on this subject. **Compared with expectant management until 42 weeks, induction of labor at 38 completed weeks in women with insulin-dependent diabetes (>90% gestational) is associated with similar incidence of CD, and reduced incidence of macrosomia and less mild shoulder dystocia.**[23] There is insufficient evidence to assess any other maternal or perinatal morbidity.

In women requiring medication, management is usually more similar to that of the pregestational diabetic, where delivery is advocated in the 39th week. Assessment of fetal lung maturity is not necessary if delivery occurs ≥ 39 weeks in a well-dated, well-controlled patient. If delivery occurs prior to this time, and is unrelated to maternal or obstetric indications, documentation through amniocentesis of mature lung indices is advocated, using a phosphatidylglycerol level of ≥ 3%. While recognizing that macrosomia remains a difficult antenatal diagnosis both clinically and by ultrasound, delivery via cesarean section is suggested for fetuses estimated to be > 4500 g[8] (see also Chapter 40). Operative deliveries should be avoided in women with fetuses estimated to be > 4000 g and prolonged second stage of labor.

Intrapartum glucose management

Intrapartum management requires frequent assessment of blood glucose levels during labor. For patients who have required insulin therapy, hourly assessments of blood sugars are suggested to maintain them between 70 and 120 mg/dl. IV insulin may need to be instituted to maintain the above glucose levels, but it is seldom required in these patients. Patients managed with diet alone may not need as frequent evaluations during labor and can have every 4-hour assessments.

Anesthesia

No specific adjustments are necessary, unless the woman is obese.

Postpartum/breastfeeding

In the postpartum period, women with GDM do not in general require medication to control their blood sugars. Checking a fasting and postprandial value prior to discharge can be employed. Owing to the increased frequency of developing frank diabetes in these women, **screening with a 75 g glucose challenge or other non-pregnant tests** (see Table 4.1) is advocated when the woman is **6–8 weeks postpartum**. This can be accomplished by either the obstetrician with referral if values are abnormal, or even better by referral for the screening to a medicine specialist. Breastfeeding, diet, and exercise should be encouraged in these women, particularly if they are obese. All forms of contraception can be employed without contraindication in this population.

Patients should be informed that they are at increased risk for developing diabetes during their lifetime, up to 50% over the next 30 years. Women with obesity, early GA at diagnosis, and worse abnormalities on screening during and after pregnancy have the highest chance of adult-onset diabetes.

Counseling regarding diet and exercise, maintenance of normal BMI, and surveillance with periodic screening are indicated.

References

1. Galerneau F, Inzucchi SE. Diabetes mellitus in pregnancy. Obstet Gynecol Clin North Am 2004; 31: 907–33. [review]
2. Expert Committee on the Diagnosis and Classification of Diabetes Mellitus. Report of the expert committee on the diagnosis and classification of diabetes mellitus. Diabetes Care 2000; 23(Suppl 1): S4–S19. [review, guideline]
3. ACOG Practice Bulletin. Pregestational diabetes mellitus. Obstet Gynecol 2005; 105: 675–84. [review]
4. American Diabetes Association. Gestational diabetes mellitus. Diabetes Care 2004; Suppl 1: S88–90. [review]
5. Korenbrot CC, Steinberg A, Bender C, Newberry S. Preconception care: a systematic review. Matern Child Health J 2002; 6: 75–88. [review of seven studies addressing the value of preconception care in the diabetic patient]
6. Walkinshaw SA. Very tight versus tight control for diabetes in pregnancy. Cochrane Database Syst Rev 2007; 1. [meta-analysis: 2 RCTs, *n* = 182]
7. Sanchez-Ramos L, Bernstein S, Kaunitz AM. Expectant management versus labor induction for suspected fetal macrosomia: a systematic review. Obstet Gynecol 2002; 100: 997–1102. [meta-analysis]
8. ACOG Practice Bulletin. Gestational diabetes. Obstet Gynecol 2001; 98: 525–38. [review]
9. Crowther CA, Hiller JE, Moss JR, et al. Effect of treatment of gestational diabetes mellitus on pregnancy outcomes. N Engl J Med 2005; 352: 2477–86. [RCT, *n* = 1000. Impaired glucose tolerance (defined following 75 g OGTT as fasting < 7.0 mmol/L, 2 hours between 7.8 mmol/L and 11.0 mmol/L). Diet, glucose monitoring, and insulin as needed vs routine care]
10. Brody SC, Harris R, Lohr K. Screening for gestational diabetes: a summary of the evidence for the U.S. Preventive Services Task Force. Obstet Gynecol 2003; 101: 380–92. [review]
11. Tuffnell DJ, West J, Walkinshaw SA. Treatments for gestational diabetes and impaired glucose tolerance in pregnancy. Cochrane Database Syst Rev 2007; 1. [meta-analysis: 3 RCTs, *n* = 223 – now one more added Crowther 2005, Ref 9]
12. Bancroft K, Tuffnell DJ, Mason GC, Rogerson LJ, Mansfield M. A randomised controlled pilot study of the management of gestational impaired glucose tolerance. BJOG 2000; 107(8): 959–63. [RCT, *n* = 68. Impaired glucose tolerance (defined following 75 g OGTT as fasting < 7.0 mmol/L, 2 hours between 7.8 mmol/L and 11.0 mmol/L – same as Crowther). Monitored group was given standard dietary advice, glucose metabolism was monitored by capillary glucose series 5 days a week, Hgb A$_{1c}$ was measured monthly (insulin was introduced if 5 or more capillary measurements > 7.0 mmol/L in 1 week), serial ultrasound for growth and amniotic fluid, Doppler studies, CTG monitoring. Unmonitored group received dietary advice, Hgb A$_{1c}$ monthly but no capillary glucose measurements]
13. Ford FA, Bruce CB, Fraser RB. Preliminary report of a randomised trial of dietary advice in women with mild abnormalities of glucose tolerance in pregnancy. Personal communication, 1997. [RCT, *n* = 29. Impaired glucose tolerance (defined following a 75 g OGTT as 2-hour plasma glucose level between 8 mmol/L and 11 mmol/L – similar to Crowther. Dietary treatment group was given specific 'diabetic type' advice (i.e. 'high-fiber, high-carbohydrate, low-fat, and appropriate energy'). No mention of insulin therapy. The control

group received no specific dietary advice. Both groups attended clinic weekly and performed plasma glucose profiles]

14. Langer O, Anyaegbunam A, Brustman L, Divon M. Management of women with one abnormal oral glucose tolerance test value reduces adverse outcome in pregnancy. Am J Obstet Gynecol 1989; 161: 593–9. [RCT, *n*=126. Inclusion criteria: one abnormal value following 100 g OGTT (according to National Diabetes Data Group values fasting >105 mg/dl, 1-hour >190 mg/dl, 2-hour >165 mg/dl, 3-hour >145 mg/dl). Three groups in this study – 'treated', 'untreated', and a control group of women with normal screening/OGTT results. (Data for this group is not included in this review.) All participants monitored capillary blood glucose 7 times/day. (This was just for a 4-week period for the untreated group.) Treated group was managed according to diabetic protocol, including dietary advice (determined by prepregnancy BMI), insulin treatment based on 0.7 units per kg of body weight measured in pregnancy. The untreated group continued normal eating patterns]

15. Coustan DR, Widness JA, Carpenter MW, et al. Should the 50-gram, one-hour plasma glucose screening test for gestational diabetes be administered in the fasting or fed state? Am J Obstet Gynecol 1986; 154: 1031–5. [II-2, *n*=72]

16. Murphy NJ, Meyer BA, O'Kell RT, Hogart ME. Carbohydrate sources for gestational diabetes mellitus screening. J Reprod Med 1994; 39: 977–81. [RCT, *n*=108]

17. Lamar ME, Kuehl TJ, Cooney AT, et al. Jelly beans as an alternative to a fifty gram glucose beverage for gestational diabetes screening. Am J Obstet Gynecol 1999; 181: 1154–7. [RCT, *n*=160]

18. Bung P, Bung C, Artal R, et al. Therapeutic exercise for insulin-requiring gestational diabetics: effects on fetus – results of a randomized prospective longitudinal study. J Perinat Med 1993; 21: 125–37. [RCT]

19. Jovanovic-Peterson L, Durak EP, Peterson CM. Randomized trial of diet versus diet plus cardiovascular conditioning on glucose levels in gestational diabetes. Am J Obstet Gynecol 1989; 161: 415–19. [RCT, *n*=19]

20. Avery MD, Leon AS, Kopher RA. Effects of a partially home-based exercise program for women with gestational diabetes. Obstet Gynecol 1997; 89: 10–15. [RCT, *n*=33]

21. de Veciana M, Major CA, Morgan MA, et al. Postprandial versus preprandial blood glucose monitoring in women with gestational diabetes mellitus requiring insulin therapy. N Engl J Med 1995; 333: 1237–41. [RCT, *n*=66]

22. Langer O, Conway DL, Berkus MD, et al. A comparison of glyburide and insulin in women with gestational diabetes. N Engl J Med 2000; 343: 1134–8. [RCT, *n*=404]

23. Kjos SL, Henry OA, Montoro M, Buchanan TA, Mestman JH. Insulin-requiring diabetes in pregnancy: a randomized trial of active induction of labor and expectant management. Am J Obstet Gynecol 1993; 169: 611–15. [RCT, *n*=200]

5

Hypothyroidism*

Alisa B Modena

KEY POINTS

- **Hypothyroidism** is characterized by inadequate thyroid hormone production, and usually requires **elevated thyrotropin or thyroid-stimulating hormone (TSH), and low free thyroxine (T_4)** (or free tryiodothyronine [T_3]) for diagnosis.
- **Subclinical hypothyroidism** usually requires **elevated TSH but normal free T_4 for diagnosis.**
- **Hashimoto's thyroiditis** is the most common cause of hypothyroidism in pregnancy, with thyroid peroxidase (TPO) antibodies found in > 90% of these women.
- Untreated or partially treated hypothyroidism is associated with an increased risk of **pre-eclampsia, abruption, preterm birth, low birth weight, fetal death,** and long-term **impaired psychomotor function in the child.**
- All physiological changes and placental transfer should be known by the physician caring for thyroid disease in pregnancy (see Table 5.1).
- **Women at high risk for hypothyroidism** should be **screened** with TSH and **free T_4 (FT_4).**
- **The goal of** levothyroxine **treatment** in pregnancy is maternal serum TSH 0.5–2.0 µIU/ml, and free T_4 in the upper third of normal range. **Most** women **need an increase in the thyroxine replacement dose during pregnancy.**
- **Iodine supplementation** in a population with high levels of endemic cretinism results in a reduction in deaths during infancy and early childhood, with decreased endemic cretinism at the age of 4 years and better psychomotor development scores between 4 and 25 months of age.
- **TSH and free T_4 levels** should be checked **preconceptionally, at first prenatal visit in first trimester,** 4 weeks after altering the doses (therefore, **every 4 weeks until TSH is normal,** especially in the first 20 weeks), **and at least every trimester in pregnancy.**
- Every woman with a thyroid nodule should have fine-needle aspiration of the nodule, and TSH checked.

DEFINITIONS

TSH is thyroid-stimulating hormone or thyrotropin; T_4 is thyroxine; T_3 is triodothyronine; FT_4 stands for free T_4.

(Clinical or overt) hypothyroidism

Inadequate thyroid hormone production of any cause that usually requires **elevated TSH and low free T_4 (or free T_3).**

Subclinical hypothyroidism

Usually requires elevated TSH and normal free T_4. Elevated TSH reflects the sensitivity of the hypothalamic–pituitary axis to small decreases in thyroid hormone; as the thyroid gland fails, the TSH level may rise above the upper limit of normal while the free T_4 is still within the normal range.

INCIDENCE

There is a 1% incidence in the general population and 1/1600–2000 in pregnant women.[1] General screening of obstetric patients reveals an incidence of 2.5% elevated serum TSH.[2] There is an increased incidence with concurrent autoimmune disease, i.e. 5–8% incidence in patients with type 1 diabetes.[3] In the USA, 10–15% of pregnant women are iodine deficient (urinary iodine concentration < 5 µg/dl).[4]

SIGNS/SYMPTOMS

Hypothyroidism may be masked by the hypermetabolic state of pregnancy.

---

*Includes thyroid nodule and postpartum thyroiditis.

Table 5.1   *Thyroid physiology changes in pregnancy and transplacental passage*

	Change in pregnancy	Placental transfer
Thyrotropin-releasing hormone (TRH)	–	++
Thyroid-stimulating hormone (TSH)	–	–
Resin tri-iodothyronine uptake (RT₃U)	↓	–
Thyroxine-binding globulin (TBG)	↑	+
Total thyroxine (TT₄)	↑	– (minimal)
Total tri-iodothyronine (TT₃)	↑	–
Free thyroxine (FT₄)	–	++
Free tri-iodothyronine (FT₃)	–	++
Thyroid-stimulating immunoglobulin (TSI)	–	++
Antithyroid peroxidase antibody	↓	++
Iodide	↓	++
Levothyroxine replacement	NA	– (minimal)
Thioamide (propylthiouracil [PTU] or methimazole) therapy	NA	++

NA, not applicable

The most common signs include dry skin, weakness, facial puffiness, and mild to moderate weight gain.[5] Fatigue, constipation, cold intolerance, muscle cramps, insomnia, hair loss, goiter, prolonged relaxation phase of deep tendon reflexes, carpal tunnel syndrome, intellectual slowness, voice changes, myxedema, and (extremely rarely) coma are less common.

PATHOPHYSIOLOGY

The thyroid maintains the metabolism in cells by stimulating transcription and translation. It also stimulates oxygen consumption and regulates lipid and carbohydrate metabolism, and is necessary for normal growth and maturation. The thyroid is under the control of TSH from the anterior pituitary. TSH induces thyroid growth, differentiation, and iodine metabolism.

The majority (> 99%) of cases of hypothyroidism are due to primary thyroid abnormality, with a small number of cases caused by hypothalamic dysfunction.

Hashimoto's thyroiditis is the most common cause of hypothyroidism in pregnancy. It is a chronic autoimmune lymphocytic thyroiditis, characterized by antithyroid antibodies (thyroid peroxidase [TPO] antibodies 90%, thyroglobulin antibodies 20–50%), and usually goiter as a presenting symptom.[6] Less common causes are subacute viral thyroiditis; iodine deficiency (median urinary iodine level < 100 µg/L); 'burned-out' Graves' disease, after radioiodine therapy, thyroidectomy, or antithyroid drugs; other head and neck surgery; other radiation therapy to the head, neck, or chest area; medications – lithium, iodine, amiodarone; rarely hypothalamic dysfunction, i.e. Sheehan's syndrome.

COMPLICATIONS

Untreated or partially treated clinical hypothyroidism is associated with increased risk of:[7,8] infertility, **pre-eclampsia** (44%), **abruption** (19%), **preterm birth, low birth weight** (31%), and **fetal death** (12%). Fetal goiter is unusual in women with hypothyroidism, unless they had previous hyperthyroidism and thyroid-stimulating immunoglobulins (TSI) are still > 200%. Infants whose mothers had serum FT₄ below the 10th percentile may have a high incidence of **impaired psychomotor function**.[9] Untreated subclinical hypothyroidism may be associated with a significantly lower IQ in children compared with normal controls.[10]

MANAGEMENT
Pregnancy considerations
Anatomy/radiology

In pregnancy, moderate glandular hyperplasia and increased vascularity in the thyroid are physiological effects. Thyroid volume measured with ultrasound increases by a mean of 18%.[4,11] **Any significant goiter requires further evaluation.**

Physiology

Several changes in thyroid physiology occur, as shown in Table 5.1. **Thyroxine-binding globulin** (TBG) increases about 200% secondary to estrogen-stimulated hepatocyte production and altered glycosylation, which inhibits degradation. **High levels**

Table 5.2   *Thyroid-stimulating hormone (TSH) percentiles (in μIU/ml) according to gestational age in singleton pregnancies*

Gestational age (week)	2.5th percentile	50th percentile	97.5th percentile
6	0.23	1.36	4.94
7	0.14	1.21	5.09
8	0.09	1.01	4.93
9	0.03	0.84	4.04
10	0.02	0.74	3.12
11	0.01	0.76	3.65
12	0.01	0.79	3.32
13	0.01	0.78	4.05
14	0.01	0.85	3.33
15	0.02	0.92	3.40
16	0.04	0.92	2.74
17	0.02	0.98	3.32
18	0.17	1.07	3.48
19	0.22	1.07	3.03
20	0.25	1.11	3.20
21	0.28	1.21	3.04
22	0.26	1.15	4.09
23	0.25	1.08	3.02
24	0.34	1.13	2.99
25	0.30	1.11	2.82
26	0.20	1.07	2.89
27	0.36	1.11	2.84
28	0.30	1.03	2.78
29	0.31	1.07	3.14
30	0.20	1.07	3.27
31	0.23	1.06	2.81
32	0.31	1.07	2.98
33	0.31	1.20	5.25
34	0.20	1.18	3.18
35	0.30	1.20	3.41
36	0.33	1.31	4.59
37	0.37	1.35	6.40
38	0.23	1.16	4.33
39	0.57	1.59	5.14
>40	0.38	1.68	5.43

Adapted from Dashe et al.[12] Values are in μIU/mL.

of human chorionic gonadotropin (HCG), which peak at 10–12 weeks, have some TSH-like activity and stimulate thyroid hormone secretion, which in turn **suppresses TSH**. Normal TSH levels in pregnancy are shown in Table 5.2. TSH suppression is even more marked for twins.[12] Peripheral metabolism of thyroid hormones is also altered by placental deiodinases, more in the second half of pregnancy.[13] Throughout pregnancy there is an approximately 30–50% increase in thyroxine (T_4) requirement.[14,15] Pregnancy does not appear to alter the course of thyroid cancer.[16]

Fetal thyroid physiology

In the fetus, the small amount of thyroxine that crosses the placenta provides all the thyroid hormone until 10–12 weeks. Upon the beginning of activation of the fetal hypothalamic–pituitary–thyroid axis at this gestational age (GA), the fetal thyroid begins to concentrate iodine and synthesize iodothyronines. At 18–20 weeks, the fetal thyroid is controlled by fetal pituitary TSH and mature hormone synthesis begins. Fetal TSH, T_4, and T_3 all begin to increase throughout gestation, as there seems to be minimal negative feedback mechanism.[17]

Placental physiology (see Table 5.1)

It is important to be aware of which molecules cross the placenta and can affect the fetus. FT_4, FT_3, TRH, iodine, TSI, and anti-TPO cross the placenta.[18] TSH does not cross the

Table 5.3   *Screening for hypothyroidism in pregnancy[6]*
Symptomatic (see Signs/symptoms section)
Previous therapy for hyperthyroidism
History of high-dose neck irradiation
Goiter/palpable thyroid nodules
Family history of thyroid disease
Suspected hypopituitarism
Type I diabetes mellitus[3]
Hyperlipidemia
Medications (iodine, amiodarone, lithium, dilantin [phenytoin], rifampin)

Table 5.4 *Primary vs secondary hypothyroidism*	
Primary hypothyroidism	
TSH	↑
FT_4	↓
Antithyroglobulin	+/−
Anti-thyroid peroxidase	+/−
Secondary hypothyroidism:	
TSH	↓
FT_4	↓

placenta. The placenta rapidly deiodinates maternal T_4 and T_3 to the inactive reverse-T_3.

Screening/diagnosis

Universal screening for maternal hypothyroidism is not usually recommended,[19] even if some have proposed it.[10] **Women at high risk for hypothyroidism should be screened** (Table 5.3).[20] Tests used for screening and diagnosis: **TSH** (most sensitive),[21,22] and **FT_4**. Elevated TSH, and low either free T_4 or free T_3 is consistent with clinical hypothyroidism (Table 5.4). In the first trimester, even a TSH level > 2.5 μIU/mL may be abnormal. Elevated TSH, and normal free T_4 (thyroid deficiency) are consistent with **subclinical hypothyroidism.**

Thyroid peroxidase antibody (TPO) is present in 90% of women with Hashimoto's thyroiditis, but also present in 10% of euthyroid women at 12 weeks. TPO crosses the placenta, may increase incidence of spontaneous abortion,[23] and increases the incidence of postpartum thyroid dysfunction.[24] Measuring TPO or thyroglobulin antibodies is important for diagnosis, but serial levels are usually not indicated since treatment does not alter them.

Treatment
Goal

Maternal serum TSH 0.5–2.0 μIU/ml and FT_4 in upper third of normal range.

Thyroxine replacement
Dose

Pre-existing hypothyroidism.   Approximately **45–85% of women need an increase in thyroxine replacement dose** up to 45% during pregnancy, owing to weight gain, increased T_4 pool, high serum TBG, placental deiodinase activity, and transfer of T_4 to the fetus.[25,26] Some clinicians advocate increasing replacement by 30% as soon as pregnancy is confirmed, but outcome data are not available.[14]

New diagnosis.   Levothyroxine can be started at 0.1–0.15 mg/day, adjusted by monitoring TSH levels. Thyroxine replament will need to be increased as in pre-existing disease. Ferrous sulfate interferes with T_4 absorption and should be taken at a different time of day from thyroxine therapy.[27] It takes approximately 4 weeks for thyroxine therapy to alter the TSH level. Under-replacement (see above) but also over-replacement (associated with pregnancy loss, low birth weight) should be avoided.[28]

Levothyroxine

This drug is the recommended thyroid replacement. Desiccated thyroid preparation such as Armour Thyroid (at 30 mg/day initial dose, then increased incrementally by 15 mg every 2–3 weeks until maintenance dose of 60–120 mg/day) is an alternative only if levothyroxine is unavailable.

Iodine supplement

Iodine supplementation in a population with high levels of endemic cretinism results in a reduction of the condition with no apparent adverse effects.[29] Iodine supplementation in areas of endemic cretinism is associated with a reduction in deaths during infancy and early childhood, with decreased cretinism at 4 years and better psychomotor development scores between 4 and 25 months of age. 10–15% of the US population has iodine deficiency, which can manifest as subclinical hypothyroidism, or with normal TSH and low T_4; 200 mg of iodine is the recommended daily dose during pregnancy.

Subclinical hypothyroidism

Screening and treatment for subclinical hypothyroidism are controversial: at present they are recommended by endocrinologists[30] but not by obstetricians.[19] Maternal subclinical hypothyroidism was associated with a 19% incidence of IQ < 85 at 7–9 years old, vs 5% in children of euthyroid mothers in a controversial study.[10] Subclinical hypothyroidism has been associated with an increased incidence of preterm birth, abruption, respiratory distress syndrome (RDS), and admission to NICU.[31] **There is insufficient evidence (no trials) to assess if treatment of maternal subclinical hypothyroidism with thyroid hormone replacement affects any outcome of the offspring.** Women with subclinical hypothyroidism and thyroid antibodies (e.g. TPO) frequently progress to overt hypothyroidism, and may develop hyperlipidemia and atherosclerotic heart disease.[32]

Antepartum management

- **TSH and free T$_4$ levels** should be checked **preconceptionally, at first prenatal visit in first trimester, 4 weeks after altering the doses (therefore every 4 weeks until TSH is normal, especially in the first 20 weeks), and at least every trimester in pregnancy.**
- Assess fetal heart rate at each visit by doptone to rule out fetal bradycardia < 120 beats/min.
- Antepartum testing is not recommended if euthyroid; weekly NSTs, beginning at 32–34 weeks, for clinically hypothyroid patients.
- Special ultrasound is not recommended if euthyroid; monthly ultrasound for fetal growth, thyroid circumference,[33] fetal heart rate are recommended if clinically hypothyroid.
- It is important to inform the pediatrician at time of delivery.

Congenital hypothyroidism

Iodine-deficient hypothyroidism/cretinism occurs in 1/4000 births, 5% identified at birth by clinical symptoms, others by newborn screening. The USA screens all newborns. If the condition is discovered and treated within the first few weeks of life, near-normal growth and intelligence can be expected.[34,35] The majority of cases are the result of agenesis/dysgenesis of fetal thyroid, dyshormonogenesis, or iodine deficiency. Fetuses are protected in utero by the small quantity of maternal T$_4$ which crosses the placenta. Neonatal issues include neurological abnormalities, respiratory difficulties, growth failure, lethargy and hypotonia, and myxedema of the larynx and epiglottis.

Postpartum

Immediately post-delivery, the maternal dosage of levothyroxine should be reduced to the prepregnancy dose, and TSH levels should be measured 6–8 weeks postpartum, with follow-up by a medical doctor or endocrinologist.

THYROID NODULE
Incidence

It is found that 5–10% of thyroid tumors are malignant. Thyroid cancer occurs in 1/1000 pregnant women with palpable thyroid nodule.

Diagnosis

Ultrasound is used to define a dominant nodule, followed by **fine-needle aspiration**, which has a 95% diagnostic accuracy in pregnancy.[36] Radioisotope scanning is contraindicated in pregnancy. Serum **TSH** and free T$_4$ should be checked.

Thyroid surgery

For malignancy diagnosed on fine-needle aspiration, neck exploration should be performed either in the second trimester or postpartum.[36] Neck irradiation for malignancy should be deferred if possible until after pregnancy.

POSTPARTUM THYROIDITIS
Definition

Autoimmune inflammation of the thyroid gland that presents as new-onset painless hypothyroidism, transient thyrotoxicosis, or thyrotoxicosis followed by hypothyroidism **within 1 year postpartum.**

Incidence

The condition occurs in 5% of women in the USA who do not have a history of thyroid disease,[37] and may occur after either delivery or pregnancy loss.

Risk factors

Postpartum depression, high serum thyroid peroxidase antibody concentration, history of Graves's disease, or type I diabetes.

Etiology

Subacute lymphocytic thyroiditis or postpartum exacerbation of chronic lymphocytic thyroiditis.

Diagnosis

Documentation of new-onset abnormal levels of TSH and/or FT$_4$ within the first postpartum year. All women with symptoms of thyroid dysfunction or who develop a goiter postpartum should be evaluated with TSH and FT$_4$. If the diagnosis is unclear, an anti-TPO antibody level should be measured.

Three clinical presentations

1. Transient hyperthyroidism followed by recovery – 28%.
2. Transient hyperthyroidism, followed by transient or rarely permanent hypothyroidism – 28%.
3. Transient or permanent hypothyroidism – 44%.

Management

Most women do not require treatment unless they have symptoms. If symptomatic, thyrotoxicosis should be treated with a beta-adrenergic antagonist drug. Transient hypothyroidism is treated with thyroxine, with attempts made to wean the patient off thyroid replacement within 6 months.

Recurrence risk

Risk of recurrence is 70%.[38]

REFERENCES

1. Montoro MN. Management of hypothyroidism during pregnancy. Clin Obstet Gynecol 1997; 40(1): 65–80. [II-2]
2. Klein RZ, Haddow JE, Faix JD, et al. Prevalence of thyroid deficiency in pregnant women. Clin Endocrinol (Oxf) 1991; 35(1): 41–6. [II-2]
3. Alvarez-Marfany M, Roman SH, Drexler AJ, Robertson C, Stagnaro-Green A. Long-term prospective study of postpartum thyroid dysfunction in women with insulin dependent diabetes mellitus. J Clin Endocrinol Metab 1994; 79(1): 10–16. [II-2]
4. Hollowell JG, Staehling NW, Hannon WH, et al. Iodine nutrition in the United States. Trends and public health implications: iodine excretion data from National Health and Nutrition Examination Surveys I and III (1971–1974 and 1988–1994). J Clin Endocrinol Metab 1998; 83(10): 3401–8. [II-2]
5. Rakel RE. Textbook of Family Practice, 6th edn. Philadelphia: WB Saunders; 2002. [review]
6. Weetman AP, McGregor AM. Autoimmune thyroid disease: developments in our understanding. Endocr Rev 1984; 5(2): 309–55. [III]
7. Leung AS, Millar LK, Koonings PP, Montoro M, Mestman JH. Perinatal outcome in hypothyroid pregnancies. Obstet Gynecol 1993; 81(3): 349–53. [II-2]
8. Davis LE, Leveno KJ, Cunningham FG. Hypothyroidism complicating pregnancy. Obstet Gynecol 1988; 72(1): 108–12. [II-3]
9. Pop VJ, Kuijpens JL, van Baar AL, et al. Low maternal free thyroxine concentrations during early pregnancy are associated with impaired psychomotor development in infancy. Clin Endocrinol (Oxf) 1999; 50(2): 149–55. [II-2]
10. Haddow JE, Palomaki GE, Allan WC, et al. Maternal thyroid deficiency during pregnancy and subsequent neuropsychological development of the child. N Engl J Med 1999; 341(8): 549–55. [II-2]
11. Rasmussen NG, Hornnes PJ, Hegedus L. Ultrasonographically determined thyroid size in pregnancy and post partum: the goitrogenic effect of pregnancy. Am J Obstet Gynecol 1989; 160(5 Pt 1): 1216–20. [II-3]
12. Dashe JS, Casey BM, Wells CE, et al. Thyroid-stimulating hormone in singleton and twin pregnancy: importance of gestational age-specific reference ranges. Obstet Gynecol 2005; 106: 753–7. [II-3]
13. Glinoer D, de Nayer P, Bourdoux P, et al. Regulation of maternal thyroid during pregnancy. J Clin Endocrinol Metab 1990; 71(2): 276–87. [II-3]
14. Alexander EK, Marqusee E, Lawrence J, et al. Timing and magnitude of increases in levothyroxine requirements during pregnancy in women with hypothyroidism. N Engl J Med 2004; 351(3): 241–9. [II-2, n=19]
15. Glinoer D. The regulation of thyroid function in pregnancy: pathways of endocrine adaptation from physiology to pathology. Endocr Rev 1997; 18(3): 404–33. [III]
16. Moosa M, Mazzaferri EL. Outcome of differentiated thyroid cancer diagnosed in pregnant women. J Clin Endocrinol Metab 1997; 82(9): 2862–6. [II-2]
17. Burrow GN, Fisher DA, Larsen PR. Maternal and fetal thyroid function. N Engl J Med 1994; 331(16): 1072–8. [III]
18. Bajoria R, Fisk NM. Permeability of human placenta and fetal membranes to thyrotropin-stimulating hormone in vitro. Pediatr Res 1998; 43(5): 621–8. [II-3]
19. ACOG. Thyroid disease in pregnancy. ACOG Practice Bulletin, No. 37, 2002. [review]
20. Gharib H, Cobin RH, Dickey RA. Subclinical hypothyroidism during pregnancy: position statement from the American Association of Clinical Endocrinologists. Endocr Pract 1999; 5(6): 367–8. [review, guideline]
21. American Association of Clinical Endocrinologists. AACE clinical practice guidelines for evaluation and treatment of hyperthyroidism and hypothyroidism. Jacksonville, Florida: AACE; 1996. [review, guideline]
22. Ladenson PW, Singer PA, Ain KB, et al. Thyroid Association guidelines for detection of thyroid dysfunction. Arch Intern Med 2000; 160(11): 1573–5. [review, guideline]
23. Stagnaro-Green A, Roman SH, Cobin RH, et al. Detection of at-risk pregnancy by means of highly sensitive assays for thyroid autoantibodies. JAMA 1990; 264(11): 1422–5. [II-3]
24. Kuijpens JL, Pop VJ, Vader HL, Drexhage HA, Wiersinga WM. Prediction of post partum thyroid dysfunction: can it be improved? Eur J Endocrinol 1998; 139(1): 36–43. [II-2]
25. Mandel SJ, Larsen PR, Seely EW, Brent GA. Increased need for thyroxine during pregnancy in women with primary hypothyroidism. N Engl J Med 1990; 323(2): 91–6. [II-2]
26. Kaplan MM. Management of thyroxine therapy during pregnancy. Endocr Pract 1996; 2(4): 281–6. [III]
27. Brent GA. Maternal hypothyroidism: recognition and management. Thyroid 1999; 9(7): 661–5. [III]
28. Anselmo J, Cao D, Karrison T, Weiss RE, Refetoff S. Fetal loss associated with excess thyroid hormone exposure. JAMA 2004; 292: 691–5. [II-3]

29. Mahomed K, Gulmezoglu AM. Maternal iodine supplements in areas of deficiency. Cochrane Database Syst Rev 2007; 1. [meta-analysis: 3 RCTs, $n=1551$]

30. Gharib H, Tuttle RM, Baskin J, et al. Consensus statement #1: subclinical thyroid dysfunction: a joint statement on management from the American Association of Clinical Endocrinologists, the American Thyroid Association, and the Endocrine Society. Thyroid 2005; 15: 24–8. [III]

31. Casey BM, Dashe JS, Wells CE, et al. Subclinical hypothyroidism and pregnancy outcomes. Obstet Gynecol 2004; 105: 239–45. [II-2]

32. Pearce EN, Farwell AP, Braverman LE. Thyroiditis. N Engl J Med 2003; 348: 2646–55. [III]

33. Ranzini AC, Ananth CV, Smulian JC et al. Ultrasonography of the fetal thyroid: nomograms based on biparietal diameter and gestational age. J Ultrasound Med 2001; 20(6): 613–17. [II-2]

34. Glorieux J, Dussault J, Van Vliet G. Intellectual development at age 12 years of children with congenital hypothyroidism diagnosed by neonatal screening. J Pediatr 1992; 121(4): 581–4. [II-2]

35. Rovet JF, Ehrlich RM, Sorbara DL. Neurodevelopment in infants and preschool children with congenital hypothyroidism: etiological and treatment factors affecting outcome. J Pediatr Psychol 1992; 17(2): 187–213. [II-2]

36. Tan GH, Gharib H, Goellner JR, van Heerden JA, Bahn RS. Management of thyroid nodules in pregnancy. Arch Intern Med 1996; 156(20): 2317–20. [II-2]

37. Gerstein HC. How common is postpartum thyroiditis? A methodologic overview of the literature. Arch Intern Med 1990; 150(7): 1397–400. [III]

38. Lazarus JH, Ammari F, Oretti R, et al. Clinical aspects of recurrent postpartum thyroiditis. Br J Gen Pract 1997; 47(418): 305–8. [II-3]

6

Hyperthyroidism*

Alisa B Modena

KEY POINTS

- Graves' disease accounts for 95% of women with hyper-thyroidism.
- Untreated hyperthyroidism is associated with increased risks of **spontaneous pregnancy loss, preterm birth, pre-eclampsia, fetal death, fetal growth restriction (FGR), neonatal Graves' disease,** as well as maternal **congestive heart failure** and **thyroid storm.**
- **Hyperemesis gravidarum (HG)** can be associated with **gestational transient biochemical thyrotoxicosis** (low, usually undetectable thyroid stimulating hormone [TSH] and/or elevated thyroxine [T$_4$]), but this biochemical change always resolves spontaneously. Therefore, there should be **no testing, follow-up, or treatment for bio-chemical thyrotoxicosis in women with HG.**
- Clinical hyperthyroidism is **diagnosed** by **suppressed TSH** and **elevated serum free T$_4$ (FT$_4$).** Thyroid-stimulating immunoglobulin (TSI) can be obtained, as positive TSI is consistent with Graves' disease, and values $\geq$ 200–500% indicate a higher risk for fetal/neonatal hyperthyroidism.
- The goal of treatment is to keep FT$_4$ in high normal range. **Measure TSH and FT$_4$** every 4 weeks until FT$_4$ is consis-tently in the high normal range, and then every trimester.
- Treatment is with **either propylthiouracil (PTU) or methimazole.** Because of the very rare teratogenic effects of methimazole, and the dual mechanism of action of PTU, PTU has been recommended as the thioamide of choice in pregnancy, but methimazole is an effective alternative.
- Radioiodine is absolutely contraindicated in pregnancy.
- **Thyroid storm** is initially dignosed clinically, and treated aggressively with PTU, SSKI (saturated solution of potassium iodide), dexamethasone, and propranolol.

DEFINITIONS

Hyperthyroidism: Hyperfunctioning thyroid gland that results in thyrotoxicosis. It usually implies low thyroid-stimulating hormone (TSH), and high thyroxine (T$_4$) (or tri-iodothyroxine [T$_3$]).

Graves' disease: Autoimmune disease characterized by production of thyroid-stimulating immunoglobulin (TSI) or thyroid-stimulating hormone-binding inhibitory immunoglobulin (TBII) (coexists with TSI 30% of the time),[1] that stimulate or inhibit the thyrotropin receptor.

Thyrotoxicosis: Clinical and biochemical state that results from an excess production or exposure to thyroid hormone, of any etiology.

Gestational thyrotoxicosis: Human gonadotropin-induced suppression of TSH by stimulation of T$_4$ production. Biochemical tests consistent with hyperthyroidism, but no disease.

Thyroid storm: Severe, acute, life-threatening exacerba-tion of the signs/symptoms of hyperthyroidism.

Subclinical hyperthyroidism: Sustained TSH $< 0.1\,\mu$IU/ml with normal free T$_4$ (FT$_4$) and free T$_3$ (FT$_3$), in the absence of non-thyroidal illness.

SIGNS/SYMPTOMS

Symptoms

Symptoms may mimic the hypermetabolic state of preg-nancy: nervousness, tremor, frequent stools, excessive sweating, heat intolerance, insomnia, palpitations, and decreased appetite.

---

*Includes thyroid storm.

Physical examination

Hypertension, goiter, tachycardia (>100 beats/min that does not decrease with Valsalva), wide pulse pressure, weight loss, ophthalmopathy (lid lag, lid retraction), and dermopathy (localized, pretibial myxedema). Goiter occurs only with iodine deficiency or thyroid disease, and must be considered pathological.

INCIDENCE

Hyperthyroidism is found in 0.2% of pregnancies.

ETIOLOGY

Graves' disease, which accounts for 95% of women with hyperthyroidism, is characterized by TSI (usually) and/or TBII. It can have a diffuse thyromegaly and infiltrative ophthalmopathy. Non-Graves' hyperthyroidism accounts for 5% of women with hyperthyroidism, and can be associated with toxic nodular and multinodular goiter, hyperfunctioning thyroid adenoma, subacute thyroiditis, extrathyroid source of thyroid hormone, or viral thyroiditis.

BASIC PHYSIOLOGY/ PATHOPHYSIOLOGY

(See also Chapter 5.) Ninety-five percent of cases of hyperthyroidism are caused by TSI stimulating excess thyroid hormone production by the thyroid gland (Graves' disease); 40–50% of women with Graves' disease have remission of the disease in 12–18 months.[2]

COMPLICATIONS

Untreated hyperthyroidism is associated with increased risks of **spontaneous pregnancy loss, preterm birth, pre-eclampsia, fetal death, fetal growth restriction (FGR),** maternal **congestive heart failure,** and **thyroid storm.**[3–6] **Neonatal Graves' disease** can affect neonates of women with Graves' disease. Long-term uncontrolled hyperthyroidism, even subclinical, is associated with increased maternal risk for atrial fibrillation, dementia, Alzheimer's disease, and hip fractures.

MANAGEMENT

Pregnancy considerations

(See also Chapter 5, including tables.) **High levels of human chorionic gonadotropin (HCG),** which peak at 10–12 weeks, have some TSH-like activity and stimulate thyroid hormone secretion, which in turn **suppresses TSH.** Normal TSH levels in pregnancy are shown in Table 5.2. TSH suppression is even more marked for twins.

Hyperemesis gravidarum (HG) is diagnosed by nausea and vomiting associated with ≥5% weight loss (see Chapter 8). **Gestational transient biochemical thyrotoxicosis** (low, usually undetectable TSH, and/or elevated T_4) may be related to high serum HCG, and can occur in 3–11% of normal pregnancies, especially during the period of the highest serum HCG concentrations (10–12 weeks).[7] Therefore, **no testing, follow-up, or treatment for thyroid disease in women with HG should be initiated,** since there is no true thyroid disease, and the biochemical hyperthyroidism resolves spontaneously. Women with signs or symptoms of hyperthyroidism from before pregnancy should be tested, regardless of HG.

Gestational trophoblastic disease: 50–60% of women with hydatidiform mole or choriocarcinoma may have severe hyperthyroidism, which is primarily treated with evacuation of the mole or chemotherapy directed against the choriocarcinoma.

Following thyroid surgery/ablation, women who continue to produce antibodies (i.e. TSI) warrant assessment of maternal TSI level, as these antibodies are associated with fetal/neonatal Graves' disease.[8] Because of the physiological changes of pregnancy, **hyperthyroidism typically ameliorates during the third trimester, but may worsen postpartum.**

Screening/diagnosis

Women with signs/symptoms consistent with hyperthyroidism should be screened with serum **TSH and FT$_4$.**[9,10] **Clinical hyperthyroidism is diagnosed by suppressed TSH and elevated serum FT$_4$.** FT$_3$ is measured in thyrotoxic patients with suppressed TSH but normal FT$_4$ measurements (5% of hyperthyroid women). FT$_3$ elevation indicates T_3 thyrotoxicosis. **TSI** can be obtained in women with clinical hyperthyroidism at the first visit and/or at 28–30 weeks.[8,11] A positive TSI is consistent with Graves' disease. Values ≥ 200–500% indicate a higher risk for fetal/neonatal hyperthyroidism, and can be useful for fetal and neonatal management. Unfortunately, there is no standard test for TSI, often making comparisons between different laboratories or studies impossible.

Routine measurements of thyroid function are **not** recommended in patients with HG unless other overt signs of hyperthyroidism are evident.

Treatment

Goal

The goal is to control symptoms of hyperthyroidism without causing fetal hypothyroidism, keeping **FT$_4$ in the high normal range** and TSH in the low normal range, with the lowest possible dose of thionamide. Propylthiouracil (PTU) > 200 mg/day may result in fetal goiter,[12] whereas keeping the FT_4 in the high normal range minimizes the risk of fetal hypothyroidism. **It may be helpful to measure TSH and FT_4 every 4 weeks until FT_4 is consistently in the high normal range**; then, measurements every trimester may be obtained. Dosing may need to be decreased as pregnancy advances, and about 30% of patients can discontinue antithyroid therapy and still remain euthyroid.

Thionamides

Propylthiouracil
Can be started at 100 mg every 8 hours, and the dose adjusted according to laboratory values and symptoms. It might take 6–8 weeks to obtain an adequate effect, with the initial clinical response in as little as 2–3 weeks. The usual dose of PTU is 50–150 mg every 8 hours, with requirements usually inversely proportional to gestational age (decrease as pregnancy advances).

Methimazole
Can be started at 20 mg once a day, modified as needed according to laboratory values and symptoms. It is an acceptable alternative, as it is equally effective. The teratological risks of aplasia cutis and esophageal and choanal atresia (9 cases in literature) are extremely rare.[13–16] There is no significant difference between PTU and methimazole in normalizing maternal TSH or in neonatal thyroid function, which might imply that transplacental transfer is similar.[14] **Because of the very rare teratogenic effects of methimazole, and the dual mechanism of action of PTU, PTU has been recommended as the thioamide of choice in pregnancy.**[2] There is no trial comparing the two in pregnancy, and methimazole may be preferred because of once a day dosing. **Methimazole is a very reasonable alternative**, and can also be used when there is an allergic reaction to PTU.

Mode of action
Both thionamides compete for peroxidase, blocking organification of iodide, and so decreasing thyroid hormone synthesis. PTU also inhibits peripheral $T_4 \rightarrow T_3$ conversion, and is thought to work faster than methimazole.

Side effects
Maternal. Agranulocytosis (granulocytes < 250/ml) is the most serious side effect, and occurs in 0.1–0.4% of cases. Risk factors are older gravidas, and higher doses. It presents with fever, sore throat, malaise, and gingivitis. If hyperthyroid women treated with thioamides present with sore throat and fever, discontinue therapy and check a complete blood count. Other side effects (all with incidence of < 5%) are thrombocytopenia, hepatitis, lupus-like syndrome, vasculitis, rash, pruritus, nausea, arthritis, anorexia, drug fever, and loss of taste or smell.

Fetal/neonatal. As PTU and methimazole both cross the placenta, they may cause **fetal hypothyroidism**. Transient hypothyroidism may cause goiter secondary to suppression of the fetal pituitary–thyroid axis. This, however, rarely requires therapy. IQ scores of children exposed to thionamide in utero are normal compared with non-exposed siblings. [17,18]

Radioiodine

This therapy **is absolutely contraindicated in pregnancy.** Fetal thyroid tissue will be ablated after 10 weeks. If given prior to 10 weeks, radioiodine does not appear to cause congenital hypothyroidism.[19,20] If given after 10 weeks, termination should be presented as an option. Breastfeeding should be avoided for 120 days after this therapy. The half-life for radioiodine is 8 days.

Beta-blockers

Propranolol 20–40 mg orally every 8–12 hours, or atenolol 50–100 mg orally once a day, are useful for rapid control of adrenergic symptoms of thyrotoxicosis, until thionamide takes effect (4–6 weeks). This therapy does **not** alter synthesis or secretion of thyroid hormone. The goal is to keep the maternal heart rate at 80–90 beats/min, without palpitations. Prolonged therapy can lead to fetal side effects such as FGR, fetal bradycardia, hypoglycemia, and subnormal response to hypoxemic stress.

Surgery

Thyroidectomy is usually indicated for women who cannot tolerate thionamide therapy, with other indications similar to non-pregnant women.

Iodine

Short-term use is safe for symptomatic relief,[21] whereas use for > 2 weeks may cause fetal goiter.[22]

Antepartum testing

- The **fetal heart rate** can be assessed for at least 1 minute at each visit by doptone to rule out fetal tachycardia > 180 beats/min.
- Thyroid function testing with **TSH and FT_4** should be performed at least every trimester.
- Weekly non-stress tests (**NSTs**) can begin at 32–34 weeks, especially in women with uncontrolled hyperthyroidism or elevated TSI.
- **Ultrasound** can assess fetal heart rate, thyroid (for goiter), and growth. If clinically hyperthyroid, ultrasounds every

4 weeks for growth may be indicated. If FGR or fetal tachycardia are present, fetal thyroid circumference can be assessed.[23]

- The fetus is at risk from either hypothyroidism from transplacental passage of antithyroid drugs, or from hyperthyroidism from TSI. The presence of a fetal goiter would point to fetal thyroid dysfunction, but not distinguish between these two possibilities. **Fetal blood sampling** is rarely indicated, but can be considered if high maternal TSI ($\geq$ 200–500% normal), with fetal signs suggestive of severe thyroid disease, i.e. fetal hydrops, goiter, tachycardia, cardiomegaly, FGR, or a history of prior fetus with hyperthyroidism.[24,25] Fetal hyperthyroidism should not be feared or tested for if TSI < 130% (normal range). If the fetus is hypothyroid, injection of thyroxine in amniotic fluid is a possible intervention. If the fetus is hyperthyroid, maternal treatment with thionamide to prevent fetal effects may be indicated even if the maternal T_4 is low or normal.[26]
- It is important to **inform the pediatrician** at the time of delivery of maternal diagnosis and drug therapy.

Neonate

Neonates born to mothers with Graves' disease should be followed closely by a pediatrician for the possibility of transient neonatal hyperthyroidism. **Neonatal Graves' disease** can affect 1–5% of neonates of women with Graves' disease, unrelated to maternal thyroid function, secondary to transplacental transfer TSI or TBII. The risk is high if the TSI index is $\geq$ 5, or TSI $\geq$ 200–500%.[27] Signs are tachycardia (> 160 beats/min), goiter, FGR, advanced bone age, craniosynostosis, hydrops, later motor difficulties, hyperactivity, and failure to thrive.[27] Neonates of women who have been treated surgically or with radioactive iodine before pregnancy and still gave TSI are at highest risk for neonatal Graves' disease since thioamide therapy is not present to counteract this effect. On the other hand, fetal and neonatal complications can also arise from thioamide treatment of the disease, as, when this is excessive, signs of hypothyroidism can occur.

Postpartum

Both PTU and methimazole are considered safe. Only small amounts of PTU cross into breast milk, while higher amounts of methimazole are present in breast milk.[28,29]

THYROID STORM

Incidence

Rare hypermetabolic state, which occurs in 1% of hyperthyroid women.

---

1. *Propylthiouracil* (PTU), 600–800 mg orally, immediately, even before laboratory results are back; then, 150–200 mg orally every 4–6 hours. If oral administration is not possible, use methimazole rectal suppositories.

2. Starting 1–2 hours after PTU administration, a saturated solution of *potassium iodide* (SSKI), 2–5 drops orally every 8 hours, or sodium iodide, 0.5–1.0 g intravenously every 8 hours, or Lugol's solution, 8 drops every 6 hours, or lithium carbonate, 300 mg orally every 6 hours.

3. *Dexamethasone*, 2 mg intravenously or intramuscularly every 6 hours for four doses.

4. *Propranolol*, 20–80 mg orally every 4–6 hours, or propranolol, 1–2 mg intravenously every 5 minutes for a total of 6 mg, then 1–10 mg intravenously every 4 hours.

5. If the patient has a history of severe bronchospasm:
   - reserpine, 1–5 mg intramuscularly every 4–6 hours
   - guanethidine, 1 mg/kg orally every 12 hours
   - diltiazem, 60 mg orally every 6–8 hours.

6. Phenobarbital, 30–60 mg orally every 6–8 hours as needed for extreme restlessness.

Figure 6.1
Treatment of thyroid storm in pregnant women. (Adapted from ACOG Practice Bulletin No. 37.[28])

Precipitating factors

Labor, infection, pre-eclampsia, and surgery.

Signs/symptoms

Fever, tachycardia disproportionate to fever, mental status change, vomiting, diarrhea, cardiac arrhythmia, and rarely seizures, shock, stupor, and coma.

Diagnosis

Diagnosis of thyroid storm, initially, should be made **clinically** with a combination of signs and symptoms. Confirmatory laboratory tests include increased FT_4 (or increased FT_3), and very low TSH.

Treatment

PTU, SSKI (saturated solution of potassium iodide), dexamethasone, and propranolol should be given as shown in Figure 6.1.[28] SSKI blocks the release of thyroid hormone from the gland. Dexamethasone decreases thyroid hormone release and peripheral conversion of T_4 to T_3. Propranolol inhibits the adrenergic effects of excessive thyroid hormone. Supportive measures include intravenous (IV) fluids with glucose, acetaminophen (as antipyretic), and oxygen, as needed. Fetal monitoring and maternal cardiac monitoring are recommended.[11] Delivery in the presence of thyroid storm should be avoided if at all possible, with maternal treatment leading to in-utero fetal resuscitation. The underlying cause, e.g. infection, should be treated.

REFERENCES

1. Amino N, Izumi Y, Hidaka Y, et al. No increase of blocking type anti-thyrotropin receptor antibodies during pregnancy in patients with Graves' disease. J Clin Endocrinol Metab 2003; 88(12): 5871–4.
2. Cooper DS. Antithyroid drugs. N Engl J Med 2005; 352: 905–17. [III, review]
3. Davis LE, Lucas MJ, Hankins GD, Roark ML, Cunningham FG. Thyrotoxicosis complicating pregnancy. Am J Obstet Gynecol 1989; 160(1): 63–70. [II-2]
4. Mestman JH. Diagnosis and management of maternal and fetal thyroid disorders. Curr Opin Obstet Gynecol 1999; 11(2): 167–75. [III, review]
5. Millar LK, Wing DA, Leung AS, et al. Low birth weight and preeclampsia in pregnancies complicated by hyperthyroidism. Obstet Gynecol 1994; 84(6): 946–9. [II-2]
6. Phoojaroenchanachai M, Sriussadaporn S, Peerapatdit T, et al. Effect of maternal hyperthyroidism during late pregnancy on the risk of neonatal low birth weight. Clin Endocrinol (Oxf) 2001; 54(3): 365–70. [II-3]
7. Yeo CP, Khoo DH, Eng PH, et al. Prevalence of gestational thyrotoxicosis in Asian women evaluated in the 8th to 14th weeks of pregnancy: correlations with total and free beta human chorionic gonadotrophin. Clin Endocrinol (Oxf) 2001; 55(3): 391–8. [II-2]
8. Weetman AP. Graves' disease. N Engl J Med 2000; 343(17): 1236–48. [III, review]
9. American Association of Clinical Endocrinologists. AACE clinical practice guidelines for evaluation and treatment of hyperthyroidism and hypothyroidism. Jacksonville, Florida: AACE; 1996.
10. Ladenson PW, Singer PA, Ain KB, et al. Thyroid Association guidelines for detection of thyroid dysfunction. Arch Intern Med 2000; 160(11): 1573–5.
11. Ecker JL, Musci TJ. Thyroid function and disease in pregnancy. Curr Probl Obstet Gynecol Fertil 2000; 23: 109–122. [III]
12. Hamburger JI. Thyroid nodules in pregnancy. Thyroid 1992; 2(2): 165–8. [III]
13. Wing DA, Millar LK, Koonings PP, Montoro MN, Mestman JH. A comparison of propylthiouracil versus methimazole in the treatment of hyperthyroidism in pregnancy. Am J Obstet Gynecol 1994; 170 (1 Pt 1): 90–5. [II-2]
14. Momotani N, Noh JY, Ishikawa N, Ito K. Effects of propylthiouracil and methimazole on fetal thyroid status in mothers with Graves' hyperthyroidism. J Clin Endocrinol Metab 1997; 82(11): 3633–6. [II-2]
15. Clementi M, Di Gianantonio E, Pelo E, et al. Methimazole embryopathy: delineation of the phenotype. Am J Med Genet 1999; 83(1): 43–6. [III]
16. Di Gianantonio E, Schaefer C, Mastroiacovo PP, et al. Adverse effects of prenatal methimazole exposure. Teratology 2001; 64(5): 262–6. [II-2]
17. Burrow GN, Klatskin EH, Genel M. Intellectual development in children whose mothers received propylthiouracil during pregnancy. Yale J Biol Med 1978; 51(2): 151–6. [II-2]
18. Eisenstein Z, Weiss M, Katz Y, Bank H. Intellectual capacity of subjects exposed to methimazole or propylthiouracil in utero. Eur J Pediatr 1992; 151(8): 558–9. [II-2]
19. Berg GE, Nystrom EH, Jacobsson L, et al. Radioiodine treatment of hyperthyroidism in a pregnant women. J Nucl Med 1998; 39(2): 357–61. [II-3]
20. Evans PM, Webster J, Evans WD, Bevan JS, Scanlon MF. Radioiodine treatment in unsuspected pregnancy. Clin Endocrinol (Oxf) 1998; 48(3): 281–3. [II-3]
21. Nohr SB, Jorgensen A, Pedersen KM, Laurberg P. Postpartum thyroid dysfunction in pregnant thyroid peroxidase antibody-positive women living in an area with mild to moderate iodine deficiency: is iodine supplementation safe? J Clin Endocrinol Metab 2000; 85(9): 3191–8. [II-2]
22. Momotani N, Hisaoka T, Noh J, Ishikawa N, Ito K. Effects of iodine on thyroid status of fetus versus mother in treatment of Graves' disease complicated by pregnancy. J Clin Endocrinol Metab 1992; 75(3): 738–44. [II-2]
23. Ranzini AC, Ananth CV, Smulian JC, et al. Ultrasonography of the fetal thyroid: nomograms based on biparietal diameter and gestational age. J Ultrasound Med 2001; 20(6): 613–17. [II-2]
24. Nachum Z, Rakover Y, Weiner E, Shalev E. Graves' disease in pregnancy: prospective evaluation of a selective invasive treatment protocol. Am J Obstet Gynecol 2003; 189(1): 159–65. [II-2]
25. Kilkpatrick S. Umbilical blood sampling in women with thyroid disease in pregnancy: Is it necessary? Am J Obstet Gynecol 2003; 189: 1–2. [III]
26. Peleg D, Cada S, Peleg A, Ben-Ami M. The relationship between maternal serum thyroid-stimulating immunoglobulin and fetal and neonatal thyrotoxicosis. Obstet Gynecol 2002; 99(6): 1040–3. [II-2]
27. Becks GP, Burrow GN. Thyroid disease and pregnancy. Med Clin North Am 1991; 75(1): 121–50. [III, review]
28. Thyroid disease in pregnancy. ACOG Practice Bulletin. No. 37, August 2002. [Review]
29. Briggs GG, Freeman RK, Yaffe SJ. Drugs in Pregnancy and Lactation, 6th edn. Philadelphia: Lippincott Williams & Wilkins; 2001. [II-2]

7

Prolactinoma

Vincenzo Berghella

KEY POINTS

- Diagnosis: ↑ prolactin and MRI (magnetic resonance imaging)-proven pituitary adenoma.
- Preconception: treat with dopamine agonist (bromocriptine or cabergoline) aiming to normalize prolactin and decrease size of adenoma, continuing therapy up to positive pregnancy test. Discourage pregnancy until those aims have been achieved, and any neurological or visual symptoms or suprasellar involvement have been resolved.
- Maternal risk is adenoma enlargement; this occurs in pregnancy in 1–5% of microadenomas and about 15–35% of macroadenomas.
- Bromocriptine (and probably cabergoline) have been shown to be safe for the fetus.
- Compared with cabergoline, bromocriptine has the advantages of being cheaper and having more pregnancy safety data, but the disadvantages of twice-daily (vs twice-weekly) dosing and more side effects.
- Management depends on size of adenoma:
  - Microadenoma (< 1 cm): consider stopping dopamine agonist in pregnancy, especially if normal prolactin and stable microadenoma ≥ 2 years pre-pregnancy. During the pregnancy, the woman should be asked about headaches and changes in vision at each visit (at least every 3 months). Prolactin levels should not be checked in pregnancy, since they physiologically increase (10-fold) in pregnancy.
  - Macroadenoma (≥ 1 cm): dopamine agonist should be continued. Monitoring as per microadenoma, plus formal visual field testing every 3 months. Transsphenoidal surgery suggested only if maximal dopamine agonist therapy is ineffective.

DIAGNOSIS/DEFINITION

Pituitary adenomas producing prolactin (prolactinomas, or lactotroph adenomas) are diagnosed preconception by sustained elevation of serum prolactin (usually > 40 μg/L × 2; normal prolactin non-pregnant: < 20 μg/L) and radiographic (best is magnetic resonance imaging [MRI]) evidence of pituitary adenoma. Rule out other causes of prolactinemia.[1]

SYMPTOMS

Before pregnancy: galactorrhea, 80% of women; irregular menses (e.g. oligomenorrhea).

EPIDEMIOLOGY/INCIDENCE

Prolactinomas account for about 40% of pituitary tumors.

ETIOLOGY/BASIC PATHOPHYSIOLOGY

These adenomas produce prolactin. Outside of pregnancy, prolactin levels parallel tumor size fairly closely. Increased prolactin usually causes infertility because of the inhibitory effect of prolactin on secretion of gonadotropin-releasing hormone (GNRH), which in turn inhibits the release of luteinizing hormone (LH) and follicle-stimulating hormone (FSH), so impairing gonadal steroidogenesis and ovulation, and thereby conception. Sometimes the mass effect of a macroadenoma can also lead to infertility.

CLASSIFICATION

- Microadenoma < 10 mm.
- Macrodenoma ≥ 10 mm.

COMPLICATIONS
Mother

The principal risk is the increase in adenoma size sufficient to cause neurological symptoms, most importantly visual impairment and also headaches. In women with lactotroph adenomas who become pregnant, the hyperestrogenemia of pregnancy may increase the size of the adenoma. This should be distinguished from increase in pituitary (overall) size (physiological effect in pregnancy). The risk that the adenoma increase will be clinically important depends upon the size of the adenoma *before* pregnancy. The risk of a clinically important increase in the size of a lactotroph microadenoma during pregnancy is small. Because of enlargement, about 1–5% of pregnant women with *micro*adenomas develop neurological symptoms, such as headaches and/or a visual field abnormality; and about 1% diabetes insipidus. With *macro*adenomas, neurological symptoms occur in ≥ 13–36% of pregnant women, and diabetes insipidus in about 1–2%.[2,4] Long-term hyperprolactinemia may lead to **decrease in bone density**, which again increases (not back to normal levels) after normal levels are re-established.[1]

Fetus

The main potential risk to the fetus is from dopamine agonist treatment of hyperprolactinemia. Administration of *bromocriptine* during the first month of pregnancy does not harm the fetus (over 1000 pregnancies reported).[5,6] There are less data available about the use of bromocriptine later in pregnancy, but no adverse events have been reported. *Cabergoline* use in pregnancy is probably safe, too (about 300 pregnancies reported), but less experience is reported.[7,8]

PREGNANCY CONSIDERATIONS

The ability to treat prolactinomas successfully with dopamine agonists in > 90% of patients allows most women with this disorder to become pregnant. The theoretical basis for an **increase in size of the pituitary** during pregnancy is that hyperestrogenemia causes lactotroph hyperplasia. Secondary to estrogen causing lactotroph hyperplasia, there is a progressive increase in pituitary size, as assessed by MRI, throughout pregnancy, so that the volume during the third trimester is more than double that in non-pregnant women.[9]

PREGNANCY-RELATED MANAGEMENT

Principles

Effect of pregnancy on disease

The whole pituitary enlarges in pregnancy. The prolactinoma can enlarge. Prolactin levels are physiologically elevated, and cannot be used for management.

Effect of disease on pregnancy

No obstetric effects unless major surgery is needed.

Work-up (Figure 7.1)

- **Prolactin** levels are not helpful in pregnancy.
- **MRI** is more effective in revealing small tumors and the extension of large tumors compared with computed tomography (CT) scan.[1]

Treatment (see Figure 7.1)

Dopamine antagonists

The primary therapy for all prolactinomas is a dopamine agonist. The dopamine agonists approved in the USA are bromocriptine and cabergoline.

Bromocriptine (Parlodel)

Dose. **Start at 0.625 mg po qhs** with snack × 1w. Then, add 1.25 mg qam × 1w, then increase by 1.25 mg. So at 4 weeks, a total of 5 mg (split **2.5 mg q12h**) is reached and prolactin rechecked. Usually, a total of 5–7.5 mg (split q12h) total dose is required (to normalise prolactin in non-pregnant women). *Can also use intravaginally* (same dose, less side effects, minimal vaginal irritation).

Mechanism of action. Dopamine agonist (dopamine inhibits lactotroph receptors, so less prolactin is produced, size of tumors is decreased); ergot derivative.

Evidence for effectiveness. See below.

Safety in pregnancy. Safe (Food and Drug Administration [FDA] category B). Breastfeeding is contraindicated.

Side effects. Nausea, hypotension, depression (less if therapy is initiated at night).

Cabergoline (Dostinex)

Dose. Start at 0.25 mg twice weekly, increase monthly until normal prolactin (before pregnancy). Usual required dose: 0.25–0.5 twice weekly; max dose: 1 mg twice weekly.

Mechanism of action. Dopamine agonist (see above); non-ergot; high affinity for lactotroph dopamine receptors.

Evidence for effectiveness. See below.

Safety in pregnancy. Safe (FDA category B). Breastfeeding is contraindicated.

Side effects. Minimal.

Preconception counseling

Treatment of women with lactotroph adenomas outside of pregnancy is based on the size of the tumor, the

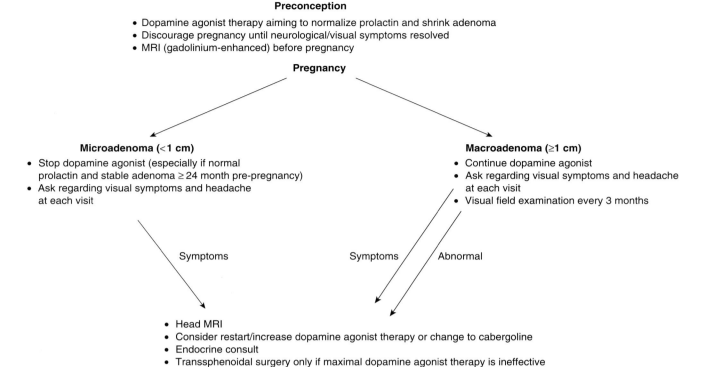

Figure 7.1
Management of prolactinoma in pregnancy.

presence/absence of gonadal dysfunction, and the woman's desire regarding fertility.[1] Treatment should begin before conception with advice to the woman and her partner about the risks of pregnancy to her and the fetus. When a dopamine agonist is needed to lower the serum prolactin concentration to permit ovulation, counseling should include the fact that bromocriptine has larger safety data, whereas cabergoline (Dostinex) has less data in pregnancy (all reassuring so far). Bromocriptine normalizes prolactin levels in >80% of women with microadenomas, restoring menses and fertility in >90%. Compared with cabergoline, bromocriptine has the advantages of being cheaper and having more pregnancy safety data, but the disadvantages of twice-daily (vs twice-weekly) dosing and more side effects. If a woman cannot tolerate bromocriptine, cabergoline should be recommended: 70% of patients who do not have a response to bromocriptine respond to cabergoline. Pergolide should not be recommended because it is not FDA-approved to treat hyperprolactinemia, has not been studied during pregnancy, and has been associated with cardiac valvular defects.[10]

Microadenomas

A woman who has a lactotroph microadenoma should be told that the risk of clinically important enlargement of her adenoma during pregnancy is very small (1–5%) and that it **should not be a deterrent to becoming pregnant**. She should also be told that bromocriptine or cabergoline will probably be effective if symptoms do occur. If she is willing to take this small risk of enlargement, she should be given bromocriptine or cabergoline before pregnancy in whatever dosage is necessary to lower her serum prolactin concentration to normal. Bromocriptine is the drug with the greater experience. When the serum prolactin concentration is normal and menses have occurred regularly for a few months, the woman can attempt to become pregnant. Before pregnancy, the dopamine agonist should be tapered to the lowest effective dose, and can be discontinued before pregnancy if used for ≥24 months with normal prolactin levels, as about 25% of patients maintain normal levels even off medication; most need to eventually restart it, though.

Macroadenomas

A woman who has a lactotroph macroadenoma should be advised of the relatively higher risk of clinically important tumor enlargement during pregnancy.[2–4] A macroadenoma is an **absolute indication for therapy** (dopamine agonist, followed together with endocrinologist), in non-pregnant or pregnant women. Doses of dopamine agonists sufficient to control the macroadenoma are usually higher (bromocriptine 7.5–10 mg/daily; cabergoline 0.5–1 mg twice weekly) than with microadenomas. Before pregnancy, the dopamine agonist should be carefully tapered to the lowest effective dose: this may take weeks to years. Advice and monitoring depend upon how large the adenoma is.

- If the macroadenoma does not elevate the optic chiasm or extend behind the sella, treatment with bromocriptine or cabergoline for a sufficient period to shrink it substantially should reduce the chance of clinically important enlargement during pregnancy.[2,11] Once this has occurred, the woman can attempt to become pregnant.
- If the adenoma is very large or elevates the optic chiasm, pregnancy should be strongly discouraged until the adenoma has been adequately treated. If the macroadenoma extends behind the sella, the woman should undergo visual field examination and testing of anterior pituitary function. Transsphenoidal surgery may be necessary and, perhaps postoperatively, radiation. Postoperative treatment with bromocriptine or cabergoline may also be helpful in reducing adenoma size further and lowering the serum prolactin concentration to normal. Such a regimen reduces the chance that symptomatic expansion will occur during pregnancy,[2,3] but it may still occur.
- Pregnancy should also be discouraged in a woman whose macroadenoma is unresponsive to bromocriptine and cabergoline, even if it is not elevating the optic chiasm, until the size has been greatly reduced by transsphenoidal surgery, because medical treatment is not likely to be effective if the adenoma enlarges during pregnancy.

Prenatal care

See also above regarding preconception counseling.

Microadenoma

Bromocriptine, and probably cabergoline, are safe in pregnancy. They can be discontinued as soon as pregnancy has been confirmed if the patient who has a normal prepregnancy prolactin and a recent reassuring (adenoma < 1 cm) MRI so desires. During the pregnancy, the woman should be asked about headaches and changes in vision at each visit (or at least every 3 months). A formal visual field test can be performed every 3 months, but this is not absolutely necessary. Prolactin levels should not be checked, since they physiologically increase (about 10-fold) in pregnancy. If no symptoms occur, serum prolactin can be measured 2 months after delivery or cessation of nursing, and if it is similar to the pretreatment value, the drug can be resumed.

Macroadenoma

The **dopamine agonist should be continued during pregnancy** in most cases. In these patients, discontinuation of the drug usually leads to expansion of the adenoma.[1] Monitoring during pregnancy should be similar to that described above for women with microadenomas, except for the fact that formal visual field testing every 3 months should be performed.

General

A perceived change in vision should be assessed by a neuro-ophthalmologist, and an MRI (gadolinium-enhanced) scan, more effective than CT scan,[1] should be performed if an abnormality consistent with a pituitary adenoma is confirmed. If the adenoma has enlarged to a degree that could account for the symptoms, the woman should be treated with higher doses of bromocriptine throughout the remainder of the pregnancy, which will usually decrease the size of the adenoma and alleviate the symptoms.[12,13] If the adenoma does not respond to bromocriptine, cabergoline may be successful.[14] If cabergoline is not successful, transsphenoidal surgery could be considered in the second trimester if vision is severely compromised; in comparison, surgery for persistent visual symptoms in the third trimester should be deferred until delivery if possible. **Surgery is recommended *only* if medical therapy is ineffective.**

Antepartum testing

None is needed (except if other indications are present).

Delivery

No special precautions.

Anesthesia

No special precautions.

Postpartum

A prolactin level and a gadolinium-enhanced MRI can be performed 6–8 weeks postpartum. All women with macroadenomas and those with microadenomas and elevated prolactin should be continued/started on dopamine agonist therapy, with endocrine follow-up.

Breastfeeding

A microadenoma is not a contraindication to nursing. If the woman has no neurological symptoms at the time of delivery, nursing should not be of substantial risk. If she does have neurological symptoms at the time of delivery or if they develop during nursing, she should be treated with a dopamine agonist. Since the dopamine agonists suppress lactation, the woman on these drugs should be advised against breastfeeding.

REFERENCES

1. Schlechte JA. Prolactinoma. N Engl J Med 2003; 349: 2035–41. [III, review]
2. Gemzell C, Wang CF. Outcome of pregnancy in women with pituitary adenoma. Fertil Steril 1979; 31: 363–72. [A survey of 25 physicians in 1979 revealed that they had seen a total of 91 pregnancies in 85 women with lactotroph microadenomas and 46 women with lactotroph macroadenomas were followed during 56 pregnancies]
3. Molitch ME. Management of prolactinomas during pregnancy. J Reprod Med 1999; 44: 1121–6. [III, review]
4. Kupersmith MJ, Rosenberg C, Kleinberg D. Visual loss in pregnant women with pituitary adenomas. Ann Intern Med 1994; 121: 473–7. [II–3]
5. Turkalj I, Braun P, Krupp P. Surveillance of bromocriptine in pregnancy. JAMA 1982; 247: 1589–91. [The manufacturer of bromocriptine surveyed physicians known to prescribe bromocriptine. The survey evaluated 1410 pregnancies in 1335 women who took the drug during pregnancy, primarily during the first month. The incidence of spontaneous abortions (11.1%) and major (1%) and minor (2.5%) congenital malformations was similar to that in the general population. Only eight women had taken bromocriptine after the second month of pregnancy]
6. Molitch M. Pregnancy and the hyperprolactenemic woman. N Engl J Med 1985; 23: 1364–70. [II-3, safety of bromocriptine]
7. Robert E, Musatti L, Piscitelli G, et al. Pregnancy outcome after treatment with the ergot derivative, cabergoline. Reprod Toxicol 1996; 10: 333–7. [II-3, $n=226$]
8. Ricci E, Parazzini F, Motta T, et al. Pregnancy outcome after cabergoline treatment in early weeks of gestation. Reprod Toxicol 2002; 16: 791–3. [II-3, cabergoline safety proven in 61 pregnancies]
9. Gonzalez JG, Elizondo G, Saldivar D, et al. Pituitary gland growth during normal pregnancy: an in vivo study using magnetic resonance imaging. Am J Med 1988; 85: 217–20. [II-3]
10. Flowers CM, Racoosin JA, Lu SL, Beitz JG. The US Food and Drug Administration's registry of patients with pergolide-associated valvular heart disease. Mayo Clin Proc 2003; 78: 730–1. [II-3]
11. Ahmed M, Al-Dossary E, Woodhouse NJ. Macroprolactinomas with suprasellar extension: effect of bromocriptine withdrawal during one or more pregnancies. Fertil Steril 1992; 58: 492–7. [II-2]
12. Konopka P, Raymond JP, Merceron RE, Seneze J. Continuous administration of bromocriptine in the prevention of neurological complications in pregnant women with prolactinomas. Am J Obstet Gynecol 1983; 146: 935–8. [II-3]
13. Van Roon E, van der Vijver JC, Gerretsen G, Hekster RE, Wattendorff RA. Rapid regression of a suprasellar extending prolactinoma after bromocriptine treatment during pregnancy. Fertil Steril 1981; 36: 173–7. [II-3]
14. Liu C, Tyrrell JB. Successful treatment of a large macroprolactinoma with cabergoline during pregnancy. Pituitary 2001; 4: 179–85. [II-3]

8

Nausea/vomiting of pregnancy and hyperemesis gravidarum

Vincenzo Berghella

KEY POINTS

- Diagnosis of hyperemesis gravidarum (HG) is *nausea and vomiting ≥ 3 times/day*, with *large ketones in urine* or acetone in blood, *and weight loss of >3 kg or >5% of prepregnancy weight*, having excluded other diagnoses.
- Do not test for thyroid stimulating hormone (TSH) in women with nausea/vomiting or HG, unless they have a pre-existing history/symptoms of hyperthyroidism.
- **For prevention, start prenatal vitamins before conception.**
- Start treating nausea and vomiting to prevent HG.
- **Safe therapies proven to improve nausea, vomiting, and HG are** (in approximate order of invasiveness/potency):

  - acupressure/acustimulation wrist band
  - acupuncture
  - ginger capsules
  - vitamin B_6
  - doxilamine (suggest use in combination with vitamin B_6)
  - promethazine
  - trimethobenzamine
  - ondansetron.

DIAGNOSIS/DEFINITION

Hyperemesis gravidarum (HG) is **nausea and vomiting ≥ 3 times/day, with large ketones in urine** or acetone in blood (dehydration, fluid, and electrolytes changes), *and* **weight loss of >3 kg or >5% of prepregnancy weight**, having excluded other diagnoses (diagnosis of exclusion).

EPIDEMIOLOGY/INCIDENCE

About 75% of pregnant women have nausea and/or vomiting (25% are unaffected): 50% have both nausea and vomiting (n/v), while 25% have nausea only; 18% have more than once/day vomiting; **0.5–1% have true HG.** HG is possibly more common in mothers carrying a female fetus.[1] The onset is about 4–6 weeks, peak 8–12 weeks, resolution <20 weeks. Doubt the diagnosis if the symptoms start >9 weeks. Not usually just 'morning sickness'.[2]

GENETICS

More common in first-degree relatives (daughters, sisters).

ETIOLOGY

Hypotheses:

1. Gastrointestinal (GI) motility decreases in pregnancy (but not particularly in HG; probably secondary phenomenon).
2. Hormones – (human chorionic gonadotropin (HCG), thyroxine, cortisol, etc). – trigger chemoreceptor trigger zone (CTZ) in the brainstem–vomiting center.
3. CTZ is more sensitive to hormones.
4. *Helicobacter pylori*: immunoglobulin G (IgG) present in 90.5% of HG patients; 47.5% of controls.[3]
5. Associated with unwanted, unplanned pregnancies (and conversion disorder).[4] 85% of women with HG report poor support by partner.

Some clinicians have also postulated that n/v is evolutionary, to protect the fetus from teratogenic exposures.

CLASSIFICATION

Classification is not clinically useful,[5] since management is based mostly on the woman's perception of severity and her desire for treatment.

RISK FACTORS/ASSOCIATIONS

Obesity, nulliparity, prior HG (recurrence about 67%), female fetus, history of motion sickness, and history of migraines. Associated with high HCG levels (larger placental mass, as in multiple pregnancy, molar pregnancy). Associated with high estradiol levels (if n/v on oral contraceptive pills [OCP], woman will probably get n/v in pregnancy). Smoking is associated with lower levels of HCG and estradiol, and therefore smokers have lower incidence of HG.

Ptyalism

Very little is known regarding **ptyalism** (aka sialorrhea, excessive salivation); diagnosis is salivation > 1900 ml/day; etiological hypothesis is the stimulation by starch (possibly pica). It is characterized by an inability to swallow, not excessive production. No therapy (gum, lozengers, small meals, anticholenergics, ganglion-blocking agents, oxyphenonium bromide, etc.) has been studied appropriately, or been shown to be efficacious in pregnancy. Check hydration, nutrition, psychological status, and other issues as per n/v.[6]

COMPLICATIONS

Maternal: minimal in mild cases of n/v. For HG: diminished quality of life may lead to a decision for termination (2.9% in Sweden;[7] never a US study); depression. Rare: Wernicke's encephalopathy (vitamin B_1 deficiency; permanent neurological disability or maternal death); splenic avulsion, esophageal rupture, pneumothorax, acute tubular necrosis. In extreme and very rare cases of HG, maternal death can occur.

Fetal/neonatal: minimal in mild cases of n/v; not increased fetal growth restriction (FGR) or higher incidence of congenital anomalies. Severe HG, usually necessitating parenteral nutrition, is associated with FGR and fetal death.

HG is also associated with lower pregnancy loss incidence (secondary to robust placental synthesis) and high healthcare costs (time lost from work).

PREGNANCY MANAGEMENT
Principles

Prevention is better than treatment: i.e. **intervene early on n/v to prevent worsening.**[8] HG is a diagnosis of exclusion. Nausea and vomiting tends to be undertreated by some physicians and some patients, whereas there are many safe and effective therapies.

Work-up

Work-up is aimed at ruling out differential diagnostic possibilities such as GI (gallbladder disease, hepatitis, pancreatitis, appendicitis, inflammatory bowel disease), genitourinary, ovarian torsion, thyrotoxicosis, diabetic ketoacidosis, Addison's disease, brain tumor, migraine, vestibular lesion, pseudotumor cerebri, food/drug poisoning/toxicity, acute fatty liver/pre-eclampsia, etc.

History and review of systems

Special attention to severity of weight loss, prior GI diagnosis, and dietary, physical, and psychological stressors.

Physical examination

Special attention to vital signs, signs of dehydration, goiter, abdominal, neurological exam.

Laboratory tests

Serum
Electrolytes, glucose, liver function tests (LFTs), amylase, lipase, acetone (quantitative HCG not helpful in management).

Urine
Ketones, specific gravity.

Thyroid
No need to send TSH (60–70% of HG have 'transient biochemical hyperthyroidism of pregnancy' with ↓ TSH and ↑ free thyroid index; this is secondary to HCG simulating thyroxine synthesis from pituitary; always resolves spontaneously in 1–10 weeks;[9,10] only test if pregnant woman has a history of thyroid disease or goiter).

Radiological

Fetal ultrasound (to assess for molar pregnancy, multiple gestation, etc.).

Consults

Occasionally consider psychiatry consult, depending on history.

Therapy
Prevention

Prenatal multivitamins before/at conception.[11] Intervene early on n/v.

Suggested step-wise approach

A combination of interventions are often necessary

Outpatient nausea and vomiting

Lifestyle/dietary changes.   Avoid odor/food triggers. Stop medications (e.g. iron, large vitamins) producing n/v. Counsel regarding safety and efficacy of treatment; provide reassurance regarding outcomes (see above). There is no evidence that rest improves n/v. Diet: small meals; eat only one spoonful, wait, eat again, etc.; avoid an empty stomach; avoid fatty greasy spicy foods; ginger ale; prefer protein, but a high protein diet is associated with higher incidences of preterm birth and fetal death.

Treat any underlying/concomitant GI disorder (reflux, ulcer, anorexia, etc.) appropriately.

Drugs/other interventions.   The following drugs/interventions in *italics* have been evaluated at least in one trial showing efficacy (starting with a non-pharmacological intervention).

Acupressure/acustimulation wrist bands.   [(P6 'Neiguan' point) acupressure[12–20] or acustimulation.[21] (Relief Band Device, Woodside Biomedical – www.reliefband.com, or Seaband.) Wear the band all the time until n/v, HG resolved. No pregnant safety or breastfeeding concerns.

If still n/v, add

Ginger.   350 mg po tid[22–28] (can also substitute for vitamin B_6 if vitamin B_6 not effective)

If still n/v, add/substitute

Vitamin B_6.   (thiamine) 10–25 mg po tid/qid[29–30] ($\downarrow$n, not decreased vomiting – both benefit)

If still n/v, add

Doxylamine.   (Unisom) 25 mg qhs and 12.5 mg bid (adjust dose to symptoms);[31–34] antihistamine H_1 receptor blocker. With vitamin B_6 (=Bendectin) it is safe (proven with over 170 000 exposures) and effective (>70% decrease in nausea). Also, can use/add other antihistamines, e.g. *dimenhydrinate* (Dramamine) 50–100 mg po/pr/IV q4–6h (not to exceed 400 mg/day, or 200 mg/day if also doxylamine).

If still n/v, add

Promethazine.   (Phenergan) 12.5–50 mg po/pr/IM q4–6h, 12.5–25 mg IV q4–6h in IV fluids, or

Prochlorperazine.   (Compazine) 10 mg po q6h, 25 mg pr q12h (derivative of Phenergan). Both are phenothiazines (antipsychotics, too). Side effects: $\downarrow$BP, sedation, Parkinson's tremors, rash, anticholinergic side effects, tardive dyskinesia)

and/or

Trimethobenzamide.   (Tigan) 200 mg pr/IM tid/qid, 250 mg po tid (dopamine antagonist directly to emetic center CTZ)

and/or

Metoclopramide.   (Reglan) 10–30 mg po qid and hs 30 minutes before meals, 5–10 mg IV/IM q8h (dopamine antagonist).

If above interventions or combination thereof not effective, add/substitute

Ondansetron.   (Zofran) 4–12 mg po q6–8h; 8–10 mg IV q8h – serotonin (5-hydroxytryptamine) 3 receptor antagonist. Side effects: headache, mild sedation. Safety data not large. At least as effective as Phenergan 50 mg q8h, but probably better.[35]

Other therapies.   There are also no trials of efficacy for scopolamine, droperidol/haloperidol (maternal risk of prolonged QT interval), and diphenhydramine (Benadryl) (25–50 mg IV/IM/po q6h as alternative for other antihistamine).

In general, **do *not* use steroids to treat HG or just n/v** of pregnancy, or use only as last resort for maximum of 3 days. Usual dosing: methylprednisolone 16 mg po/IV tid, or prednisolone 20 mg po bid. Safety data: possible increased incidence of oral cleft if used < 10 weeks. Significant maternal side effects. (Adrenocorticotropic hormone [ACTH] is not beneficial;[36] methylprednisolone is more effective than promethazine;[37] prednisone is not beneficial;[38] IV then po methylprednisolone is not better than placebo.[39])

Do *not* use diazepam, a category D drug, because of possible fetal effects, despite one trial on its efficacy.[40] One trial of **acupuncture** was as effective in treating nausea of pregnancy as a sham procedure,[41] but a larger trial showed that acupuncture is an **effective treatment** for women with n/v in pregnancy.[42]

Inpatient HG

(See outpatient guideline above as well.) Admit only if HG diagnosis is confirmed as above, woman is not tolerating oral intake, and failed outpatient management. Some suggest just brief emergency room (ER) visits for severe cases needing emergent hydration. Home infusion services should be used as much as safely possible. Admission by itself does not improve HG, and should be limited.

- Diet: nothing per mouth (NPO) at first; with improvement, advance to small dry meals (see above).
- IV fluids can be used if dehydration is present (no studies on best IV fluid). Add thiamine 100 mg qd for 2–3 days, then multivitamins to IV fluids.
- Can use combination antiemetic therapy as above.
- First IV/IM therapy around the clock, then IV only prn, then oral therapy when tolerated. Acupressure is not effective for inpatient treatment of HG.[43]
- If persistent weight loss or dehydration (e.g. over 5–7 days despite aggressive inpatient therapy), consider consulting gastroenterology, and either parenteral or enteral nutrition.

Parenteral nutrition

Several catheters and regimens are possible; individualize and consult nutrition. Generally, parenteral nutrition (PN) is associated with a high incidence of catheter complications, e.g. infection, leading to sepsis, thrombosis/occlusion, and dislodgement. Peripheral catheters have high morbidity, and central catheters have central access complications. Other complications include pneumothorax, cholestasis, preterm birth, fetal death. This is an expensive therapy.

Enteral nutrition: nasogastric tube

There are several types of nasogastric (NG) tubes (e.g. 8 Fr Dobbhoff).

- Mechanism: avoid contact/smell of food. This intervention is best used for persistent n/v, with no response to antiemetic therapy. There are no trials of comparison between PN or NG tube. Since PN is associated with several possible complications, consider NG tube first if tolerated.[5]
- Nutrition (Harris–Benedict equation):

  $655 + (9.6 \times$ wt [kg]$) + (1.8 \times$ ht [cm]$) - (4.7 -$ age [years]$)$

- Order enteric nutrition in consultation with nutrition service. Basal energy expenditure + 300 cal (pregnancy); divide by 24 h. Start at 25 ml/h, increase by 25 ml/h until goal. Then give over 8–12 hours overnight.[44]
- Complications: poorly tolerated by some women; NG tube occlusion.

Other issues

Consider psychiatric consult in severe, refractory-to-therapy cases. Psychotherapy has not been evaluated in any trial. Hypnosis decreased vomiting in one non-randomized study.[45] The woman can be discharged home on IV fluids and/or PN as long as stable, not losing weight, etc.

REFERENCES

1. Askling J, Erlandsson G, Kaijser M, Akre O, Ekbom A. Sickness in pregnancy and sex of child. Lancet 1999; 354: 2053. [II-3]
2. Lacroix R, Eason E, Melzack R. Nausea and vomiting during pregnancy: a prospective study of its frequency, intensity, and patterns of change. Am J Obstet Gynecol 2000; 182: 931–7. [II-3]
3. Frigo P, Lang C, Reisenberger K, Kolbl H, Hirschl AM. Hyperemesis gravidarum associated with *Helicobacter pylori* seropositivity. Obstet Gynecol 1998; 91: 615–17. [II-3]
4. El-Mallakh RS, Liebowitz NR, Hale MS. Hyperemesis gravidarum as conversion disorder. J Nerv Ment Dis 1990; 178: 655–9. [II-3]
5. American College of Obstetrics and Gynecology. Nausea and vomiting of pregnancy. ACOG Practice Bulletin 52. Obstet Gynecol 2004; 103: 803–15. [review]
6. Van Dinter MC. Ptyalism in pregnant women. JOGNN 1991; 20: 206–9. [review]
7. Jarnfelt-Samsioe A, Eriksson B, Waldenstrom J, Samsioe G. Some new aspects on emesis gravidarum. Relations to clinical data, serum electrolytes, total protein and creatinine. Gynecol Obstet Invest 1985; 19: 174–86.
8. Brent R. Medical, social, and legal implications of treating nausea and vomiting of pregnancy. Am J Obstet Gynecol 2002; 186: S262–6. [review]
9. Goodwin TM, Montoro M, Mestman JH. Transient hyperthyroidism and hyperemesis gravidarum: clinical aspects. Am J Obstet Gynecol 1992; 167: 648–52. [II-3]
10. Goodwin TM, Mestman J. Transient hyperthyroidism of hyperemesis gravidarum. Contemp Obstet Gynecol 1996; 116: 65–78. [II-3, and review]
11. Czeizel AE, Dudas I, Fritz G, et al. The effect of periconceptional multivitamin–mineral supplementation on vertigo, nausea and vomiting. Arch Gynecol Obstet 1992; 251: 181–5. [RCT, $n=48$]
12. Murphy PA. Alternative therapies for nausea and vomiting of pregnancy. Obstet Gynecol 1998; 91: 149–55. [meta-analysis: 10 RCTs, 7 RCTs on acupressure]
13. Dundee JW, Sourial FB, Ghaly RG, Bell PF. P6 acupressure reduces morning sickness. J Royal Soc Med 1988; 81(8): 456–7. [RCT]
14. Hyde E. Acupressure therapy for morning sickness. A controlled clinical trial. J Nurse Midwifery 1989; 34(4): 171–8. [RCT]
15. de Aloysio D, Penacchioni P. Morning sickness control in early pregnancy by Neiguan point acupressure. Obstet Gynecol 1992; 80(5): 852–4. [RCT]
16. Evans AT, Samuels SN, Marshall C, Bertolucci LE. Suppression of pregnancy-induced nausea and vomiting with sensory afferent stimulation. J Reprod Med 1993; 38: 603–6. [RCT, $n=23$]
17. Bayreuther J, Lewith GT, Pickering R. A double-blind cross-over study to evaluate the effectiveness of acupressure at pericardium 6 (P6) in the treatment of early morning sickness (EMS). Complem Ther Med 1994; 2: 70–6. [RCT, $n=23$]
18. Belluomini J, Litt RC, Lee KA, Katz M. Acupressure for nausea and vomiting of pregnancy: a randomized, blinded study. Obstet Gynecol 1994; 84(2): 245–8. [RCT]
19. O'Brien B, Relyea MJ, Taerum T. Efficacy of P6 acupressure in the treatment of nausea and vomiting during pregnancy. Am J Obstet Gynecol 1996; 174: 708–15. [RCT]
20. Werntoft E, Dykes AK. Effect of acupressure on nausea and vomiting during pregnancy. J Reprod Med 2001; 46: 835–9. [RCT, $n=60$]
21. Rosen T, de Veciana M, Miller HS, et al. A randomized controlled trial of nerve stimulation for relief of nausea and vomiting in pregnancy. Obstet Gynecol 2003; 102: 129–35. [RCT, $n=230$]
22. Fischer-Rasmussen W, Kjaer SK, Dahl C, Asping U. Ginger treatment of hyperemesis gravidarum. Eur J Obstet Gynecol Reprod Biol 1991; 38: 19–24. [RCT, $n=27$]
23. Vutyavanich T, Kraisarin T, Ruangsri R. Ginger for nausea and vomiting in pregnancy: randomized, double-masked, placebo-controlled trial. Obstet Gynecol 2001; 97: 577–82. [RCT, $n=70$]
24. Keating A, Chez RA. Ginger syrup as an antiemetic in early pregnancy. Altern Ther Health Med 2002; 8: 89–91. [RCT]
25. Willetts C, Ekanganki A, Eden JA. Effect of a ginger extract on pregnancy-induced nausea: a randomized trial. Austr NZ J Obstet Gynecol 2003; 43: 139–44. [RCT]
26. Sripramote M, Lekhyananda N. A randomized comparison of ginger and vitamin B_6 in the treatment of nausea and vomiting in pregnancy. J Med Assoc Thai 2003; 86: 846–53. [RCT, n=138]
27. Smith C, Crowther C, Willson K, Hotham N, McMillian V. A randomized controlled trial of ginger to treat nausea and vomiting in pregnancy. Obstet Gynecol 2004; 103: 639–45 [RCT, $n=291$]
28. Borrelli F, Capasso R, Aviello G, Pittler MH, Izzo AA. Effectiveness and safety of ginger in the treatment of pregnancy-induced nausea and vomiting. Obstet Gynecol 2005; 105: 849–56. [meta-analysis: 6 RCTs, $n=675$]
29. Sahakian V, Rouse D, Sipes S, Rose N, Niebyl N. Vitamin B_6 is effective therapy for nausea and vomiting of pregnancy: a randomized double-blind placebo-controlled study. Obstet Gynecol 1991; 78: 33. [RCT, $n=59$; vitamin B_6 25 mg orally q8h × 72 hours vs placebo]
30. Vutyavanich T, Wongtrangan S, Ruangsri RA. Pyridoxine for nausea and vomiting of pregnancy: a randomized, double-blind, placebo-controlled trial. Am J Obstet Gynecol 1995; 173: 881–4. [RCT, $n=342$; vitamin B_6 30 mg orally q8h vs placebo]

31. Geiger CJ, Fahrenbach DM, Healey FJ. Bendectin in the treatment of nausea and vomiting in pregnancy. Obstet Gynecol 1959; 14: 688–90. [RCT, *n*=110]
32. Wheatley D. Treatment of pregnancy sickness. Br J Obstet Gynecol 1977; 84: 444–7. [RCT, *n*=56]
33. McGuinness BW, Binns DT. 'Debendox' in pregnancy sickness. J R Coll Gen Pract 1971; 21: 500–3. [RCT, *n*=81]
34. Jewell D, Young G. Interventions for nausea and vomiting in early pregnancy. Cochrane Database Syst Rev 2007; 1. [meta-analysis: general reference]
35. Sullivan CA, Johnson CA, Roach H, et al. A pilot study of intravenous ondansetron for hyperemesis gravidarum. Am J Obstet Gynecol 1996; 174: 1565–8. [RCT, *n*=30; ondansetron 10 mg IV vs promethazine 50 mg IV, both q8h]
36. Ylikorkala O, Kauppila A, Ollanketo ML. Intramuscular ACTH or placebo in the treatment of hyperemesis gravidarum. Acta Obstet Gynecol Scand 1979; 58(5): 453–5. [RCT, *n* = 32]
37. Safari HR, Fassett MJ, Souter IC, Alsulyman OM, Goodwin TM. The efficacy of methylprednisolone in the treatment of hyperemesis gravidarum: a randomized, double-blind, controlled study. Am J Obstet Gynecol 1998; 179: 921–4. [RCT, *n*=40]
38. Nelson-Piercy C, Fayers P, de Swiet M. Randomised, double-blind, placebo-controlled trial of corticosteroids for the treatment of hyperemesis gravidarum. BJOG 2001; 108(1): 9–15. [RCT, *n*=24]
39. Yost NP, McIntire DD, Wians FH, et al. A randomized, placebo-controlled trial of corticosteroids for hyperemesis due to pregnancy. Obstet Gynecol 2003; 102: 1250–4. [RCT, *n*=126]
40. Ditto A, Morgante G, la Marca A, De Leo V. Evaluation of treatment of hyperemesis gravidarum using parenteral fluid with or without diazepam. A randomized study. Gynecol Obstet Invest 1999; 48(4): 232–6. [RCT, *n*=50]
41. Knight B, Mudge C, Openshaw S, et al. Effect of acupuncture on nausea of pregnancy: a randomized, controlled trial. Obstet Gynecol 2001; 97: 184–8. [RCT, *n*=55]
42. Smith C, Crowther C, Beilby J. Acupuncture to treat nausea and vomiting in early pregnancy: a randomized controlled trial. Birth 2002; 29: 1–9. [RCT, *n*=593]
43. Heazell A, Thornaycroft J, Walton V, Etherington I. Acupressure for the in-patient treatment of nausea and vomiting in early pregnancy: a randomized controlled trial. Am J Obstet Gynecol 2006; 194: 815–20. [RCT, *n*=80]
44. Hsu JJ, Clark-Glena R, Nelson DK, Kim CH. Nasogastric enteral feeding in the management of hyperemesis gravidarum. Obstet Gynecol 1996; 88: 343–6. [II-3]
45. Apfel RJ, Kelly SF, Frankel FH. The role of hypnotizability in the pathogenesis and treatment of nausea and vomiting of pregnancy. J Psychosom Obstet Gynecol 1986; 5: 179–86. [II-3]

9

Intrahepatic cholestasis of pregnancy

Vincenzo Berghella

KEY POINTS

- The diagnosis of intrahepatic cholestasis of pregnancy (ICP) is **pruritus** and **elevated serum bile acids.**
- A bile acid level of ≥ 40 mmol/L represents severe disease.
- **Complications of untreated, usually severe ICP** include spontaneous preterm birth, meconium, non-reassuring fetal heart rate tracing (NRFHT), fetal death, neonatal death, and postpartum hemorrhage. Fetal deaths occur mostly ≥ 37 weeks, and no perinatal deaths have occurred in recent series with treatment and delivery by 37–38 weeks.
- Ursodeoxycholic acid (UDCA) **is the current treatment of choice for cholestasis of pregnancy.**
- **Vitamin K** 10 mg once per day at onset of ICP or 34 weeks has been suggested for prevention of postpartum hemorrhage, but there is insufficient evidence for a strong recommendation.
- There are several reports of sudden fetal death within 24 hours of a reactive non-stress test (NST), and insufficient evidence for a recommended fetal testing protocol.
- Especially in severe cases, **delivery should occur by 37–38 weeks.**

HISTORIC NOTES

'Benign jaundice of pregnancy' is the old name for intrahepatic cholestasis of pregnancy, and should not be used anymore.

DIAGNOSIS/DEFINITION

Pruritus (100% of patients) **and elevated serum bile acids** (≥ 14 mmol/L in > 90%), in the absence of other liver disease, and which resolves after pregnancy. If bile acids are normal, some clinicians accept as diagnostic pruritus plus abnormal transaminases.[1] Other accepted names are gestational cholestasis or obstetric cholestasis.

SYMPTOMS

Pruritus is usually over the whole body, most severe on the palms and soles.

EPIDEMIOLOGY/INCIDENCE

Incidence is 0.01–0.5% in the USA; 5% Hispanics; 10% in Chile. ICP most commonly occurs in third trimester, rapidly resolves after delivery, and is associated with adverse pregnancy outcome.

GENETICS

It is found that 15–30% of ICP have a family history of intrahepatic cholestasis (IC), but most cases of ICP are not related to known mutations of familial IC.

ETIOLOGY/BASIC PATHOPHYSIOLOGY

The metabolic demands of pregnancy stress the liver and exceed the capacity for cholesterol metabolism in susceptible individuals. Bile acids such as glycocholic acid and taurocholic acid increase in serum and cause the symptom of itching.[2]

CLASSIFICATION

A bile acid level of ≥ 40 mmol/L represents severe disease, which constitutes about 20% of cases of ICP. Complications occur mainly with severe ICP.[3]

RISK FACTORS/ASSOCIATIONS

Associated with family history of IC, multiple pregnancies, winter season, and selenium deficiency.

COMPLICATIONS

Complications without treatment (especially of severe ICP) are spontaneous preterm birth (SPTB) 15%, meconium 45%, non-reassuring fetal heart rate testing (NRFHT) 5–15%, fetal death 2–10%, neonatal death 1–2%, and postpartum hemorrhage 20–22%. SPTB occurs mostly at 32–36 weeks, as for other SPTB. Fetal deaths occur mostly ≥ 37 weeks.[4] Etiology of fetal deaths is unclear, but taurocholate is toxic to cardiomyocytes.[5] Complications occur almost only in severe cases. No perinatal deaths have occurred in recent series with treatment and delivery by 37–38 weeks.[1,6]

PREGNANCY CONSIDERATIONS

Up to 50% of women recall pruritus during pregnancy, but few have elevated bile acids. Bile acids may be normal at first, and increase later (usually increase an average of 3 weeks after the symptoms of pruritus); 80–86% of ICP diagnoses are made after 30 weeks.

PREGNANCY MANAGEMENT
Principles

Severe ICP is associated with perinatal complications, so that the largest series has proposed no intervention for milder cases (i.e. bile acids < 40 mmol/L).[3]

Work-up

- **Bile acids:** repeat serially if initially negative and high clinical suspicion.
- **Transaminases:** aspartate aminotransferase (AST) and alanine aminotransferase (ALT) are elevated 60% of times.
- Gamma-glutamyltransferase (GGT) (is elevated 30% of times).
- Consider checking right upper quadrant ultrasound (10% have cholelithiasis).
- Urine culture.
- Other hepatic work-up, including hepatitis A, B, and C.

Management
Prevention

No preventive measures have been proposed.

Therapy

There is limited evidence to assess the effect of different treatments for cholestasis of pregnancy. The two therapies best studied are ursodeoxycholic acid (UDCA) and S-adenosyl-L-methionine (SAMe).

Ursodeoxycholic acid (UDCA; ursodiol)
Mechanism of action. Hydrophilic bile acid which inhibits intestinal absorption of other bile acids, enhances excretory hepatocyte function and choleretic activity, stabilizing the hepatocyte cell membrane and diluting the more toxic bile acids in the enterohepatic circulation.[6] It may also allow for transport of bile acids out of the fetal compartment.

Dose. 10–25 mg/kg divided in 2 doses daily. Usually start at 300–450 bid.

Side effects. Diarrhea.

Effectiveness. Compared with placebo, UDCA is associated with a minimal decrease in pruritus, **greater reductions in bile salts and liver enzymes, fewer preterm births,** and no difference in incidence of NRFHT.[7] The outcome of fetal death is generally uncommon, but indirect evidence correlates lower bile acids with less fetal deaths and other complications. **Compared with SAMe, UDCA has a similar effect on pruritus, a significantly greater reduction of bile acids and transaminases, with non-statistically lower incidences of preterm birth, meconium, and admission to ICN.** [6,7] Compared with dexamethasone, UDCA is associated with a greater reduction in bile acids and liver enzymes, with improvement in pruritus only in women with severe ICP.[8]

S-adenosyl-L-methionine (SAMe)
Mechanism of action. SAMe has similar mechanism of action and side effects as UDCA.

Dose. 500 mg orally twice per day.

Effectiveness
Compared with placebo, only one trial showed significantly **greater improvements in pruritus, bile salts, and liver enzymes** with SAMe.[7]

Other trials

Guar gum
Compared with placebo, there are no differences in pruritus, bile salts, or fetal/neonatal outcomes observed.[7]

Activated charcoal
Compared with no treatment, the reduction in bile salts was greater with charcoal, but there was no difference in pruritus relief, or fetal/neonatal outcomes.[7]

UDCA and SAMe
Compared with placebo or UDCA alone, UDCA and SAMe resulted in greater improvements in pruritus, bile salts, and selected liver function assays in a small trial; UDCA and SAMe vs SAMe resulted in greater improvements in bile salts and ALT only.[7]

Conclusion

Given the above results, and the greater experience with UDCA, **UDCA is the current treatment of choice for cholestasis of pregnancy.** No treatments were found to be unsafe. No study had enough data to properly assess the effect on fetal/neonatal outcomes.

Other treatment

Given the low effect of UDCA or SAMe on itching, other antipruritic therapy may be required.

Vitamin K

10 mg once per day at onset of ICP or 34 weeks has been suggested for prevention of postpartum hemorrhage, but there is insufficient evidence for a strong recommendation.

Antepartum testing

No study specifically addresses fetal surveillance and its frequency in ICP. Kick counts daily, and non-stress tests (NSTs) once/week starting at diagnosis (usually on or after 32 weeks) have been proposed, but **there are several reports of sudden fetal death within 24 hours of a reactive NST.**

Delivery

Especially in severe cases (bile acid level of ≥ 40 mmol/L), **consider delivery by 37–38 weeks.**[3,6,7] The pregnancy can be delivered earlier if amniocentesis is positive for fetal lung maturity (FLM) or meconium. Women with mild (< 40 μmol/L) ICP can probably be managed expectantly.[3]

REFERENCES

1. Kenyon AP, Piercy CN, Girling J, et al. Obstetric cholestasis, outcome with active management: a series of 70 cases. BJOG 2002; 109: 282–8. [II-3]
2. Traunder M, Meier PJ, Boyer JL. Molecular pathogenesis of cholestasis. N Engl J Med 1998; 339: 1217–27. [review; non-pregnant]
3. Glantz A, Marschall HU, Mattsson LA. Intrahepatic cholestasis of pregnancy: relationships between bile acid levels and fetal complication rates. Hepatology 2004; 40(2): 467–74. [II-3, n = 693 – largest series]
4. Williamson C, Hems LM, Goulis DG, et al. Clinical outcome in a series of cases of obstetric cholestasis identified via a patient support group. BJOG 2004; 111(7): 676–81. [II-3, n = 352]
5. Gorelik J, Shevchuk A, de Swiet M, et al. Comparison of the arrhythmogenic effects of tauro- and glycoconjugates of cholic acid in an in vitro study of rat cardiomyocytes. BJOG 2004; 111(8): 867–70. [II-2]
6. Roncaglia N, Locatelli A, Arreghini A, et al. A randomized controlled trial of ursodeoxycholic acid and S-adenosyl-L-methionine in the treatment of gestational cholestasis. BJOG 2004; 111: 17–21. [RCT, n = 46]
7. Burrows RF, Clavisi O, Burrows E. Interventions for treating cholestasis in pregnancy. Cochrane Database Syst Rev 2005; 4. [meta-analysis: 9 RCTs, n = 227. UDCA vs placebo: 3 RCTs, n = 56. UDCA vs SAMe: 3 RCTs, n = 82. SAMe vs placebo: 4 RCTs, n = 82. Guar gum: 1 RCT, n = 48. Activated charcoal: 1 RCT, n = 20. UDCA + SAMe vs placebo, UDCA or SAMe: 1 RCT, n = 32 (8/group). Sample sizes of individual studies were small, the largest study included 48 women and five of the nine studies included 20 women or fewer]
8. Glantz A, Marschall HU, Lammert F, Mattsson LA. Intrahepatic cholestasis of pregnancy: a randomized controlled trial comparing dexamethasone and ursodeoxycholic acid. Hepatology 2005; 2(6): 1399–405. [RCT, n = 130]

10

Pregnancy after liver transplantation

Fabrizio di Francesco, Cataldo Doria, and Ignazio R Marino

KEY POINTS

- Pregnancy does not alter hepatic allograph function.
- The best candidates for pregnancy after liver transplantation are patients in good general health ≥ 1 year after transplant, with no or minimal proteinuria (< 1 g/24 hours), and creatinine < 1.3 mg/dl, with no or well-controlled hypertension, no evidence of recent graft rejection, and stable immunosuppression regimen and liver function.

HISTORIC NOTES

The first human liver transplant was performed in 1963 by Thomas Starzl (University of Colorado).[1] Through the years, great improvements have been made in the field, owing to a better understanding of the tissue compatibility and organ storage, the immune system, earlier detection and treatment of rejection, and better prevention and management of infections. As a result, among liver transplant recipients, a higher survival rate and a return to a good quality of life have been achieved. The first known post-transplantation pregnancy in a liver transplant recipient was reported in 1978.[2]

In 1991, the National Transplantation Pregnancy Registry (NTPR) was established at Thomas Jefferson University Hospital in Philadelphia with the aim of collecting and analyzing data about pregnancy and delivery in graft recipients.

DIAGNOSIS/DEFINITION

Orthotopic liver transplantation (OLTx) is the treatment of choice for all non-neoplastic end-stage liver diseases and for selected patients with non-resectable hepatic malignancies.

End-stage liver disease (ESLD) is any hepatic disease that jeopardizes the survival or that seriously modifies the quality of life of the patient, and for which the transplant is the only therapy, since no other medical or surgical treatment exists that is able to provide a reasonable chance of recovery.

SYMPTOMS

Before undergoing OLTx some patients remain in quite good clinical condition. There may be huge individual differences in terms of hospital care requirements. As the liver disease progresses, symptoms such as encephalopathy, weakness, and lethargy become more frequent. Intractable ascites, peripheral edema, anorexia, jaundice, pruritus and cholestasis, peritonitis and pneumonia may also develop. Often there is a severely depleted nutritional state.

INDICATIONS

The main indications for OLTx are reported in Table 10.1. Although chronic hepatitis C virus infection represents the leading indication for OLTx in the USA, autoimmune hepatitis is probably the most frequent reason for transplantation among recipients who become pregnant afterwards. The reason is based on the fact that autoimmune hepatitis is a more common indication for transplantation in younger reproductive-age patients.[3,4]

EPIDEMIOLOGY/INCIDENCE

Approximately one-third of all patients who have undergone OLTx are women, and about 75% of female recipients are of reproductive age.[3]

BASIC PATHOPHYSIOLOGY

Patients with end-organ failure experience hypothalamic–pituitary–gonadal dysfunction and decreased ovulation or sperm maturation.[5] Amenorrhea or menstrual abnormalities with decreased fertility occur in up to 50% of women with chronic liver disease.[4,6] A successful transplant almost uniformly leads to a prompt return to normal menstrual cycles and to reproductive functions due to the recovery of gonadotropic function.[7,8] This is an important component on

Table 10.1 *Main indications for liver transplant*
Acute liver failure
Post-inflammatory cirrhosis
Post-alcoholic cirrhosis
Primary biliary cirrhosis
Secondary biliary cirrhosis
Primary sclerosing cholangitis
Autoimmune cirrhosis
Cirrhosis of unknown etiology
Inborn errors of metabolism
Biliary atresia
Congenital hepatic fibrosis
Cystic fibrosis
Budd–Chiari syndrome
Hepatic cysts
Hepatic trauma
Benign tumors
Primary malignant tumors

the restoration of normality of life for patients who are still in childbearing age, and it is evidenced by the increasing number of post-transplantation pregnancies reported worldwide.[9]

PRECONCEPTION COUNSELING

It is universally recognized that, although pregnancy in graft recipients seems to be well tolerated and associated with a good outcome, it must be considered high risk, requiring close surveillance by a coordinated team.[6] Therefore, since a return to fertility is the rule after OLTx, gynecologists and a transplant team should extensively counsel reproductive-age transplant patients before and after transplantation, and appropriate contraceptive plans should be recommended. For patients wishing to avoid pregnancy, there are limited data on appropriate contraception following transplantation. Barrier methods are preferred. Oral contraceptives are relatively contraindicated because of many theoretical complications such as the risk of thromboembolism, cholestasis, exacerbated hypertension, and interference in cyclosporine metabolism. While intrauterine devices may initially minimally increase the risks of infection, especially in immunocompromised women,[5] their use is probably safe and recommended.

Ideally, patients should be vaccinated prior to transplantation against influenza, pneumococcus, hepatitis B, and tetanus. Alternatively, they should be vaccinated prepregnancy (see also Chapter 37).

TIMING OF PREGNANCY

The shortest interval from OLTx to conception reported in the literature is 3 weeks.[10] Several authors recommend **waiting at least 1–2 years after OLTx**, based on rejection risks, and to allow stabilization of allograft function and of immunosuppressive regimen. However, the current opinion is that the advice to wait 2 years after a successful transplant may be too restrictive, because the new immunosuppressive strategies have decreased rejection rates in the first post-transplant year.

When choosing the timing of pregnancy after OLTx, several individual factors should be considered. These are detailed below.

1. *Good general health ≥ 1 year following transplant:*
   - risk of acute graft rejection
   - risk of acute infection that might impact the fetus (cytomegalovirus [CMV] acute infection is most common within 6–12 months post transplant).
2. *Proteinuria and creatinine level:*
   - no or minimal proteinuria ($< 1\,g/24$ hours)
   - creatinine $< 1.3\,mg/dl$.
3. *Rejection and immunosuppression:*
   - no evidence of recent graft rejection (in the past year)
   - stable immunosuppression regimen (stable dosing).
4. *Stable liver function:*
   - patients with stable liver function have a low risk for opportunistic infections.
5. *Maternal age.*
6. *Medical non-compliance.*

COMORBIDITIES/RISK FACTORS

In the presence of stable allograft and renal function, pregnancies following OLTx are generally well tolerated with a good maternal and neonatal outcome.

However, several comorbidity factors may influence pregnancy outcomes.

Etiology of original disease

Recurrent liver disease, especially viral hepatitis, appears to be one of the most serious risks for both mother and child.

Vertical transmission occurs in 10–20% of hepatitis B surface antigen (HBsAg)-positive (hepatitis B e antigen [HB$_e$Ag]-negative) non-transplant mothers without immunoprophylaxis. For prevention of vertical transmission, all neonates, born to women with HBsAg positive, should receive immunoprophylaxis (HBIg) and HB vaccine within 12 hours of birth. This combination prevents > 90% of neonatal hepatitis B virus (HBV) infection.[11] Therefore, the incidence of vertical transmission to the child of HBV carriers who underwent OLTx presumptively could be quite similar.

Also, the rate of maternal–fetal hepatitis C (HCV) transmission in OLTx recipients is unclear, requiring additional analysis. The vertical infection rate in pregnant HCV RNA positive subjects is around 3–5% (in the absence of other viral co-infections).[12] A well-documented risk factor for HCV vertical transmission is maternal high viral load. Therefore, special attention should be given to patients with high viral load post-transplant (see also Chapters 29 and 30).

Hypertension

Often in the post-transplantation population there is an increased incidence of hypertension and renal insufficiency caused by cyclosporine and, in smaller measure, by tacrolimus. In fact, it is known that both immunosuppressive regimens can induce endothelial cell dysfunction and decrease endogenous nitric oxide production, causing renal dysfunction and hypertension. This could explain the increased incidence of pre-eclampsia among pregnant women after OLTx.[4,6]

Mild renal insufficiency or hypertension can be well controlled with the same treatment (calcium channel blocker) used in the non-transplant population.[13]

Diabetes

New-onset diabetes mellitus (NODM) develops in approximately 15% of liver transplant recipients and a similar proportion of patients have diabetes prior to transplantation.[14]

Pre-existing diabetes and probably NODM are associated with increased mortality and risk of infection. Controversial data exist concerning the impact of immunosuppressive therapy on the development of post-transplantation diabetes mellitus. Corticosteroid exposure should be limited as much as possible. Reduction of calcineurin inhibitor dose is advised. The management of NODM is essentially similar to that of diabetes in the non-transplant population. Numerous studies have established a direct relationship between maternal glycemic control and neonatal outcomes for all types of diabetes. Evidence indicates that intrauterine exposure to type 1 and 2 diabetes increases the risk of obesity, insulin resistance, insulin secretory defect, and subsequent development of type 2 diabetes in the offspring. Early diagnosis, patient education, proper follow-up, and postpartum testing will certainly decrease poor perinatal outcomes, enabling also a secondary prevention of type 2 diabetes in the long term. Modern treatment protocols during pregnancy emphasize strict glycemic control by a combination of diet and medication. Traditionally, insulin therapy has been considered the gold standard for management of diabetes, because of its efficacy in achieving tight glucose control and the fact that it does not cross the placenta[15] (see Chapter 4).

Cytomegalovirus acute infection

CMV acute infection is the most common type of infection within 6–12 months post transplant. It is particularly dangerous in early pregnancy. CMV infection is a causative agent of congenital malformation (microcephaly, cerebral palsy, sensorineural deafness) or congenital liver disease. Such abnormalities are seen in approximately 10–15% of infected pregnancies. CMV infection is the leading cause of neonatal death in post-OLTx pregnancy series. The use of antiviral agents in the management of CMV infection during pregnancy is still controversial[6] (see also Chapter 41).

Rejection

Most reported cases of graft rejection occur during the earlier phase of pregnancy. If the transplanted organ is functioning well before the recipient becomes pregnant, there does not seem to be a greater risk of rejection during pregnancy. It is universally recognized that inappropriate reduction of the immunosuppression therapy during pregnancy leads to rejection of the transplanted organ. The reported incidence of biopsy-proven acute rejection in pregnancy is about 10%.[6] When acute rejection is suspected, percutaneous liver biopsy is not contraindicated in pregnant patients, although ultrasound visualization is recommended to reduce the risk of complications. Evaluation of rejection includes liver Doppler ultrasound to exclude an anatomic source of graft dysfunction. Although rejection is a concern, it can be successfully managed with adjustment of immunosuppressive medications. For more serious cases the use of steroids as antirejection therapy is safe. On the other hand, safety of antilymphocyte globulins and rituximab is still unknown. There have been some reports of lower birth weights and premature births in mothers who had experienced rejection during pregnancy.

Infrarenal aortic graft

Particular attention should be paid to patients with infra-aortic grafts for hepatic arterial flow. One death as a result of clotting of the aortic graft by external compression from the gravid uterus has been reported.[13] Therefore, patients with infra-aortic graft should be monitored with color Doppler ultrasonography during pregnancy.

PREGNANCY COMPLICATIONS

Pregnancy does not seem to deteriorate allograft function in OLTx recipients.

Although pregnancies in liver-transplanted women are generally associated with good outcomes, they are considered high risk due to the higher rate of complications, requiring close surveillance by transplant clinicians, gynecologists, and obstetricians.

Pregnancy complications include the following conditions.

Table 10.2 *Immunosuppressive agents and their side effects*	
Immunosuppressant	Side effect
Prednisone[a]	Glucose intolerance
Azathioprine[a]	Leukopenia
Cyclosporine[ab]	Hypertension, nephrotoxicity
Tacrolimus[ab]	Hypertension, nephrotoxicity, neurotoxicity, glucose intolerance, myocardial hypertrophy
Mycophenolate mofetil	Gastrointestinal disturbance; animal studies raise concern regarding potential for human teratogenicity

[a]These have no known teratogenic effects.
[b]Follow with blood levels.

Preterm birth and low birth weight

Children born to female transplant recipients are more likely to be premature and/or small for gestational age. The risk of prematurity is up to 50% and the mean gestational age at delivery ranges between 36 and 37 weeks.[4–6,9] The consequences of decreased gestational age at delivery, particularly under 34 weeks' gestation, may include neonatal morbidity, mortality, and long-term morbidities. (See Chapter 15 in *Obstetric Evidence Based Guidelines*.)

Intrauterine growth restriction

The risk of intrauterine growth restriction (IUGR) is around 20%. IUGR is associated with perinatal morbidity and mortality, with long-term health implications. The management of IUGR is to achieve the delivery of the newborn in the best-possible condition, balancing the risks of prematurity against those of continued intrauterine existence. (See Chapter 39.)

Pre-eclampsia

Hypertension and occurrence of pre-eclampsia are more common in OLTx recipients, with an incidence of 20%. These complications are more common in patients taking cyclosporine, probably because of the related endothelial cell dysfunction, and are less common with tacrolimus.[3,4,6,13] The management of pre-eclampsia is the same as in the non-transplant population. (See Chapter 1.)

Blood chemistry tests and liver function

Pruritus and cholestasis occur frequently. Elevated alkaline phosphatase levels are found in approximately 35% of normal pregnancies after OLTx. Graft rejection needs to be considered in all cases and differentiated from other conditions. Hemolysis, elevated liver enzymes, low platelet count (HELLP) syndrome and anemia have been reported.[4]

IMMUNOSUPPRESSIVE AGENTS COMMONLY USED AND THEIR POTENTIAL SIDE EFFECTS (TABLE 10.2)

The potential risks of the exposure of infants to immunosuppressive medications are not very well known. Presumably these medications may interfere with fetal thymic development. Also, the teratogenic effects are not very clear. Tacrolimus is the most common and effective of these agents.

WORK-UP

Close surveillance by the maternal–fetal medicine and liver transplant teams is recommended.

- Baseline laboratory tests should include the following:
  a. bilirubin, creatinine
  b. liver function test
  c. cyclosporine/tacrolimus levels
  d. 24-hour urinary protein and creatinine clearance
  e. urine analysis and urine culture
  f. CMV, HSV (herpes simplex virus), and Toxoplasmosis immunoglobulins IgM and IgG; HBsAg, HBsAb, HepCAb.
  Repeat lab testing (a–e) will occur at a minimum of once every trimester until 32 weeks. After 32 weeks, obtain labs (a–d) every other week or as needed.
  Elevations of liver function tests and/or bilirubin could be indicative of rejection (<10% incidence in pregnancy).

Evaluation of rejection includes liver ultrasound with Doppler to exclude anatomic sources of graft dysfunction. Liver biopsy to diagnose rejection is not contraindicated in pregnancy.

- Because of an increased risk of carbohydrate intolerance caused by the administration of prednisone or tacrolimus, patients should be screened with glucose tolerance tests in the first trimester, followed by routine screening between 24 and 28 weeks. There are several drugs that interact with cyclosporine (Table 15.4 in Chapter 15).

ANTEPARTUM TESTING

A dating **ultrasound** will be performed in the first trimester. A detailed anatomy ultrasound will be performed in the second trimester. During the third trimester, assessment of fetal growth will be accomplished with serial (as needed) ultrasound examinations.

Weekly non-stress tests will begin at 32 weeks, unless medical or obstetric complications indicate earlier testing.

LABOR AND DELIVERY ISSUES

Patients who have received steroids during the antepartum period should receive 'stress dose' steroids (i.e. hydrocortisone 100 mg IV every 8 hours × 24 hours). Cesarean delivery should be performed only for obstetric indications.

BREASTFEEDING

In general, not enough data are available to make a formal recommendation. However, breastfeeding is contraindicated in patients on cyclosporine.

REFERENCES

1. Starzl TE, Marchioro TL, Von Kaulla KN, et al. Homotransplantation of the liver in humans. Surg Gynecol Obstet 1963; 117: 659–76. [II-3]
2. Walcott WO, Derick DE, Jolley JJ, et al. Successful pregnancy in a liver transplant patient. Am J Obstet Gynecol 1978; 132(3): 340–1. [II-3]
3. Jabiry-Zieniewicz Z, Cyganek A, Luterek K, et al. Pregnancy and delivery after liver transplantation. Transplant Proc 2005; 37(2): 1197–200. [II-2]
4. Nagy S, Bush MC, Berkowitz R, et al. Pregnancy outcome in liver transplant recipients. Obstet Gynecol 2003; 102(1): 121–8. [II-2]
5. McKay DB, Josephson MA, Armenti VT, et al. Reproduction and transplantation: report on the AST Consensus Conference on Reproductive Issues and Transplantation. Am J Transplant 2005; 5(7): 1592–9. [review]
6. Armenti VT, Herrine SK, Radomski JS, et al. Pregnancy after liver transplantation. Liver Transpl 2000; 6(6): 671–85. [II-2]
7. Cundy TF, O'Grady JG, Williams R. Recovery of menstruation and pregnancy after liver transplantation. Gut 1990; 31(3): 337–8. [II-3]
8. Parolin MB, Rabinovitch I, Urbanetz AA, et al. Impact of successful liver transplantation on reproductive function and sexuality in women with advanced liver disease. Transplant Proc 2004; 36(4): 943–4. [II-3]
9. Armenti VT, Radomski JS, Moritz MJ, et al. Report from the National Transplantation Pregnancy Registry (NTPR): outcomes of pregnancy after transplantation. Clin Transpl 2004; 103–14. [II-2]
10. Laifer SA, Darby MJ, Scantlebury VP, et al. Pregnancy and liver transplantation. Obstet Gynecol 1990; 76(6): 1083–8. [II-2]
11. Lai CL, Ratziu V, Yuen MF, et al. Viral hepatitis B. Lancet 2003; 362: 2089–94. [review]
12. Ferrero S, Lungaro P, Bruzzone BM, et al. Prospective study of mother-to-infant transmission of hepatitis C virus: a 10-year survey (1990–2000). Acta Obstet Gynecol Scand 2003; 82(3): 229–34. [II-2]
13. Jain AB, Reyes J, Marcos A, et al. Pregnancy after liver transplantation with tacrolimus immunosuppression: a single center's experience update at 13 years. Transplantation 2003; 76(5): 827–32. [II-2]
14. Marchetti P. New-onset diabetes after liver transplantation: from pathogenesis to management. Liver Transpl 2005; 11(6): 612–20. [review]
15. Homko CJ, Sivan E, Reece AE. Is there a role for oral antihyperglycemics in gestational diabetes and type 2 diabetes during pregnancy? Treat Endocrinol 2004; 3(3): 133–9. [review]

11

Maternal anemia

Karen Feisullin

KEY POINTS

- Anemia in pregnancy is defined as a **hemoglobin** level (Hgb) < **11 g/dl**.
- The most **common cause** of maternal anemia is **iron deficiency**.
- **All pregnant women** should have an **Hgb** and mean corpuscular volume (**MCV**) evaluated.
- **All** individuals of **African ancestry** should have a **hemoglobin electrophoresis**.
- **Work-up** of anemia in pregnancy is described in **Figure 11.4**. MCV, **ferritin** level, and **hemoglobin electrophoresis** are key laboratory tests.
- Iron-deficiency anemia:

  - **Iron and folate supplementation** before or in pregnancy **prevent low hemoglobin at birth or at 6 weeks postpartum.** There is insufficient long-term and outcome data, but the largest trial reported **decreased perinatal mortality** with selective iron supplementation (compared with routine).
  - **Therapy** of iron-deficiency anemia with oral iron treatment in pregnancy is associated with a **reduction in the number of women with hemoglobin** concentration < **11 g/dl** and a **greater mean hemoglobin level**, but again there are **insufficient data on clinically relevant outcomes.** Compared with standard oral preparations, **controlled-release iron preparations are associated with a diminished frequency of constipation.**

For sickle cell disease, see Chapter 12; for von Willebrand disease, see Chapter 13; for care of the Jehovah's Witness pregnant woman, see Chapter 14.

DEFINITION

Hemoglobin (Hgb) < 11 g/dl. Other clinicians have defined it as Hgb < 10.5 g/dl.

SYMPTOMS

Women are usually asymptomatic, unless hemoglobin < 6–7 g/dl.

INCIDENCE

Incidence depends on etiology of anemia. Iron deficiency anemia occurs in > 20–30% of women, even in developed countries if iron supplementation is not provided.

GENETICS

See below and Figures 11.1–11.3 and Table 11.1 for thalassemias. *Cis* α-thalassemia is more common in Southeast Asian ancestry; β-thalassemia is more common in women of Mediterranean, Asian, Middle Eastern, Hispanic, and West Indian ancestry.[1] Ethnicity is not a good predictor of risk, as ethnic background is often mixed and many individuals marry outside their ethnic group.

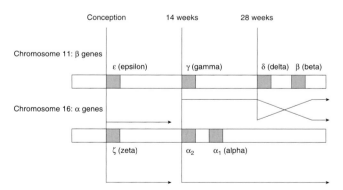

Figure 11.1
Developmental sequence of hemoglobin chains.

α-thalassemia silent carrier (asymptomatic)	α α / α −
	(heterozygous α$^+$-thalassemia)
α-thalassemia trait (mild anemia)	α − / α − (*trans*)
	(homozygous α$^+$-thalassemia)
	or
	− − / α α (*cis*)
	(heterozygous α^0-thalassemia)
α-thalassemia major (Hgb H disease)	α − / − −
(mostly Hgb H hemolytic anemia)	(α$^+$-thalassemia/ α^0-thalassemia)
Hydrops fetalis	− − / − −
(80% Hgb Bart's/20% Hgb H)	(homozygous α^0-thalassemia)

Figure 11.2
Types of α-thalassemias. Because there are two α chains on each chromosome 16, the possibility exists for four different disease states (unlike β-thalassemias, where only two disease states are found).

β^0: absence of β-chain production → causes more severe anemia		
β$^+$: decrease in β-chain production → causes milder anemia		
β-thalassemia trait: one β chain affected	β / β^0	may be o or +
Cooley's anemia: both β chains affected	β^0 / β^0	may be o or +

Figure 11.3
Types of β thalassemias.

ETIOLOGY/PATHOPHYSIOLOGY

The most common cause of maternal anemia is iron deficiency. Some degree of iron deficiency (i.e. Hgb 11–12 g/dl) is physiologic in pregnancy: the red blood cell (RBC) mass and plasma both increase, but the plasma increase (40–60%) is much more than the RBC increase (15–30%), causing a lowering of the Hgb level (see Chapter 2 of *Obstetric Evidence Based Guidelines*). Etiology of other causes of anemia depends on diagnosis. See below, and Figures 11.1–11.3 and Table 11.1 for thalassemias.

RISK FACTORS

For iron-deficiency anemia: multiple gestations, low socio-economic status, malnutrition, history of heavy menses, short interconception period, etc.

COMPLICATIONS

For iron-deficiency anemia: preterm birth (PTB), low birth weight, possible need for transfusion, etc.

Table 11.1	*Types of hemoglobins*		
Abbreviations	Composition		Description
Hgb A$_1$	2 α chains	2 β chains	Major adult hemoglobin
Hgb A$_2$	2 α chains	2 δ chains	Minor adult hemoglobin
Hgb F	2 α chains	2 γ chains	Fetal hemoglobin
Hgb H	−	4 β chains	α-thalassemia major (−/−α)
Hgb Barts	−	4 γ chains	Hydrops fetalis (−/−)
Hgb Gower	2 ε chains	2 ζ chains	Embryonic hemoglobin

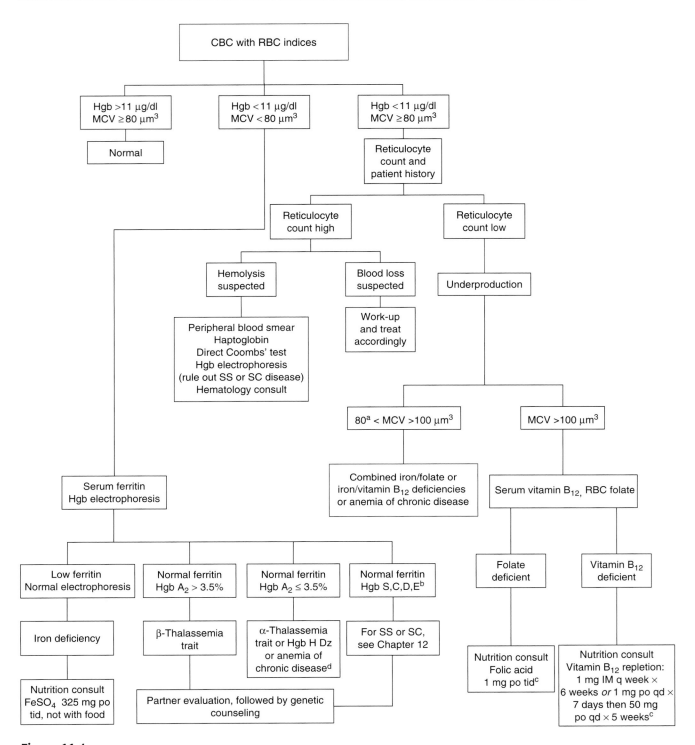

Figure 11.4
Work-up for maternal anemia – algorithm. CBC, complete blood count; RBC, red blood cells; MCV, mean corpuscular volume; Hgb, hemoglobin; SS and SC anemia (sickle cell disease); RDW, red cell distribution width; Dz, disease.

[a] MCV > 80 μm^3 does not rule out α-thalassemia silent carriers ($\alpha\alpha$ / α –). Microcytic anemia: low RDW $\rightarrow$ thalassemia; high RDW $\rightarrow$ iron deficiency.
[b] Hemoglobins S, C, D, and E are β-chain variants caused by different mutations.
[c] Should see reticulocyte response within 3–10 days of therapy.
[d] DNA testing for α hemoglobin chain is available and should be offered to couples of Southeast Asian ancestry.

Table 11.2 *Laboratory reference ranges*

Ferritin 20–150 ng/ml

Folate 3–18 ng/ml

Vitamin B$_{12}$ (cobalamin) 250–1200 pg/ml

Mean corpuscular volume (MCV) 80–100 μm^3

Normal hemoglobin electrophoresis

    Hgb A$_1$ > 95%

    Hgb A$_2$ ≤ 3.5%

    Hgb F < 1%

MANAGEMENT

Work-up

(See Figure 11.4 and Table 11.2.)

- Initial evaluation: complete blood count (CBC) with indices (**hemoglobin [Hgb]** and **mean corpuscular volume [MCV]**). These two indices should be **checked** in **all pregnant women**:

  - If Hgb < 11 g/dl and MCV < 80 μm^3: obtain Hgb electrophoresis and serum ferritin, follow algorithm.
  - If Hgb < 11 g/dl and MCV ≥ 80 μm^3: check reticulocyte count to determine if anemia is secondary to underproduction or hemolysis and obtain a history to identify any evidence of active bleeding, chronic disease, glucose-6-phosphate dehydrogenase (G6PD) deficiency, or a family history of RBC disorders if high reticulocyte count (≥ 3% RBC), then anemia is secondary to hemolysis or blood loss. Consider: (1) peripheral blood smear and haptoglobin (decreased); (2) direct Coombs test (suggests autoimmune hemolytic anemia); (3) Hgb electrophoresis to rule out SS or SC anemia (sickle cell disease); and (4) hemoccult or other tests if other sources of blood loss are suggested by history.
  - If low reticulocyte count (< 3% RBC), then anemia is secondary to underproduction and should be evaluated according to the algorithm.

- **All** individuals of **African ancestry** should have a **hemoglobin electrophoresis**. Solubility testing is inadequate for screening since it fails to identify other important hemoglobinopathies.[1]
- Anemia of chronic disease is usually associated with normocytic anemia (about 20% are associated with microcytic anemia). Causes include chronic liver disease, thyroid disease, uremia, chronic infections, and malignancies. A reasonable work-up is liver function tests (LFTs), blood urea nitrogen (BUN), creatinine, thyroid-stimulating hormone (TSH), and any tests for malignancy or chronic infection indicated by patient history and risk factors. Also check serum iron, serum vitamin B$_{12}$, and RBC folate to rule out combined deficiencies.

- A nutrition consult should be obtained for patients with vitamin B$_{12}$, folate, and iron deficiencies.
- If documented results from a prior hemoglobin electrophoresis can be obtained, this test should not be repeated.
- A **genetic consult** should be obtained for all patients with inherited disorders. Attempt to obtain a blood sample for hemoglobin electrophoresis from the father of the baby prior to the genetic consult. DNA testing for α-globin abnormalities is available.

Prevention

Iron

There is no evidence to advise against a **policy of routine iron and folate supplementation in pregnancy**. Iron supplementation appears to **prevent low hemoglobin at birth and at 6 weeks postpartum**.[2,3] There is very little information on pregnancy outcomes for either mother or baby. Iron supplementation raised or maintained the serum ferritin above 10 mg/L. It resulted in a substantial reduction of women with a hemoglobin level below 10 or 10.5 g in late pregnancy. Iron supplementation, however, had no detectable effect on any substantive measures of either maternal or fetal outcome.[2,3]

In one trial, with the largest number of participants, selective supplementation was associated with an increased likelihood of cesarean section and postpartum blood transfusion, but a **lower perinatal mortality rate** (up to 7 days after birth) compared with routine supplementation.[2,4,5] There are few data derived from communities where iron deficiency is common and anemia is a serious health problem.

Folate

Compared with placebo or no supplementation, folate supplementation is associated with increased or maintained serum folate levels and red cell folate levels.[6] Folate supplementation is associated with a reduction in the proportion of women with low hemoglobin level in late pregnancy and megaloblastic erythropoiesis. Compared with placebo, folate supplementation is associated with similar incidences of pre-eclampsia, PTB, perinatal mortality, and a possible reduction in the incidence of low birth weight. Owing to limited data, there is **insufficient evidence** to assess if folate supplementation has any substantial effect on maternal or neonatal outcomes.[6]

Therapy

There is insufficient evidence on the criteria for treating iron-deficiency anemia in pregnancy, and on its effects, due to the shortage of good-quality trials. Compared with placebo, oral iron treatment in pregnancy is associated with a **reduction in the number of women with hemoglobin < 11 g/dl** and a **greater mean hemoglobin level**.[7] There are **no data on clinically relevant outcomes**. Side effects include nausea, vomiting, constipation, and abdominal cramps. These gastrointestinal side effects are more common with oral iron treatments than with other preparations. Compared with standard oral preparations, **controlled-release iron preparations are associated with a diminished frequency of constipation**.

When comparing different iron treatments, the **intravenous (IV) route** of administration was associated with an increased risk of venous thrombosis.[7] Two more recent trials have reported that IV iron sucrose (calculated as: weight before pregnancy (kg) × 110 g/L – actual hemoglobin [g/L] × 0.24 + 500 mg) treated iron-deficiency anemia and restored iron stores faster and more effectively than oral iron polymaltose complex (300 mg elemental iron) daily[8] or oral iron sulfate 240 mg daily,[9] without serious side effects but again with insufficient data on important maternal or perinatal outcomes.

There are insufficient data to assess the effects of other forms of prevention or therapy, including self-donation in pregnancy.

Antepartum testing

No specific precautions, except a growth ultrasound in the third trimester.

Delivery and anesthesia

No specific precautions, except for minimizing blood loss and availability of blood for possible transfusion.

Postpartum/breastfeeding

There is **insufficient evidence** to assess different therapies for postpartum anemia. When compared with iron therapy only, erythropoietin increased the likelihood of lactation at discharge from hospital in a very small trial.[10] There was no apparent effect on the need for blood transfusions, although the randomized controlled trials (RCTs) may have been of insufficient size to rule out important clinical differences. Hematological indices (hemoglobin and hemocrit) showed some increases when erythropoietin was compared with iron only, and iron and folate, but not when compared with placebo. An iron-rich diet has not been studied as an intervention. **Most clinical outcomes have not been studied**.[10]

Given that postpartum anemia is associated with several complications, including less ability to fully engage in childcare, household tasks, and exercise, as well as altered cognition, mood, and productivity, preventive measures for iron-deficiency postpartum anemia are recommended.[11]

REFERENCES

1. American College of Obstetrics and Gynecology. Hemoglobinopathies in pregnancy. ACOG Practice Bulletin No. 64, 2005. [review].
2. Mahomed K. Iron supplementation in pregnancy. Cochrane Database Syst Rev 2007; 1. [meta-analysis: 20 RCTs, $n => 6000$]
3. Mahomed K. Iron and folate supplementation in pregnancy. Cochrane Database Syst Rev 2007; 1. [meta-analysis: 8 RCTs, $n = 5449$]
4. Hemminki E, Rimpela U. A randomized comparison of routine vs selective iron supplementation during pregnancy. J Am Coll Nutr 1991; 10: 3–10. [RCT, $n = 2694$]
5. Hemminki E, Merilainen J. Long term follow-up of mothers and their infants in a randomized trial on iron prophylaxis during pregnancy. Am J Obstet Gynecol 1995; 173(1): 205–29. [RCT, $n = 2694$]
6. Mahomed K. Folate supplementation in pregnancy. Cochrane Database Syst Rev 2007; 1. [meta-analysis: 21 RCTs, $n => 3100$]
7. Cuervo LG, Mahomed K. Treatments for iron deficiency anaemia in pregnancy. Cochrane Database Syst Rev 2007; 1. [meta-analysis: 5 RCTs, $n = 1234$]
8. Al RA, Unlubilgin E, Kandemir O, et al. Intravenous versus oral iron for treatment of anemia in pregnancy: a randomized trial. Obstet Gynecol 2005; 106: 1335–40. [RCT, $n = 90$]
9. Bayoumeu F, Subiran-Buisset C, Baka N-E, et al. Iron therapy in iron deficiency anemia in pregnancy: intravenous route versus oral route. Am J Obstet Gynecol 2002; 186: 518–22. [RCT, $n = 50$]
10. Dodd J, Dare MR, Middleton P. Treatment for women with postpartum iron deficiency anaemia. Cochrane Database Syst Rev 2007; 1. [meta-analysis: 6 RCTs, $n = 411$]
11. Bodnar LM, Cogswell ME, McDonald T. Have we forgotten the significance of postpartum iron deficiency? Am J Obstet Gynecol 2005; 193: 36–44. [review]

12

Sickle cell disease

Jolene Seibel-Seamon

KEY POINTS

- **Sickle cell disease** is an **autosomal recessive** disease resulting from an alteration in the structure of hemoglobin, producing HbS. It is characterized by hemolysis and vaso-occlusive phenomena.
- The most severe forms are **HbSS** (**sickle cell anemia**), HbS-β⁰, and only some cases of HbSC.
- Diagnosis is made by **hemoglobin electrophoresis.**
- Complications may include pregnancy loss, fetal growth restriction (FGR), anemia, painful crises, urinary tract infection (UTI) and other infections, preterm birth (PTB), pre-eclampsia, acute chest syndrome (ACS), alloimmunization, antepartum admissions, postpartum infections, and maternal mortality.
- **Pneumococcal vaccine** is an important prevention intervention.
- **Painful crises** are managed with narcotics (preferably **morphine**) therapy, and intravenous (**IV**) **fluids**. Antibiotics should be added if the woman is febrile, has an infection, or has ACS; oxygen should be added if the woman has low oxygen saturation.
- Prophylactic blood transfusions are not beneficial. **Blood transfusions are indicated for symptomatic or orthostatic anemia, hemoglobin <6 g/dl or hematocrit <25%, acute stroke, ACS, or multiple organ failure.**
- In the 10% of sickle cell disease women with ACS, a chest X-ray is necessary. Antibiotics (usually cephalosporin and erythromycin), aimed at infectious pathogen(s) in the pulmonary tree, and bronchodilators are the mainstays of therapy.

HISTORIC NOTES

Sickle cell disease was first described in 1910 by Herrick. In 1949, Linus Pauling described the molecular structure of sickle cell hemoglobin by protein electrophoresis. In 1956, Ingram and Hunt discovered the single amino acid change in sickle cell hemoglobin.[1]

DEFINITION

Sickle cell disease is an inherited disorder resulting from an **alteration in the structure of hemoglobin, producing HbS.** It is characterized by **hemolysis and vaso-occlusive** phenomena. Sickle cell disease is associated with a mild to moderate chronic anemia. Sickle cell disease can occur with **hemoglobin SS (HbSS or sickle cell anemia)**, β-thalassemia (HbS/β⁰), hemoglobin C (HbSC disease), hereditary persistence of fetal hemoglobin (HbS/HPHP), and hemoglobin E (HbS/HbE). The clinical manifestations vary among these genotypes, with HbS/β⁰ usually having a similar severe phenotype to HbSS; HbSC intermediate disease; and very mild or symptom-free for HbS/β⁺, HbS/HPHP, and HbS/HbE.[1,2]

DIAGNOSIS

The diagnosis is made by **hemoglobin (Hgb) electrophoresis**, according to the definition above.

EPIDEMIOLOGY/INCIDENCE

Sickle cell disease occurs in about 1 in 600 African-Americans. The sickle cell trait occurs in 1 in 12 African-Americans. It is more common in West Africa, in the Mediterranean countries, and in Saudi Arabia, India, South and Central America, and Southeast Asia.[1,2]

GENETICS/INHERITANCE

Sickle cell disease is an **autosomal recessive** disorder characterized by a single nucleotide substitution (GTG for GAG) in the 6th codon of the β-globin gene (making it an HbS gene) in chromosome 11, leading to substitution of valine for glutamic acid on the β-globin chain, and resulting in β^S globin. Inheriting one HbS gene results in the sickle cell trait. Inheriting two HbS genes results in sickle cell disease.

If both parents carry one HbS gene, the fetus has a 25% chance of having sickle cell anemia, a 50% chance of having sickle cell trait, and a 25% chance of being unaffected.[2]

PATHOPHYSIOLOGY

Hemoglobin provides the oxygen-carrying capacity of erythrocytes. It contains four heme groups (pyrrole rings + iron) attached to four globin polypeptides. The globin polypeptides are characterized as alpha (α), beta (β), gamma (γ), delta (δ), epsilon (ϵ), and zeta (ζ). In adults, hemoglobin is primarily HbA1 (α_2/β_2). HbA2 (α_2/δ_2) is present in minor concentrations. HbS occurs when valine is substituted for glutamine in the β-globin gene. This defective hemoglobin forms long rod-like structures, resulting in sickle-shaped red blood cells. Sickle-shaped cells block vessels, causing oxygen deprivation, which results in the clinical manifestations of the disease. The life span of a sickle cell is about 10–20 days compared with the 120-day life span of a normal red blood cell. This chronic hemolysis contributes to the anemia.[1–3] Dehydration, infection, decrease in oxygen tension, and acidosis are common triggers of crisis. Vaso-occlusion causes small bone infarcts, which then cause pain. As vaso-occlusion can occur in any vessel, this is a systemic disease that can affect any organ.

SYMPTOMS

1. Chronic hemolytic anemia

- Fatigue, pallor, shortness of breath.
- Aplastic crisis presents with severe anemia and reticulocytopenia. It is the most common hematological crisis during pregnancy.

2. Acute vaso-occlusive episodes

- Pain involving the chest, lower back, abdomen, head, and bones/extremities.
- Exacerbated by cold, infection, stress, dehydration, alcohol, and fatigue.

3. Infections

- Urinary tract infections, pneumonia, osteomyelitis, endometritis.
- Organisms include *Streptococcus pneumoniae*, *Haemophilus influenzae*, *Staphylococcus*, Gram-negative organisms, *Salmonella*, and *Mycoplasma*.

4. Cardiac

- Systolic murmur, cardiomegaly, high-output failure.

5. Pulmonary

- Acute chest syndrome (ACS) presents with chest pain, dyspnea, tachypnea, fever, cough, leukocytosis, and pulmonary infiltrates. It is usually a result of infection, vaso-occlusion, or bone marrow embolization.

6. Gastrointestinal

- Right upper quadrant syndrome presents with abdominal pain, fever, hepatomegaly, hyperbilirubinemia, and increased liver function tests. Splenomegaly is common.

7. Renal

- Hematuria, papillary necrosis, nephrotic syndrome, renal infarction, pyelonephritis, hyposthenuria, and renal medullary carcinoma.

8. Neurological

- Transient ischemic attacks, cerebrovascular accidents, seizures, coma, hemiparesis, hemianesthesia, visual field changes, and cranial nerve palsy.
- Moyamoya disease is a progressive occlusive process of the cerebral vasculature that results in the formation of collateral vessels with the appearance of 'puffs of smoke' (*moyamoya* in Japanese) on angiography.

9. Skeletal

- Avascular necrosis most often occurs in the humeral and femoral heads and is characterized by pain.

COMPLICATIONS

Effects of SS disease on pregnancy.

- ## Pregnancy loss

  HbSS: the rate of pregnancy loss, most commonly in the first trimester, ranges from 7 to 36%.[4–6]
  HbSC: the rate of pregnancy loss is about 9%.[6]

- ## Fetal death

  HbSS & HbSC: no significantly increased rate of fetal death in recent series.[4,5]

- ## Fetal growth restriction (FGR)

HbSS: 4.9 times more likely.[4]
HbSC: 2.2 times more likely.[4]

- ## Small for gestational age (SGA)

HbSS: About 21%.[7] Pre-eclampsia and acute anemia episodes are risk factors for SGA. High hemoglobin F levels are protective for fetal growth.[7]
HbSC: not at increased risk for SGA.[7]

- ## Acute anemia

HbSS: 4%.[7]
HbS/β^0: 15%.[7]

- ## Painful crisis

HbSS: 20–50%.[4,5,7] There is no difference in the rate of painful episodes before, during, and after pregnancies.[7]
HbSC: 19–26%.[4,7]

- ## Urinary tract infections

HbSS: 15%.[5]

- ## Preterm birth

HbSS: 2.8 times more likely. The mean gestational age at delivery is 34–37 weeks.[4,7]
HbSC: no increased risk for preterm birth.[4]

- ## Pre-eclampsia

HbSS & HbSC: no increased risk for pre-eclampsia.[4]

- ## Acute chest syndrome

HbSS: 7–20%.[5,7]

- ## Alloimmunization

Any woman with sickle cell disease is at increased risk for rhesus (Rh) and other antibodies if she has had blood transfusions in the past.

- ## Antepartum admissions

Because of all the above complications, in particular painful crises, and increased incidences of infections in general, women with sickle cell disease in pregnancy are at increased risk for hospitalization.
HbSS: 6.8 times more likely.[4]
HbSC: 2.8 times more likely.[4]

- ## Postpartum complications

HbSS & HbSC: more likely to have postpartum infections secondary to endomyometritis or pyelonephritis. No increased risk for postpartum hemorrhage.[4,5]

- ## Maternal mortality

HbSS: the mortality rate ranges from 0.45 to 2.1%.[5,7] Life expectancy for HbSS women is about 50 years old. Causes of mortality include ACS (see below), thromboembolism (pulmonary embolism, stroke), etc.

PREGNANCY MANAGEMENT
Principles

Multidisciplinary, involving hematologist, blood bank, primary care physician, obstetrician, and any other involved healthcare workers (e.g. pain and drug dependency services, social, supportive, etc.).

Work-up

- For diagnosis: hemoglobin electrophoresis.
- For a crisis: hemoglobin, hemoglobin electrophoresis, urine culture, and culture of any other possible infectious source; blood gas if hypoxia is present.

Preventive care

Pneumococcal vaccine.

Preconception care

Patients are no longer counseled to avoid pregnancy. Counseling should include increased risk of complications, as described above.

Prenatal care

1. Initial visit: medical (assess for chronic organ damage), obstetric, transfusion, and social history; nutritional assessment; discuss precipitating factors for painful crises and prior successful pain management. Counseling regarding risks, as described above.

2. Initial laboratory studies: complete blood count (CBC), reticulocyte count, Hgb electrophoresis, serum iron studies, bilirubin, liver function tests (LFTs), hepatitis A, B, C, human immunodeficiency virus (HIV), blood urea nitrogen (BUN), creatinine, antibody screen, rubella antibody titer, venereal disease research laboratory (VDRL), tuberculosis skin test, Papanicolaou (Pap) smear as appropriate, *Chlamydia* and gonorrhea cultures.
3. Test the father of the baby (CBC, hemoglobin electrophoresis). Offer genetic counseling if father is positive for sickle cell. If father is positive for sickle cell, direct DNA analysis is available by polymerase chain reaction (PCR) via chorionic villus sampling (CVS) or amniocentesis.
4. Serial urine cultures every 6–8 weeks.
5. CBC every trimester.
6. Folate supplementation 1 mg daily. Ferrous sulfate 325 mg orally bid only if iron deficient.
7. Pneumococcal vaccine. The safety of the vaccine during the first trimester has not been evaluated; however, no adverse outcomes have occurred in newborns whose mothers were inadvertently vaccinated.[8]
8. Ultrasound at 18–20 weeks, and then growth scan at 32 weeks.

Antenatal testing

There are no prospective studies on the use of antepartum testing in sickle cell disease women.[6] Fetal monitoring can be started at 32 weeks, with weekly non-stress test/amniotic fluid index (NST/AFIs), especially if fetus is SGA.[2]

Therapy

Painful crisis

Narcotics

Morphine is the preferred agent. Consider using a patient-controlled analgesia (PCA) system for severe pain. Oral controlled-release morphine is as effective as intravenous (IV) morphine in non-pregnant adults. Ask women regarding which narcotic or pain management works best for them, and implement as appropriate. After 28–32 weeks, avoid non-steroidal anti-inflammatory drugs (NSAIDs), which are safe and effective earlier in pregnancy. Prescribe stool softeners with narcotic use.[9]

Intravenous fluids

Effective in non-pregnant adults. Adequate fluid intake is 60 ml/kg/24 hours in adults.[9] Consider 150 ml/h. Monitor fluid balance.

Antibiotics

Broad-spectrum antibiotics should be used if patient is febrile (temperature >38°C), or if there is evidence of infection. Add a macrolide (e.g. erythromycin) if chest symptoms are present.[9]

Oxygen

Ineffective in providing clinical benefit in non-pregnant adults. Use only for ACS or if O_2 saturation is less than patient's known state or <95%.[9]

Labor and delivery

There is no need to alter general recommendations for labor and delivery in women in sickle cell crisis. A crisis is not an indication for cesarean delivery or other special intervention. Close monitoring of mother and fetus for adequate oxygenation is paramount. Caution with maternal narcotic use for pain control is suggested, as is warning of the neonatologist for the probable opioid withdrawal syndrome in the neonate.

Anemia

Transfusions

In non-pregnant adults, prophylactic transfusions are not recommended, except in special circumstances. There is limited evidence to assess the efficacy of prophylactic blood transfusions for pregnant women with sickle cell disease. Compared with transfusion only for Hgb <6 g/dl, transfusion (or exchange transfusion) with two units of red blood cells (RBCs) every week for 3 weeks, or until the hemoglobin level is 10–11 g/dl or hemoglobin S <35%, is associated with no significant difference in perinatal outcome.[10] Prophylactic transfusions decreased the number of painful crises (14% vs 50%). Disadvantages of prophylactic transfusion include increase in costs, number of hospitalizations, and risk of alloimmunization.[10] Therefore, **prophylactic blood transfusions are not indicated universally for pregnant women with sickle cell disease.**

Indications for transfusions are any woman who is **symptomatic or orthostatic from anemia, and/or with a hemoglobin of <6 g/dl or hematocrit (Hct) <25%, or with acute stroke or chest syndrome or multiple organ failure.** Sickle cell crisis is not an absolute indication for transfusion. Persistent crises are an indication for transfusion to avoid recurrence, with patient counseling. If blood transfusion is indicated, it should always be leukodepleted and matched for Rh and Kell antigens. Counseling regarding potential side effects of blood transfusion is indicated. The goals of transfusion are usually hematocrit >35%, HbA_1 >40%, and HbS <35%.

There is insufficient evidence to compare exchange vs regular blood transfusions for sickle cell disease in pregnancy. For Hct <15%, a direct transfusion is always preferable.

Hydroxyurea

Avoid use of hydroxyurea in pregnancy, as it is unsafe for the fetus. It is effective as a preventing agent in reducing crisis rate, use of transfusions, and incidence of ACS in non-pregnant adults.

Alloimmunization

If the antibody screen is positive, follow guideline as in Chapter 47. The antigen status of the father of the pregnancy should be tested, as he often does not carry the offending antigen, with the maternal antibody usually acquired by prior transfusions. Bilirubin level (delta optical density at 450 nm [delta OD450]) in amniotic fluid is unreliable for detecting fetal anemia, as maternal hemolysis and hyperbilirubinemia increase fetal and amniotic fluid bilirubin levels. MCA PSV (middle cerebral artery peak systolic velocity) by Doppler ultrasound is reliable, and should be used if screening for fetal anemia is necessary.

Delivery

It is safe for patients to deliver vaginally. Inductions and cesarean sections should be reserved for obstetric indications. There is one case report of a sickle cell crisis triggered by induction of labor with a prostaglandin.[11]

Anesthesia

There are no contraindications to anesthesia (IV, regional, or general).

Postpartum

During the postpartum period, early ambulation and adequate hydration is encouraged. Compression boots and incentive spirometry should be used during bed rest. Anemia should be assessed and transfusion only if indicated (see above). Breastfeeding is encouraged. Low-dose oral contraceptives, Depo-Provera (medroxyprogesterone) injections, and intrauterine devices are all safe in preventing pregnancy.[12]

ACUTE CHEST SYNDROME
Definition

New pulmonary infiltrate of at least one complete lung segment with alveolar consolidation and excluding atelectasis; and presence of chest pain, temperature >38.5°C, tachypnea, wheezing, or cough. Hypoxia, decreasing Hgb levels, and progressive pneumonia are frequent. ACS is mostly associated with pulmonary fat embolism and pulmonary infection, with a 3–10% chance of death, related to pulmonary embolus (PE) and pneumonia.

Incidence

ACS develops in about 10% of women with sickle cell disease.

Basic pathophysiology

The cause of ACS remains mainly unknown. Infection leading to sickle crisis, anemia, hypoxia, and vaso-occlusion with ischemic damage is the most common association.

Symptoms

Chest pain, pain in arms and legs, dypnea, fever, etc.

Complications

ACS is one of the most common causes of death in patients with sickle cell disease (3–10%). Neurological complications, probably secondary to central nervous system (CNS) hypoxia, occur in about 20% of patients. Pulmonary emboli and infarction can also occur.

Work-up

For ACS, chest X-ray; sputum culture, nasopharyngeal sample, and/or bronchoscopy washings culture (*Chlamydia pneumoniae* and *Mycoplasma pneumoniae* are the most common pathogens).

Therapy

Antibiotics (usually cephalosporin and erythromycin) aimed at infectious pathogen(s) in the pulmonary tree and bronchodilators (even if no evidence of reactive airway disease). Blood transfusions (especially in hypoxic and/or anemic women), oxygen (15% need mechanical ventilation), and pain control as needed.[13]

SICKLE CELL TRAIT

Pregnant women with the sickle cell trait in pregnancy should be screened with a hemoglobin electrophoresis if this has not been done before. They are at increased risk of **urinary tract infections** (UTIs), and therefore should have a urine culture at first prenatal visit and every trimester, with asymptomatic bacteriuria adequately treated.

HBSC DISEASE

HbC is the result of a single nucleotide substitution (A for G) in the 6th codon of the β-globin gene (making it an HbC gene) in chromosome 11, leading to substitution of lysine for glutamic acid on the β-globin chain, and resulting in β^c globin. One percent of African-Americans are carriers (trait). Diagnosis is by electrophoresis. No disease with trait only.

HbSC disease occurs in about 1/833 African-americans. About 40–60% have the same clinical course as HbSS disease, whereas others have a milder disease. Preventive and prenatal management should be as for HbSS.

SICKLE β-THALASSEMIA DISEASE (HBS-βTHAL)

Diagnosis by hemoglobin electrophoresis: HbS > HbA; ↑ HbA_2, ↑ HbF. Prognosis and management are as for HbSS.

HEMOGLOBIN E

Hemoglobin E is prevalent in South-East Asia. There is no increase in morbidity and mortality, except a possible slight decrease in birth weight and an increase in abruption.

REFERENCES

1. Rust OA, Perry KG Jr. Pregnancy complicated by sickle hemoglobinopathy. Clin Obstet Gynecol 1995; 38(3): 472–84. [review]

2. Rappaport VJ. Hemaglobinopathies in pregnancy. Obstet Gynecol Clin North Am 2004; 31(2): 287–317. [review]

3. Stuart MJ, Nagel RL. Sickle-cell disease. Lancet 2004; 364: 1343–60. [review; non-pregnant]

4. Sun PM, Wilburn W, Raynor BD, Jamieson D. Sickle cell disease in pregnancy: twenty years of experience at Grady Memorial Hospital, Atlanta, Georgia. Am J Obstet Gynecol 2001; 184(6): 1127–30. [II-2]

5. Serjeant GR, Loy LL, Crowther M, Hambleton IR, Thame M. Outcome of pregnancy in homozygous sickle cell disease. Obstet Gynecol 2004; 103(6): 1278–85. [II-2]

6. Milner PF, Jones BR, Dobler J. Outcome of pregnancy in sickle cell anemia and sickle cell-hemoglobin C disease. An analysis of 181 pregnancies in 98 patients, and a review of the literature. Am J Obstet Gynecol 1986; 138: 239–45. [II-3]

7. Smith JA, Espeland M, Bellevue R, et al. Pregnancy in sickle cell disease: experience of the Cooperative Study of Sickle Cell Disease. Obstet Gynecol 1996; 87(2): 199–204. [II-2]

8. www.cdc.org [II-3]

9. Refs DC, Olujohungbe AD; Parkher NE, et al. Guidelines for the management of the acute painful crisis in sickle cell disease. Br J Haematol 2003; 120: 744–52. [guideline]

10. Koshy M, Burd L, Wallace D, Moawed A, Baron J. Prophylactic red-cell transfusions in pregnant patients with sickle cell disease. A randomized cooperative study. N Engl J Med 1988; 319(22): 1447–52. [RCT, n=72]

11. Faron G, Corbisier C, Tecco L, Vokaer A. First sickle cell crisis triggered by induction of labor in a primigravida. Eur J Obstet Gynecol Reprod Biol 2001; 94(20): 304–6. [II-3]

12. Freie HM. Sickle cell disease and hormonal contraception. Acta Obstet Gynecol Scand 1983; 62: 211–17. [II-3]

13. Vichinsky EP, Neumayr LD, Earles AN, et al. Causes and outcomes of the acute chest syndrome in sickle cell disease. N Engl J Med 2000; 342: 1855–65. [II-3]

13

von Willebrand disease

Vincenzo Berghella

KEY POINTS

- **Ensure correct diagnosis.** Be aware of **physiological increase of factor VIII and von Willebrand factor (vWF) levels in pregnancy.**
- Key **laboratory tests: factor VIII, von Willebrand factor antigen (vWFAg), ristocetin cofactor activity, and bleeding time.**
- Test DDAVP (1-deamino-8-D-arginine; desmopressin) **responsiveness** in second or third trimester.
- **Therapy for most common type (I) if factor VIII < 40% of normal is DDAVP.**

HISTORIC NOTES

First described in 1926 by Finnish pediatrician Erik von Willebrand.

DIAGNOSIS/DEFINITION

Diagnosis (send all four laboratory tests) [of type I]: (1) prolonged **bleeding time**, (2) low levels of **factor VIII**, (3) decreased **vWF:Ag** (von Willebrand factor antigen; an immunoreactive protein), and (4) decreased **ristocetin cofactor activity** (binding of vWF:Ag to the platelet membrane glycoprotein Iba, mediated by the antibiotic ristocetin). Can have normal prothrombin time (PT) and partial thromboplastin time (PTT), and normal bleeding time (rarely). In pregnancy, many of these values are normal, and diagnosis cannot be made reliably. For distinguishing types: (5) multimeric analysis and (6) factor VIII binding assay. Factor VIII levels are best (but not very good) at predicting surgical/soft-tissue bleeding.

SYMPTOMS

Abnormal bleeding. Ask for detailed personal history (menstruation, injuries, surgeries, etc.) and family history.

EPIDEMIOLOGY/INCIDENCE

Incidence about 1%; most common congenital hemorrhagic disease.

GENETICS

Usually autosomal dominant. vWF is a large multimeric glycoprotein encoded on chromosome 12. There are over 250 mutations known.

ETIOLOGY/BASIC PATHOPHYSIOLOGY

Decrease (quantitative: types I and III) in von Willebrand factor (vWF; also known as factor VIII cofactor) or (qualitative: type II) its function. This cofactor is critical for normal platelet adhesion at site of vascular injury (Figure 13.1[1]).

CLASSIFICATION

- **Type I.** (60–85%) Autosomal dominant. Partial quantitative decrease. **Mild–moderate decrease in vWF.** Also **decreased factor VIII** 5–30 (normal 50–150 IU/dl); **decreased vWF:Ag, decreased vWF: activity** – measured by **ristocetin**-induced **cofactor** assay.
- **Type II.** (10–30%) Autosomal dominant. Qualitative defect of vWF. **Normal vWF but dysfunction:**

  A: decreased vWF function
  B: decreased vWF function, causing increased binding of platelets and so **decreased platelets** by platelet agglutination.
  M, N: Type II M and type II N are uncommon.

- **Type III.** (1–5%) Autosomal recessive. Quantitative decrease. **No vWF** and very low factor VIII. Severe symptoms, and **do not respond to DDAVP.**

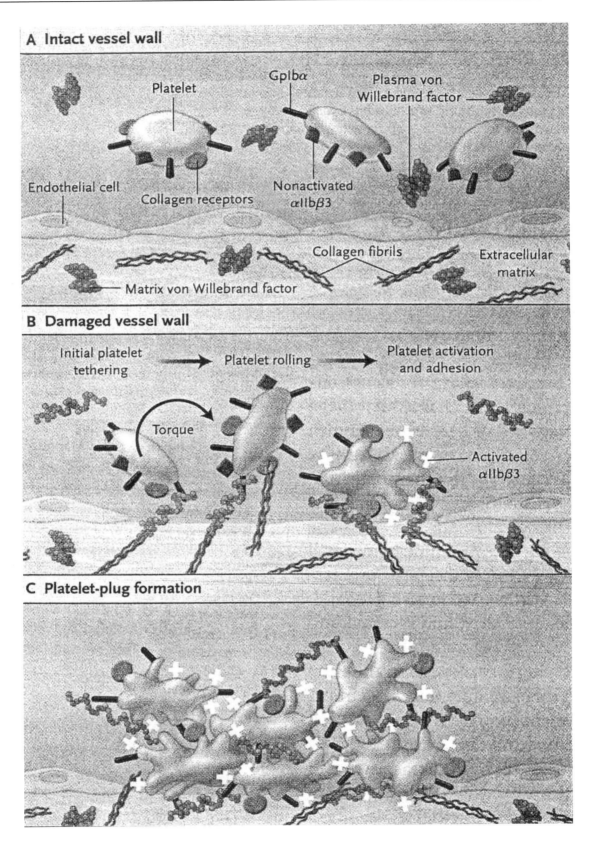

Figure 13.1

Normal platelet adhesion at site of vascular injury. (A) Intact vessel wall. (B) Damaged vessel wall. (C) Platelet-plug formation. Reprinted with permission, from[1].

COMPLICATIONS

Intra- and postpartum hemorrhage. Does not impair fertility or increase pregnancy loss.

PREGNANCY CONSIDERATIONS

Factor VIII and vWF levels rise in pregnancy, so they might be normal at term even with vW disease.

PREGNANCY MANAGEMENT

Principles

Treat as you would in non-pregnant adult.

Work-up

See diagnosis above.

Management

Preconception counseling

Obtain history, type of vW, records, etc.; hematology and genetic counseling consult as necessary; baseline laboratory tests (see work-up above); hepatitis B vaccine. If vW type I with factor VIII levels < 50 IU/dl, type II or III, or history of severe bleeding, consider care in a high-risk center, with close collaboration with hematologist.

Prenatal care

First trimester: see 'preconception counseling' if not done yet. Prenatal diagnosis, including chorionic villus sampling (CVS), is possible (give DDAVP [desmopressin] or other prophylaxis as appropriate per type – see below). Second/third trimester: anesthesia consult; test response to DDAVP. Third trimester: monitor laboratory tests; birth plan (anesthesia, DDAVP, etc.). Aim to achieve factor VIII levels of ≥ 50 IU/dl, associated with very low risk of any bleeding complications.[2]

Therapy

Type I
DDAVP (desmopressin; i.e. 1-deamino-8-D-arginine vasopressin; synthetic vasopressin [antidiuretic hormone] analog) 0.3 μg/kg IV over 30 minutes. Works within 1 hour. Also available subcutaneous (SQ) (0.3 μg/kg) or nasal inhalation (300 μg in adults). Mechanism of action is promoting release of vWF and factor VIII from endothelial cells; thus, increases ristocetin cofactor activity, and increases × 3 vWF:Ag level, and factor VIII procoagulant level (FVIII:C). Can give test dose, and then **check factor VIII and ristocetin cofactor activity at peak – 1 hour – and clearance – 4 hours. It lasts up to 10 hours; so repeat q12h, max 2–4 doses. DDAVP is first-line therapy for type I, second-line therapy for type IIA, and is contraindicated for type IIB.**

Safe in pregnancy for mother and fetus (does not cross placenta),[2] and during breastfeeding.

If not responsive to DDAVP: **Alphanate** (factor VIII and vWF mixed). This is better than cryoprecipitate because there are no infectious disease issues. Otherwise, use **Humate-P** (purified factor VIII); or **cryoprecipitate** (fibrinogen and vWF), or fresh frozen plasma (**FFP;** watch volume overload). Applies to all above: limited data, but probably safe. Counsel regarding blood product precautions.

Type IIa
Factor VIII/vWF concentrates (as Alphanate, Humate-P, etc.).

Type IIb
No treatment is available.

Type III
Without alloantibodies, factor VIII/vWF concentrates; with alloantibodies, recombinant factor VIII.

Antepartum testing

Not indicated unless other complications present (no known direct fetal risks).

Delivery

Types I and II: measure (1) bleeding time, (2) **factor VIII,** (3) vWFAg, and (4) ristocetin cofactor activity. **If factor VIII levels are > 30–40% of normal (or ≥ 50 IU/dl), there is very low risk of bleeding with vaginal or cesarean delivery. If lower, prophylactically administer DDAVP (if DDAVP responder) or concentrates/blood products** (see above, according to type) *at time of delivery (if possible 1 hour before),* **and 12 hours thereafter** (then as needed).

Type III: do not measure factor VIII, as always low. Treat daily as above, starting before delivery.

Given that the fetus has up to a 50% chance (depending on type) of having vW disease, scalp lead, scalp pH, and operative vaginal delivery should be avoided if possible. Oxytocin dose should be carefully monitored, since fluid retention can be a side effect of both oxytocin and DDAVP, and lead to life-threatening hyponatremia.

Anesthesia

Regional anesthesia is safe if normal partial thromboplastin time (PTT), factor VIII levels of ≥ 50 IU/dl, and normal ristocetin cofactor activity.

Postpartum/breastfeeding

Measure factor VIII 1–2 weeks postpartum, since increased level during pregnancy will again physiologically decrease in vW disease. Risk of postpartum bleeding in fact continues for about 2–4 weeks, so that additional doses of DDAVP and close monitoring are required. Consider oral contraception.

FUTURE

vWF produced by recombinant DNA techniques.

RARE/RELATED

Glanzmann disease (congenital thrombasthenia): congenital bleeding disorder defined by defective or quantitatively abnormal glycoprotein (GP) IIb/IIIa receptors (see Figure 13.1). Diagnosis: bleeding and abnormal platelet aggregation in response to stimuli, prolonged bleeding times, normal platelet counts;[3] 4 pregnancies in the world's literature up to 1978, very few if any after.

REFERENCES

1. Mannucci P. Treatment of von Willebrand disease. N Engl J Med 2004; 351: 683–94. [review]
2. James AH. Von Willebrand disease. Obstet Gynecol Surv 2006; 61: 136–45. [review]
3. Newman PJ, Seligsohn U, Lyman S, et al. The molecular genetic basis of Glanzmann thrombasthenia in the Iraqi-Jewish and Arab populations in Israel. Proc Natl Acad Sci USA 1991; 88: 3160–4. [II-3]

14

Care of the Jehovah's Witness pregnant woman

Regina L Arvon

KEY POINTS

- Members of the Jehovah's Witness faith **refuse blood transfusions** because they believe that **accepting them violates God's law,** and would lead to excommunication and eternal damnation.
- Refusal of blood can lead to an **increased risk of maternal** (and at times therefore fetal) **death,** especially in cases of obstetric hemorrhage.
- All obstetric providers are responsible for **asking each woman at her first prenatal visit** (or preconceptionally) **if she has any objection to receiving any blood product in case of necessity.**
- The woman's wishes should be **respected,** following the principle of **autonomy.**
- After counseling, the patient should be asked to sign the **consent for blood products,** as well as the **Health Care Power of Attorney.**
- The third stage should be managed actively, and postpartum hemorrhage prevented as much as possible. The use of cell saver is safe and effective in pregnancy.

HISTORIC NOTES

That is why I have said to the sons of Israel: 'No soul of you must eat blood and no alien resident who is residing as an alien in your midst should eat blood

(Holy Bible: Leviticus 17:12).

Charles Russell started the Jehovah's Witness Christian sect in Pennsylvania in 1872.

DIAGNOSIS/DEFINITION

Members of the Jehovah's Witness faith **refuse blood transfusions** because they believe that **accepting them violates God's law,** and would lead to excommunication and eternal damnation, as to take literally the statement from the Bible.

COMPLICATIONS

The risk of **obstetric hemorrhage** is approximately 6% in Jehovah's Witness women.[1] The risk of **maternal death** is about 0.5%, a 44-fold increase compared with non-Jehovah's Witness controls.[1]

MANAGEMENT

There are no trials to assess the efficacy of interventions specifically in Jehovah's Witness women (see Chapters 8 and 22 of *Obstetric Evidence Based Guidelines* for third stage and abnormal third stage, respectively, for general recommendations).

Preconception counseling

Counsel regarding complications and management of blood loss in pregnancy.

Prenatal care

All obstetric providers are responsible for asking each woman at her first prenatal visit (or preconceptionally) if she has any objection to receiving any blood product in case of necessity. The woman who states she would decline blood transfusion even if medically necessary and/or is a Jehovah's Witness should be managed as follows:

- Counsel the woman and any family member present regarding the reasons and the risks of blood product refusal, including the possibility of maternal and fetal death. The counseling should be documented on the medical record. The patient might want to consult with the 'elders' before signing informed refusal. **Her wishes should be respected, following the principle of autonomy.** A physician has the right of refusing to provide care for a Jehovah's Witness only if an alternative caregiver agrees to accept and care for the patient.[2]

Blood Product Consent for Jehovah's Witness Patients

I hereby consent to the blood products marked below:

- ____Whole Blood
- ____Fresh Frozen Plasma
- ____Cryoprecipitate
- ____Albumin
- ____Erythropoietin
- ____Immune globulins (blood fraction, Rhogam)
- ____Clotting factors
- ____PolyHeme (human hemoglobin), Hemopure products (bovine hemoglobin)
- ____Recombinant Factors (VII, VIIa, VIII, IX)
- ____Platelet cell fractions (Platelet Gel)
- ____Other surgical procedures, medical tests, or current therapy using my own blood, i.e. tagged red cells, white cells, blood patching
- ____Hemodialysis equipment (nonblood primed)
- ____Intraoperative blood salvage ("cell saver")
- ____Intraoperative hemodilution

_____
Patient's name—please print

_____
Patient's Signature

_____
Date

Figure 14.1
Consent form for Jehovah's Witness patients.

- After counseling, the patient should be asked to sign the **consent for blood products** (Figure 14.1), as well as the **Health Care Power of Attorney**.[2] These two consents should be kept in the medical record and be available at labor and delivery. Approximately 39% of Jehovah's Witness pregnant women accept a variety of donated blood products, and 55% accept either intraoperative normovolemic hemodilution or transfusion of their own blood obtained by a cell saver.[3]
- Consider including a copy of this guideline in the medical record, for reference.
- Selected high-risk patients, e.g. those with hemoglobin < 9 mg/dl, may be considered for appropriate replacement of iron, folic acid, and erythropoietin, which can be coordinated by a maternal fetal medicine and/or a hematologist specialist.
- A routine consult with the Maternal–Fetal Medicine service is not required, but can be considered, especially if the woman is at risk for obstetrical hemorrhage (e.g. placenta previa or accreta, or bleeding disorders).
- A routine ethics consult is not indicated, but can be considered in specific cases.

Antepartum testing

No specific antepartum testing is indicated.

Delivery

- Consents: upon admission and prior to the surgery/delivery, all Jehovah's Witness patients should have signed the two consent forms above. If consents have not been previously signed or are not available, the patient should be recounseled and consents signed.
- **The third stage should be managed actively, and postpartum hemorrhage prevented as much as possible** (see Chapters 8 and 22 of *Obstetric Evidence Based Guidelines*). Oxytocin, methylergonovine, 15-methyl-prostaglandin $F_{2\alpha}$, misoprostol, and other medical, and, if necessary, surgical therapies should be employed.[4]
- If an operative delivery or bleeding disorder is anticipated, if the patient has a history of a low-lying placenta or a placenta previa, or if an operative delivery is to occur, a **cell saver** can be on standby in the Labor and Delivery unit throughout the patient's labor and delivery. Use of the cell saver is safe in obstetrics.[5]

Anesthesia

An anesthesiology consult should be obtained. The anesthesiologist will review the patient's medical record and consents, including consent or refusal for blood products.

REFERENCES

1. Singla AK, Lapinski RH, Berkowitz RL, Saphier CJ. Are women who are Jehovah's Witnesses at risk of maternal death? Am J Obstet Gynecol 2001; 185: 893–5. [II-2, *n*=332]
2. Gyamfi C, Gyamfi MM, Berkowitz RL. Ethical and medicolegal considerations in the obstetric care of a Jehovah's Witness. Obstet Gynecol 2003; 102: 173–80. [review]
3. Gyamfi C, Berkowitz RL. Responses by pregnant Jehovah's Witnesses on health care proxies. Obstet Gynecol 2004; 104: 541–4. [II-3]
4. Singla AK, Berkowitz RL, Saphier CJ. Obstetric hemorrhage in Jehovah's Witnesses. Contemp Obstet Gynecol 2002; 4: 32–43. [review]
5. Catling S, Joels L. Cell salvage in obstetrics: the time has come. BJOG 2005; 112: 131–2. [review]

15

Renal disease

Alisa B Modena

KEY POINTS

- Frequency of complications in pregnancies with maternal renal disease is directly proportional to the initial creatinine level.
- Complications include **preterm birth, pre-eclampsia, fetal growth restriction, low birth weight**, and **perinatal mortality**. In women with **creatinine ≥ 1.4 mg/dl**, about 10% will have progressive **renal deterioration.**
- **Work-up** includes serum **creatinine, blood urea nitrogen (BUN), and electrolytes**, as well as **24-hour urine collection for protein and creatinine clearance.**
- Hypertension is commonly associated with renal disease, and should be treated so as to **keep the diastolic blood pressure below 90 mmHg.**
- Women on **dialysis** (end-stage renal disease [ESRD]) should be counseled **preconceptionally** that they **should receive a renal transplant** and **then wait 1–2 years** before attempting pregnancy. Women on dialysis should be maintained on **effective contraception.** Pregnancy counseling should include a review of the very **high rates of** the above **complications.**
- There is an overall **incidence** of live births in women after **renal transplantation** of >90%.
- **Pelvic floor exercises** during and after pregnancy **decrease the incidence of urinary incontinence in the third trimester and postpartum.**

HISTORIC NOTES

'Children of women with renal disease used to be born dangerously or not at all – not at all if their doctors had their way.'[1]

DIAGNOSIS/DEFINITIONS

- **Chronic renal insufficiency** (CRI): the early stage, when the kidneys no longer function properly but do not yet require dialysis. CRI can be difficult to diagnose as

symptoms are not usually apparent until kidney disease has progressed significantly.
- **Chronic renal failure** (CRF): irreversible, progressive impaired kidney function. CRF generally progresses to ESRD.
- **End-stage renal disease** (ESRD): Patients with ESRD no longer have kidney function adequate to sustain life and **require dialysis or kidney transplantation.** Without proper treatment, ESRD is fatal.
- **Nephrotic syndrome** (NS): a condition caused by any disease that damages the kidneys' filtering system, the glomeruli. NS is associated with hypoalbuminemia, edema, and hypercholesterolemia. In pregnancy, it is usually defined as ≥ 5 g of protein in a 24-hour urine specimen.

SYMPTOMS

Symptoms of renal disease vary according to etiology. However, they often include frequent need to urinate and swelling, as well as possible anemia, fatigue, weakness, headaches, and loss of appetite. As renal disease progresses, other symptoms, such as nausea, vomiting, bad breath, and itchy skin may develop, as toxic metabolites that are normally filtered out by the kidneys build up to harmful levels in the bloodstream.

EPIDEMIOLOGY/INCIDENCE

The overall incidence of renal disease in the general obstetric population is **0.03–0.12%.**[2–4]

PHYSIOLOGIC RENAL CHANGES IN PREGNANCY

Glomerular filtration rate (GFR) increases shortly after conception and serum levels of creatinine and urea decrease to

Table 15.1 *Classification of renal Insufficiency*

Category	Serum creatinine, μmol/L (mg/dl)
Preserved/mildly impaired renal function	< 125 (< 1.4)
Mildly impaired renal function	< 125 (1.1–1.3)
Moderate renal insufficiency	125–250 (1.4–2.8)
Severe renal insufficiency	> 250 (> 2.8)

Adapted from references 6 and 7.

Table 15.2 *Rate of complications (%) according to degree of renal insufficiency*

Creatinine (mg/dl)	PTB	Pre-eclampsia	HTN	FGR	Live birth
<1.4	20	11	25	24	> 90
1.4–2.8	36–60	42	56	31–37	> 90
>2.8	73–86	86	56	43–57	> 90
Dialysis	60–90	60–80	80–100	50–80	40–70
Renal transplant	52–57	23–37	47–63	20–66	74–80

PTB, preterm birth; HTN, hypertension; FGR, fetal growth restriction.
Data from references 9, 14, 15, 18 and 25.

mean values of 0.6 mg/dl and 9 mg/dl, respectively. Near term a 15–20% decrement in GFR occurs.[5] Ideally, evaluation of renal function in pregnancy should be based on GFR, but creatinine clearance is an adequate surrogate of GFR. There is an increase in the size of the kidneys and urinary collecting system. Kidney length increases approximately 1 cm and volume increases 30%. The entire collecting system is dilated. Functionally, there is an increased renal plasma flow (peak 60–80% in the second trimester, then falls to 50–60% during the third trimester). Glomerular filtration rate increases 30% during the first trimester, and peaks at 50% above prepregnancy values in the second trimester. (See also Chapter 2 in *Obstetric Evidence Based Guidelines.*)

CLASSIFICATION

See Table 15.1.[6,7]

RISK FACTORS/PRECONCEPTION COUNSELING

As renal functional loss progresses, the risks to mother and fetus increase substantially.[6] The goal is to optimize prepregnancy health.

Specific diseases. Patients with scleroderma and polyarteritis nodosa should be discouraged from pregnancy.[6,8,9]

Patients with lupus nephritis do well when the disease is in remission for 6 months prior to conception, with a live birth rate of up to 95%.[10] Overall rates of preterm delivery and pre-eclampsia are based on degree of renal insufficiency, and the total live birth rate for all lupus patients is 58–95%.[10, 11]

Mild renal insufficiency. Patients experience usually a successful pregnancy, with no adverse affect on the course of their disease.[12]

Moderate and severe renal insufficiency. The prognosis is more guarded; 43% of these pregnancies are associated with deterioration in renal function, of which 10% did not reverse postpartum.[13]

COMPLICATIONS

Prognosis is directly related to the degree of renal insufficiency (Table 15.2).[9,14,15]

General

Best outcomes are in women with preconception serum creatinine levels < 1.4 mg/dl and diastolic blood pressure of ≤ 90 mmHg.[3,6] Creatinine clearance < 70 ml/min prior to conception is associated with worse outcome, even when serum levels show only mildly impaired renal function.[16]

Poorer prognosis is associated with the need for more than one antihypertensive medication.[12]

Infertility

Conception with GFR < 25 ml/min is rare secondary to alterations in the hypothalamic–pituitary–ovarian (HPO) axis.[17]

Hypertension

Incidence of hypertension increases from 28% at baseline to approximately 50% by the third trimester,[13] and depends on degree of renal insufficiency (Table 15.2).

Proteinuria

Urinary protein excretion > 3 g in 24 hours increases from approximately 25% to 41%.[13]

Pre-eclampsia

Increased incidence, and diagnosis is difficult (Table 15.2).

Preterm labor

Incidence as high as 85%[18] (Table 15.2).

Low birth weight (LBW)

As high as 66%[18] (Table 15.2 for FGR).

Perinatal mortality

About 10–20%[12,13] overall (Table 15.2).

Cost

Women with chronic renal disease have increased median cost of pregnancy.[2]

PREGNANCY CONSIDERATIONS

Pregnancy does not appear to adversely affect the natural history of renal disease in patients with mild dysfunction; however, 10% with moderate to severe disease will suffer irreversible deterioration during pregnancy.[3,13,19]

WORK-UP

Serum creatinine, blood urea nitrogen (BUN), and electrolytes as well as **24-hour urine collection for protein and creatinine clearance.** Renal biopsy should be reserved for patients whose diagnosis is in question.

PREVENTION

Aim to preserve whatever renal function remains.

MANAGEMENT

Patients with moderate or severe renal insufficiency should be managed with a **multidisciplinary approach,** in conjunction with a perinatologist, nephrologist, and neonatologist.

Prenatal care
Prenatal visits

Women should be seen every 2–4 weeks until 32 weeks' gestation, after which they should be seen weekly due to the increased risk for severe pre-eclampsia. Careful monitoring of blood pressure for early detection of hypertension and superimposed pre-eclampsia should be performed at every visit.

Laboratory tests

Evaluation of renal function by **24-hour creatinine clearance and protein excretion** frequently, e.g. on approximately a monthly basis. Frequent (e.g. monthly) **urine culture** should be done for early detection of asymptomatic bacteriuria or confirmation of urinary tract infection. Maternal anemia should be corrected with iron supplementation or Epogen (epoetin alfa) if severe.

Antenatal testing

- Frequent (e.g. monthly) ultrasound for fetal growth.
- Biophysical assessment (e.g. non-stress tests [NSTs], biophysical profile, Doppler of umbilical artery) of fetal well-being weekly after ≥ 32 weeks.

Patient education

The symptoms of preterm labor and pre-eclampsia should be reviewed with women who have chronic renal disease.

Therapy

Hypertension

Hypertension should be treated aggressively in obstetric patients with underlying renal dysfunction to preserve kidney function longer. The goal is to **keep diastolic blood pressure below 90 mmHg.** Use of antihypertensive medication in pregnancy is discussed in chapter 1.

Pre-eclampsia

Magnesium is not contraindicated, but should be **used with extreme caution,** begun at 1 g/h, possibly without a bolus, or just given as boluses as needed. Evaluation for magnesium side effects should occur at least hourly, and magnesium levels should be checked often (e.g. every 2 hours) in labor to adjust dose. Calcium gluconate should be at the bedside. An alternative is to use phenytoin 15–20 mg/kg IV (intravenous). There is insufficient evidence to recommend the use of low-dose aspirin in the second trimester for women with renal insufficiency or renal failure.[20]

Preterm labor

Magnesium and indomethacin should be used with caution, as they are renally excreted.

Asymptomatic bacteriuria

Bacteriuria should be treated for 1–2 weeks, and suppression should be given for the remainder of the pregnancy.[20]

Delivery

Delivery should be performed at a tertiary care center. Mode of delivery should be for standard obstetric indications. Deliberate preterm delivery may be necessary in the face of worsening maternal renal function, severe pre-eclampsia, or worsening fetal status.

Postpartum/breastfeeding

Little is known about the quantities of immunosuppressive agents in breast milk. Whereas small series have shown little toxicity, caution should be used when recommending breastfeeding to patients taking these agents.[21]

Long-term renal prognosis

When kidney dysfunction is mild, pregnancy does not appear to adversely alter the natural history, with the possible exception of scleroderma and polyarteritis nodosa.[12] **In women with moderate to severe renal insufficiency** (maternal serum creatinine ≥ 1.4 mg/dl), a significant proportion (10% of patients) will have progressive renal deterioration at 12 months.[13]

SPECIAL CONSIDERATIONS IN PREGNANCY

Dialysis

Principles/counseling

Women on dialysis (ESRD) have impaired fertility secondary to suppression of hypothalamic–pituitary–adrenal (HPA) axis function → anovulation, amenorrhea. Fertility rates are improving with advances in dialysis, overall decreased serum creatinine levels, and improvement of azotemia. Published rates of fertility range from 1 to 7%. Dialysis-dependent patients with ESRD should be **offered contraception.**[22]

Women on dialysis (ESRD) who desire pregnancy should be counseled preconceptionally that they should receive a renal transplant and then wait 1–2 years before attempting pregnancy. If a woman becomes pregnant while on dialysis, the key is **coordination of multidisciplinary care** to maintain blood pressure control, fluid balance, and adequate nutrition. There is an overall > 50–70% likelihood of fetal survival.[23] Live births in women with dialysis during pregnancy have improved from 23%,[24] to about 50% in 1994,[14] to 79% in 1998,[23] to 92% in 2002.[22]

Complications

Stillbirth (8–50%), **neonatal death** (9–25%), **preterm delivery** (48–84%), **severe pre-eclampsia** (11%),[18,25] **polyhydramnios,** fetal growth restriction (**FGR**) (50–80%), **hypertension** (100%), **anemia** (100%), and even **maternal death** despite recent improved overall outcomes.[22] Most of the morbidity occurs secondary to prematurity. The risk of congenital anomalies does not appear to be increased.

Pregnancy management

Counseling

- Owing to the high incidence of complications, termination may be discussed, as well as the opportunity for possibly a better outcome after renal transplantation.
- Dialysis:[22]
  - Intensive hemodialysis **6–7 times/week** is recommended for patients with ESRD. There appears to be a trend toward better infant survival in women who receive dialysis ≥ 20 hours per week.[18]
  - Prepregnancy dialysis regimen should be increased by approximately 50%.

- **Hemodialysis** (HD) is probably superior to peritoneal dialysis (PD), but this has not been studied in any trial in pregnancy. One study reported that women undergoing HD had a successful pregnancy rate of 79%, vs 33% with PD.[23] There does not appear to be any advantage to peritoneal dialysis, and the risk of peritonitis is too high to introduce this modality in the pregnant patient population.[18,25]
- Aggressively use HD to decrease azotemia to improve pregnancy outcomes. Keep BUN low (7–10 mg/dl), so no osmotic diuresis in fetus. Maintain serum urea < 60 mg/dl.
- Avoid maternal hypotension during HD. Keep blood pressure 130–150/80–90 mmHg.
- Avoid excessive fluid shifts; ensure minimal fluctuations and limit volume changes.
- Alter heparin regimen near delivery if possible.
- Use maternal dry weight to base HD volume.
- No studies suggest fetal surveillance is necessary during HD.
- Altering HD rates to achieve maximal volume control may decrease incidence of polyhydramnios.
- Nutritional consult.[26]
- Other metabolic changes:
    keep bicarbonate 22–26 mmol/L
    keep hemoglobin 11–12 g/dl with Epogen (safe, does not cross placenta)
    replace calcium (≥ 2 g/day) and phosphorus dialysate – may need more potassium, less calcium.

Other management issues

- Adequate calorie and protein supply needs to be assured.
- Ensure good blood pressure control.
- Maintain attention towards signs and symptoms of preterm labor.
- Maintain normal calcium levels.
- Maternal serum screening for aneuploidy is unreliable in this group of patients.[22,27]
- Indocin may worsen kidney function. Magnesium should be avoided if possible, or used cautiously with frequent levels.
- Close antepartum fetal surveillance is warranted due to risk of FGR and non-reassuring fetal heart rate testing (NRFHT).
- Consider delivery at 34–36 weeks.
- There are insufficient data to assess the effects of antenatal steroids, and the risk of gestational diabetes (GDM) in HD patients.

Antepartum care should otherwise be similar to those patients with chronic renal disease.

Postpartum
Most women return to prepregnancy dialysis regimens and have uncomplicated postpartum recoveries. Postpartum care must address contraception. Future pregnancies should follow renal transplant.

Renal transplantation

Principles

Management should occur at a center with a **transplant nephrologist. Serial assessment of renal function, diagnosis and treatment of rejection, blood pressure control, and control of anemia** should be achieved with a multidisciplinary team. There is an overall **success** of pregnancy (live births) in women after renal transplantation of **>90%**.[28] If graft function is adequate and stable, pregnancy does not cause accelerated graft demise.[29] However, one case-control study suggested that graft function is adversely affected by pregnancy.[30] At 10-year follow-up, graft survival was 69% of pregnant women vs 100% of non-pregnant controls.

Complications

Increased incidences of FGR, premature rupture of membranes, preterm delivery, pre-eclampsia and perinatal death (Table 15.2).

Preconception counseling

The ideal candidate for pregnancy is a woman with:

1. Good general health for 2 years post-transplant before attempting conception.
2. Minimal (ideally < 300 mg, or at least < 1000 mg/24 hours) proteinuria.
3. Absence (ideal) or at least good control of hypertension.
4. No evidence of graft rejection.
5. Absence of pelvicaliceal distention on intravenous pyelography (IVP).
6. Stable renal function (maternal serum creatinine < 1.4 mg/dl, or best < 1.1 mg/dl).
7. Stable immunosuppressive regimen.
8. If possible, drug therapy should be reduced to maintenance levels: prednisone < 15 mg/day, azathioprine < 2 mg/kg/day, and cyclosporine < 5 mg/kg/day.[20]

Prenatal care

Attempt to obtain operative records from transplant surgery (to identify location of kidney). Be aware of side effects of immunosuppressive agents (Table 15.3). A common immunosuppressive drug is currently tacrolimus (Prograf). It crosses the placenta, but has not been associated with an increase in congenital anomalies. Avoid nephrotoxic drugs. Be aware of significant drug interactions with cyclosporine (Table 15.4).

Table 15.3 *Immunosuppressive agents commonly used and their side effects*	
Agent	Side effect
• Prednisone[a]	Glucose intolerance
• Azathioprine[a]	Leukopenia
• Cyclosporine[ab]	Hypertension, nephrotoxicity (watch for drug interactions – see below)
• Tacrolimus[ab]	Hypertension, nephrotoxicity, neurotoxicity, glucose intolerance, myocardial hypertrophy
• Mycophenolate mofetil	GI disturbance; animal studies raise concerns regarding potential for human teratogenicity

[a]These drugs have no known teratogenic effects.
[b]Follow with blood levels.

Antenatal visits

These visits should be every 2–4 weeks up to 32 weeks, and weekly thereafter.

Laboratory tests

These tests include monthly assessment of complete blood count (CBC), **BUN, serum creatinine, electrolytes, serum urate, 24-hour creatinine clearance and protein** levels, and urine specimen for **culture.** Initial labs should also include serum serologies for **cytomegalovirus (CMV), toxoplasmosis,** and **herpes simplex** virus (immunoglobulins IgM and IgG for each) and liver function tests **(LFTs). Levels of immunosuppressive agent** (tacrolimus, cyclosporine, etc.) should be obtained at least every trimester. If the patient is on prednisone or tacrolimus, obtain fasting and 2-hour postprandial blood sugars upon presentation. If these values are normal, perform a glucose challenge test at 24 weeks.

Antepartum testing

Fetal surveillance should follow the recommendations for chronic renal disease.

Labor management

Management should include careful monitoring of maternal fluid balance, cardiovascular status, and temperature. Cesarean delivery should be for obstetric indications only. Women who have received steroids for a long period during the antepartum period should be considered for 'stress dose' steroids. Notification of the use of immunosuppressants to the pediatrician is important for proper follow-up of the neonate.

Renal graft rejection

Renal graft rejection occurs in 4–9% of pregnant allograft recipients and is difficult to diagnose. Factors that increase risk include increased number of episodes of rejection during the year prior to conception, maternal serum creatinine >2 mg/dl and proteinuria >500 mg/dl, and graft

dysfunction during pregnancy.[29] Clinical hallmarks include fever, oliguria, deteriorating renal function, renal enlargement, and tenderness. **Renal ultrasound** and **biopsy** for diagnosis are necessary before aggressive antirejection therapy is begun.

Postpartum/breastfeeding

In general, not enough data are available to make a formal recommendation regarding the safety of immunosuppressive medications during breastfeeding. However, breastfeeding is contraindicated in patients on cyclosporine[21].

Resources

USA National Transplant Pregnancy Registry (www.temple.edu/ntpr).

Urinary tract infections

Screening

All pregnant women should be screened at the first prenatal visit for asymptomatic bacteriuria. Women with risk factors for urinary tract infections, such as diabetes mellitus (DM), GDM, neurogenic bladder, prior frequent urinary tract infections (UTIs), and sickle cell disease, should be screened every trimester.

Complications

Pregnant women with asymptomatic bacteriuria are at increased risk for symptomatic infection and **pyelonephritis.** There is also a direct relationship between untreated bacteriuria and **low birth weight,** and **preterm birth.** Other complications of UTIs or pyelonephritis include fetal mortality, possibly long-term mental retardation and developmental delay,[31] pre-eclampsia, anemia, and pulmonary and renal insufficiency. Treatment of asymptomatic bacteriuria

Table 15.4 *Drug interactions with cyclosporine*	
Drugs that exhibit nephrotoxic synergy	
Gentamicin	Cimetidine
Tobramycin	Ranitidine
Vancomycin	Diclofenac
Amphotericin B	Trimethoprim with sulfamethoxazole
Ketoconazole	Azapropazone
Melphalan	
Careful monitoring of renal function should be practiced when cyclosporine is used with nephrotoxic drugs.	
Drugs that alter cyclosporine levels	
Cyclosporine is extensively metabolized by the liver. Therefore, circulating cyclosporine levels may be influenced by drugs that affect hepatic microsomal enzymes, particularly the cytochrome P-450 system. Substances known to inhibit these enzymes will decrease hepatic metabolism and increase cyclosporine levels. Substances that are inducers of cytochrome P-450 activity will increase hepatic metabolism and decrease cyclosporine levels. Monitoring of circulating cyclosporine levels and appropriate cyclosporine dosage adjustment are essential when these drugs are used concomitantly.	
Drugs that *increase* cyclosporine levels	
Diltiazem	Danazol
Nicardipine	Bromocriptine
Verapamil	Metoclopramide
Ketoconazole	Erythromycin
Fluconazole	Methylprednisone
Intracondazole	
Drugs that *decrease* cyclosporine levels	
Rifampin	Phenobarbital
Phenytoin	Carbamazepine
Other drug interactions	
Reduced clearance of prednisolone, digoxin, and lovastatin has been observed when these drugs are administered with cyclosporine. In addition, a decrease in the apparent volume of distribution of digoxin has been reported after cyclosporine administration. Severe digitalis toxicity has been seen within days of starting cyclosporine in several patients taking digoxin. Cyclosporine should not be used with potassium-sparing diuretics because hyperkalemia can occur. During treatment with cyclosporine, vaccination may be less effective: and the use of live vaccines should be avoided. Myositis has occurred with concomitant lovastatin, frequent gingival hyperplasia with nifedipine, and convulsions with high-dose methylprednisolone.	

prevents these complications (see Chapters 1 and 15 of *Obstetric Evidence Based Guidelines*).

Prevention

Cranberry juice (10–16 oz daily) decreases the incidence of recurrent *Escherichia coli* UTIs. *Lactobacillus GG* drink does not have a benefit.[32]

Diagnosis

A threshold of $\geq 100\,000$ colony-forming units (CFUs) is an indication for treatment. Group B streptococcus in the urine should be appropriately treated at any concentration (see Chapter 15 of *Obstetric Evidence Based Guidelines*). It is important to avoid contamination by cleansing the perineum and then collecting 'mid-stream' urine.

Treatment

Check allergies and urine drug sensitivities. If appropriate, treat with **nitrofurantoin** 100 mg orally twice per day for 7 days. If not effective, oral alternatives are cephalexin 250 mg every 6 hours, amoxicillin 250 mg every 8 hours, or trimethoprim–sulfamethoxazole 160/800 mg orally every 12 hours for 7 days.

Follow-up

A **test of cure** is necessary. If positive, repeat antibiotic regimen (consider different, sensitive regimen) and assess compliance. Suppressive therapy (once a day – bedtime – of any of nitrofurantoin 50 mg, amoxicillin 250 mg, or cephalexin 250 mg) is indicated after two UTIs or one pyelonephritis.

Pyelonephritis

Incidence

The incidence of pyelonephritisis is 1–2% in pregnancy.[33]

Diagnosis

UTI with costovertebral angle tenderness (CVAT), accompanied usually by systemic symptoms such as fever. So positive urine culture is necessary for diagnosis.

Management

- **Urine culture sensitivity is crucial to assure adequate antibiotic coverage.**
- Work-up should include CBC, electrolytes, creatinine, and LFTs.
- Usually inpatient treatment, especially if before 24 weeks. Outpatient therapy can be considered for uncomplicated women with pyelonephritis after IV ceftriaxone.[34,35]
- **IV antibiotics** for 24–48 hours or at least until the patient is > 24 hours afebrile:
  - Ancef (cefazolin) 1 g every 6–8 hours, or
  - ampicillin 1–2 g every 6 hours, with gentamicin 1.5 mg/kg every 8 hours, or
  - ceftriaxone 1–2 g every 24 hours, or
  - trimethoprim–sulfamethoxazole 160/800 mg every 12 hours.
- If not afebrile within 48 hours with appropriate regimen, or if recurrent pyelonephritis, consider renal ultrasound.
- Once IV therapy is completed, oral therapy should be continued for 10–14 days, followed by suppression and frequent urine cultures (see above).

Urinary nephrolithiasis

Incidence

About 0.03–0.4% (about 1/2000). Up to 12% of the general population has a urinary stone during their lifetime, with recurrence rates approaching 50%.[36] Nephrolithiasis is also called renal calculi or stones.

Risks

More common in Caucasians, second and third trimester, right side,[37] recurrent UTIs, gout, prior renal stones, family history.

Pregnancy considerations

The incidence of renal stones may be higher in pregnancy because of hormonal changes, urinary tract dilatation, and obstruction leading to urinary stasis.

Diagnosis

The best imaging technique in the non-pregnant adult is unenhanced helical computed tomography (**CT**) **scan** of the abdomen and pelvis, with a 96% sensitivity and 100% specificity.[36] If CT is unavailable, a plain abdominal X-ray should be performed, since 75–90% of urinary stones are radiopaque. **Ultrasonography** has only a sensitivity of 11–24% with > 90% specificity in non-pregnant adults, but because of a sensitivity of about 67% in pregnancy is currently the **first-line screening test in pregnancy**. If the ultrasound is initially negative, an MRU (magnetic resonance urography)[38] should be considered, or, if unavailable, probably an X-ray second and a CT scan third. It is important to know that mild to moderate hydronephrosis is physiologic in pregnancy and is usually worse on the right kidney.

Management

Composition, location, and size of stone should be assessed. Determine upper tract anatomy and the woman's preferences. Urgent intervention is indicated with obstructed, infected upper urinary tract, impending renal deterioration, intractable pain or vomiting, anuria, or high-grade obstruction of a solitary or transplanted kidney.

There are no trials in pregnancy or even in non-pregnant adults for **pain control**. Ketorolac and diclofenac appear to be as effective as narcotics. All are used acutely intravenously.

Usually increasing fluids and movement are used as initial interventions in pregnancy as well as in non-pregnant adults. Over 70% of stones in pregnancy resolve with conservative management. A urinary stone seen by ultrasound (or CT) but not X-ray is probably a uric acid stone: 20 mmol of potassium citrate orally 2–3 times daily (aim to alkalinize urine to pH 6.5–7.0) can be an effective medical therapy for dissolution of this type of stone.

After initial conservative management, insertion of **stents** is a safe intervention in pregnancy. Percutaneous nephrostomy is needed only rarely, but is safe in pregnancy. Ureteroscopy is also a more and more popular and safe intervention. If the non-pregnant woman so desires, shock wave lithotripsy or ureteroscopy can be performed.[36] Shock wave lithotripsy is considered a first-line therapy for proximal ureteral stones < 1 cm in non-pregnant adults. Inadvertent lithotripsy in pregnancy is not a cause for concern, but it is not recommended in pregnancy.[39]

Prevention of urinary incontinence

Incidence

Urinary incontinence has been reported to occur in 5–40% of pregnant and postpartum women.

Prevention

Pelvic floor exercises *during pregnancy* **decrease the incidence of urinary incontinence in the third trimester and postpartum,** up to 6 months after birth.[40–42] Pelvic floor muscle strength is also significantly higher. Group training with a physiotherapist for 60 minutes once per week and twice daily at home 8–12 times for a period of 12 weeks between 20 and 36 weeks, holding the pelvic floor muscle contraction 6–8 seconds each time with rest periods of 6 seconds, is one accepted and effective intervention.[42]

Pelvic floor muscle training *after childbirth* is **effective in prevention and treatment of urinary incontinence.**[43–47]

Postpartum urinary retention

Definition

Absence of spontaneous micturition 6 hours after vaginal delivery or 6 hours after catheter removal (after cesarean delivery). A residual < 50 ml is normal, whereas a residual > 200 ml is abnormal.[48]

Incidence

The incidence of postpartum urinary retention is 0.5–3%.

Risk factors

Nulliparity, prolonged stages of labor, epidural anesthesia, operative or cesarean delivery.

Management

There are no trials to assess any intervention. Oral analgesia, standing and walking, warm bath, and immersing hands in cold water may help. An ultrasound for bladder volume may be helpful. If bladder volume by ultrasound is < 400 ml, wait; if > 400 ml, **intermittent catheterization every 4–6 hours until the woman is able to void and then the first residual volume is < 150 ml** is usually recommended, and preferred to indwelling catheterization. Pharmacological treatment should be avoided. If the woman has still retention upon discharge and/or after 48 hours, self-catherization should be taught. Prophylactic antibiotics are indicated in women who require catheterization. There are no clear long-term sequelae of postpartum urinary retention.

REFERENCES

1. Anonymous. Pregnancy and renal disease. Lancet 1975; 2(7939): 801–2. [review]
2. Fink JC, Schwartz SM, Benedetti TJ, Stehman-Breen CO. Increased risk of adverse maternal and infant outcomes among women with renal disease. Paediatr Perinat Epidemiol 1998; 12(3): 277–87. [II-2]
3. Bar J, Ben-Rafael Z, Padoa A, et al. Prediction of pregnancy outcome in subgroups of women with renal disease. Clin Nephrol 2000; 53(6): 437–44. [II-2]
4. Fischer MJ, Lehnerz SD, Hebert JR, Parikh CR. Kidney disease is an independent risk factor for adverse fetal and maternal outcomes in pregnancy. Am J Kidney Dis 2004; 43(3): 415–23. [II-3]
5. Milne JE, Lindheimer MD, Davison JM. Glomerular heteroporous membrane modeling in third trimester and postpartum before and during amino acid infusion. Am J Physiol Renal Physiol 2002; 282(1): F170–5. [II-2]
6. Lindheimer MD, Davison JM, Katz AI. The kidney and hypertension in pregnancy: twenty exciting years. Semin Nephrol 2001; 21(2): 173–89. [review]
7. Modena A, Hoffman M, Tolosa JE. Chronic renal disease in pregnancy: a modern approach to predicting outcome. Am J Obstet Gynecol 2005; 193: s86. [II-2]
8. Jungers P, Houillier P, Forget D, Henry-Amar M. Specific controversies concerning the natural history of renal disease in pregnancy. Am J Kidney Dis 1991; 17(2): 116–22. [III]
9. Jones DC. Pregnancy complicated by chronic renal disease. Clin Perinatol 1997; 24(2): 483–96. [III]
10. Huong DL, Wechsler B, Vauthier-Brouzes D, et al. Pregnancy in past or present lupus nephritis: a study of 32 pregnancies from a single centre. Ann Rheum Dis 2001; 60(6): 599–604. [II-2]
11. Hayslett JP. The effect of systemic lupus erythematosus on pregnancy and pregnancy outcome. Am J Reprod Immunol 1992; 28(3–4): 33: 199–204. [II-2]
12. Jungers P, Chauveau D, Choukroun G, et al. Pregnancy in women with impaired renal function. Clin Nephrol 1997; 47(5): 281–8. [II-2]
13. Jones DC, Hayslett JP. Outcome of pregnancy in women with moderate or severe renal insufficiency. N Engl J Med 1996; 335: 226–32. [II-2]
14. Hou SH. Frequency and outcome of pregnancy in women on dialysis. Am J Kidney Dis 1994; 23(1): 60–3. [II-3]
15. Armenti VT, Radomski JS, Moritz MJ, et al. Report from the National Transplantation Pregnancy Registry (NTPR): outcomes of pregnancy after transplantation. Clin Transpl 2001; 97–105. [II-2]
16. Abe S. An overview of pregnancy in women with underlying renal disorders. Am J Kidney Dis 1991; 17(2): 112–15. [II-3]

17. Holley JL, Bernardini J, Quadri KM, Greenberg A, Laifer SA. Pregnancy outcomes in a prospective matched control study of pregnancy and renal disease. Clin Nephrol 1996; 45(2): 77–82. [II-2]

18. Okundaye I, Abrinko P, Hou S. Registry of pregnancy in dialysis patients. Am J Kidney Dis 1998; 31(5): 766–73. [II-2]

19. Cunningham FG, Cox SM, Harstad TW, Mason RA, Pritchard JA. Chronic renal disease and pregnancy outcome. Am J Obstet Gynecol 1990; 163: 352–9. [II-3]

20. Hou S. Pregnancy in chronic renal insufficiency and end-stage renal disease. Am J Kidney Dis 1999; 33(2): 235–52. [II-3]

21. Nyberg G, Haljamae U, Frisenette-Fich C, Wennergren M, Kjellmer I. Breast-feeding during treatment with cyclosporine. Transplantation 1998; 65(2): 253–5. [II-3]

22. Chao AS, Huang JY, Lien R, et al. Pregnancy in women who undergo long-term hemodialysis. Am J Obstet Gynecol 2002; 187(1): 152–6. [II-3]

23. Romao JE Jr, Luders C, Kahhale S, et al. Pregnancy in women on chronic dialysis. A single-center experience with 17 cases. Nephron 1998; 78(4): 416–22. [II-3]

24. Registration Committee of the European Dialysis and Transplant Association. Successful pregnancies in women treated by dialysis and trasnplantation. BJOG 1980; 87: 839–45. [II-3]

25. Chan WS, Okun N, Kjellstrand CM. Pregnancy in chronic dialysis: a review and analysis of the literature. Int J Artif Organs 1998; 21(5): 259–68. [II-3]

26. Hou S. Pregnancy in chronic renal insufficiency and end-stage renal disease. Am J Kidney Dis 1999; 33: 235–52. [II-2]

27. Cheng PJ, Liu CM, Chang SD, Lin YT, Soong YK. Elevated second-trimester maternal serum hCG in patients undergoing haemodialysis. Prenat Diagn 1999; 19(10): 955–8. [II-3]

28. Armenti VT, Radomski JS, Moritz MJ, et al. Report from the National Transplantation Pregnancy Registry (NTPR): outcomes of pregnancy after transplantation. Clin Transpl 2002; 121–30. [II-2]

29. Armenti VT, McGrory CH, Cater JR, Radomski JS, Moritz MJ. Pregnancy outcomes in female renal transplant recipients. Transplant Proc 1998; 30(5): 1732–4. (level II-2)

30. Salmela K, Kyllonen, L, Homberg C. Gronhagen-Riska C. Impaired renal function after pregnancy in renal transplant recipients. Transplantation 1993; 56: 1372–5. [II-2]

31. McDermott S, Callaghan W, Szwejbka L, Mann H, Daguise V. Urinary tract infections during pregnancy and mental retardation and developmental delay. Obstet Gynecol 2000; 96: 113–19. [II-2]

32. Kontiokari T, Sundqvist K, Nuutinen M, et al. Randomised trial of cranberry-lingonberry juice and *Lactobacillus GG* drink for the prevention of urinary tract infections in women. BMJ 2001; 322: 1571. [RCT, 150 non-pregnant women]

33. Hill JB, Sheffield JS, McIntire DD, Wendel GD. Acute pyelonephritis in pregnancy. Obstet Gynecol 2005; 105: 18–23. [II-3, *n* = 440 cases of pyelonephritis]

34. Millar LK, Wing DA, Paul RH, Grimes DA. Outpatient treatment of pyelonephritis in pregnancy: a randomized controlled trial. Obstet Gynecol 1995; 86: 560–4. [RCT, *n* = 120]

35. Wing DA, Hendershott CM, DeBuque L, Millar LK. Outpatient treatment of acute pyelonephritis in pregnancy after 24 weeks. Obstet Gynecol 1999; 94: 683–8. [RCT, *n* = 92]

36. Teichman JMH. Acute renal colic from ureteral calculus. N Engl J Med 2004; 350: 684–93. [non-pregnant adult review]

37. Lewis DF, Robichaux AG, Jaekle RK, Marcum NG, Stedman CM. Urolithiasis in pregnancy: diagnosis, management and pregnancy outcome. J Reprod Med 2003; 48: 28–32. [II-3, *n* = 86]

38. Spencer JA, Chahal R, Kelly A, et al. Evaluation of painful hydronephrosis in pregnancy: magnetic resonance urographic patterns in physiological dilatation versus calculus obstruction. J Urol 2004; 171: 256–60. [II-3]

39. Asgari MA, Safarinejad MR, Hosseini SY, Dadkhah F. Extracorporeal shock wave lithotripsy of renal calculi during pregnancy. BJU Int 1999; 84: 615–17. [II-3]

40. Sampselle CM, Miler JM, Mims BL, et al. Effect of pelvic muscle exercise on transient incontinence during pregnancy and after childbirth. Obstet Gynecol 1998; 91: 406–12. [RCT, n = 46]

41. Reilly ET, Freeman RM, Waterfield MR, et al. Prevention of postpartum stress incontinence in primigravidae with increased bladder neck mobility: a randomized controlled trial of antenatal pelvic floor exercises. BJOG 2002; 109: 68–76 [RCT]

42. Morkved S, Bo K, Schei B, Salvesen KA. Pelvic floor muscle training during pregnancy to prevent urinary incontinence: a single-blind randomized controlled trial. Obstet Gynecol 2003; 191: 313–19. [RCT, *n* = 301]

43. Morkved S, Bo K. The effect of postpartum pelvic floor muscle exercise in the prevention and treatment of urinary incontinence. Int Urogynecol J 1997; 8: 217–64. [RCT]

44. Morkved S, Bo K. Effect of postpartum pelvic floor muscle training in prevention and treatment of urinary incontinence: a one-year follow up. BJOG 2000; 107: 1022–8. [RCT follow-up]

45. Wilson PD, Herbison GP. A randomized controlled trial of pelvic floor muscle exercises to treat postnatal urinary incontinence. Int Urogynecol J Pelvic Floor Dysfunct 1998; 9: 257–64. [RCT]

46. Chiarelli P. Female urinary incontinence in Australia: prevalence and prevention in postpartum women [dissertation]. Callaghan, Australia: The University of Newcastle; 2001. [RCT]

47. Glazener CMA, Herbison GP, Wilson PD, et al. Conservative management of persistent postnatal urinary and faecal incontinence: randomised controlled trial. BMJ 2001; 323: 593–6. [RCT]

48. Yip SK, Sahota D, Pang MW, Day L. Postpartum urinary retention. Obstet Gynecol 2005; 106: 602–6. [review]

16

Seizures

Meriem K Bensalem Owen and Franca Cambi

KEY POINTS

- **Epilepsy** is a chronic neurological condition in which recurrent (≥2) seizures occur unprovoked by systemic or neurological insults. The most important diagnostic tool is the **history**.
- There is an **increase in seizure frequency** in 25–33% of women with epilepsy during pregnancy. **Fetal loss**, peri-natal death, **congenital anomalies** (4–8%, or about twice the baseline risk), **neonatal hemorrhage** from vitamin K deficiency, **low birth weight**, **prematurity**, **induction**, **developmental delay**, and **childhood epilepsy** have been reported in the past to be more frequent, but more recent data do not confirm an increase in these complications.
- **Supplemental folic acid (up to 4 mg/day)** should be given to all women of childbearing age taking **antiepileptic drugs (AEDs)** and be continued during pregnancy.
- **Counsel** women with seizures or epilepsy about the risk of AED-associated teratogenicity and neurodevelop-mental delay, the necessity of folic acid supplementation, possible changes in seizure frequency during pregnancy, importance of medication compliance and AED level monitoring, inheritance risks for seizures, vit-amin K supplementation in the last month of pregnancy especially for women taking enzyme-inducing AEDs, and the benefits of breastfeeding.
- **Monotherapy at the lowest possible dose of the AED most efficient in controlling seizures** should be **the goal**.
- **Optimize AED therapy and complete AED changes** if possible **at least 6 months before planned conception**.
- **Stopping or changing an AED during pregnancy for the sole purpose of reducing teratogenicity is not advised.**
- **Prenatal testing** should include first trimester ultrasound, **maternal alpha-fetoprotein (AFP) levels, anatomy and echocardiographic ultrasounds,** and (if needed) amnio-centesis for amniotic fluid AFP and acetylcholinesterase.
- As pregnancy progresses, both total and non-protein bound plasma concentrations of AEDs decline; therefore, both total and free **AED levels should be monitored**. Monitor AED levels through the 8th postpartum week.

- Because there is a decrease in vitamin-K-dependent clotting factors, **10 mg/day of vitamin K should be pre-scribed orally from 36 weeks' gestation until delivery.**
- **Encourage breastfeeding** and monitor for sedation or feeding difficulties, which can be caused by certain AEDs, usually those with low protein binding.

Recommendations and guidelines presented in this chapter are in large part based on the Practice Parameters of the American Academy of Neurology.[1]

DIAGNOSES/DEFINITIONS

- **Seizures** result from an abnormal paroxysmal discharge of a group of cerebral neurons.
- **Epilepsy** is a chronic neurological condition in which recurrent (≥2) seizures occur unprovoked by systemic or neurological insults.

HISTORY

The most important diagnostic tool is the **history**. The examination is very often normal unless the patient has a structural brain lesion.

The history should include the following information:

- The presence or absence of an aura, which is a recurrent stereotypic abnormal sensation or experience. The aura is a simple partial seizure.
- Seizure description by an eye witness, including duration.
- Postictal phase, description and duration.
- Exacerbating factors.
- Birth history, especially when the seizure onset is in the neonatal period or early childhood.
- History of febrile convulsions, central nervous system infections, or head trauma with loss of consciousness.
- Family history.

Ancillary tests include electroencephalogram (EEG), laboratory tests as indicated by the history, and imaging of the brain. Magnetic resonance imaging (MRI) **of the head** is more sensitive than computed tomography (CT) scan for detecting subtle lesions.

EEG and MRI of the head pose no risk to the fetus, so that work-up for diagnosis should proceed in pregnancy just as in non-pregnant adults.

SYMPTOMS

The particular site of the brain affected usually determines the clinical expression of the seizure.

EPIDEMIOLOGY/INCIDENCE

Epilepsy occurs in 0.5–0.8% of the general population, with 5% of people reporting a seizure at some time in their life. The incidence of epilepsy in pregnant women is about **0.5%** in the USA. One-quarter to one-third of women with epilepsy have an increase in seizure frequency during pregnancy, and this occurs in about 30% of patients during their first trimester. Over 90% of women with epilepsy have successful pregnancies and deliver healthy babies.

ETIOLOGY/BASIC PATHOPHYSIOLOGY

Paroxysmal discharges of neurons occur when the threshold for firing of neuronal membranes is reduced. The pathophysiology of epileptic disorders is not very well understood. Structural abnormalities of neuronal transmitter receptors, channelopathies, excessive excitatory activity, cortical remodeling, and loss of inhibitory neuronal activity have all been implicated as possible mechanisms.

CLASSIFICATIONS

Depending on their onset, seizures are classified as either **partial** (focal) or **generalized**. The prototype for generalized seizures is the generalized tonic clonic (GTC) seizure. Partial seizures can be further subdivided into **simple partial** or **complex partial** seizures. During simple partial seizures awareness is preserved and the patient can either experience focal motor manifestations or experience a subjective feeling, called an aura. **Auras** can be olfactory, gustatory, sensory, auditory, visual, vertiginous sensations or psychic experiences (such as "déjà vu'). **Complex partial seizures** (CPS) are characterized by impairment of awareness; these seizures can secondarily generalize.

RISK FACTORS/ASSOCIATIONS

Difficult birth or complicated pregnancy, head trauma, central nervous system infections, family history, and complicated febrile convulsions.

COMPLICATIONS

Epileptic women of childbearing age should be informed of the risks associated with antiepileptic drug (AED) use prior to conception, and that seizures may be harmful to mother and fetus.

Maternal complications

About 25–33% of women with epilepsy have an **increase in seizure frequency** during pregnancy. Women can injure themselves during seizures, especially in the case of CPS or GTC seizures.

Fetal complications

GTC seizures increase the risk of hypoxia and acidosis as well as injury from blunt trauma. Generalized seizures but not partial seizures occurring during labor can affect fetal heart rate. **Fetal loss** (1.3–14%) and **perinatal death** (1.3–7.8%), **congenital malformations/anomalies** (4–8%, or about twice the baseline risk), **neonatal hemorrhage** from vitamin K deficiency, **low birth weight** (7–10%), **prematurity** (4–11%), **induction, developmental delay,** and **childhood epilepsy** are associated with in-utero exposure to AEDs. Most common congenital malformations, which differ for different AEDs, are cardiac, neural tube, craniofacial, fingers, and others. The largest series did not confirm these increased risks, except the risk of induction.[2] Bleeding occurs internally during the first 24 hours of life due to deficiency of vitamin-K-dependent clotting factors, and this complication is often associated with the use of enzyme-inducing AEDs (Table 16.1), which are competitive inhibitors of prothrombin precursors.[1,3]

Table 16.1 *Enzyme-inducing AEDs*	
Barbiturates	
Carbamazepine	
Oxcarbazepine	
Phenytoin	
Primidone	
Topiramate (with doses > 200 mg/day)	

AEDs, antiepileptic drugs.

Table 16.2	Pharmacokinetic profile of the most commonly used AEDs			
	Mechanism	Pregnancy category	Protein binding (%)	Adverse effects
First-generation AEDs				
Phenytoin (Dilantin)	Na	D	90	Rash, ataxia, hirsutism, gingival hypertrophy, osteoporosis
Carbamazepine (Tegretol)	Ca, GABA	D	75	Rash, diplopia, sexual function, osteoporosis
Valproic acid (Depakote, Depakene)	Na, GABA	D	85–95	Weight gain, tremor, hair loss, encephalopathy, hepatotoxicity, pancreatitis, polycystic ovaries
Ethosuximide (Zarontin)	T-type Ca	C	0	Nausea, vomiting, anorexia, rash
Second-generation AEDs				
Gabapentin (Neurontin)	?	C	0	Weight gain, edema, myoclonus
Pregabalin (Lyrica)	GABA transporter	C	0	Increased appetite, confusion, somnolence
Lamotrigine (Lamictal)	Na, Glutamate	C	55	Rash
Levetiracetam (Keppra)	?	C	0	Behavioral changes, asthenia
Oxcarbazepine (Oxcarbamazepine)	Na, Ca	C	40	Hyponatremia, diplopia rash
Tiagabine (Gabitril)	GABA reuptake	C	96	Encephalopathy, status epilepticus
Topiramate (Topamax)	Multiple	C	10	Renal stones, speech difficulties, paresthesias, weight loss, acidosis, closed-angle glaucoma
Zonisamide (Zonegran)	Na, T-type Ca	C	40–60	Renal stones, weight loss, paresthesias, contraindicated if history of allergy to sulfa drugs

AEDs, antiepileptic drugs; GABA, γ-aminobutyric acid L; Na, sodium channel; Ca, calcium channel.

MANAGEMENT

Principles

Effect of pregnancy on disease

About 25–30% of women with epilepsy have an increase in seizure frequency during pregnancy, and this occurs in about 30% of patients during their first trimester, especially if not well controlled. Increase in hepatic cytochrome P450 enzyme activity and renal clearance causes the **concentration** of some **AEDs to fall** (see Table 16.1). Decreased protein binding results **in higher levels of unbound biologically active AEDs** and may cause toxicity (Table 16.2). About 50% of women have no change in seizure activity, while about 25% experience a decrease in seizure activity.

Effect of disease on pregnancy

See complications above.

Preconception counseling

- Conception should be deferred until seizures are well controlled on minimum dose of medication. Monotherapy is preferable. Good compliance with AEDs is essential to avoid any seizures.

- If the patient has been seizure-free for ≥ 2 years and has a normal EEG,[1,4] consult with neurology regarding the possibility of stopping anticonvulsant medications. The patient should be observed for 6–12 months off AED before attempting conception. The risk of seizure relapse is 12% and 32% at 6 and 12 months, respectively.
- Patients should take **folic acid** supplementation preconceptionally (3 months) and continue it through the first trimester.[1,5] The appropriate dose of folic acid has not been determined. However, women on anticonvulsant medications associated with an increased risk of neural tube defects (carbamazepine and valproic acid) should receive **4 mg/day**. The dose can be decreased to 1 mg/day after 8 weeks. Women on anticonvulsant medications not specifically associated with an increased risk of neural tube defects can receive 1 mg/day.
- Inform patients that women with epilepsy receiving anticonvulsant medications have a 4–8% risk of having a baby with a congenital malformation.
- Driving privileges should be suspended for several months after a seizure; the exact length varies depending on the State.
- Home/work: avoid baths; take showers instead. No manipulation of heavy machinery or working at heights.
- Enzyme-inducing AEDs (see Table 16.1) enhance the metabolism of oral contraceptives, therefore decreasing their efficacy. Pregnancies should be planned.
- Emphasize that 90% of women with epilepsy have successful pregnancies and deliver healthy babies.

Prenatal counseling

At the first prenatal visit and during pregnancy as necessary, counsel women with seizures or epilepsy regarding all of the above preconception issues.[1,5] In addition, discuss:

- The possible change in seizure frequency during pregnancy.
- The risk of AED-associated teratogenicity and neuro-development delay.
- The importance of medication compliance and AED level monitoring during pregnancy. AED levels decline as a result of enhanced AED hepatic metabolism, changes in volume distribution, and increase in glomerular filtration rate, which leads to increased renal clearance and decreased protein binding. Therefore, levels should be measured on highly protein-bound AEDs.
- The pros and cons of breastfeeding.
- Inheritance risks for seizures.
- Child care issues.

Prenatal care

- Supplemental **folic acid** (at least 1 mg/day) should be given to all women of childbearing age taking AEDs and continued during pregnancy.

- A first trimester ultrasound is indicated for exact dating.
- Prenatal testing for neural tube defects with **alpha-feto-protein (AFP)** levels at 15–18 weeks' gestation (up to 21 weeks) – especially those being treated with carbamazepine, divalproex sodium, and valproic acid.
- If appropriate, amniocentesis for amniotic fluid AFP and acetylcholinesterase levels.
- **Ultrasound at 18–20 weeks'** gestation to assess for anatomic anomalies.
- Fetal **echocardiogram** at about 22 weeks.
- An ultrasound for growth at ≥ 32 weeks is not mandatory, but reserved for regular obstetric indications.
- Prescribe 10 mg/day of **vitamin K**[1] in the last month of pregnancy (from 36 weeks on) for patients taking enzyme-inducing AEDs (see Table 16.1). Neonates should receive vitamin K, 1 mg intramuscular (IM) at birth. Given this routine neonatal therapy with vitamin K for all neonates in many countries, the benefit of prenatal maternal vitamin K therapy is unknown, with no trial available for assessment.

Therapy (see Table 16.2)

- **Multidisciplinary** communication between the primary care provider, obstetrician, geneticist and neurologist/epileptologist for counseling and management of seizures and epilepsy during pregnancy is crucial.
- **There is no trial that indicates which AED is safest during pregnancy.** The best choice is the AED that best controls the seizures. All the AEDs are FDA (Food and Drug Administration) category C, except for the following AEDs which are category D: carbamazepine, phenobarbital, primidone, phenytoin and valproate. These five AEDs should therefore be avoided if possible, by using a different therapy beginning in the preconception period. Switching and abruptly stopping of AEDs are to be avoided.
- Regarding AED therapy, at the beginning of pregnancy it is recommended that the patient is on **monotherapy** with the AED of choice for the seizure type, achieving optimal seizure control at the lowest effective dose.
- **Monitor AED levels** (free levels) at the beginning of each trimester and in the last month of pregnancy. AED levels are expected to decline during pregnancy. For highly protein-bound AEDs, such as phenytoin and valproic acid, **free and total levels** should be measured. Free levels (serum or saliva) are available for carbamazepine, valproic acid, phenobarbital, and phenytoin. Avoid high peak levels by spreading out the total daily dose into multiple smaller doses.
- AEDs have effects on sodium, potassium, or calcium channels. They also can affect neurotransmitters, enhancing the inhibitory neurotransmitter γ-aminobutyric acid (GABA) or inhibiting the excitatory glutamate.

- AED Pregnancy Registry:
  - Phone 1-888-233-2334
  - www.aedpregnancyregistry.org

Delivery

AED medication should be continued in labor and in the immediate postpartum period.

Postpartum/breastfeeding

Breastfeeding is encouraged. The greater the protein binding of AED (see Table 16.2), the lower is its concentration in breast milk. Breastfeeding is not contraindicated in patients on anticonvulsant medications unless excess neonatal sedation occurs. **Monitor newborns** or infants for sedation when breastfeeding mothers with seizures take low protein-bound AEDs.[1]

For most AEDs, the pharmacokinetics in the mother will return to prepregnancy levels within 10–14 days after delivery. **Monitor AED levels** through the 8th postpartum week and adjust doses accordingly to avoid toxicity.[1] Sleep deprivation may exacerbate seizures, and should therefore be avoided. Women with epilepsy should not bathe their child while they are alone at home, should avoid stair climbing while carrying the baby; a portable changing pad placed on the floor should be used. New mothers should avoid using a carrier in front or on their back. A portable carrier with handles is a safer alternative in the event of a seizure and subsequent fall. Women taking AEDs that are enzyme inducers (see Table 16.1) who desire oral contraceptives should receive formulations containing $\geq 50\ \mu g$ of estrogen.[1]

REFERENCES

1. Practice parameters: management issues for women with epilepsy (summary statement). Report of the Quality Standards Subcommittee of the American Academy of Neurology. Neurology 1998; 51: 944–8. [guideline]
2. Richmond JR, Krishnamoorthy P, Andermann E, Benjamin A. Epilepsy and pregnancy: an obstetric perspective. Am J Obstet Gynecol 2004; 190: 371–9. [II-2]
3. Penovich PE, Eck KE, Economou VV. Recommendations for the care of women with epilepsy. Cleve Clin J Med 2004; 71 (Suppl 2): S49–57. [guideline]
4. McAuley JW, Anderson GD. Treatment of epilepsy in women of reproductive age: pharmacokinetic considerations. Clin Pharmacokinet 2002; 41: 559–79. [II-3]
5. Zahn CA, Morrell MJ, Collins SD, Labiner DM, Yerby MS. Management issues for women with epilepsy: a review of the literature. Neurology 1998; 51: 949–56. [review]

17

Headache

Tarvez Tucker

KEY POINTS

- **New-onset headache in pregnancy** should initiate a **thorough neurological evaluation** that may include **neuroradiographic studies or cerebrospinal fluid analysis.**
- Several worrisome conditions that cause headache occur more commonly in pregnant women. These include subarachnoid hemorrhage, stroke, pituitary tumor or apoplexy, and cerebral venous thrombosis.
- **Most causes of headache in pregnancy** are not due to ominous causes, but are **due to migraine or tension-type headache.**
- **Education about avoiding specific food, caffeine, and alcohol triggers** for migraine may reduce reliance on both preventive and acute medications. Pregnant patients with headache should **avoid skipping meals, should regularize their sleep and exercise habits, partake of a low tyramine diet,** and consider **magnesium supplementation** (plain over-the-counter magnesium 250–750 mg/day) as an adjunctive migraine preventive.
- **Acute and preventive medication should be used, as in non-pregnant women,** but with caution in pregnancy, since most are not absolutely contraindicated. Certain medicines are safer during specific trimesters.
- **Most** patients with migraine without aura, and many with migraine with aura, **enjoy improvement or remission of headache during pregnancy,** particularly during the second and third trimester.
- Patients who are unknowingly pregnant and who have taken medications early in pregnancy in the non-steroidal anti-inflammatory class or the triptan class can be reassured that drugs of these classes have not been shown to increase the incidence of teratogenicity.
- For **acute treatment** of primary headache, **acetaminophen, alone (preferably), or with codeine,** should be the first choice during all trimesters. **Naproxen and**

ibuprofen are safe and well-tolerated in pregnancy up to **28 weeks.** Severe unrelenting migraine responds well to parenteral antiemetics such as metoclopramide and prochlorperazine. **Propranolol is the prophylactic medication of choice** for the pregnant patient whose headache frequency requires daily preventive medication, and for whom non-pharmacological approaches to headache prophylaxis have failed.

BACKGROUND/EPIDEMIOLOGY

The relationship between headache and pregnancy has long been a focus of concern among clinicians for two significant reasons. First, benign, or primary headache types are far more common in women than men, and the impact of headache in women is directly affected by reproductive-life events. Migraine headache, which afflicts 18% of women in the USA, has an incidence that peaks at the time of menarche in young girls, has its highest prevalence in the reproductive years of 20–50, is commonly exacerbated by menses, influenced by use of the birth control pill and hormone replacement therapy, and is often improved following menopause. Pregnancy generally improves migraine, particularly migraine without aura, and the postpartum period often exacerbates migraine. Secondly, pregnancy has long been an exclusion criterion for controlled clinical trials. Therefore, data on the safety of drugs used for primary headache types in pregnant women, such as migraine and tension-type headache, is scant. Yet in a survey by the World Health Organization of drug utilization, 86% of pregnant women took some form of medication.

Clinicians should be particularly vigilant regarding headaches of secondary, worrisome causes, as several ominous conditions such as stroke, pituitary tumors, and subarachnoid hemorrhage occur more frequently in women who are pregnant than those who are not.[1]

DIAGNOSTIC CONSIDERATIONS FOR HEADACHE IN PREGNANCY

Causes

Secondary (ominous) causes of headache

- Cortical venous thrombosis or cranial sinus thrombosis
- Subarachnoid hemorrhage
- Pre-eclampsia or eclampsia associated with elevated blood pressure
- Stroke
- Idiopathic intracranial hypertension (pseudotumor cerebri)
- Pituitary tumor and pituitary apoplexy
- Headache associated with trauma to the head or neck, or to infection or disease of the meninges, sinuses, eyes or ears.

Primary (benign) causes of headache

- Migraine with and without aura
- Ocular migraine
- Tension-type headache
- Trigeminal autonomic cephalgias.

A classification of headache disorders is given in Table 17.1.

Diagnosis and symptoms of ominous headache

- The first or the worst headache of a patient's life
- Strictly unilateral headache (*always* occurs on one side)
- Headache associated with fever, meningeal signs, papilledema or focal neurological signs, including inco-ordination
- Headache that progressively worsens over time
- Headache that escalates with maneuvers which increase intracranial pressure such as Valsalva, lifting heavy weights, or bending over.

EPIDEMIOLOGY/BASIC PATHOPHYSIOLOGY

Eighteen percent of women and 6% of men experience **migraine** headache, but nearly half of these patients remain undiagnosed. It is estimated that an even greater number of women, approximately 40%, suffer from episodic or chronic tension-type headache. Migraine is generally improved during pregnancy, but it is important to note that a first migraine can occur during pregnancy, usually in the first

Table 17.1 *International Headache Society criteria for the diagnosis of headache disorders*

Migraine without aura
A. At least 5 attacks fulfilling criteria B–D
B. Headache duration of 4–72 hours
C. Headache with at least two of the following:
   a. Unilateral location
   b. Pulsating quality
   c. Moderate or severe pain intensity
   d. Aggravation by routine physical activity
D. During headache at least one of the following:
   a. Nausea and/or vomiting
   b. Photophobia and phonophobia
 	
Migraine with aura
A. Aura consisting of at least one of the following:
   a. Fully reversible visual symptoms (flickering lights or spots) or loss of vision
   b. Fully reversible sensory symptoms (paresthesias or numbness)
   c. Fully reversible speech disturbance
B. Aura develops gradually over ≥5 minutes and lasts ≤ 60 minutes
 	
Tension-type headache
A. At least 10 episodes occurring less than one day per month on average and fulfilling criteria B–D
B. Headache lasting from 30 minutes to 7 days
C. Headache that has at least two of the following characteristics.
   a. Bilateral location
   b. Pressing/tightening (non-pulsatile) quality
   c. Mild or moderate intensity
   d. Not aggravated by routine physical activity

Adapted from ICHD-2, *International Classification of Headache Disorders* 2nd edn., published in *Cephalalgia* vol. 24, Supplement 1, 2004, Blackwell Publishing, Edinburgh, UK.

trimester. The elevated and sustained levels of plasma estrogens are felt to be protective during pregnancy and the fall in estrogen at the onset of menses a factor in menstrually-associated migraine. Estrogens are known to increase pain thresholds in animal studies[2] and endogenous opioids also increase as pregnancy progresses. Migraine returns rapidly after delivery, usually within 3–6 days.

Blood vessels within the brain, particularly at the circle of Willis, are pain-sensitive, as are the venous sinuses within the dura. Therefore it is not surprising that subarachnoid hemorrhage from a ruptured aneurysm, or vessel distention from a venous thrombosis, would produce head pain. Intracerebral and subarachnoid blood acts as an irritant, setting up an inflammatory reaction and potentially interfering with cerebrospinal fluid reabsorption, causing hydrocephalus.

The pathophysiology of migraine is complex and incompletely understood. Even less is known about the genesis of tension-type headache. Functional magnetic resonance imaging (MRI) studies of patients with migraine show that a period of hyperemia precedes the oligemia present during the migraine aura and the headache itself can begin before hyperemia, while blood flow in the cerebral cortex is still reduced. These studies thereby challenge the older theories of migraine pathophysiology of aura caused by vasoconstriction and headache caused by vasodilation. The roles of neurogenic inflammation, of central sensitization in the trigeminal pathways of the brainstem, and of spreading neuronal depression during headache are currently under study.

GENETICS

The vast majority of migraine patients have a first-degree relative with the disorder. However, the only migrainous syndrome for which we have some genetic understanding is familial hemiplegic migraine, which has an autosomal dominant mode of inheritance. The gene for most families with this syndrome, which causes reversible hemiparesis with headache attacks, has been identified on the short arm of chromosome 19p13.

PREGNANCY CONSIDERATIONS
Effect of pregnancy on the disorder

There have been several retrospective studies of the course of migraine in pregnancy.[3,4] **Most (58–79%) women note improvement or complete remission** of their headaches, generally by the second and third trimester. Women whose migraines began during the menarche and **those with menstrually associated migraine are more likely to have headaches recede during pregnancy.**[3] Women with migraine without aura experience improvement in headache during pregnancy more than women with migraine with aura.[5]

Some migraineurs will have increased head pain during the first trimester. A small percentage of women with migraine in these studies developed worse headache during pregnancy. Most of these women had migraine with aura.

Effect of the disorder on pregnancy

Patients with migraine do not have an increased incidence of teratogenicity, pre-eclampsia, stillbirth, or miscarriage compared with controls.[6] However, one study from Denmark reported that women with migraine had a higher incidence of low-birth-weight infants than women without migraine.[7]

EVALUATION OF HEADACHE IN PREGNANCY

Headache in pregnancy should be evaluated in the same manner as headache without pregnancy. The clinician should be alert to the warning signs of ominous headache, as listed above. Again, certain conditions that cause worrisome headache are more common in pregnancy. Headache that presents in a sudden (thunderclap) fashion may indicate subarachnoid hemorrhage, particularly if associated with a change in consciousness or focal neurological signs. Sudden headache can also accompany pre-eclampsia or pituitary apoplexy. Venous or sinus thrombosis, associated with the puerperium, can present with seizure, precipitous headache, vomiting, or focal signs and, if intracranial pressure is elevated, papilledema.

Whether or not to obtain a computed tomography (CT) or MRI scan as part of the evaluation of headache in pregnancy depends on the degree of suspicion for an ominous cause of headache. Generally speaking, **head CT and MRI are safe in pregnancy**, although the decision to obtain the study should be based on the risk of missing a structural or serious cause of headache without the study. **Gadolinium**, used as a contrast agent for MRI scanning, does cross the placenta.[8] However, if an intracerebral bleed, mass lesion, or meningitis is suspected, the benefit of CT, MRI or magnetic resonance angiography (MRA) far outweighs the potential risks, including the risk of gadolinium, which was deemed **safe** by the European Society of Radiology, since no effect on the fetus has been reported in the literature after gadolinium contrast media.[9] Lumbar puncture to diagnose meningitis or hemorrhage should not be performed without first obtaining a CT of the brain without contrast to avoid the risk of herniation if a mass, or cerebral edema, is present.

ACUTE THERAPY FOR HEADACHE (FIGURE 17.1)

Long-standing therapies for the treatment of acute, primary headache in non-pregnant women include short-acting analgesics such as acetaminophen, aspirin, non-steroidal anti-inflammatory drugs (NSAIDs), opioids, ergot alkaloids, isometheptene, and caffeine–barbiturate combinations. Newer migraine-specific medications belong to the triptan class, heralded by the entry of the first triptan, sumatriptan, in the USA in the early 1990s.

Fortunately, most primary headaches tend to improve as pregnancy progresses. However, in the first trimester, when headache can be volatile, concern arises as to the potential effect of analgesics on embryogenesis. The situation is particularly poignant as many women, unknowingly pregnant, will have used acute short-acting medications to treat

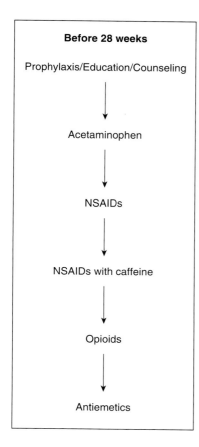

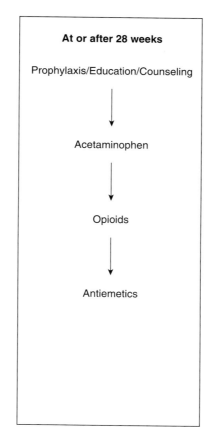

Figure 17.1

Proposed algorithm for management of primary headache in pregnancy, based on gestational age. NSAIDs, non-steroidal anti-inflammatory drugs.

migraine or tension-type headache in the very early days or weeks after conception.

Most simple analgesics are FDA (Food and Drug Administration) Pregnancy Risk Category C (risk to humans has not been ruled out). These include aspirin (Category D in the late third trimester), codeine, propoxyphene, butalbital, and all the triptans. Category B drugs (no evidence of risk in humans, but without controlled human studies) include **acetaminophen, caffeine, ibuprofen, indomethacin, and naproxen** (note **the latter three are Category D in the third trimester**). NSAID use has been associated with premature closure of the ductus arteriosus and pulmonary hypertension in the neonate when given late in pregnancy.[10]

Meperidine and morphine are FDA Category C in pregnancy, but their use should be restricted late in pregnancy.[3] Prednisone, which can be used to treat 'status migrainosus,' is preferred over dexamethasone because the latter more readily crosses the placenta.

Ergotamines and dihydroergotamine are Category X, and should never be used in pregnant women. Ergots are abortifacients and have been shown to cause fetal distress and birth defects (class III).

Interestingly, the antiemetic medicines, such as **metoclopramide, chlorpromazine, and prochlorperazine,** are effective parenterally for the head pain itself, as well as the

nausea and vomiting that can accompany migraine, and are generally considered safe in pregnancy. Intravenous or intramuscular antiemetics, with fluid replacement, are very effective in aborting status migrainosus, or severe headache in the Emergency Room or Urgent Care Center.

Although aspirin is labeled Category C, it is unique in that some clinical trials have studied aspirin during pregnancy for conditions other than headache, for example, in patients with antiphospholipid syndrome.[11] Recommended dosing of aspirin is high, at 500–1000 mg per headache attack.[5]

The triptans are serotonin (5-hydroxytryptamine; 5-HT) 1B/1D receptor agonists that are singularly effective in treating migraine headache and the accompanying symptoms of photosensitivity, nausea, and vomiting. Studies of sumatriptan use in pregnant women have recently been reviewed by Loder[12] and describe the favorable clinical outcome of pregnancies in women exposed in the first trimester to sumatriptan. The triptan class is Category C and, as such, is not recommended for pregnant migraineurs. However, based on the pregnancy registry, if a patient has unwittingly taken **sumatriptan**, prior to knowledge of her pregnancy, **reassurance is appropriate given the probable lack of teratogenicity of this drug**. It is not known whether this positive outcome may also be extrapolated to other medications in the triptan class.

HEADACHE PROPHYLAXIS IN PREGNANCY

Since primary headaches generally diminish in the second and third trimester, clinicians should be encouraged to treat headaches in early pregnancy with short-acting agents such as acetaminophen, or low doses of codeine. **Preventive therapy should be reserved for those few pregnant patients whose headaches continue to worsen throughout pregnancy.** There are no prospective randomized clinical trials of migraine prophylactic drugs in pregnant women.

Non-pharmacological therapies should be initiated first. **Relaxation training, thermal biofeedback** combined with relaxation techniques, and **cognitive behavioral therapies** have been subjected to rigorous well-designed randomized clinical trials in non-pregnant adults and show efficacy in migraine prevention.[13] In contradistinction, evidence based therapy recommendations for acupuncture, hypnosis, and chiropractic manipulation for headache prevention are not as yet available.

Whenever a second comorbid condition exists with migraine, it is advisable to use one drug to treat both conditions. Examples include migraine and epilepsy, wherein an anticonvulsant may be effective to treat both conditions, and migraine and depression, for which an SSRI (selective serotonin reuptake inhibitor) such as fluoxetine (Category B) may similarly permit monotherapy.

Propranolol is probably the safest drug to use in later pregnancy as a preventive intervention for headache, as it has not been known to have a teratogenic effect.[5] Verapamil (calcium channel blocker) may also be beneficial.[14] Valproic acid should be avoided for headache prophylaxis, due to its potential for causing neural tube defects. The use of topiramate and gabapentin should be restricted for headache prophylaxis in view of their potential association with fetal defects, although these drugs can be very effective for non-pregnant migraineurs.

Education about avoiding specific food, caffeine, and alcohol triggers for migraine may reduce reliance on both preventive and acute medications. Pregnant patients with headache should **avoid skipping meals, should regularize their sleep and exercise habits, partake of a low tyramine diet**, and consider **magnesium supplementation** (plain over-the-counter magnesium 250–750 mg/day) as an adjunctive migraine preventive.

REFERENCES

1. Silberstein SD. Headaches in pregnancy. Neurol Clin 2004; 22(4): 727–56. [review]
2. Dawson-Basoa MB, Gintzler AR. 17-Beta-estradiol and progesterone modulate an intrinsic opioid analgesic system. Brain Res 1993; 601: 241–5. [II-3]
3. Aube M. Migraine in pregnancy. Neurology 1999; 53 (4 Suppl 1): S26–8.
4. Silberstein SD, Lipton RB, Goadsby PJ. Headache in Clinical Practice. London: Martin Dunitz; 2002. [review]
5. Fox AW, Diamond ML, Spierings ELH. Migraine during pregnancy. CNS Drugs 2005 19(6):465–81. [review]
6. Wainscott G, Volans GN. The outcome of pregnancy in women suffering from migraine. Postgrad Med J 1978; 54: 98–102. [II-2]
7. Olesen C, Steffensen FH, Sorensen HT, Nielsen GL, Olsen J. Pregnancy outcome following prescription for sumatriptan. Headache 1999; 40: 20–4. [II-3]
8. Schwartz RB. Neurodiagnostic imaging of the pregnant patient. In: Deinsky O, Feldmann E, Hainline B, eds. Neurologic Complications of Pregnancy. New York: Raven Press; 1994: 243–8. [review]
9. Webb JAW, Thomsen HS, Morcos SK. The use of iodinated and gadolinium contrast media during pregnancy and lactation. Eur Radiol 2005; 15: 1234–40. [review]
10. Morris JL, Rosen DA, Rosen KR. Nonsteroidal anti-inflammatory agents in neonates. Paediatr Drugs 2003; 5: 385–405. [review]
11. Vainio M, Kujansuu E, Iso-Mustajarvi J, Maenpaa J. Low dose acetylsalicyclic acid in prevention of pregnancy-induced hypertension and intrauterine growth retardation in women with bilateral uterine artery notches. BJOG 2002; 109: 161–7. [II-2]
12. Loder E. Safety of sumatriptan in pregnancy: a review of the data so far. CNS Drugs 2003; 17(1): 1–7. [review]
13. Campbell JK, Penaien DB, Wall EM, and the US Headache Consortium. Evidenced-based guidelines for migraine headache: behavioral and physical treatments. In: AOA.net (online). Available at: www.aoanet.org/MembersOnly/hcnonpharnpdf, Accessed February 25, 2006. [review]
14. Silberstein SD. Migraine. Lancet 2004; 363: 381–91. [review]

18

Spinal cord injury

Leonardo Pereira

KEY POINTS

- Pregnancies in women with spinal cord injury (SCI) are associated with increased risks of **urinary tract infections, preterm birth, and anemia. The most worrisome, potentially fatal** complication is **autonomic dysreflexia (ADR).**
- Antenatal management of women with pre-existing SCI includes **frequent urinary cultures** *or* **antibiotic suppression (self-intermittent catheterization** is preferred); **stool softeners** and a **high fiber diet**; routine **skin examinations**; and **frequent position changes.** In women with lesions above the level of T5, baseline and serial pulmonary function tests (PFTs) are used to assess vital capacity. There are insufficient data at this time to recommend universal thromboprophylaxis.
- ADR affects **up to 85% of women with lesions at or above the level of T6.** The most common sign of ADR is **systemic hypertension.** Symptoms are synchronous with uterine contractions. Prevention involves avoidance of triggers (constipation, catheterization, examinations, etc.), and **early epidural anesthesia.** Antihypertensive therapy for ADR includes **nitroprusside, amyl nitrate, trimethaphan,** and **hydralazine.**
- Several **prophylactic procedures** are necessary for **labor and delivery** in the SCI woman. Among these, **continuous hemodynamic monitoring during labor by maternal electrocardiogram, pulse oximetry, and arterial line** should be performed in patients with **baseline pulmonary insufficiency.**

DIAGNOSIS/DEFINITION

Spinal cord injury (SCI) is diagnosed neurologically. It can occur following trauma to the spinal cord but also occurs as a result of a variety of pathologies (e.g. neural tube defect, congenital anomaly, infectious, and transverse myelitis).

EPIDEMIOLOGY/INCIDENCE

About 1000 new spinal cord injuries per year occur in women aged 16–30 years old in the USA. SCI diagnosed during pregnancy is rare. SCI pre-existing pregnancy is relatively more common.

CLASSIFICATION

SCI is classified by its etiology, and, especially, by the level of the lesion. The higher is the functional level of the lesion, the worse are the disease and prognosis.

COMPLICATIONS

For women with pre-existing SCI: **asymptomatic bacteriuria, lower urinary tract infections** (up to 35% incidence),[1] and **pyelonephritis** are common. The risk of preterm birth is between 8 and 13%.[1-4] Anemia can occur in 12% of women with SCI, especially with history of chronic pyelonephritis, decubitus, and/or renal failure. The most worrisome, potentially fatal complication is **autonomic dysreflexia (ADR).**

PREGNANCY MANAGEMENT
Preconception counseling

Women with pre-existing SCI who are contemplating pregnancy should be referred for preconception counseling. If the spinal cord lesion is congenital or hereditary in origin, genetic counseling is warranted. Women with congenital spinal lesions such as meningomyelocele should be made aware of the increased risk of spinal cord lesions to their offspring and placed on 4 mg/day of folic acid.[5] All other SCI women should take at least 400 μg of folic acid preconceptionally.

Patients with pre-existing SCI are probably at no greater risk than the general obstetric population for either congenital malformations or fetal death.[6-8] In contrast to patients with SCI antecedent to pregnancy, patients who suffer traumatic SCI during pregnancy may be at risk for **spontaneous abortion, fetal malformation, abruptio placentae, or direct fetal injury.**[9] A fetal malformation rate of 11% has been reported in 45 patients who suffered spinal cord injuries during pregnancy.[8]

Prenatal care

Acute spinal cord injury during pregnancy

Acutely, SCI results in neurogenic shock or 'spinal shock' due to the loss of sympathetic innervation. This typically presents with hypotension, bradycardia, and hypothermia due to parasympathetic effects. Adequate volume resuscitation and pressor support should be administered. Direct measurements of pulmonary capillary wedge pressure with a pulmonary artery catheter will assist clinical management. Internal hemorrhage should be identified and treated with the aid of a trauma surgeon if possible.

In the setting of acute SCI, initial stabilization of the neck and spinal column should occur immediately and airway patency should be secured. This may require a jaw thrust maneuver, nasal trumpet, or nasal intubation. Administration of methylprednisolone within 8 hours of SCI may improve neurological recovery in select cases.[10] The risk of deep venous thrombosis and pulmonary embolism is greatest within 8 weeks of traumatic SCI.[11] Prophylactic anticoagulation should be considered during this period.

Antenatal management of pre-existing spinal cord injury

Urinary
Frequent urinary cultures *or* **antibiotic suppression.**[12–14] **Self-intermittent catheterization** (every 4–6 hours, and more frequently in the third trimester) is preferred to continuous indwelling catheterization. The perineum should be cleaned before catheterization.

Gastrointestinal
Stool softeners and a **high-fiber diet** are used to prevent constipation.

Dermatology
Routine **skin examinations** for any evidence of decubitus ulcers at each visit, and **frequent position changes.** Wheelchairs may need to be resized or fitted with extra padding.

Pulmonary
In patients with high thoracic or cervical spine lesions, usually above the level of T5, baseline and serial **pulmonary function tests** (PFTs) to assess vital capacity (VC), and, especially if VC < 13 ml/kg, **possible need for ventilatory assistance** in labor are recommended.[12,14] Supine tilted positioning is suggested for labor.

Thromboembolic
Despite a theoretical increased risk of venous thromboembolism, there are **insufficient data at this time to recommend universal thromboprophylaxis** during pregnancy. Each case should be addressed individually. Women suffering acute SCI during pregnancy should receive thromboprophylaxis for at least 8 weeks post trauma based on the high rate of deep venous thromboses reported in non-pregnant patients during this time period.[11]

Hematology
Screen for and treat anemia aggressively.

General support
Focus on range of motion exercises in lower extremities, elevation of legs, exercises to increase upper body strength, and social support services.

Autonomic dysreflexia

ADR is the most serious complication impacting obstetric management, affecting **up to 85% of patients with lesions at or above the level of T6**[2] (above sympathetic outflow and above the upper level of greater splanchnic flow). It is potentially fatal. It is attributed to loss of hypothalamic control over sympathetic spinal reflexes of somatic or visceral sensory impulses still active distal to the level of the lesion.[15] **The most common sign of ADR is systemic hypertension** (vasoconstriction), which is often severe. Maternal clinical manifestations include hyperthermia, piloerection, diaphoresis, increased extremity spasticity, pupil dilation, nasal congestion, respiratory distress, bradycardia (most common) or tachycardia or cardiac arrhythmia, extreme fear and anxiety, headache, loss of consciousness, intracranial bleed, convulsions, and even death. **Symptoms are synchronous with uterine contractions.** Blood pressure rises with contractions, then normalizes in between.

General
ADR may be mistaken for preeclampsia, but several findings may help differentiate the two conditions (Table 18.1).

Triggers
Afferent stimuli (usually distention) from hollow viscus (bladder, bowel, uterus) or skin (irritation or temperature change) below level of the spinal cord lesion. These include uterine contractions, cervical manipulation/pelvic examinations, cold stirrups, insertion of speculum, manipulation of urinary catheters, catheter obstruction, constipation, and decubitus ulcers.

Preventive management of autonomic dysreflexia in susceptible patients
1. Routine bladder catheterization with topical anesthetic.
2. Avoidance of constipation with bowel regimen.

Table 18.1	*Differentiating ADR from pre-eclampsia*				
Disease	Symptoms	Hematological	Hepatic function	Urinalysis	Treatment
Pre-eclampsia	Independent of uterine contractions	Decreased platelets	Elevated uric acid and/or liver function tests	Proteinuria	Intravenous prophylactic $MgSO_4$ and delivery (Chapter 1)
ADR	Synchronous with uterine contractions	Normal	Normal	Norepinephrine	Remove stimulus; antihypertensive therapy

$MgSO_4$, magnesium sulfate; ADR, autonomic dysreflexia.

3. Pelvic examinations: consider pudendal block or topical anesthetic (lidocaine) prior to examination. Avoid cold stirrups or speculums if possible.
4. Prophylactic **antihypertensive therapy** (as necessary to prevent *recurrent* ADR) with oral nifedipine (10–20 mg), or terazosin (1–10 mg qhs) or clonidine.[16]
5. **Epidural anesthesia** at the onset of labor.

Treatment of autonomic dysreflexia
1. Remove offending stimulus. Expedite delivery if in second stage with forceps or vacuum or perform cesarean delivery (discuss this with patient prior to labor).
2. Positioning: blood pressure may be lowered by tilting head upward.
3. Antihypertensive therapy – rapid onset:
   - **Nitroprusside** (0.5 µg/kg/min intravenously, titrate to blood pressure), or sublingual sodium nitroglycerin (0.3–0.6 ml).
   - **Amyl nitrate** (1 capsule crushed for inhalation).
   - Ganglionic blocking agent: **trimethaphan** (Arfonad), 1 ampule in 500 ml D5W at 3–4 mg/min continuous intravenously.
   - α-Adrenergic blocking agent (guanethidine).
   - Direct vasodilator: **hydralazine**, 10 mg orally, or nifedipine, bite and swallow tablet 10–20 mg.
4. Anesthesia – **regional** (preferred), or general anesthesia can treat ADR.

Antepartum testing

No specific testing is recommended.

Ascertainment and preparation for (preterm or term) labor

Women with spinal cord transection above T10, especially above T6, may have **painless labor**, and are at risk for unattended delivery. Even with lower levels, if transection is complete, patients may not feel contractions. Symptoms which are related through the sympathetic nervous system may alert patients to labor. These should be reviewed with patients as they near term: abdominal or leg spasms, shortness of breath, and increased spasticity. **Uterine palpation techniques** should be reviewed with patients. Consider inpatient hospitalization, especially if patients are dilated and have high (above T6) lesions (because of possible unattended delivery with ADR).

Women with SCI should have an anesthesia consult before term, with plan for epidural at onset of labor.

Delivery

Patients with spinal cord transection above the level of T10 are at risk for unattended delivery secondary to unrecognized contractions. Consider inpatient hospitalization for patients with advanced cervical dilation because of the risk of unattended delivery, or patients with spinal cord lesions above the level of T6 because of the high risk of ADR.[1,14,17]

Labor is the period during which ADR is most likely to occur; therefore, there should be a plan for delivery in a unit capable of invasive hemodynamic monitoring. **Appropriate antihypertensive therapy should be available at the patient's bedside during labor.** If induction is necessary, women with cervical ripening should have continuous blood pressure monitoring, and possibly an epidural. **Continuous hemodynamic monitoring during labor by maternal electrocardiogram, pulse oximetry, and arterial line** should be performed in patients with **baseline pulmonary insufficiency.**[14,17] Body temperature should be closely monitored, without assuming that temperature increases are due to intra-amniotic infection (may be caused by underlying thermodysregulation). A Foley catheter may be placed during labor to avoid bladder distention or repeated catheterizations. Patients should change position and have a skin examination every 2 hours to prevent decubitus ulcer formation. Episiotomy should be avoided, not only because it is not beneficial in general but also because it is a possible trigger for ADR.

The rate of spontaneous vaginal delivery and need for assisted vaginal delivery depends on the level of the spinal cord lesion. Approximately 30% of SCI patients will be delivered by cesarean section[1,2,4] (Table 18.2).

Table 18.2 *Mode of delivery stratified by level of SCI*[a]

Delivery mode	≥ T6 level (%)	< T6 level (%)	All SCI (%)
SVD	13 (29)	18 (46)	31 (37)
AVD	19[b] (42)	7 (18)	26 (31)
CD	13 (29)	14 (36)	27 (32)
Total	45 (100)	39 (100)	84 (100)

SCI, spinal cord injury; SVD, spontaneous vaginal delivery; AVD, assisted vaginal delivery; CD, cesarean delivery.
[a]Combined data from Wanner et al,[1] Verduyn,[2] and Hughes et al.[4]
[b]Majority of assisted vaginal deliveries performed because of autonomic dysreflexia.

Anesthesia

Epidural anesthesia should be administered early in labor.[18,19] This is to prevent ADR, with a goal for T10 level. Prehydration is very important, as these patients tend to be hypotensive.

Postpartum/breastfeeding

In the postpartum period, bladder distention and constipation should be avoided. The use of thromboprophylaxis of SCI patients during the puerperium is controversial. Breastfeeding should be encouraged. Oral contraceptive pills appear to be safe,[2,20] although some authors discourage their use.[21] Progesterone-only pills, transdermal patches, intramuscular medroxyprogesterone injections, condoms and spermicide, and intrauterine devices are all acceptable alternatives.

RESOURCES

SCI patients and non-medical personnel may be referred to www.spinalcord.org/resource, posted by the NSCIA (National Spinal Cord Injury Association), for more information.

REFERENCES

1. Wanner MB, Rageth CJ, Zach GA. Pregnancy and autonomic hyperreflexia in patients with spinal cord lesions. Paraplegia 1987; 25: 482–90. [II-3]
2. Verduyn WH. Spinal cord injured women, pregnancy and delivery. Paraplegia 1986; 24: 231–40. [II-3]
3. Westgren N, Hultling C, Levi R, Westgren M. Pregnancy and delivery in women with a traumatic spinal cord injury in Sweden, 1980–1991. Obstet Gynecol 1993; 81: 926–30. [II-3]
4. Hughes SJ, Short DJ, Usherwood MM, Tebbutt H. Management of the pregnant woman with spinal cord injuries. Br J Obstet Gynaecol 1991; 98: 513–18. [II-3]
5. Center for Disease Control. Recommendations for the use of folic acid to reduce the number of cases of spina bifida and other neural tube defects. MMWR Morb Mortal Wkly Rep 1992; 41: 1. [review, based on RCTs; see also Chapter 1 of *Obstetric Evidence Based Guidelines]*
6. Burns AS, Jackson AB. Gynecologic and reproductive issues in women with spinal cord injury. Phys Med Rehabil Clin N Am 2001; 12: 183–99. [review]
7. McGregor JA, Meeuwsen J. Autonomic hyperreflexia: a mortal danger for spinal cord-damaged women in labor. Am J Obstet Gynecol 1985; 151: 330–3. [III; case report of intraventricular hemorrhage due to autonomic hyperreflexia during labor]
8. Göller H, Paeslack V. Pregnancy damage and birth-complications in the children of paraplegic women. Paraplegia 1972; 10: 213–17. [II-3]
9. Atterbury JL, Groome LJ. Pregnancy in women with spinal cord injuries. Orthop Nurs 1998; 33: 603–13. [review]
10. Gilson GJ, Miller AC, Clevenger FW, Curet LB. Acute spinal cord injury and neurogenic shock in pregnancy. Obstet Gynecol Surv 1995; 50: 556–60. [II-3]
11. Sugarman B. Medical complications of spinal cord injury. Q J Med 1985; 54: 3–18. [II-3]
12. Obstetric management of patients with spinal cord injuries. ACOG Committee Opinion No. 275. American College of Obstetricians and Gynecologists. Obstet Gynecol 2002; 100: 625–7. [review]
13. Young BK, Katz M, Klein SA. Pregnancy after spinal cord injury: altered maternal and fetal response to labor. Obstet Gynecol 1983; 62(1): 59–63. [II-3]
14. Greenspoon JS, Paul RH. Paraplegia and quadriplegia: special considerations during pregnancy and labor and delivery. Am J Obstet Gynecol 1986; 155: 738–41. [III]
15. Berghella V, Spector T, Trauffer P, Johnson A. Pregnancy in patients with preexisting transverse myelitis. Obstet Gynecol 1996; 87: 809–12. [III; case reports of transverse myelitis]
16. Vaidyanathan S, Soni BM, Sett P, et al. Pathophysiology of autonomic dysreflexia: long-term treatment with terazosin in adult and paediatric spinal cord injury patients manifesting recurrent dysreflexic episodes. Spinal Cord 1998; 36: 761–70. [II-2]
17. Robertson DNS. Pregnancy and labour in paraplegics. Paraplegia 1972; 10: 209–12. [III]
18. Baker ER, Cardenas DD. Pregnancy in spinal cord injured women. Arch Phys Med Rehabil 1996; 77: 501–7. [review]
19. Pope CS, Markenson GR, Bayer-Zwirello LA, Maissel GS. Pregnancy complicated by chronic spinal cord injury and history of autonomic hyperreflexia. Obstet Gynecol 2001; 97: 802–3. [III; 1 new case report and review]
20. Jackson AB, Wadley V. A multicenter study of women's self-reported reproductive health after spinal cord injury. Arch Phys Med Rehabil 1999; 80: 1420–8. [II-2]
21. Sipski ML. The impact of spinal cord injury on female sexuality, menstruation and pregnancy: a review of the literature. J Am Paraplegia Soc 1991; 14: 122–6. [review]

19

Cancer

Elyce Cardonick

KEY POINTS

- **Avoid delay in diagnosis**, by performing the necessary diagnostic studies in a timely and adequate fashion as in non-pregnant adults, with rare exceptions.
- Avoid unnecessary radiological studies unless results will alter cancer treatment or patient decisions during pregnancy.
- Avoid iatrogenic preterm deliveries.
- When choosing a particular **chemotherapeutic regimen** for a particular cancer, **choose one based on the most experience of use and proven safety during pregnancy**, as long as it will offer a **similar chance of cure** for the pregnant patient. **Administer the same doses of chemotherapy as given to non-pregnant women.**
- Send **placental pathology** for all cancers, especially in cases of melanoma.
- Close multidisciplinary management, especially with **medical and radiation oncologists, maternal–fetal specialist and neonatalogist**, is vital to optimize outcomes.

INCIDENCE/EPIDEMIOLOGY

Cancer complicates approximately 1/1000 pregnancies, and 1 out of every 118 malignancies is associated with pregnancy.[1] There is no increased incidence of malignancy in pregnant women. Upon reviewing the literature, almost 400 pregnant women have been diagnosed and treated for cancer during pregnancy. The most common cancers that occur during pregnancy are breast, cervical, leukemia, lymphoma, thyroid, and melanoma.[2]

GENERAL CANCER IN PREGNANCY CONSIDERATIONS

There are no specific trials regarding management of cancer in pregnancy. **Delay in diagnosis should be avoided** by performing the necessary diagnostic studies in a timely and adequate fashion as in non-pregnant adults. **Diagnostic measures** should not be delayed when a pregnant patient presents with a suspicious sign or symptom. Staging measures, however, can often be delayed until after delivery if the results would not change the course of treatment or patient decisions during pregnancy. Chemotherapy regimens should be comparable to those used in non-pregnant patients; however, using the newest agents is not recommended in the absence of safety data even if favored for non-pregnant patients; for example, non-pregnant women may be treated for breast cancer with Adriamycin (doxorubicin)/Cytoxan (cyclophosphamide), idarubicin/Cytoxan, or epirubicin/ Cytoxan. Although the latter regimen may be better tolerated in non-pregnant patients, the first regimen has the most reported cases in the pregnancy literature, and so this regimen with the most experience of use during pregnancy should be chosen, until more information accumulates. Different drugs in the same class of chemotherapy agents may have different properties that allow more placental transfer. **Once the regimen is chosen, the pregnant woman should be given the same doses of chemotherapy as given to a non-pregnant woman for the same cancer type and stage**, to ensure best treatment and outcomes. If dosage is based on patient weight, the woman's changing weight during pregnancy should be used, not the ideal body weight. **Close multidisciplinary management, especially with an oncologist and a maternal–fetal specialist knowledgeable on cancer and pregnancy special considerations, is vital to optimize outcomes.** Obstetric management rarely needs to be altered, and evidence based interventions proven beneficial in pregnancy should be available to all women with cancer in pregnancy. Moreover, non-proven interventions such as iatrogenic preterm deliveries should be avoided. **Placental pathology** should be sent for all cancers, especially in cases of melanoma. **For most cancers, termination of pregnancy does not improve or affect outcome.** If the patient wishes to continue the pregnancy, she and her physician must decide whether the cancer treatment can be delayed until postpartum without compromising the woman's chance of cure. If not, one can discuss the option of receiving chemotherapy during the second and third trimester of pregnancy. This option must balance what is best for maternal survival yet not harmful to the developing fetus.

GENERAL CHEMOTHERAPY CONSIDERATIONS

Chemotherapy often cannot and should not be delayed solely due to pregnancy if such a delay would decrease the maternal chance of cure. Chemotherapy given during the first trimester has the highest chance of causing malformations, as the majority of organogenesis occurs between 3 and 8 weeks postconception. Many chemotherapeutic agents are safe for the fetus, especially after 12 weeks of pregnancy, even though the brain continues to develop for the remainder of the pregnancy.[3] **If one controls for the gestational age at delivery, fetal growth restriction does not appear to be increased in most cases, especially with solid tumors.** Patients with systemic disease such as leukemia are at risk for increased perinatal morbidity and mortality, including an increased risk for growth restriction and intrauterine fetal demise.

Transplacental studies of different chemotherapy agents during pregnancy are very few, and at times conflicting. Doxorubicin was not detectable in amniotic fluid, placental tissue, fetal brain, or the gastrointestinal (GI) tract but was detectable in fetal liver, kidney, and lung 15 hours after intravenous (IV) administration.[4,5] Umbilical blood sampling 2 and 5 weeks post-multiagent chemotherapy for maternal leukemia showed that fetal hematopoiesis was normal each time.[6]

Long-term follow up

Long-term follow up of children exposed to chemotherapy is limited. A case series of neurodevelopmental follow-up for a mean of 18 years on 84 children exposed in utero to various types of chemotherapy for maternal hematological malignancy shows that clinical health status is comparable to their unexposed siblings. No cancer has been diagnosed in any of the children, and 12 children exposed in utero have now had their own children. All second-generation children were normal in appearance, but did not undergo the same rigorous testing as their parents.[7] A single case of malignancy (papillary thyroid cancer at 11 years old, neuroblastoma at 14 years old) was diagnosed in a 14-year-old boy who was exposed in utero to multiple chemotherapeutic agents for maternal leukemia. His fraternal twin (exposed to the same agents) is healthy.[8] He was also born with congenital anomalies, including esophageal atresia, abnormal inferior vena cava (IVC), and a right arm deformity.

BREAST CANCER
General

Breast cancer is one of the most common cancers complicating pregnancy. Seven to 15% of premenopausal cases occur during pregnancy. The histology of breast cancer diagnosed during pregnancy is no different from the non-pregnant patient population. There is no survival difference between women diagnosed with breast cancer during pregnancy and age- and stage-matched non-pregnant women.[1,9–11] Pregnant women may be more likely to be diagnosed at stage II compared with non-pregnant women (74 vs 37%), and less likely to be diagnosed with early-stage disease (21 vs 54%).[12] Women < 40 years old are more likely to be diagnosed with stage II disease than women > 40 years old. When matched for stage of disease, women < 40 years old have a statistically worse 5-year survival compared with women > 40 years old at diagnosis (55% vs 75%). According to these data, **the age of the reproductive-age woman may have a stronger influence on survival than pregnancy.**[12] Nodal status is a highly significant predictor, whereas pregnancy is not.[11]

Delay in diagnosis

Studies show both patients and physicians follow a breast mass longer in pregnant women before performing a biopsy. Other factors contributing to a possible delay in diagnosis are that masses found on examination are ascribed to 'normal breast changes' of pregnancy and malignancy is not suspected. Pregnant women therefore are often diagnosed with larger tumors at later stages than non-pregnant women. A **delay in diagnosis obviously worsens prognosis, and is inexcusable.**

Diagnostic tests and safety in pregnancy

Mammography has less sensitivity for screening in pregnancy, owing to the increased overall density, vascularity, cellularity, and water content of the breast, which leads to less contrast during pregnancy. The fetal exposure to mammography is not a concern (0.4 rad). **During pregnancy, breast ultrasound has a better accuracy than mammography and should be performed for palpable masses.** The work-up of a solitary mass should continue as in non-pregnant women, with **fine-needle aspiration**, core biopsy or excision. False-positive cytological findings can occur in pregnancy, owing to the highly proliferative state of the breast.[13] As in premenopausal nonpregnant women, most tumors in pregnant women are estrogen-receptor negative.[14] Receptor assays for estrogen and progesterone should be done with immunohistochemistry, not competitive binding assays, which may give false-negative results due to the saturation with endogenous steroid hormone during pregnancy.[15]

Effects on pregnancy

Breast cancer itself (excluding therapy) does not directly affect perinatal outcome.

Termination of pregnancy

Routine termination of pregnancy does not appear to offer a survival advantage for pregnant women diagnosed with breast cancer of any stage.[12,16,17] It is difficult to determine, from studies comparing survival for women who terminate their pregnancies with women who carry to term, if women with advanced or aggressive disease were encouraged to terminate their pregnancy whereas women with earlier-stage disease were not. This is because stage of disease at diagnosis was not reported, but rather survival for the group who terminated the pregnancy was compared with women who continued beyond 24 weeks. However, no study has demonstrated improved survival for women who terminate the pregnancy.

Staging during pregnancy

Mammography is indicated once breast cancer is diagnosed during pregnancy, to exclude multifocal disease in the affected breast or cancer in the contralateral breast. A chest X-ray (with abdominal shielding) is recommended to exclude pulmonary metastasis and can be safely performed with fetal exposure of 0.06 mrad. If further evaluation is necessary, magnetic resonance imaging (MRI) of the thorax is recommended.[18] For early stage disease, if CBC, chemistries and check x-ray are normal, and there are no other suspicions present based on physical exam, no further imaging is needed. The risk of bony metastasis with stage I or II breast cancer is 3–7%. A bone scan can be safely deferred until after pregnancy for asymptomatic patients with early-stage disease. If a patient is symptomatic, or has advanced-stage disease, a bone scan can be performed with a Foley catheter in place and intravenous hydration to promote washout of the excreted radiopharmaceutical from the patient's bladder. A dose of 10 mCi rather than 20 mCi of technetium-99m (Tc-99m) MDP (methylene disphosphonate) and doubling the imaging time reduce fetal radiation exposure.[19] MRI of the skeleton can detect 80% of metastatic deposits. A brain scan is of little yield unless the patient has neurological symptoms and findings. An abdominal MRI is recommended as an alternative to contrast-enhanced CT if liver metastases are suspected or patient has advanced disease. Abdominal ultrasound can also be performed.

Surgery during pregnancy

Breast conservation surgery or mastectomy can be safely performed at any gestational age during pregnancy, with attention paid to avoiding the supine position after 20 weeks' gestation. One must consider that after breast conservation surgery, radiation therapy is standard after chemotherapy is concluded. This is not usually necessary after a modified radical mastectomy (unless there is node positive disease, large tumor size or positive margins). The time delay between completing chemotherapy and beginning radiation therapy that will not compromise the woman's prognosis is unknown; however, there is not usually a prolonged delay for non-pregnant women. Therefore, if a patient is diagnosed early in pregnancy and would complete chemotherapy by 30 weeks of gestation (usually 4 cycles given 2–3 weeks apart), at least 6 weeks of delay would occur before radiation therapy would start without an iatrogenic preterm delivery before 36 weeks. For patients who are diagnosed early in pregnancy, consider mastectomy rather than breast conservation surgery so as to avoid an extended period of time between completing chemotherapy during pregnancy and starting radiation postpartum.

Radiation has been safely given during pregnancy for other cancers, but not usually for breast cancer. Other than this concern about the time delay between finishing chemotherapy and local radiation to the chest wall postpartum, there is no contraindication to breast conservation surgery for pregnant women diagnosed with breast cancer. It is recommended that all pregnant patients delay reconstruction after mastectomy until postpartum, because of the inherent changes that will occur in the unaffected breast due to pregnancy, postpartum atrophy, and possibly breastfeeding. Cosmetic results will be better if one delays reconstruction until after the postpartum period to match the unaffected breast.

Sentinel node biopsy

Sentinel node mapping and biopsy are commonly used for young non-pregnant women to avoid the complications of lymphedema after complete axillary lymphadenectomy. Sentinel node biopsy can be safely performed in pregnancy with Tc-99m sulfur colloid, which identifies the first draining node(s) relative to the site of the primary invasive tumor.[20] For sentinel node imaging, only a minimal dose (500–600 μCi) of double-filtered Tc-99 m sulfur colloid is injected at the site of the breast tumor. The entire radioisotope stays trapped at the site of injection or within the lymphatics until decay occurs (half-life = 6 hours).[18] There is limited information on the use of blue dyes such as lymphazurin for sentinel node mapping in pregnancy and the current recommendation is to use the Tc-99m rather than any dye injection.

Treatment during pregnancy

The majority of women reported in the literature were treated with Adriamycin (doxorubicin) and Cytoxan (cyclophosphamide), with or without 5-fluouracil (5-FU). Currently, doxorubicin is the preferred anthracycline to use during pregnancy, given its safety and use in over

120 cases during pregnancy for various types of cancer. With epirubicin, 3 fetal/neonatal losses have been reported among 14 cases, so the use of epirubicin during pregnancy should occur with caution, even if this anthracycline has lower myelotoxic and cardiotoxic properties than doxorubicin.[21] Transient neonatal cardiomyopathy has been reported after idarubicin exposure and the use of this anthracycline is not recommended during pregnancy. Nonpregnant women with positive nodes are treated with taxane therapy, usually after completing Cytoxan, and an anthracycline, with or without 5-FU. Studies in animals, however, raise concerns about taxane use during pregnancy, and human case reports are rare and currently insufficient for an evidence based recommendation[3]. There have been no reported adverse effects in human pregnancies exposed to taxanes. One could consider giving the taxane after delivery if it can be safely delayed.

HODGKIN'S DISEASE
General

The mean age of diagnosis for Hodgkin's disease is 32 years old.[22] Pregnant women are not more likely to be diagnosed at a higher stage than non-pregnant women.[23] Pregnancy does not adversely affect survival. The ABVD regimen (Adriamycin [doxorubicin], bleomycin, vinblastine, dacarbazine) has been used safely during pregnancy. Chemotherapy during organogenesis in the first trimester will increase the risk for malformations (see treatment below).

Diagnostic tests and safety in pregnancy

The clinical behavior of Hodgkin's disease during pregnancy does not appear to differ from non-pregnant women. Pregnant women can present with a cough, night sweats, and weight loss. A patient with such complaints should have a complete physical examination and clavicular adenopathy can be safely biopsied during pregnancy. A chest X-ray can be performed safely with minimal fetal exposure. (An abdominal shield is still indicated for all radiological studies during pregnancy.) A bone marrow biopsy can also be safely performed. Surgeons should be advised of the safety of narcotic use for pregnant women undergoing surgical procedures to avoid patient discomfort.

Effects on pregnancy

Hodgkin's disease does not directly affect perinatal outcome. Infants born to women with Hodgkin's disease do not seem to have a higher risk for prematurity or intrauterine growth restriction.[23]

Termination of pregnancy

Therapeutic termination of a pregnancy does not improve the course of disease.[24]

Surgery during pregnancy

At times, a histological examination of a lymph node is inconclusive. In such cases, if mediastinal adenopathy is evident on X-ray or CT of the chest, a guided biopsy may be indicated to confirm a diagnosis.

Staging during pregnancy

The staging of Hodgkin's disease is based on history and physical examination, hematological and biochemical testing, bone marrow biopsy, and radiological imaging. A staging laparotomy and splenectomy are no longer routinely performed in non-pregnant patients. Gallium scanning is not routine anymore, even in non-pregnant patients.

Currently, women with stages I and II receive combined modality treatment, so full staging during pregnancy is unlikely to change the recommended treatment during the course of pregnancy, and can be delayed to the postpartum period. Image staging in non-pregnant patients includes a chest X-ray and CT. In the pregnant woman, a two-view chest X-ray is suggested. Fetal exposure is negligible with abdominal shielding. A chest MRI can assess lymphadenopathy, and the information gained is comparable to a CT.[18] MRI can also evaluate the bone marrow and detect splenic involvement that may be undetectable with CT.

Treatment during pregnancy
Chemotherapy

The ABVD regimen for Hodgkin's lymphoma has been reported to be safe in pregnancy, although dacarbazine is the least-studied agent. Similar doses should be given to the pregnant patient with adjustment for weight gain during pregnancy.

Radiotherapy

Radiotherapy for Hodgkin's disease during pregnancy has been reported to be safe for the fetus.[25] Exposure of the fetus to radiation is determined by the internal scatter, leakage from the tube head, and scatter from the collimator. Internal scatter depends on the source of radiation, the distance of the fetus from the source, and the size of treatment fields. Blocks are not recommended in pregnancy because of the additional scatter they create. During radiotherapy, shielding will not stop scatter radiation. Exposure of the fetus can be estimated with simulated measurements, which have shown that treatment with a 6MV linear accelerator exposes the fetus to less radiation than treatment with cobalt 60.[25] The highest risk of brain damage and mental retardation is between 8 and 15 weeks' gestation.[26] Radiation for Hodgkin's disease is usually reserved for cases progressing despite chemotherapy, the lymphocyte predominant type, or if chemotherapy is not an option.

NON-HODGKIN'S LYMPHOMA
General

Non-Hodgkin's lymphoma (NHL) is rarely reported during pregnancy, as this generally occurs in an older age group (mean age at diagnosis is 42 years old). Pregnant women present with an aggressive histology,[22,27] but the response to treatment, failure, and progression rates are similar to non-pregnant patients. Symptoms can vary widely, with many complaints similar to symptoms in normal pregnancy, which can lead to a delay in diagnosis of NHL in pregnancy.

Avoid delay in diagnosis

Pregnant women with NHL can present with breast or ovarian masses, misleading the initial diagnosis to a gynecological malignancy. When masses are bilateral and massive in size, one should suspect NHL (see treatment below).

Effects on pregnancy

NHL does not directly affect pregnancy. However, pregnancy can affect the presentation of NHL, and some authors report a progression of NHL postpartum. [27–29] NHL can present with lymphadenopathy, as with non-pregnant patients; however, pregnant patients can have involvement of the breasts, ovaries, and uterus. A hormonal influence of pregnancy on the progression of NHL is suggested by the frequent and massive involvement of such organs during pregnancy, which are otherwise unusually involved with lymphoma in non-pregnant patients.[27]

Treatment during pregnancy

Thirty-five cases of non-Hodgkin's lymphoma were treated during pregnancy with multiple regimens, most including doxorubicin, cyclophosphamide, and vincristine. No malformations occurred, even with first trimester treatment in 11 cases. Breast or ovarian masses should not be removed after biopsy confirms lymphoma. The masses will respond to systemic chemotherapy.

LEUKEMIA (ACUTE AND CHRONIC)
General

Leukemia is rarely diagnosed during pregnancy as affected women are usually amenorrheic. Acute leukemia, which usually occurs in young women, is more common than chronic leukemia during pregnancy.

Avoid delay in diagnosis

Pregnant women with leukemia can present with severe anemia, thrombocytopenia, infection or sepsis, fever, bone pain, or bleeding.

Diagnostic tests and safety in pregnancy

Bone marrow biopsy can be safely performed during pregnancy.

Termination of pregnancy

Termination of pregnancy has not been shown to improve prognosis. Patients newly diagnosed with acute leukemia are too ill to safely undergo a dilatation and curettage procedure when termination is elected. If a patient elects termination, induction chemotherapy should still be given during the pregnancy to induce remission so that the procedure can be safely performed; otherwise, the patient is at too high a risk for the complications of sepsis, hemorrhage, and disseminated intravascular coagulation (DIC).

Effect on pregnancy

Acute leukemia is one of the cancers which can affect perinatal outcome. The earlier the diagnosis in pregnancy, the higher the perinatal mortality. Pregnancy complications include miscarriage, preterm labor, and low birth weight, regardless of therapy.[30,31] Suspected etiologies include maternal anemia, DIC or leukemia cells affecting blood flow and nutrient exchange in the intervillous spaces of the placenta and decreased oxygen transport to the fetus.[31]

Treatment during pregnancy

Aggressive hematological and obstetric management is advocated when acute leukemia is diagnosed. The prognosis for both mother and fetus is poor when acute leukemia is not treated during pregnancy. When intensive chemotherapy is given in pregnancy, complete remission is achieved in

75% of patients.[30] Without therapy, maternal death may occur within 2 months.[31] Chemotherapy treatment during pregnancy is associated with higher maternal and fetal/neonatal survival compared with chemotherapy postponed until postpartum.[31] All cases with anomalies occurred with first trimester exposure to cytarabine or 6-thioguanine, alone or in combination with an anthracycline. Cytarabine and 6-thioguanine should be avoided in the first trimester if possible. Combinations including vincristine, 6-MP (6-mercaptopurine), doxorubicin or daunorubicin, cyclophosphamide, prednisone, and methotrexate were used in all trimesters without anomalies. Transient myelosuppression can occur in neonates, especially if delivered within 3–4 weeks of chemotherapy.[32] More rarely, transient neonatal cardiomyopathy has been reported. Cardiomyopathy occurred mostly after use of idarubicin.[33] Iatrogenic preterm deliveries or elective inductions should be avoided before remission is attempted, as the patient with acute leukemia is at risk for hemorrhage, DIC, and sepsis during labor and delivery if lacerations or endometritis occurs.

Chronic leukemia rarely occurs during pregnancy, as the average age at diagnosis is in the 5th or 6th decade. Hydroxyurea or busulfan appear safe for use during pregnancy if necessary, although in the majority of cases treatment can be delayed without consequence until after delivery. Leukophoresis can be a temporizing measure to reduce white blood cells (WBCs) and spleen size if necessary.[34,35]

MELANOMA

General

One-third of women diagnosed with malignant melanoma are of childbearing age.[36] When pregnant patients are matched to non-pregnant controls for prognostic factors such as tumor thickness, there is **no significant difference in survival rates** for women with stage I melanoma.[37–40] One study reported that pregnancy at diagnosis was significantly associated with **metastatic disease** when controlling for tumor site, thickness, and Clark level, but survival was not significantly decreased for pregnant patients.[41,42]

Avoid delay in diagnosis

Pregnant women are diagnosed with **thicker tumors** compared with non-pregnant women. This (as well as the increase in metastatic disease) has been ascribed in the literature to a delay in diagnosis due to changes in mole appearance during pregnancy. Hyperpigmentation can occur secondary to an increased secretion of melanocyte-stimulating hormone (MSH); however, the color of the mole should still be uniform. The maximum increase/decrease in the size of melanocytic nevi in pregnancy is 1 mm.[43,44] During pregnancy, one must still look for signs of melanoma, listed below, which should *not* be ascribed to normal changes in pregnancy. These include the ABCD signs: A for asymmetry; B for notched, irregular, or indistinct borders; C for an uneven color; D for diameter > 6 mm.

Effects on pregnancy

Melanoma is one of the rare cancers that can **metastasize to the placenta**. Most reported cases have occurred in patients with metastatic spread to the lymph nodes at diagnosis. The placenta should be sent for pathological evaluation in all cases of melanoma diagnosed during pregnancy. If melanoma is found in the placenta, the neonate should be followed closely for 1 year with frequent skin evaluations.

Termination of pregnancy

No advantage in prognosis or survival has been demonstrated with elective pregnancy termination in patients with stage I melanoma.

Surgery during pregnancy

Wide local excision is the only cure for melanoma, and can be safely performed during pregnancy at any gestational age. Patients should be positioned with uterine displacement after 20 weeks' gestation.

Staging and sentinel node biopsy

Wide local excision is the only cure for melanoma, and should be done after a biopsy is suspicious for melanoma. Sentinel node mapping can be safely performed during pregnancy, with Tc-99 sulfur colloid. Intradermal injection of Tc-labeled sulfur colloid causes negligible ionizing radiation to the fetus (see sentinel node biopsy under breast cancer for safety). The majority of the dose stays localized to the injection site or within the lymphatics until decay occurs. For stage I or II melanoma, a chest X-ray is indicated for staging if the melanoma is > 1.0 mm thick. For stage III disease, an MRI of the chest and abdomen, with or without the pelvis, is recommended in addition to the chest X-ray for evaluation of lymphadenopathy or evidence of liver metastases. MRI of the brain and skeleton are also recommended.

Treatment during pregnancy

Surgery is the only effective treatment for early stage melanoma, and chemotherapy has not been shown to significantly prolong survival. Postpartum, patients with advanced disease can enroll in clinical trials using interferon or melanoma vaccinations. (Chapter 3)

INVASIVE CERVICAL CANCER

General

Invasive carcinoma of the cervix occurs in approximately 1/2200 pregnancies, but this incidence is declining due to widespread and improved Papanicolaou (Pap) screening.[45,46] (see also Chapter 30 in *Obstetric Evidence Based Guidelines*.) Tumor characteristics and maternal survival are not adversely affected by pregnancy.[46] Unlike non-pregnant patients, presenting symptoms are more likely to be abnormal Pap screens rather than bleeding. The predominant histological type is squamous cell. The prognosis is comparable with non-pregnant patients.[46–48]

Avoid delay in diagnosis

Pregnant women are more likely to be diagnosed with early-stage disease as cervical screening is routine during prenatal care in most countries.[46]

Diagnostic tests and safety in pregnancy

The cytobrush can be safely used during pregnancy to obtain an adequate Pap smear during prenatal care. Pregnant patients should be warned of the possibility of bleeding afterwards. Directed biopsies are performed if a lesion is visible at colposcopy during any trimester. The risk of a missed diagnosis outweighs the risk (e.g. bleeding) of the biopsy. A cone biopsy is rarely necessary for diagnosis in pregnancy. (see also Chapter 30 in *Obstetric Evidence Based Guidelines*.)

Effect on pregnancy

Cervical cancer does not adversely affect pregnancy directly; however, cancer treatment affects future fertility if hysterectomy is indicated.

Termination of pregnancy

A spontaneous loss of the pregnancy may occur when treatment for cervical cancer is initiated for patients diagnosed prior to 18 weeks' gestation (see surgery).

Treatment during pregnancy

Non-pregnant patients with stages IB/IIA can have surgery or radiotherapy for cervical cancer. The gestational age at diagnosis determines the treatment recommendations. For all stages of cervical cancer diagnosed before 18 weeks, immediate treatment is recommended. A cone biopsy is rarely performed in pregnancy unless a patient is early in gestation and desires to continue the pregnancy when microinvasion is suspected. (See also Chapter 30 in *Obstetric Evidence Based Guidelines*.) For early stage (IB/IIA), a radical hysterectomy or radiotherapy can be performed with the fetus in situ. Often a spontaneous miscarriage will occur within a short time after radiotherapy. For patients with advanced-stage disease, external radiotherapy and chemotherapy with the fetus in situ is suggested. Spontaneous abortion often follows radiotherapy; however, hysterotomy to facilitate brachytherapy may be required if this does not occur.[49]

Patients diagnosed with early stage disease after 18 weeks' gestation can delay surgical treatment for cervical cancer in order to improve fetal maturity and survival. When treatment for cervical cancer is intentionally delayed for 6–17 weeks, fetal outcome is markedly improved, and maternal survival is not adversely affected.[50–53] If a patient is diagnosed with stage IA or IB invasive cervical cancer at 18 weeks' gestation or later, an intentional delay until 34 weeks will improve fetal survival without an apparent maternal risk, understanding that only approximately 60 patients have been reported with this approach. Patients with more advanced disease than IB can receive platinum-based chemotherapy during the second and third trimesters.

Staging during pregnancy

Imaging for staging includes evaluation of regional lymph node chains, as lymphadenopathy has prognostic and therapeutic implications. MRI can detect depth of stromal invasion and evaluate the parametria. MRI can also identify a dilated collecting system and enlarged lymph nodes. A two-view chest X-ray with proper shielding can be performed if indicated clinically.

Treatment during pregnancy

Treatment for invasive cervical cancer involves either surgery, radiation, or both, depending on the stage at diagnosis. The safe use of neoadjuvant platinum-based chemotherapy has been reported.[54,55] (see also surgery for cervical cancer).

Mode of delivery

When the pregnant patient with invasive cervical cancer stages IB/IIA is to deliver, the recommended procedure is a cesarean section/radical hysterectomy. Patients with more advanced-stage disease would still be delivered by cesarean section with postpartum radiotherapy. A classical cesarean delivery is recommended to avoid extension into the lower uterine segment.[56] At the time of cesarean section, pelvic and para-aortic nodes should be sampled, and an oophoropexy can be performed to move the ovaries out of the radiation field. Episiotomy site recurrences of cervical cancer have been reported after vaginal delivery.[57]

THYROID CANCER

General

The mean age of diagnosis for thyroid cancer is between 30 and 34 years of age, with most cases in pregnancy presenting as a solitary nodule.[58] There is no evidence that pregnancy changes the clinical course of the disease, and no evidence that thyroid cancer adversely affects pregnancy outcome. The prognosis of differentiated thyroid cancer is the same in pregnant and non-pregnant women.[59] No endocrine association between maternal hormonal changes and thyroid cancer has been found. Treatment depends on histological subtype, degree of differentiation, stage, and gestational age at diagnosis.

Avoid delay in diagnosis

The thyroid can enlarge during normal pregnancy, but solitary nodules should be evaluated.

Diagnostic tests and safety in pregnancy

Biopsy of a solid nodule can be safely performed during pregnancy at any gestational age.

Termination of pregnancy

No survival advantage is known for elective termination of pregnancy for thyroid cancer.

Surgery during pregnancy

The type of thyroid cancer and the gestational age at diagnosis determine if thyroidectomy is necessary during pregnancy, or can be safely postponed until postpartum (see treatment).

Treatment during pregnancy

Differentiated types of thyroid cancer such as papillary, follicular, or mixed types are slow growing and surgery can be postponed until postpartum for patients diagnosed after 12 weeks' gestation. Prior to 12 weeks, a subtotal thyroidectomy is recommended.[60] If a nodule is noted[59] to enlarge during pregnancy, the surrounding tissues are fixed, or lymphatic invasion is seen on the original biopsy, surgery should not be delayed to postpartum, regardless of the gestational age at diagnosis. Patients who delay treatment due to pregnancy should be advised to undergo surgery within 1 year of diagnosis.[60]

Medullary or anaplastic types of thyroid cancer are more aggressive, and surgery should not be postponed. A total thyroidectomy may be necessary. If the lesion is compromising the airway, radiotherapy may be necessary during pregnancy. During total thyroidectomy, parathyroid tissue is often inadvertently removed as well. For the remainder of the pregnancy and during preterm or term deliveries (uterine muscle is working), the calcium balance should be watched carefully. Magnesium for preterm labor or pre-eclampsia should be used with caution for this reason.

COMPLICATIONS OF CANCER THERAPY DURING PREGNANCY

During chemotherapy, side effects such as nausea and vomiting may occur, and may compound the nausea related to the pregnancy. Patients should be well hydrated before, during, and after chemotherapy sessions. Ondansetron, metoclopramide, Kytril (granisetron), and Benadryl (diphenhydramine) can be safely given in pregnancy for nausea. Decadron (dexamethasone) can also be given, and may enhance the effectiveness of antiemetics. Given the relative immunosuppression of pregnancy, combined with the bone marrow suppression with chemotherapy, pregnant women are at risk for infection, and therefore the fetuses are at risk for exposure as well. If neutropenia occurs, Neupogen (filgrastim) can be given safely in pregnancy. Epogen (epoetin alfa) is safe during pregnancy, if anemia occurs. Complications can include poor maternal weight gain due to either nausea and vomiting, or chemotherapy-induced stomatitis. Patients should increase caloric and protein intake in the weeks preceding and following chemotherapy. Nutritional supplementation is sometimes necessary.

MATERNAL SURVEILLANCE

Prechemotherapy studies: an echocardiogram is preferred over multigated equilibrium radionuclide cineangiography (MUGA) to evaluate baseline cardiac function prior to anthracycline therapy. This can provide the necessary information regarding cardiac function and valvular disease. Patients who have any fevers during chemotherapy require comprehensive evaluations for presence of infection, especially during the nadir period. Monitor weight gain throughout pregnancy.

FETAL SURVEILLANCE AND TIMING OF DELIVERY

Often, Decadron is given with chemotherapy to enhance the effectiveness of antiemetics. If the patient requires tocolysis for preterm labor, and has received intravenous Decadron with chemotherapy after 24 weeks, steroids such as betamethasone may not be necessary to stimulate fetal lung maturity. The fetal/neonatal safety of repeated doses of steroids has not been demonstrated and repeated courses of steroids are not currently recommended.

The preterm infant cannot metabolize chemotherapy agents as well as the term infant; therefore, iatrogenic preterm deliveries should be avoided in patients receiving chemotherapy, and preterm labor should be treated aggressively. Chemotherapy may need to be temporarily delayed if the patient has preterm labor. Growth ultrasounds in the late second and third trimesters (26–28 weeks) are suggested when women receive chemotherapy or radiotherapy during pregnancy, especially for patients diagnosed with acute leukemia, given the increased risk of intrauterine growth restriction.

Transient bone marrow suppression of the neonate can occur if delivery is within 3–4 weeks of treatment. Delivery should be avoided during this nadir period if possible. To ensure this, chemotherapy should not be given after 34 weeks, as the patient could potentially go into spontaneous labor during the nadir period. If additional treatment is still required, early induction may be considered, so that the interval between the last treatment and postpartum treatment is not greater than 6 weeks. (For example, if last treatment is 33 weeks, consider induction at 38 weeks; so 1 week afterwards, the patient can continue with chemotherapy with a 6-week interval between the last treatment during pregnancy and the postpartum treatment.)

NEONATAL EVALUATION AFTER CHEMOTHERAPY DURING PREGNANCY

The **placenta should be sent for pathology examination in all cases** of women diagnosed with cancer during pregnancy, regardless of cancer treatment. A complete blood count (CBC) with differential is recommended on both the cord blood and the neonate when chemotherapy has been given during pregnancy. Additional long-term follow-up on the children exposed to cancer and its treatment in utero is necessary. A Cancer and Childbirth Registry has been established to follow all children of women diagnosed with cancer during pregnancy. The women are also followed yearly. Information about cancer diagnosis, treatment, pregnancy outcomes, and long-term survival is collected and kept confidential.

Contact the Cancer and Pregnancy Registry at 856-757-7876, 856-342-2491 or www.cancerinpregnancy.com; www.cancerandpregnancy.com.

REFERENCES

1. Donegan W. Cancer and pregnancy. CA Cancer J Clin 1983; 33(4): 194–214. [review]
2. Weisz B, Meirow D, Schiff E, Lishner M. Impact and treatment of cancer during pregnancy. Expert Rev Anticancer Ther 2004; 4(5): 889–902. [II-2]
3. Cardonick E, Iacobacci A. Use of chemotherapy during human pregnancy. Lancet Oncol 2004; 5(5): 283–91. [review]
4. Barni S, Ardizzoia A, Zanetta G, et al. Weekly doxorubicin chemotherapy for breast cancer in pregnancy. A case report. Tumori 1992; 78(5): 349–50. [II-2]
5. d'Incalci M, Broggini M, Buscaglia M, Parki G. Transplacental passage of doxorubicin. Lancet 1983; 75: 8314–15. [II-2]
6. Morishita S, Imai A, Kawabata I, Tamaya T. Acute myelogenous leukemia in pregnancy: fetal blood sampling and early effects of chemotherapy. Int J Gynaecol Obstet 1994; 44(3): 273–7. [II-2]
7. Aviles A, Neri N. Hematological malignancies and pregnancy: a final report of 84 children who received chemotherapy in utero. Clin Lymphoma 2001; 2(3): 173–7. [II-2]
8. Zemlickis D, Lishner M, Erlich R, Koren G. Teratogenicity and carcinogenicity in a twin exposed in utero to cyclophosphamide. Teratog Carcinog Mutagen 1993; 13: 139–43. [II-2]
9. Gallenberg MM, Loprinzi CL. Breast cancer and pregnancy. Semin Oncol 1989; 16: 369–76. [review]
10. Gemignani ML, Petek JA. Breast cancer during pregnancy: diagnostic and therapeutic dilemmas. Adv Surg 2000; 34: 272–86. [II-2]
11. Petrek JA, Dulcoff R, Rogatko A. Prognosis of pregnancy-associated breast cancer. Cancer 1990; 67: 869–72. [II-2]
12. Nugent P, O'Connell TX. Breast cancer and pregnancy. Arch Surg 1985; 120: 1221–4. [review]
13. Finley JL, Silverman JF, Lannin DR. Fine-needle aspiration cytology of breast masses in pregnant and in lactating women. Diag Cytopathol 1989; 5: 255–8. [II-3]
14. Barnavon Y, Wallach MK. Management of the pregnant patient with carcinoma of the breast. Surg Gynecol Obstet 1990; 171(4): 347–52. [review]
15. Elledge RM, Ciocca DR, Langone G, McGuire WL. Estrogen receptor, progesterone receptor, and HER-2/neu protein in breast cancers from pregnant patients. Cancer 1993; 71: 2499–506. [II-3]
16. Clark RM, Reid J. Carcinoma of the breast in pregnancy and lactation. Int J Radiat Oncol Biol Phys 1978; 4: 693–8. [II-2]
17. Zemlickis D, Lishner M, Degendorfer P, et al. Maternal and fetal outcome after breast cancer in pregnancy. Am J Obstet Gynecol 1992; 166: 781–7. [II-2]
18. Nicklas AH, Baker ME. Imaging strategies in the pregnant cancer patient. Semin Oncol 2000; 27(6): 623–32. [II-3]
19. Baker J, Ali A, Groch MW, Fordham E, Economou SG. Bone scanning in pregnant patients with breast carcinoma. Clin Nucl Med 1987; 12(7): 519–24. [II-3]
20. Keleher A, Wendt R 3rd, Delpassand E, Stachowiak AM, Kuerer HM. The safety of lymphatic mapping in pregnant breast cancer patients using Tc-99m sulfur colloid. Breast J 2004; 10(6): 492–5. [II-3]
21. Andreadis C, Charalampidou M, Diamantopoulos N, Chouchos N, Mouratidou D. Combined chemotherapy and radiotherapy during conception and first two trimesters of gestation in a woman with metastatic breast cancer. Gynecologic Oncol 2004; 95(1): 252–5. [III]
22. Ward FT, Weiss RB. Lymphoma and pregnancy. Semin Oncol 1989; 16: 397–409. [review]
23. Lishner M, Zemlickis D, Degendorfer P, et al. Maternal and foetal outcome following Hodgkin's disease in pregnancy. Br J Cancer 1992; 65(1): 114–17. [II-2]
24. Nisce LZ, Tome MA, He S, Lee BJ III, Kutcher GJ. Management of coexisting Hodgkin's disease and pregnancy. Am J Clin Oncol 1986; 9(2): 146–51. [II-3]

25. Woo SY, Fuller LM, Cundiff JH, et al. Radiotherapy during pregnancy for clinical stages IA–IIA Hodgkin's disease. Int J Radiat Oncol Biol Phys 1992; 23(2): 407–12. [II-3]

26. Dekaban AS. Abnormalities in children exposed to x-radiation during various stages of gestation: tentative timetable of radiation injury to the human fetus. J Nucl Med 1968; 9: 471–7. [II-3]

27. Ioachim HL. Non-Hodgkin's lymphoma in pregnancy. Three cases and review of the literature. Arch Pathol Lab Med 1985; 109: 803–9. [II-3]

28. Steiner-Salz D, Yahalom J, Samuelov A, Polliack A. Non-Hodgkin's lymphoma associated with pregnancy. A report of six cases, with a review of the literature. Cancer 1985; 56(8): 2087–91. [II-3]

29. Mavrommatis CG, Daskalakis GJ, Papageorgiou IS, Antsaklis AJ, Michalas SK. Non-Hodgkin's lymphoma during pregnancy – case report. Eur J Obstet Gynecol Reprod Biol 1998; 79(1): 95–7. [II-3]

30. Reynoso EE, Shepherd FA, Messner HA, et al. Acute leukemia during pregnancy: the Toronto Leukemia Study Group experience with long-term follow-up of children exposed in utero to chemotherapeutic agents. J Clin Oncol 1987; 5: 1098–106. [II-2]

31. Catanzarite VA, Ferguson JE 2nd. Acute leukemia and pregnancy: a review of management and outcomes, 1972–1982. Obstet Gynecol Survey 1984; 39(11): 663–77. [review]

32. Okun DB, Groncy PK, Sieger L, Tanaka KR. Acute leukemia in pregnancy: transient neonatal myelosuppression after combination chemotherapy in the mother. Med Pediatr Oncol 1979; 7(4): 315–19. [II-3]

33. Achtari C, Hohlfeld P. Cardiotoxic transplacental effect of idarubicin administered during the second trimester of pregnancy. Am J Obstet Gynecol 2000; 183: 511–12. [II-3]

34. Strobl FJ, Voelkerding KV, Smith EP. Management of chronic myeloid leukemia during pregnancy with leukapheresis. J Clin Apher 1999; 14: 42–4. [II-3]

35. Fitzgerald D, Rowe JM, Heal J. Leukapheresis for control of chronic myelogenous leukemia during pregnancy. Am J Hematol 1986; 22: 213–18. [II-3]

36. Colbourn DS, Nathanson L, Belilos E. Pregnancy and malignant melanoma. Semin Oncol 1989; 16: 377–87. [review]

37. McManamny DS, Moss AL, Pocock PV, Briggs JC. Melanoma and pregnancy: a long-term follow up. Br J Obstet Gynaecol 1989; 96(12): 1419–23. [II-2]

38. Wong DJ, Strassner HT. Melanoma in pregnancy. Clin Obstet Gynecol 1990; 33: 782–91. [review]

39. Mackie RM, Bufalino R, Morabito A, Sutherland C, Cascinelli N. Lack of effect of pregnancy on outcome of melanoma. For the World Health Organisation Melanoma Programme. Lancet 1991; 337: 653–5. [II-2]

40. Lens MB, Rasdahl I, Farahmand BY, et al. Effect of pregnancy on survival of women with cutaneous malignant melanoma. J Clin Oncol 2004; 22(21): 4369–75. [II-2]

41. Slingluff CL Jr, Seigler HF. Malignant melanoma and pregnancy. Ann Plast Surg 1992; 28(1): 95–9. [review]

42. Slingluff CL Jr, Reintgen D. Malignant melanoma and the prognostic implications of pregnancy, oral contraceptives, and exogenous hormones. Semin Surg Oncol 1993; 9: 228–31. [II-2]

43. Pennoyer JW, Grin CM, Driscoll MS, et al. Changes in the size of melanocytic nevi during pregnancy [see comment]. J Am Acad Dermatol 1997; 36(3 pt 1): 378–82. [II-3]

44. Pennoyer JW, Grin CM, Driscoll MS, et al. Changes in size of melanocytic nevi during pregnancy. J Eur Acad Dermatol Venereol 2003; 17(3): 349–51. [II-3]

45. Hacker NF, Berek JS, Lagasse LD, et al. Carcinoma of the cervix associated with pregnancy. Obstet Gynecol 1982; 59: 735–46. [II-2]

46. Zemlickis D, Lishner M, Degendorfer P, et al. Maternal and fetal outcome after invasive cervical cancer in pregnancy. J Clin Oncol 1991; 9(11): 1956–61. [II-2]

47. Germann N, Haie-Meder C, Morice P, et al. Management and clinical outcomes of pregnant patients with invasive cervical cancer. Ann Oncol 2005; 16(3): 397–402. [II-2]

48. Hopkins MP, Morley GW. The prognosis and management of cervical cancer associated with pregnancy. Obstet Gynecol 1992; 80(1): 9–13. [II-2]

49. Method MW, Brost BC. Management of cervical cancer in pregnancy. Semin Surg Oncol 1999; 16(3): 251–60. [review]

50. Duggan B, Muderspach LI, Roman LD, et al. Cervical cancer in pregnancy: reporting on planned delay in therapy. Obstet Gynecol 1993; 82: 598–602. [II-3]

51. Sood AK, Sorosky JI, Krogman S, et al. Surgical management of cervical cancer complicating pregnancy: a case control study. Gynecol Oncol 1996; 63(3): 294–8. [II-2]

52. Prem KA, Makowski EL, McKelvey JL. Carcinoma of the cervix associated with pregnancy. Am J Obstet Gynecol 1996; 95: 99–108. [II-2]

53. Greer BE, Easterling TR, McLennan DA, et al. Fetal and maternal considerations in the management of stage I-B cervical cancer during pregnancy. Gynecol Oncol 1989; 34(1): 61–5. [II-2]

54. Van Calsteren K, Vergote I, Amant F. Cervical neoplasia during pregnancy: diagnosis, management and prognosis. Best Pract Rese Clin Obstet Gynaecol 2005; 19(4): 611–30. [review]

55. Marana HR, de Andrade JM, da Silva Mathes AC, et al. Chemotherapy in the treatment of locally advanced cervical cancer and pregnancy. Gynecol Oncol 2001; 80(2): 272–4. [II-2]

56. McDonald SD, Faught W, Gruslin A. Cervical cancer during pregnancy. J Obstet Gynaecol Can 2002; 24(6): 491–8. [review]

57. Cliby WA, Dodson MK, Podratz KC. Cervical cancer complicated by pregnancy: episiotomy site recurrences following vaginal delivery. Obstet Gynecol 1994; 84(2): 179–82. [II-3]

58. Morris PC. Thyroid cancer complicating pregnancy. Obstet Gynecol Clin North Am 1998; 25(2): 401–5. [review]

59. Moosa M, Mazzaferri EL. Outcome of differentiated thyroid cancer diagnosed in pregnant women. J Clin Endocrinol Metab 1997; 82(9): 2862–6. [II-3]

60. Vini L, Hyser SL, Pratt B, Harmer C. Management of differentiated thyroid cancer diagnosed during pregnancy. Eur J Endocrinol 1999; 140(5): 404–6. [II-3]

20

Smoking

Julie Takeuchi Crawford and Jorge E Tolosa

KEY POINTS

- Smoking is a **preventable risk factor** associated with **low birth weight, preterm birth, and perinatal death**.
- Smoking cessation in pregnancy reduces low birth weight, preterm birth, and perinatal death.
- **Counseling** with behavioral and educational interventions is **associated with the highest cessation rates**.
- Most pharmacotherapies are **contraindicated, or their safety and efficacy are uncertain in pregnancy**.
- Nicotine replacement therapy and **bupropion** are safe and effective in the general population, but there is **insufficient evidence** for recommending them in pregnant smokers.
- Nicotine replacement therapy is associated with known **adverse fetal effects** and nicotine is detected in breast milk.
- The greatest risk of **relapse** occurs in the **postpartum period**.
- There is **insufficient evidence** to recommend specific interventions to prevent relapse.

HISTORIC NOTES

The 20th century saw the rise of the manufactured cigarette and its popularity grew.[1] People continue to smoke despite the known adverse effects.[1]

DIAGNOSIS/DEFINITION

Tobacco dependence is a chronic addictive condition that requires repeated intervention for cessation.

EPIDEMIOLOGY/INCIDENCE

Approximately 250 million women smoke worldwide at the beginning of the 21st century.[1]

- 22% of women smoke in developed countries and 9% of women smoke in developing countries.[1]
- 25% of American women of reproductive age smoke cigarettes.[2]
- The US smoking in pregnancy incidence was 12% in 2003 (38% decrease since 1989 – 20% then). Estimated **smoking rates during pregnancy** vary in different countries from **11 to 22%**.[2]
- By age, the highest prevalence is amongst the young: 18% of smokers are < 20 years of age and 9.8% are > 35 years of age.[2]
- By race, the highest prevalence of smoking occurs among Native American and Native Alaskan women. The lowest prevalence occurs among Hispanics and Asian Pacific Islander women.[2]
- **A higher proportion of women stop smoking in pregnancy than at any other time in their lives (20–30% of women).**[3]
- Up to 40% of women stop smoking before their first antenatal visit.[3]
- **90% of those who quit smoking relapse in the first year after delivery, the majority in the first 6 weeks.**[4]

GENETICS

The maternal genotype may affect the risk of low birth weight in cigarette smokers.[5] The *CYP1A1* and *GSTTi* genes encode enzymes active in metabolism and elimination of toxic substances in cigarette smoke. Heterozygous variants of *CYP1A1* and absence of *GSTIIi* genes had significantly greater reductions in birth weight in women who smoked.

ETIOLOGY/BASIC PATHOPHYSIOLOGY

The major compounds causing harmful effects are **nicotine** and **carbon monoxide**. Other toxic compounds include ammonia, polycyclic aromatic hydrocarbons, hydrogen cyanide, vinyl chloride, and nitrogen oxides. Smoking may result in damage to fetal genetic material, with results in deletions and translocations at the chromosome 11q23 region.

Nicotine

- Crosses the placenta and can be detected in the fetal circulation at levels that exceed maternal circulation by 15%.[6]
- **Amniotic fluid levels are 88% higher than maternal plasma levels.**[6]
- Causes impaired fetal oxygen delivery: vasoconstriction and changes in capillary volume and villous membrane contribute to abnormal gas exchange within the placenta.[7]
- Results in sympathetic activation, leading to increased fetal heart rate and reduction in fetal breathing movement.

Carbon monoxide

- Crosses the placenta and can be detected in the fetal circulation at **levels that exceed maternal circulation by 15%.**[6]
- Exposure causes formation of carboxyhemoglobin. Carboxyhemoglobin is cleared slowly from the fetal circulation and diminishes tissue oxygenation via competitive inhibition with oxyhemoglobin. There is a left shift of the oxyhemoglobin dissociation curve, causing decreased availability of oxygen to the fetus.[6]

Cyanide

- Levels are higher in smokers.[6]
- The compound is toxic to rapidly dividing cells.

RISK FACTORS

Women are more likely to smoke if:

- social disadvantage and lower education
- receiving Medicaid funded maternity care
- high parity
- low levels of support and/or being without a partner
- exposure to domestic violence
- having a partner that smokes or exposure to passive smoke at home
- depression, coexisting emotional/psychiatric problems, substance abuse
- job strain
- poor coping skills (smoking can help women cope with stress)

- younger age
- fear of weight gain and unsatisfied with female body image.

Spontaneous quitters usually smoke less, are more likely to have stopped smoking before, are more likely to have a non-smoker partner or have more support and encouragement at home for quitting, and have stronger beliefs about the dangers of smoking.[3]

COMPLICATIONS
Pregnancy complications

Smoking is the **most modifiable risk factor associated with adverse pregnancy outcomes.**[8] All the risks are dose-related.

Low birth weight. Women who smoke are more likely to have a low birth weight baby (<2500 g), with a relative risk (RR) of 1.3–10. The birth weight **deficit is 200–300 g** by term.[2] Low birth weight causes the highest economic burden.[3]

Pregnancy loss. Heavy smoking of >15 cigarettes/day is associated with increased pregnancy loss, with RR 1.2–3.4.

Premature rupture of membranes (PROM). Increased risk among smokers; RR ranges from 1.9 to 4.2.

Pre-eclampsia. Smoking is associated with a *reduced* incidence of pre-eclampsia. Quitting smoking before pregnancy precludes this decrease in pre-eclampsia.

Placental abruption. Greatest among heavy smokers; RR = 1.4–2.5.

Placenta previa. RR ranges from 1.4 to 4.4.

Preterm delivery. May be due to other conditions in pregnancy, but it is mostly due to spontaneous preterm labor. Women who smoke are 1.3–2.5 times more likely to have preterm delivery. It is estimated that 10–15% of preterm birth may be due to smoking.

Fetal death. Large case-control and cohort studies suggest an RR of 1.2–1.4 in heavy smokers.

Postnatal morbidities. Increased risk of sudden infant death syndrome (SIDS), respiratory infections, reactive airway diseases, otitis media, bronchiolitis, short stature, hyperactivity, and decreased school performance.

Fetal central nervous system effects. Abnormalities in cell proliferation and differentiation lead to a decreased number of cells and eventually altered synaptic activity. Nicotine affects multiple transmitter pathways and influences the development of the fetal brain, but also affects eventual programming and synaptic competence.[9] There seems to be resolution of any growth or cognitive function early effects of smoking by about 9 years of age.[10]

Maternal lifetime complications

Atherosclerotic disease, lung cancer, chronic obstructive pulmonary disease, many forms of lung disease, increased risk of ectopic pregnancy, premature menopause, infertility, osteoporosis.

PREGNANCY CONSIDERATIONS

Pregnancy is a **unique opportunity** for medical intervention, with frequent visits, and may be the only time women seek medical attention. Concerns over the dangers of smoking to the fetus may serve as a motivation for smoking cessation. **The safety and efficacy of most pharmacotherapies are uncertain in pregnancy.**[3]

PRINCIPLES

- Goal: smoking cessation during pregnancy.
- Tobacco dependence treatments are both clinically proven and cost-effective relative to other medical disease prevention interventions.[11]
- **Smoking cessation in pregnancy can prevent** 10% of perinatal deaths, 35% of low birth weight births, and 15% of preterm deliveries.[4]
- Smoking in the third trimester has the greatest impact on birth weight.[12]
- Women who quit smoking by the third trimester have birth weights similar to those of non-smokers.[12]

MANAGEMENT

- Smoking cessation programs are helpful compared with no intervention at all.[3]
- Most smokers make many attempts to quit before success is achieved. First-time quitters need to be aware of this trend.[13]
- Explore the reasons for previous failures: assess for non-compliance and improper use of cessation aides in the past.[13]
- Assess for psychosocial comorbidities that may affect smoking cessation.[14]
- Address secondary and passive smoking.

Therapy

Assessment for intervention[13]

Assess and document tobacco use and status at every visit. This increases the likelihood of smoking-related discussions between patients and physicians and increases cessation rates.

Table 20.1   *The 5 'Rs' for smokers who are unwilling to quit smoking*

- *Relevance:* Motivational information to a patient is more effective if it is relevant to a patient's personal circumstances (i.e. smoking can cause adverse effects in pregnancy)
- *Risks:* Stress the acute and long-term risks of smoking. Try to associate it with the patient's current health or illnesses
- *Rewards:* Ask the patient to identify potential benefits of smoking
- *Roadblocks:* Identify barriers or impediments to quitting and note treatment options that could address the barriers
- *Repetition:* Repeat the motivational intervention at each visit

Table 20.2   *The 5 'As' for patients who are willing to quit smoking*

1. *Ask:* Tobacco status is inquired and documented. A multiple choice question method improves disclosure
2. *Advise:* Urge all tobacco users to quit in a clear, strong, personalized manner. Review risks associated with continued smoking
3. *Assess:* Determine the patient's willingness to quit in the next 30 days. If unwilling, the provider should ask and advise at each subsequent office visit
4. *Assist:* Provide smoking cessation materials and provide support. Help the patient develop a plan and provide practical counseling. Pharmacotherapy may be considered for the general population of smokers (unclear use in pregnancy)
5. *Arrange:* Provide follow-up contact, either in person or by telephone soon after the quit date, and further follow-up encounters as needed. Congratulate success during each visit. Review circumstances if a relapse occurred and use it as a learning experience for the patient. Consider referral or more intensive treatment. Assess pharmacotherapy use and problems

The 5-step assessment (**the 5 Rs**) can be used to address the patient who is not willing to initiate smoking cessation (Table 20.1).[11]

The 5-step intervention (**the 5 As**) is recommended in clinical practice to help pregnant women quit smoking (Table 20.2).[13] The 5 As are endorsed by the American College of Obstetricians and Gynecologists (ACOG),[15] the National Cancer Institute, and the British Thoracic Society.

Practical counseling

- Simple advice has a small but positive effect on cessation rates.[16]
- An office-based cessation counseling session of 5–15 minutes with a trained provider and provision of

Table 20.3 *Multiple choice questionnaire improves initial disclosure rates of smoking*[17]

(A) I have never smoked or I have smoked less than 100 cigarettes in my lifetime

(B) I stopped smoking before I found out I was pregnant, and I am not smoking now

(C) I stopped smoking after I found out I was pregnant, and I am not smoking now

(D) I smoke some now, but I have cut down on the number of cigarettes I smoke since I found out I was pregnant

(E) I smoke regularly now, about the same as before I found out I was pregnant

- If the patient responds to B or C, reinforce her decision to quit, congratulate her on success of quitting, and encourage her to remain smoke-free
- If the patient responds to D or E, she should be classified as a smoker.

Document in the chart and proceed to the 5 As (Table 20.2).

Table 20.4 *Smoking cessation counseling (skills training and problem-solving techniques)*

1. Identify activities that increase risk of smoking or relapse
2. Explore coping skills and describe the time and nature of withdrawal
3. Tell patients they may experience anxiety, frustration, depression, and intense cravings for cigarettes
4. Withdrawal symptoms become manageable in a few weeks
5. Make lifestyle changes to reduce stress and improve quality of life
6. Minimize time spent in the company of smokers
7. Provide as much information to the patient as possible: supplement discussions with pamphlets, booklets, videos, hotlines, internet, or support groups

pregnancy-specific educational materials increases the rate of cessation of pregnant smokers by 20%.[15]

- Disclosure rates are improved by 40% if a multiple choice questionnaire is used over the usual 'do you smoke?' question (Table 20.3).[17]
- All interventions for promoting smoking cessation in pregnancy are associated with a **6% decrease in smoking**.[3] The trials with validated **smoking cessation**, a high-intensity intervention, and a high-quality score, are associated with an absolute **decrease in continued smoking in late pregnancy of 5%**. Most studies had as intervention provision of information on risks to fetus/infant and benefits of quitting; use of written material; often teaching cognitive/behavioral strategies for quitting were included. The most effective intervention for

smoking cessation in pregnancy is **social support** and a **reward component** (23% decrease).[18,19] **Smoking cessation programs are associated with a 16% reduction in preterm birth, and a 19% reduction in low birth weight**.[3] Other outcomes (e.g. perinatal mortality) have not been adequately evaluated.

- Focus counseling on skills training and problem-solving techniques[13] (Table 20.4).
- There is a **strong dose–response relationship between the intensity of counseling and its effectiveness**.[11]
- Combined cognitive-behavioral interventions are effective methods of counseling.[3]
- More research is needed to identify the most effective and cost-effective intensity and duration of treatment for different populations of smokers.[20]
- **Group sessions** are poorly attended in most studies, but these sessions appear more effective than self-help programs.[21] **Peer counseling** by lay workers is associated with a reduced number of cigarettes smoked daily but a small non-significant decrease in cessation rates.[22]
- There is a higher success rate when patients are aware that biochemical tests for smoking (levels of nicotine/cotinine in blood, saliva, hair, etc.) will be obtained.
- Telephone hotlines (1-800-QUIT-NOW) and web information (www.smokefree.gov; www.smokefreefamilies.org) sites are helpful.

Pharmacotherapies

Nicotine replacement therapy (NRT) (Table 20.5)

- NRT includes patches, gums, inhalers, lozenges, and nasal spray.
- NRT is a part of an effective strategy to promote smoking cessation in the **general non-pregnant** population.[23]
- May help with nicotine withdrawal, but does not have a significant advantage over other types of interventions.[3]
- In the general population, the effectiveness of NRT is largely dependent on other modes of support provided to the smoker.[21]
- **Nicotine patches** during pregnancy had **no influence in smoking cessation** in women who smoked ≥10 cigarettes/day in one trial.[24]
- **Some studies show that NRT is associated with a trend for benefit**,[25–27] but more recent studies report a 60% increased rate of congenital abnormalities.[28]
- There is insufficient evidence to assure safety in pregnancy, with the ratio of risks and benefits unclear.[3]
- Class D drug with known human risk in pregnancies.
- Risk of adverse effects of nicotine on the fetus through alterations in the uterine, placental, or blood flow to the brain.[3]
- Animal studies suggest nicotine may be toxic to the developing central nervous system.[3]

Table 20.5 *Nicotine replacement therapy*[a]

Nicotine replacement	Dosing regimen	Advantages	Disadvantages
Nicotine patch: Nicoderm CQ or Nicotrol	Nicoderm CQ: 21 mg/day for 6 weeks, then 14 mg/day for 2 weeks, then 7 mg/day for 2 weeks. Nicotrol: single-dose patch for 16 hours/day for 6 weeks (no tapering recommended)	Over-the-counter, easy dosing	Pregnancy D drug. Local skin irritation in up to 50% of users, insomnia with 24 hour dosing; 30–60 minutes required for maximal effect
Nicotine gum or lozenge	Start on quit date: 2 mg tab if < 25 cigarettes per day or 4 mg tab if > 25 cigarettes per day	Over-the-counter, satisfy oral behavior	Low nicotine levels, multiple dosing
Nicotine nasal spray	1–2 doses per hour × 3 months. Most patients require from 7 to 40 sprays over 24 hours	Rapid and higher nicotine levels	Initial adverse effects may include throat and nasal irritation, discouraging use
Nicotine inhaler	10 mg cartridges used over 20 minutes; 6–16 cartridges per day	Substitutes for smoking behavior	Low nicotine levels

[a]Only recommended in the general population, as nicotine replacement therapy (NRT) is associated with congenital anomalies.
Adapted from Morales-Suarez et al.[28]

- ACOG advocates using **nicotine gum** (preferred) **or patches in pregnant women only when non-pharmacological treatments have failed.** Both the patch and the gum are preferable to smoking if there is no alternative. In these cases, the potential benefits of increased chance of smoking cessation outweigh the unknown risk of nicotine replacement with risk of concomitant smoking, but more research is strongly recommended.[15]
- Little evidence about the role of NRT for individuals who smoke less than 15 cigarettes/day.[23]
- All NRT trials look at use of nicotine patches.[3]
- Total nicotine dose is decreased in **gum**, spray, and inhalers and they are preferred to continuous formulations.[3] Blood levels of nicotine may need to be monitored with NRT in pregnancy.

Bupropion (Zyban, Wellbutrin)

- Class C drug in pregnancy and no known adverse fetal effects.
- In controlled clinical trials, this antidepressant increased cessation success for moderate to heavy smokers > 15 cigarettes/ day by 50–100% in the general population of non-pregnant smokers.[3]
- There is no benefit in light smokers < 15 cigarettes/day.[3]
- **There are no trials to assess the safety and efficacy of bupropion as a smoking cessation intervention in pregnancy.**[3] There are only two small physiology studies without recording of preterm birth.
- Dose: 300 mg/day (in two divided doses to minimize side effects). Start 2 weeks prior to anticipated quit date and continue up to 7–12 weeks.

- Advantages: non-nicotine, may be used in combination with patch for greater efficacy, provides therapy for comorbid depression.
- Disadvantages: contraindicated if history of seizures, head trauma, alcohol abuse, or anorexia. Multiple drug interactions with anti-HIV medications.

Combination therapy

- More studies are needed to determine if the use of a nicotine patch in addition to gum or spray or with bupropion is effective in smoking cessation in the general population.[29,30]
- There are no studies to address safety of this management scheme in pregnant patients.

Not recommended

Clonidine.   Limited efficacy. Superior to placebo, but not statistically significant. Side effects include drowsiness, fatigue, and dry mouth.[31]

Nortriptyline (a tricyclic agent).   Some benefit but not FDA (Food and Drug Administration) approved. Class D drug. Unsafe in pregnancy.[32]

Moclobemide (a monoamine oxidase inhibitor).   Some benefit but not FDA approved. Class C drug. Uncertain safety in pregnancy.[32]

Selective serotonin reuptake inhibitors (SSRIs).   Not effective.[33]

Opioids.   Naloxone and naltrexone. Not effective.[34]

Alternative treatments

- Acupuncture: there is no clear evidence that acupuncture, acupressure, laser therapy, or electrostimulation are more effective at smoking cessation than a placebo.[35]
- Hypnotherapy: insufficient data to perform a meta-analysis on hypnotherapy.[36]
- Interventions to increase smoking cessation among the partners of pregnant women, with the additional aim of facilitating cessation by the women themselves, has been insufficiently studied (only 1 trial).[3]
- Stages of change or feedback do not show benefit.[3]

Rewards

Incentives and competitions do not appear to enhance long-term cessation rates. Early success tends to dissipate when rewards are no longer offered.[37]

Breastfeeding

There are lower rates of breastfeeding initiation and reduced duration in smoking women. There is little evidence for association due to physiological effects of smoking on breastfeeding.[3] Breastfed infants of smoking mothers have urinary cotinine levels 50 × higher than breastfed infants of non-smoking mothers and 10 × higher than bottle-fed infants of women who smoke.[8]

Postpartum

Ninety percent of pregnant woman who quit smoking relapse in the first year after delivery,[4] probably due to a period of great stress and emotional fluctuations. There are no known effective strategies for preventing relapse.[38]

PREVENTION
Reduce initiation of smoking

Prevent sales of tobacco to young people, prohibit smoking in public places, increase tobacco taxation, workplace smoking cessation programs, ban on tobacco sponsorship of sporting and cultural events.[3]

Relapse prevention

- There is insufficient evidence to support the use of any specific interventions for helping smokers who have successfully quit for a short time to prevent relapse.[28]
- It may be more efficient to focus efforts on initial cessation attempts.[38]

- Biochemical markers may be used to monitor abstinence once cessation has occurred: carbon monoxide and urinary cotinine.[8] More research is needed to validate this method.[3]

FUTURE

More trials are needed to determine the safety and efficacy of pharmacological therapies such as bupropion.[23] The benefits of nicotine replacement therapy *may* outweigh the risks of fetal exposure to nicotine, but further studies are needed.[23] Current investigations include anti-nicotine vaccine and new pharmaceutical approaches.

REFERENCES

1. Mackay J, Eriksen M. The Tobacco Atlas. Geneva: World Health Organization; 2003. [epidemiological data]
2. U.S. Department of Health and Human Services. Women and Smoking: A Report of the Surgeon General. Rockville: U.S. Department of Health and Human Services, Public Health Service, Office of the Surgeon General; 2001. [epidemiologic data]
3. Lumley J, Oliver SS, Chamberlin C, Oakley L. Interventions for promoting smoking cessation during pregnancy. Cochrane Database Syst Rev 2007; 1. [64 trials, $n=20\,931$]
4. U.S. Department of Health and Human Services. The Health Benefits of Smoking Cessation. U.S. Department of Health and Human Services, Public Health Service, Centers for Disease Control, Center for Chronic Disease Prevention and Health Promotion, Office on Smoking and Health; 1990. [review]
5. Wang X, Zuckerman B, Pearson C, et al. Maternal cigarette smoking, metabolic gene polymorphism, and infant birth weight. JAMA 2002; 287: 195–202. [II-2]
6. Andres RL, Day MC. Perinatal complications associated with maternal tobacco use. Semin Neonatol 2000; 5: 231–41. [II-2]
7. Burton GJ, Palmer ME, Dalton KJ. Morphometric differences between the placental vasculature of non-smokers, smokers, and ex-smokers. Br J Obstet Gynaecol 1989; 96: 907–15. [II-3]
8. Uptodate: Smoking and Pregnancy Rev March 2005: www.uptodate.com [review]
9. Slotkin TA. Fetal nicotine or cocaine exposure: which one is worse? J Pharmacol Exp Ther 1998; 285(3): 931–45. [review]
10. MacArthur C, Knox EG, Lancashire RJ. Effects at age nine of maternal smoking in pregnancy: experimental and observational findings. BJOG 2001; 108: 67–73. [II-2]
11. The Tobacco Use and Dependence Clinical Practice Guideline Panel, Staff, and Consortium Representatives. Treating tobacco use and dependence: A U.S. Public Health Service Report. JAMA 2000; 283: 3244. Available on line at www.surgeongerneral.gov/tobacco/tobarqrg.htm [review]
12. Lieberman E, Gremy I, Lang JM, Cohen AP. Low birthweight at term and timing of fetal exposure to maternal smoking. Am J Public Health 1994; 84: 1127–31. [II-2]
13. Fiore MC, Bailey WC, Cohen SJ, et al. Treating tobacco use and dependence. Quick reference guide for clinicians. Rockville, MD: U.S. Department of Health and Human Services, Public Health Service; October 2000. [guideline]
14. Practice guidelines for the treatment of patients with nicotine dependence. American Psychiatric Association. Am J Psychiatry 1996; 153: 1. [guideline]

15. Smoking cessation during pregnancy. ACOG Technical Bulletin No. 260, September 2000. [review]
16. Lancaster T, Stead LF. Physician advice for smoking cessation. Cochrane Database Sys Rev 2007,1. [meta-analysis: 39 trials, $n = 31\,000$]
17. Mullen PD, Carbonari JP, Tabak E, Glenday MC. Improving disclosure of smoking by pregnant women. Am J Obstet Gynecol 1991; 165: 409–413. [II-3]
18. Sexton M, Hebel JR. A clinical trial of change in maternal smoking and its effect on birth weight. JAMA 1984; 251: 911–15. [RCT]
19. Donatelle RJ, Prows SL, Champeau D, Hudson D. Randomised controlled trial using social support and financial incentives for high risk pregnant smokers: Significant Other Supporter (SOS) program. Tobacco Control 2000; 9(Suppl 3): iii67–9. [RCT]
20. Lancaster T, Stead AF. Individual behavioural counseling for smoking cessation. Cochrane Database Syst Rev 2007,1. [meta-analysis: 21 trials, $n = 7000$]
21. Stead LF, Lancaster T. Group behaviour therapy programmes for smoking cessation. Cochrane Database Syst Rev 2007,1. [meta-analysis]
22. Marchodi CS, Oncken C, Dornelas EA, et al. The effects of peer counseling on smoking cessation and reduction. Obstet Gynecol 2003; 101: 504–10. [RCT, $n = 142$]
23. Silagy C, Lancaster T, Stead L, et al. Nicotine replacement therapy for smoking cessation. Cochrane Database Syst Rev 2007,1. [meta-analysis: 123 trials, non-pregnant adults]
24. Wisborg K, Henriksen TB, Jespersen LB, Secher NJ. Nicotine patches for pregnant smokers: a randomized controlled study. Obstet Gynecol 2000; 96: 967–71. [RCT, $n = 250$]
25. Wisborg K, Henriksen TB, Secher NJ. A prospective intervention study of stopping smoking in pregnancy in a routine antenatal care setting. Br J Obstet Gynaecol 1998; 105: 1171–6. [RCT, $n = 250$]
26. Kapur B, Hackman R, Selby P, Klein J, Koren G. Randomized, double blind, placebo-controlled trial of nicotine replacement therapy in pregnancy. Curr Ther Res 2001; 62(4): 274. [RCT, $n = 30$]
27. Hegaard H, Hjaergaard H, Moller L, Wachmann H, Ottesen B. Multimodel intervention raises smoking cessation rate during pregnancy. Acta Obstet Gynecol Scand 2003; 82: 813–19. [RCT]
28. Morales-Suarez MM, Bille C, Christensen K, Olsen J. Smoking habits, nicotine use, and congenital malformations. Obstet Gynecol 2006; 107: 51–7. [II-2]
29. Simon JA, Duncan C, Carmody TP, et al. Bupriopion for smoking cessation: a randomized trial. Arch Intern Med 2004; 164: 1797. [RCT]
30. Jorenby DE, Leischow SJ, Nides MA, et al. A controlled trial of sustained-release bupropion, a nicotine patch, or both for smoking cessation. N Engl J Med 1999; 340: 685–91. [RCT]
31. Gourlay SG, Stead LF, Benowitz NL. Clonidine for smoking cessation. Cochrane Database Syst Rev 2007,1. [meta-analysis]
32. Uptodate. Overview of smoking cessation. Rev April 2005. www.uptodate.com [review]
33. Hughes JR, Stead L, Lancaster T. Antidepressants for smoking cessation. Cochrane Database Syst Rev 2007,1. [meta-analysis]
34. David S, Lancaster T, Stead LF. Opioid antagonists for smoking cessation. Cochrane Database Syst Rev 2007,1. [meta-analysis]
35. White AR, Rampes H, Ernst E. Acupuncture for smoking cessation. Cochrane Database Syst Rev 2007,1. [meta-analysis: 22 RCTs]
36. Abbot NC, Stead LF, White AR, et al. Hypnotherapy for smoking cessation. Cochrane Database Syst Rev 2007,1. [meta-analysis]
37. Hey K, Perera R. Competitions and incentives for smoking cessation. Cochrane Database Syst Rev 2007,1. [meta-analysis: 15 RCTs]
38. Hajek P, Stead LF, West R, et al. Relapse prevention interventions for smoking cessation. Cochrane Database Syst Rev 2007,1. [meta-analysis: 40 RCTs]

21

Depression

David J Lynn and Elisabeth JS Kunkel

KEY POINTS

- Major depressive disorder (MDD) of postpartum onset (postpartum depression) is associated with maternal complications such as abuse of **alcohol**, attempt of **suicide**, and neglect of nutrition and prenatal care, as well as neonatal complications, such as **slower fetal growth and smaller infant head circumference.**
- The **Edinburgh Postnatal Depression Scale** (EPDS) should be **provided to all postpartum women** for identification.
- **The diagnosis of postpartum depression is MDD occurring within 4 weeks postpartum.**
- A **multidisciplinary approach** is a determinant for successful management.
- **Thyroid function tests, complete blood count** (CBC), **vitamin B$_{12}$, and folate** are the laboratory tests recommended.
- **Prevention: non-medical therapy** (social, support, counseling, and psychotherapy) is associated with conflicting results, with about **half of patients showing benefit.** The provision of **intensive postpartum support provided by public health nurses or midwives** (professional support), identifying mothers 'at-risk', interventions with **only a postnatal component,** and **individually based interventions,** may be more effective than other interventions. There is insufficient evidence to assess the effectiveness of **antidepressants** given immediately postpartum in preventing postnatal depression in all women or just in high-risk women. **Sertraline** (Zoloft – a selective serotonin reuptake inhibitor [SSRI]) **reduces the recurrence of postnatal depression and the time to recurrence,** whereas norethisterone enanthate, a synthetic **progestin,** is associated with a significantly **higher risk of developing postpartum depression** at 6 weeks.
- In women with **recurrent MDD in remission,** maintenance of antidepressant therapy is recommended.
- Therapy:
    - Support/psychotherapy: professional and/or social (lay person) support is associated with a

significant 66% reduction in depression. There is insufficient evidence on what are the most effective types of support. **Interpersonal therapy, psychotherapy at home,** and **non-directive counseling by nurses** are effective. It is important to **promote interaction between the mother and child,** and to involve the child's father in the therapy. Treatment of postpartum depression should **always involve some form of psychotherapy.**

- **Antidepressant medications:** It is not possible to make any recommendations for antidepressant treatment in postnatal depression, as, despite its major public impact, **there is only one small trial. The effects of depression cannot be distinguished from the antidepressant therapy effects. There are insufficient data to assess the long-term effects of the maternal depression or the antidepressant maternal therapy on the child's developing brain. A full trial of 6–8 weeks is needed before considering a trial to have failed (12 weeks for fluoxetine).** If a response is seen, the therapy should be **continued for a minimum of 6 months** after a full remission has been achieved, to avoid a relapse. For **postpartum women who are nursing,** several **medications should be continued,** because the risk of relapse induced by changing antidepressants outweighs the benefits; but if the patient is taking citalopram or doxepin or nefazodone, then either breastfeeding should be discontinued or the antidepressant should be discontinued or changed. If a postpartum patient requires **initiation of antidepressant pharmacotherapy,** the preferred drugs would be **sertraline (SSRI),** or among the tricyclic antidepressants (TCAs), nortriptyline. SSRIs and TCAs have been associated with a **neonatal withdrawal syndrome.**

- **Electroconvulsive therapy** has well-proven effectiveness in non-pregnant adults. It is not recommended as a first-line treatment, but **only after other options have failed,** and it is safe in pregnancy.

- Unproven agents such as **sedatives or nutritional supplements or antipsychotic drugs** (except for the treatment of psychotic symptoms) **cannot be recommended.**

HISTORIC NOTES

- 1930s: Electroconvulsive therapy (ECT) introduced.
- 1950s: Tricyclic antidepressants (TCAs) introduced.
- 1980: *Diagnostic and Statistical Manual of Mental Disorders*, 3rd edn (DSM-III) published, including systematic diagnostic criteria.
- 1987: First selective serotonin reuptake inhibitor (SSRI), fluoxetine, introduced in the USA.

DIAGNOSIS/DEFINITIONS

A **major depressive disorder** (MDD) is defined in the *Diagnostic and Statistical Manual of Mental Disorders*, 4th edn (DSM-IV-TR)[1] by the persistence of **at least five of the following** symptoms over a 2-week period:

1. depressed mood most of the day, nearly every day
2. markedly diminished pleasure in all, or almost all, activities most of the day, nearly every day
3. significant weight loss when not dieting, or weight gain, or decrease or increase in appetite nearly every day
4. insomnia or hypersomnia nearly every day
5. psychomotor agitation or retardation nearly every day
6. fatigue or loss of energy nearly every day
7. feelings of worthlessness or excessive or inappropriate guilt nearly every day
8. diminished ability to think or concentrate, or indecisiveness, nearly every day
9. recurrent thoughts of death, recurrent suicidal ideation without a specific plan, or a suicide attempt or a specific plan for committing suicide.

'**Postpartum blues**' are characterized as mood lability, depressed or irritable mood, and tearfulness, **beginning and remitting within 2 weeks after delivery**, even when untreated.[2] The transient mood disturbance does not affect the woman's ability to function.

Postpartum depression is defined as MDD **occurring within 4 weeks postpartum,**[1] and **can be also called MDD with postpartum onset.** Many studies include up to 3 months postpartum as definition of MDD of postpartum onset.[3] This condition is significantly underdiagnosed, and therefore undertreated.

Postpartum psychosis involves extreme disorganization of thought, bizarre behavior, unusual hallucinations, and delusions, and is usually a manifestation of bipolar disorder. This is an emergency that requires immediate psychiatric referral.

SYMPTOMS

See MDD diagnosis, above.

EPIDEMIOLOGY/INCIDENCE

It is found that **12–16% of women have a major depressive episode** (MDE) **postpartum.** Of these, 30% have thoughts of suicide or infanticide/homicide. Point prevalence of MDD in women of childbearing age is approximately 7–10%. 'Postpartum blues' are common, with an incidence of up to 75% in some studies.[2] Postpartum psychosis is rare, with an incidence of <1%.

ETIOLOGY/BASIC PATHOPHYSIOLOGY

The etiology of MDD is not clearly understood. Several biological markers have been consistently found in MDD:[4]

1. Changes in sleep architecture, including reduced rapid eye movements (REM) latency, increases in the proportion of REM sleep, increased awakenings, and reduced slow-wave sleep.
2. In about 50% of MDD patients, abnormalities in the hypothalamic–pituitary–adrenal axis functioning, demonstrated by non-suppression in the dexamethasone suppression test.
3. In approximately one-third of patients with melancholic depression, the TRH (thyrotropin-releasing hormone) stimulation test is blunted.
4. Reduced blood flow and reduced metabolism in the frontal lobes of patients with MDD are found in functional imaging studies such as single-photon emission computed tomography (SPECT) and positron emission tomography (PET).

RISK FACTORS/ASSOCIATIONS

For MDD with postpartum onset, risk factors are:
- prenatal depression
- previous postpartum psychosis
- a history of bipolar mood disorder
- past MDD with postpartum onset
- previous MDD
- unwanted pregnancy
- unemployment.

Other contributing factors can include marital instability, maternal age <19 years old, victim of violence or abuse, low self-esteem, low socioeconomic status, and other adverse life events.

COMPLICATIONS

From 10% to 15% of patients with mood disorders eventually complete **suicide**. See effects of MDD on the pregnancy and long-term effects of maternal MDD on the offspring below.

PREGNANCY CONSIDERATIONS

Effect of pregnancy on MDD

Pregnancy confers no protection to the mother against recurrences or initial episodes of MDD.

Effects of MDD on the pregnancy

Women experiencing MDD during pregnancy have been found to be more likely to abuse alcohol, to attempt suicide, and to neglect nutrition and prenatal care. They have also been reported to show **slower fetal growth, smaller infant head circumference**, and **increased risk for preterm delivery.**[4]

Long-term effects of maternal MDD on the offspring

Children born of mothers who were depressed during pregnancy have been reported to show **enduring behavioral changes**. When mothers are depressed after delivery, their infants have been reported to show reduced facial expression, reduced crying, and more irritability than other infants. In childhood, offspring of depressed mothers have been reported to show ineffective emotional regulation, slower motor development, lower self-esteem in preschool, increased fearfulness, and increased aggression compared with other children. In the long term, these offspring are reported to show suicidal behavior and emotional instability, and to require psychiatric treatment.[5]

MANAGEMENT (FIGURE 21.1)

Principles

When evaluating risks to mother and fetus, consider effects of exposure to treatment and of exposure to illness. A **multidisciplinary approach, including obstetrician, obstetric nursing, psychiatry services, psychotherapy, and counseling, and other support such as social work as appropriate, is determinant for successful management.**

Screening

MDD, most common in pregnancy with postpartum onset, is significantly underdiagnosed. **The Edinburgh Postnatal**

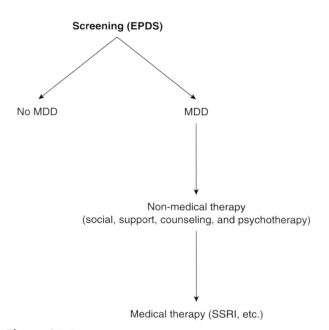

Figure 21.1
Approach to management of MDD with postpartum onset. EPDS, Edinburgh Postnatal Depression Scale; MDD, major depressive disorder; SSRI, selective serotonin reuptake inhibitor.

Depression Scale (EPDS)[6] (Table 21.1), Postpartum Depression Screening Scale (PDSS),[7] or other screening tests should be **provided to all postpartum women** for identification. The EPDS converts responses lettered 'A' with 0, 'B' with 1, 'C' with 2, and 'D' with 3. A score ≥ 10 is usually consistent with postpartum depression. The rate of detection can increase from 6% with clinical screening to 35% with the EPDS.[8] Another alternative is to ask 'Have you had a depressed mood or decreased interest or pleasure in activities most of the day nearly every day for the past 2 weeks?', and, if this is answered affirmatively, review symptoms as per MDD diagnostic criteria. The level of impairment or distress can be explored with the question: 'Has the depression made it hard for you to do your work, take care of things at home, or get along with people?'.[3]

Counseling

The woman with MDD of postpartum onset should be aware of the incidence (very common), prognosis, management, and complications of depressive postpartum disorders. Benefits and risks of interventions should be discussed.

Work-up

No clinical laboratory findings have been found to be diagnostic of MDD. **Thyroid function tests, complete blood count (CBC), vitamin B$_{12}$, folate**, and other tests are useful

| Table 21.1 *Edinburgh postnatal Depression Scale (EPDS)*[6] | |

We would like to know how you are feeling. Please circle the answer that comes closest to how you have felt in the past 7 days, not just how you feel today. When you have completed the form, please give this form to your nurse. Thank you

1. **I have been able to laugh and see the funny side of things.**
   A. As much as I always could
   B. Not quite so much now
   C. Definitely not so much now
   D. Not at all

2. **I have looked forward with enjoyment to things.**
   A. As much as I ever did
   B. Rather less than I used to
   C. Definitely less than I used to
   D. Hardly at all

3. **I have blamed myself unnecessarily when things went wrong.**
   A. No, never
   B. Not very often
   C. Yes, some of the time
   D. Yes, most of the time

4. **I have been anxious or worried for no good reason.**
   A. No, not at all
   B. Hardly ever
   C. Yes, sometimes
   D. Yes, very often

5. **I have felt scared or panicky for no good reason.**
   B. No, not much
   C. Yes, sometimes
   D. Yes, quite a lot

6. **Things have been getting on top of me.**
   A. No, I have been coping as well as ever
   B. No, most of the time I have coped quiet well
   C. Yes, sometimes I haven't been coping as well as usual
   D. Yes, most of the time I haven't been able to cope at all

7. **I have been so unhappy that I have had difficulty sleeping.**
   A. No, not at all
   B. Not very often
   C. Yes, sometimes
   D. Yes, most of the time

8. **I have felt sad or miserable**
   A. No, not at all
   B. Not very often
   C. Yes, quite often
   D. Yes, most of the time

9. **I have been so unhappy that I have been crying.**
   A. No, never
   B. Only occasionally
   C. Yes, quite often
   D. Yes, most of the time

10. **The thought of harming myself has occurred to me.**
   A. No, never
   B. Hardly ever
   C. Sometimes
   D. Yes, quiet often

in diagnosing medical disorders that can cause dysphoria. Prompt psychiatric consultation should be considered; it is especially appropriate when symptoms are severe, or when psychotic features are present. The presence of suicidal or homicidal intent or ideation is an emergency.

Prevention

Trials of **non-medical therapy** (social, support, counseling, and psychotherapy) for prevention of postpartum depression in normal women have reported conflicting results, with about **half of them showing benefit**[9–19] (Table 21.2).[20] Overall, women who receive a **psychosocial intervention are equally likely to develop postpartum depression as those receiving standard care**. The provision of **intensive postpartum support provided by public health nurses or midwives (professional support)** is associated with 32% less postpartum depression.[21] **Identifying mothers 'at-risk'** assisted the prevention of postpartum depression compared with intervening on the general population. Interventions with **only a postnatal component** appeared to be more beneficial than interventions that also incorporated an antenatal component. **Individually based interventions** may be more effective than group-based

interventions. Women who received multiple-contact intervention are just as likely to experience postpartum depression as those who received a single-contact intervention.[21]

There is insufficient evidence to assess the effectiveness of **antidepressants** given immediately postpartum in preventing postnatal depression in all women or just in high-risk women. **Sertraline** (Zoloft; an SSRI) **reduces the recurrence of postnatal depression and the time to recurrence** when compared with placebo in a very small trial.[22] Nortriptyline (a TCA) did not show any benefit over placebo.[23]

Norethisterone enanthate, a synthetic **progestin**, 200 mg IM administered once within 48 hours of delivery to unselected women is associated with a significantly **higher risk of developing postpartum depression** at 6 weeks.[24]

In women with **recurrent MDD in remission, maintenance of antidepressant therapy** at the doses which were necessary to bring about the remission is recommended.[25]

Preconception counseling

Counseling concerning risks of recurrence of MDD and risks and benefits of somatic (medications, ECT) and psychotherapeutic treatments may be helpful.

Table 21.2 *Trials on prophylactic/preventive interventions for postpartum depressions[20]*

Ref	First author	Participants	Intervention	Findings
9	Gordon	161 pregnant women	2 antenatal instruction periods with or without partner attending	Fewer postpartum 'emotional upsets', especially if partner attended also
10	Lavender	120 women pregnant for first time	Debriefing by a midwife	Less anxiety and depression
11	Small	917 women delivered by cesarean section, forceps, or vacuum extraction	Debriefing by a midwife	No effect
12	Morrell	623 women after delivery	10 home visits by a community support worker	No effect
13	Brugha	190 women depressed during pregnancy	6 antenatal classes, 2 hours per week	No effect
14	Elliott	99 women expecting first or second child	11 sessions (5 during pregnancy and 6 afterwards)	Less depression
15	Hayes	206 women pregnant for first time	Antenatal education package	No effect
16	Zlotnick	37 pregnant women	4 sessions of interpersonal therapy in groups	Less depression
17	Cooper	64 pregnant Xhosa women	2 antenatal and 20 postnatal visits by community workers	No effect on mood, but improved mother–infant interactions
18	MacArthur	2064 women after delivery	3 months of visits by midwives trained in guidelines for care	Less depression
19	Reid	1004 pregnant women	Self-help pack and one support group	No effect

Prenatal care

Nothing specific, other than appropriate support and treatment for MDD.

THERAPY

Support/psychotherapy

Treatment of postpartum depression with **professional and/or social (lay person) support is associated with a significant 66% reduction in depression** at 25 weeks after giving birth. There is insufficient evidence on what are the most effective types of support.[26] Table 21.3 reviews the trials on non-medical therapy (social, support, counseling, and psychological) for post-partum depression.[27–40] **Interpersonal therapy**, which is a time-limited psychotherapy focusing on interpersonal relationships and role transitions, was shown to be beneficial,[33] as well as **psychotherapy at home**[26,27] and non-directive counseling by nurses.[30] It is important to **promote interaction between mother and child. Involving the child's father in therapy** benefits the mother's mood, with decrease in MDD.[20]

Two defined forms of individual psychotherapy – cognitive-behavioral therapy (CBT) and interpersonal therapy (IPT) – have each been shown to be effective in mild to moderate MDD, both alone and in combination with antidepressant medications.[41] **Treatment of postpartum depression should always involve some form of psychotherapy.**[20] Policies of managed care organizations and other practical factors often limit the availability of these therapies.

Antidepressant drugs

It is not possible to make any recommendations for antidepressant treatment in postnatal depression, as, despite its major public impact, **there is only one small trial**[31] (see fluoxetine below). It is important to realize that, except for the trial, studies in pregnancy do not compare safety and effects of antidepressants in pregnant women with MDD who do or do not take antidepressants, but compare safety and effects of antidepressants in pregnant women with MDD who do take antidepressants vs women without MDD on no antidepressants, so that **the effects of depression cannot be distinguished from the antidepressant therapy effects.** As stated above, there is evidence to suggest that women

Table 21.3 *Trials on non-medical (social, support, counseling, psychological) treatment of postpartum depression*

Ref	First author	Participants	Intervention	Findings
27	Holden	50 women with postpartum depression	8 counseling visits by health visitors	Less depression
28	Fleming	142 newly delivered women	8 supportive group sessions	No effect
29	Wolman	189 primiparas without a supportive companion	Companionship during labor	Less depression
30	Wickberg	41 women with postpartum depression	6 counseling visits by nurse	Less depression
31	Appleby	61 women with postpartum depression	6 sessions of cognitive-behavioral counseling	Less depression
32	Armstrong	181 vulnerable postpartum women	Home visits by a nurse, supported by a social worker and pediatrician	Less depression and better mother–infant interaction
33	O'Hara	120 women with postpartum depression	12 weeks interpersonal psychotherapy	Less depression
34	Misri	29 women with postpartum depression	7 psychoeducational visits, involving partners	Less depression in both mothers and fathers
35	Chen	60 women with postpartum depression	4 supportive group sessions	Less depression
36	Chabrol	859 puerperal women scoring ≥9 on EPDS	A single counseling session on obstetric unit, then 5–8 home visits	Less depression
37	Honey	45 women with postpartum depression	8 psychoeducational groups	Less depression
38	Dennis	42 women with high EPDS scores	Telephone-based peer support	Less depression
39	Cooper	193 depressed mothers	3 forms of psychological treatment from 8 to 18 weeks postpartum, 5 years follow-up	Less depression and mother–infant relationship difficulties, but only in short term

EPDS, Edinburgh Postnatal Depression Scale.

with untreated depression have adverse fetal/neonatal effects, including low birth weight and developmental delay.[42] There are **insufficient data to assess long-term effects of the maternal depression or the antidepressant maternal therapy on the child's developing brain.**

All antidepressant drugs are *equally* effective and require at least 3–4 weeks to show a response – note: at least one randomized controlled trial (RCT) – in non-pregnant adults; a **full trial of 6–8 weeks is needed before considering a trial to have failed (12 weeks for fluoxetine).** If a response is seen, the therapy should be **continued for a minimum of 6 months** after a full remission has been achieved, to avoid a relapse.[3] All antidepressant drugs have been reported to **induce mania** in some patients with bipolar affective disorder, especially when used in the absence of mood-stabilizing agents. Antidepressants with proven effectiveness are sufficiently numerous and diverse that unproven agents, such as

sedatives or nutritional supplements or antipsychotic drugs (except for the treatment of psychotic symptoms), **cannot be recommended.** Even within an antidepressant drug class, failure of one antidepressant drug does not predict failure of others. Given the prevalence of adolescent pregnancy, it is important to note that the Food and Drug Administration (FDA) has mandated a warning for all antidepressant drugs when used in adolescents (and children), because pooled data have shown a doubling of suicidal ideation and behaviors (but not completed suicides) when these drugs are used in this patient group. For each drug or drug class in the following subsections, the generic name is followed by the brand name in parentheses; mechanism of action; FDA pregnancy risk category; comments on teratogenicity; comments on neonatal toxicity; comments on safety in breastfeeding; maternal side effects; and comments on drug interactions.

For **postpartum women who are nursing**, the following steps can be recommended:

1. If the patient is currently being treated successfully with fluoxetine, paroxetine, sertraline, fluvoxamine, amitriptyline, imipramine, clomipramine, desipramine, nortriptyline, maprotiline, protriptyline, amoxapine, buproprion, mirtazapine, trazodone, or venlafaxine, then this **medication should be continued**, because the risk of relapse induced by changing antidepressants outweighs the benefits.
2. If the patient is taking citalopram or doxepin or nefazodone, then either breastfeeding should be discontinued or the antidepressant should be discontinued or changed.
3. If a postpartum patient requires **initiation of antidepressant pharmacotherapy**, the preferred drugs would be **sertraline**, or among the TCAs, nortriptyline.

Selective serotonin reuptake inhibitors

All of the following SSRIs have been shown to be safe and effective for MDD in general non-pregnant use. A **neonatal withdrawal syndrome** associated with third trimester exposure to serotonin reuptake inhibitors (SSRIs – a group which includes SSRIs plus venlafaxine and duloxetine) has been described when used in pregnancy.[43–45] This syndrome includes the following transient signs in order of decreasing frequency: irritability, hypertonia, jitteriness, trouble feeding, tremor, agitation, seizures, tachypnea, posturing, crying, trouble breathing, screaming, vomiting, hypotonia, high-pitched cry, hypothermia, shivering, respiratory distress, hyperreflexia, jerkiness, and electroencephalographic (EEG) abnormalities. A database established by the WHO contains 74 total cases,[44] and a recent review 93 more cases.[45] The exact incidence is unknown, but the risk is probably < 5%, possibly < 1%.[45] **Paroxetine is the SSRI with the highest incidence of neonatal withdrawal syndrome.**[45] SSRI use after 20 weeks of pregnancy has also been associated with a 1% risk of **persistent pulmonary hypertension** of the newborn, a five-fold increase over the baseline risk of 0.2%.[46]

Fluoxetine (Prozac). Dose = 20–60 mg/day; SSRI; FDA pregnancy risk category = C;[5] teratogenicity = no difference from unexposed;[44] neonatal toxicity = behavioral syndrome (10 of 74 WHO cases);[43,47] breastfeeding = Thomson Micromedex rating 'potential risk', relative infant dose = 6.5–11,[48] ratio of infant plasma to breast milk = 0.04,[49] fluoxetine and norfluoxetine, an active metabolite, are excreted in breast milk and have been detected in infant plasma – some possible infant side effects have been reported;[50] maternal side effects = sexual dysfunction, headaches, nausea, anxiety, increased sweating, uncommonly akathisia; drug interactions – fluoxetine is an inhibitor of P450 CYPC9/10, CYP2C19, and a potent inhibitor CYP2D6.[4]

Fluoxetine (Prozac) 20 mg is, after an initial session of counseling, **as effective as a full course of cognitive-behavioral counseling** in the treatment of postnatal depression.[31]

Paroxetine (Paxil). Dose = 20–50 mg/day; SSRI; FDA pregnancy risk category = D; teratogenicity = no difference from unexposed;[44] neonatal toxicity = behavioral syndrome (51 of 74 WHO cases);[45] breastfeeding = Thomson Micromedex rating 'minimal risk', relative infant dose 1.13–1.25,[48] ratio of infant plasma to breast milk = 0.01,[49] paroxetine is excreted in breast milk to a minor extent – no detectable levels have been found in infant plasma – no infant side effects have been reported;[50] maternal side effects = sexual dysfunction, headaches, nausea, anxiety, increased sweating, uncommonly akathisia, and a transient discontinuation syndrome when abruptly stopped; drug interactions – paroxetine is a strong inhibitor of P450 CYP2D6.[4] Avoid in pregnancy if possible.

Sertraline (Zoloft). Dose = 50–200 mg/day; SSRI; FDA pregnancy risk category = C;[5] teratogenicity = no difference from unexposed;[44] neonatal toxicity = behavioral syndrome (7 of 74 WHO cases);[43] breastfeeding = Thomson Micromedex rating 'safe', relative infant dose = 0.2,[48] ratio of infant plasma to breast milk = 0.00,[49] sertraline and its weakly active metabolite norsertraline are excreted in breast milk to a low extent – detectable levels have been found in infant plasma – one case of disordered sleep may have been an infant side effect;[50] maternal side effects = sexual dysfunction, headaches, nausea, anxiety, increased sweating, uncommonly akathisia, and a transient discontinuation syndrome when abruptly stopped; drug interactions – sertraline is an inhibitor of P450 CYP2D6.[4]

Citalopram; Escitalopram (Celexa; Lexapro). Dose = 20–60 mg/day for Celexa, 10–20 mg/day for Lexapro; SSRI; FDA pregnancy risk category = C;[4] teratogenicity = no difference from unexposed;[44] neonatal toxicity = behavioral syndrome (6 of 74 WHO cases);[43] breastfeeding = Thomson Micromedex rating 'unsafe; change therapy or discontinue breastfeeding', relative infant dose = 4.4–5.1,[48] ratio of infant plasma to breast milk = 0.04,[49] citalopram and its inactive metabolite desmethylcitalopram are excreted in breast milk – some detectable levels have been found in infant plasma – one case of transient irritability, constant crying, shaking, increased tonus, convulsions, and poor food intake may have been an infant side effect;[50] maternal side effects = sexual dysfunction, headaches, nausea, anxiety, increased sweating, uncommonly akathisia and a transient discontinuation syndrome when abruptly stopped; drug interactions – citalopram is not an inhibitor of P450 enzymes.[4]

Fluvoxamine (Luvox). Dose = 50–300 mg/day; SSRI; FDA pregnancy risk category = C;[4] teratogenicity = no difference from unexposed;[44] neonatal toxicity = possible behavioral syndrome (none of 74 WHO cases);[43] breastfeeding = Thomson Micromedex rating 'potential risk', relative infant dose = 1.34–1.38,[48] ratio of infant plasma to breast milk = 0.18,[49] fluvoxamine is excreted in breast milk to a minor extent – no detectable levels have been found in infant plasma – one case of icterus is deemed unlikely to have been an infant side effect;[50] maternal side effects = sexual dysfunction, headaches, nausea, anxiety, increased sweating, uncommonly akathisia; drug interactions – fluvoxamine is an inhibitor of P450 CYP1A2, CYP2C9/10, CYP2C19, and CYP3A3/4/5.[4]

Tricyclic antidepressants

All of the following TCAs have been shown to be safe and effective for MDD in general use (note: at least one non-pregnant RCT). Risks and side effects for this group include quinidine-like cardiac effects with lethality in overdose; anticholinergic effects such as dry mouth and exacerbation of urinary obstruction; orthostatic hypotension; weight gain; and sedation.[5] Mechanisms of action may include effects on norepinephrine, serotonin, and dopamine neurotransmitter systems. For most of these agents, serum levels have been reliably linked to effectiveness and toxicity. Paroxitine should be avoided in pregnancy, if possible.

Amitriptyline (Elavil, Endep). Dose = 150–300 mg/day; TCA; FDA pregnancy risk category = unknown; teratogenicity = no difference from unexposed;[44] neonatal toxicity = not reported; breastfeeding = Thomson Micromedex rating 'potential risk', amitriptyline and its active metabolite (nortriptyline) are excreted in breast milk – some detectable levels have been found in infant plasma[49] – no infant side effects have been reported; see TCA maternal side effects above; drug interactions – amitriptyline is a substrate of P450 CYP1A2 and an inhibitor of P450 CYP2D6.[4]

Imipramine (Tofranil). Dose = 150–300 mg/day; TCA; FDA pregnancy risk category = unknown; teratogenicity = no difference from unexposed;[44] neonatal toxicity = not reported; breastfeeding = Thomson Micromedex rating 'potential risk', imipramine and its active metabolite are excreted in breast milk – some detectable levels have been found in infant plasma[49] – no infant side effects have been reported; see TCA maternal side effects above; drug interactions – imipramine is an inhibitor of P450 CYP2D6.[4]

Clomipramine (Anafranil). Dose = 150–250 mg/day; TCA; FDA pregnancy risk category = C;[5] teratogenicity = no difference from unexposed;[44] neonatal toxicity = not reported; breastfeeding = Thomson Micromedex rating 'potential risk', clomipramine and its active metabolite are excreted in breast milk – some detectable levels have been found in infant plasma[49] – no infant side effects have been reported; see TCA maternal side effects above; drug interactions – clomipramine is an inhibitor of P450 CYP2D6.[4]

Desipramine (Norpramin). Dose = 150–300 mg/day; TCA; FDA pregnancy risk category = unknown; teratogenicity = no difference from unexposed;[44] neonatal toxicity = not reported; breastfeeding = Thomson Micromedex rating 'potential risk', desipramine is excreted in breast milk – some detectable levels have been found in infant plasma[49] – no infant side effects have been reported; see TCA maternal side effects above; drug interactions – desipramine is an inhibitor of P450 CYP2D6.[4]

Nortriptyline (Pamelor, Aventyl). Dose = 75–150 mg/day; TCA; FDA pregnancy risk category = unknown; teratogenicity = no difference from unexposed;[44] neonatal toxicity = not reported; breastfeeding = Thomson Micromedex rating 'safe', nortriptyline is excreted in breast milk – lower levels than other TCAs have been found in infant plasma[49] – no infant side effects have been reported; see TCA maternal side effects above; drug interactions – nortriptyline is an inhibitor of P450 CYP2D6.[4]

Doxepin (Sinequan, Adapin). Dose = 150–300 mg/day; TCA; FDA pregnancy risk category = B; teratogenicity = no difference from unexposed;[44] neonatal toxicity = not reported; breastfeeding = Thomson Micromedex rating 'unsafe; change therapy or discontinue breastfeeding', doxepin is excreted in breast milk – some detectable levels have been found in infant plasma[49] – no infant side effects have been reported; see TCA maternal side effects above; drug interactions – doxepin is an inhibitor of P450 CYP2D6.[4]

Maprotiline (Ludiomil). Dose = 140–225 mg/day; TCA; FDA pregnancy risk category = B;[5] teratogenicity = no difference from unexposed;[44] neonatal toxicity = not reported; breastfeeding = Thomson Micromedex rating 'potential risk', maprotiline is excreted in breast milk – no data are available concerning levels in infant plasma[49] – no infant side effects have been reported; see TCA maternal side effects above; drug interactions – maprotiline is an inhibitor of P450 CYP2D6.[4]

Protriptyline (Vivactil). Dose = 15–60 mg/day; TCA; FDA pregnancy risk category = unknown; teratogenicity = no difference from unexposed;[44] neonatal toxicity = not reported; breastfeeding = Thomson Micromedex rating 'potential risk', protriptyline is excreted in breast milk – some detectable levels have been found in infant plasma[49] – no infant side effects have been reported; see TCA maternal side effects above; drug interactions – protriptyline is an inhibitor of P450 CYP2D6.[4]

Amoxapine (Asendin). Dose = 150–400 mg/day; TCA; FDA pregnancy risk category = C;[5] teratogenicity = no difference from unexposed; neonatal toxicity = not reported; breastfeeding = Thomson Micromedex rating 'potential risk', amoxapine is excreted in breast milk – no data are available concerning levels found in infant plasma[5,49] – no infant side effects have been reported; see TCA maternal side effects above, note also extrapyramidal effects, including long-term risks of tardive dyskinesia; drug interactions – amoxapine is an inhibitor of P450 CYP2D6.[4] This drug is a combination of amitriptyline and loxapine, a typical antipsychotic agent.

Other antidepressants

All of the following antidepressants have been shown to be safe and effective for MDD in general non-pregnant use (note: at least one RCT).

Buprorion (Wellbutrin). Dose = 150–450 mg/day; mechanism not clearly understood; FDA pregnancy risk category = C; teratogenicity = no difference from unexposed;[48] neonatal toxicity = none reported; breastfeeding = Thomson Micromedex rating 'potential risk', buproprion is excreted in breast milk – no detectable levels have been found in infant plasma (3 cases measured)[48] – one case of a possible infant seizure has been reported;[48] maternal side effects include increased risk of seizures; drug interactions – buproprion is an inhibitor of P450 CYP2D6.[4]

Mirtazapine (Remeron). Dose = 15–45 mg/day; mechanism is through blockade of several serotonin receptors and α_2-adrenergic receptors, increasing norepinephrine and serotonin release; FDA pregnancy risk category = C;[5] teratogenicity = no difference from unexposed;[48] neonatal toxicity = one case of persistent fetal circulation reported;[48] breastfeeding = Thomson Micromedex rating 'potential risk', mirtazapine is excreted in breast milk – no measurable levels have been found in infant plasma (1 case measured)[48] – no adverse effects have been reported; maternal side effects include weight gain, sedation, and anticholinergic effects; drug interactions – no pharmacokinetic interactions reported.[4]

Nefazodone (Serzone). Dose = 300–600 mg/day; mechanism of action not clearly understood;[5] FDA pregnancy risk category = C;[5] teratogenicity = little data available; neonatal toxicity = not reported; breastfeeding = Thomson Micromedex rating 'unsafe; change therapy or discontinue breastfeeding', nefazodone is excreted in breast milk – some detectable levels have been found in infant plasma[49] – no infant side effects have been reported; maternal side effects include rare hepatic failure, sexual dysfunction, sedation, nausea, and hypotension; drug interactions – nefazodone is an inhibitor of P450 CYP3A3/4/5.[4]

Trazodone (Desyrel). Dose = 200–300 mg/day; mechanism of action not clearly understood but involves complex agonistic and antagonistic effects on serotonergic neurotransmission;[5] FDA pregnancy risk category = C;[5] teratogenicity = no available data; neonatal toxicity = not reported; breastfeeding = Thomson Micromedex rating 'potential risk', trazodone is excreted in breast milk – no data are available on infant plasma[5,49] – no infant side effects have been reported; adult side effects include rare priapism in males, sedation, spontaneous orgasms in females, and orthostatic hypotension; drug interactions – trazodone is a substrate of P450 CYP2D6.[4]

Venlafaxine (Effexor). Dose = 150–375 mg/day; mechanism of action is through inhibition of reuptake of serotonin, norepinephrine, and dopamine; FDA pregnancy risk category = C;[5] teratogenicity = no difference from unexposed;[48] neonatal toxicity = possible behavioral syndrome (one case);[43] breastfeeding = Thomson Micromedex rating 'potential risk', relative infant dose = 5.5–7.6,[48] ratio of infant plasma to breast milk = 2.5,[49] venlafaxine is excreted in breast milk – detectable levels have been found in infant

plasma[49] – no adverse events have been described in neonates;[48] maternal side effects include sexual dysfunction, nausea, sedation, headache, increases in blood pressure, and discontinuation symptoms; drug interactions – venlafaxine is not reported to cause pharmacokinetic interactions.[4]

Monoamine oxidase inhibitors (MAOIs): phenelzine (Nardil), isocarboxazid (Marplan), tranylcypromine (Parnate). These antidepressant drugs act by inhibiting monoamine oxidase. Interactions with tyramine, a substance present in many foods, and with a wide range of sympathomimetic drugs (including TCAs, buspirone, pseudoephedrine, and venlafaxine), can produce dangerous, even fatal, hypertensive crises. Interactions with meperidine can be fatal. Interactions with serotonergic drugs, including SSRIs, fenfluramine, and tryptophan, can cause a dangerous serotonin syndrome. For all of these reasons, the utility of MAO inhibitors during pregnancy and lactation is severely limited.[5,25]

Hormonal therapy (estrogen or progesterone) for treatment of postpartum depression

There is insufficient evidence to fully assess the efficacy of hormonal therapy for postpartum depression. Estrogen therapy (24 weeks of transdermal 17β-estradiol 200 μg daily with added cyclical dehydrogesterone [10 mg daily for 12 days of each month for the last 12 weeks]) is associated with a greater improvement in depression scores than placebo among women with severe depression in a small trial.[51,52] No trials on progesterone for treatment of severe depression have been reported.

Electroconvulsive therapy

ECT has well-proven effectiveness in the treatment of MDD in non-pregnant adults, especially when **psychotic** features are present and antipsychotic medical therapy has failed (note: at least one RCT). It is not recommended as a first-line treatment, but **only after other options have failed.** Usually, treatments are given under anesthesia approximately three times per week, with a response becoming evident in 6–9 treatments. Side effects include transient memory loss, but no studies have reliably shown permanent memory loss. **ECT is safe in pregnancy.**[53]

RESOURCES

Women may find useful information at www.4woman.gov, www.chss.iup.edu/postpartum, and www.depressionafter-delivery.com.

REFERENCES

1. American Psychiatric Association. Diagnostic and Statistical Manual of Mental Disorders, 4th edn, text revision. Washington, DC: American Psychiatric Association; 2000. [review]
2. Miller LJ, Rukstalis M. Postpartum Mood Disorders. Washington, DC: American Psychiatric Publishing; 1999. [review]
3. Weisner KL, Parry BL, Piontek CM. Postpartum depression. N Engl J Med 2002; 347: 194–9. [review]
4. Hales RE, Yudofsky SC, eds. The American Psychiatric Publishing Textbook of Clinical Psychiatry, 4th edn. Washington, DC: American Psychiatric Publishing; 2003. [review]
5. Schatzberg AF, Nemeroff CB, eds. The American Psychiatric Publishing Textbook of Psychopharmacology, 3rd edn. Washington, DC: American Psychiatric Publishing; 2004. [review]
6. Cox JL, Holden JM, Sagovsky R. Detection of postnatal depression. Development of the 10-item Edinburgh Postnatal Depression Scale. Br J Psychiatry 1987; 150: 782–6. [III]
7. Beck CT, Gable RK. Further validation of the postpartum depression screening scale. Nurs Res 2001; 50: 155–64. [II-2]
8. Evins GG, Theofrastous JP, Galvin SL. Postpartum depression: a comparison of screening and routine clinical evaluation. Am J Obstet Gynecol 2000; 182: 1080–2. [II-2]
9. Gordon RE, Gordon KK. Social factors in the prevention of postpartum emotional problems. Obstet Gynecol 1960; 15: 433–8. [RCT]
10. Lavender T, Walkinshaw SA. Can midwives reduce postpartum psychological morbidity? A randomized trial. Birth 1998; 25: 215–19. [RCT]
11. Small R, Lumley J, Donohue L, Potter A, Waldenstrom U. Randomised controlled trial of midwife-led debriefing to reduce maternal depression after operative childbirth. BMJ 2000; 321: 1043–7. [RCT]
12. Morrell CJ, Spiby H, Stewart P, Walters S, Morgan A. Costs and effectiveness of community postnatal support workers: randomised controlled trial. BMJ 2000; 321: 593–8. [RCT]
13. Brugha TS, Wheatley S, Taub NA, et al. Pragmatic randomized trial of antenatal intervention to prevent post-natal depression by reducing psychosocial risk factors. Psychol Med 2000; 30: 1273–81. [RCT]
14. Elliott SA, Leverton TJ, Sanjack M, et al. Promoting mental health after childbirth: a controlled trial of primary prevention of postnatal depression. Br J Clin Psychol 2000; 39: 223–41. [RCT]
15. Hayes BA, Muller R, Bradley BS. Perinatal depression: a randomised controlled trial of an antenatal education intervention for primiparas. Birth 2001; 28: 28–35. [RCT]
16. Zlotnick C, Johnson SL, Miller IW, Pearlstein T, Howard M. Postpartum depression in women receiving public assistance: pilot study of an interpersonal-therapy-oriented group intervention. Am J Psychiatry 2001; 158: 638–40. [RCT]
17. Cooper PJ, Landman M, Tomlinson M, et al. Impact of a mother–infant intervention in an indigent peri-urban South African context pilot study. Br J Psychiatry 2002; 180: 76–80. [RCT]
18. MacArthur C, Winter HR, Bick DE, et al. Effects of redesigned community postnatal care of womens' health 4 months after birth: a cluster randomised controlled trial. Lancet 2002; 359: 378–85. [RCT]
19. Reid M, Glazener C, Murray GD, Taylor GS. A two-centred pragmatic randomised controlled trial of two interventions of postnatal support. Br J Obstet Gynaecol 2002; 109: 1164–70. [RCT]
20. Brockington I. Postpartum psychiatric disorders. Lancet 2004; 363: 303–10. [review]
21. Dennis CL, Creedy D. Psychosocial and psychological interventions for preventing postpartum depression. Cochrane Database Syst Rev 2005; 4. [meta-analysis: 15 RCTs, n = >7600]
22. Howard LM, Hoffbrand S, Henshaw C, Boath L, Bradley E. Antidepressant prevention of postnatal depression. Cochrane Database Syst Rev 2005; 4. [meta-analysis: 2 RCTs, n = 73, intention to treat analyses were not carried out in either trial]
23. Wisner KL, Perel JM, Peindl KS, et al. Prevention of recurrent postpartum depression: a randomised clinical trial. J Clin Psychiatry 2001; 62: 82–6. [RCT]
24. Lawrie TA, Hofmeyr GJ, de Jager M, et al. A double-blind randomised placebo controlled trial of postnatal norethisterone enanthate: the effect on postnatal depression and serum hormones. Br J Obstet Gynaecol 1998; 105: 1082–90. [RCT, n = 180]
25. American Psychiatric Association. Practice Guideline for the Treatment of Patients With Major Depressive Disorder, 2nd edn. Washington, DC: American Psychiatric Association; 2000. [review]
26. Ray KL, Hodnett ED. Caregiver support for postpartum depression. Cochrane Database Syst Rev 2005; 4. [meta-analysis: 2 RCTs, n = 111]
27. Holden JM, Sagovsky R, Cox JL. Counselling in a general practice setting: controlled study of a health visitor intervention of postnatal depression. BMJ 1989; 298: 223–6. [RCT]
28. Fleming AS, Klein E, Corter C. The effects of a social support group on depression, maternal attitudes and behavior in new mothers. J Child Psychol Psychiatry 1992; 33: 685–98. [RCT]
29. Wolman WL, Chalmers B, Hofmeyr GJ, Kinodem VC. Postpartum depression and companionship in the clinical birth environment: a randomized, controlled study. Am J Obstet Gynecol 1993; 168: 1388–93. [RCT]
30. Wickberg B, Hwang CP. Counselling of postnatal depression: a controlled study on a population-based Swedish sample. J Affect Disord 1996; 39: 209–16. [RCT]
31. Appleby L, Warner R, Whitton A, Faragher B. A controlled study of fluoxetine and cognitive-behavioural counseling in a treatment of postnatal depression. BMJ 1997; 314: 932–6. [RCT, n = 61; only trial in Cochrane Library on antidepressant treatment of postpartum depression].
32. Armstrong KL, Fraser JA, Dadds MR, Morris J. A randomized, controlled trial of nurse home visiting to vulnerable families with newborns. J Paediatr Child Health 1999; 35: 237–44. [RCT]
33. O'Hara MW, Stuart S, Gorman LL, Wenzel A. Efficacy of interpersonal psychotherapy for postpartum depression. Arch Gen Psychiatry 2000; 57: 1039–45. [RCT]
34. Misri S, Kostaras X, Fox D, Kostaras D. The impact of partner support in the treatment of postpartum depression. Can J Psychiatry 2000; 45: 554–8. [RCT]
35. Chen CH, Tseng YF, Chou FH, Wang SY. Effects of support group intervention in postnatally distressed women: a controlled study in Taiwan. J Psychosom Res 2000; 49: 395–9. [RCT]
36. Chabrol H, Teissedre F, Saint-Jean M, et al. [Detection, prevention and treatment of postpartum] depression: a controlled study of 859 patients. Encephal 2002; 28: 65–70. [RCT] [in French]
37. Honey KL, Bennet P, Morgan M. A brief psycho-educational group intervention for postnatal depression. Br J Clin Psychol 2002; 41; 412–19. [RCT]
38. Dennis CL. The effect of peer support on postpartum depression: a pilot randomized controlled trial. Can J Psychiatry 2003; 48: 115–24. [RCT]
39. Cooper PJ, Murray L, Wilson A, Romaniuk H. Controlled trial of the short- and long-term effect of psychological treatment of postpartum depression: 1, impact on maternal mood. Br J Psychiatry 2003; 182: 412–19. [RCT]
40. Murray L, Cooper PJ, Wilson A, Romaniuk H. Controlled trial of the short- and long-term effect of psychological treatment of postpartum depression: 2, impact on the mother–child relationship and child outcome. Br J Psychiatry 2003; 182: 420–7. [RCT]
41. Elkin I, Shea MT, Watkins JT, et al. National Institute of Mental Health Treatment of Depression Collaborative Research Program. General effectiveness of treatments. Arch Gen Psychiatry 1989; 46: 971–82. [review]
42. Mills L. Depressing observations on the use of selective serotonin-reuptake inhibitors during pregnancy. N Engl J Med 2006; 354: 636–8. [review]

43. Moses-Kolko EL, Bogen D, Perel J, et al. Neonatal signs of late in utero exposure to serotonin reuptake inhibitors: literature review and implications for clinical applications. JAMA 2005; 293: 2372–83. [review]

44. Simon GE, Cunningham ML, Davis RL. Outcomes of prenatal antidepressant exposure. Am J Psychiatry 2002; 159: 2055–61. [II-3]

45. Sanz EJ, De-las-Cuevas C, Kiuru A, Bate A, Edwards R. Selective serotonin reuptake inhibitors in pregnant women and neonatal withdrawal syndrome: a database analysis. Lancet 2005; 365: 482–7. [II-3]

46. Chambers CD, Hernandez-Diaz S, Van Marter LJ, et al. Selective serotonin-reuptake inhibitors and risk of persistent pulmonary hypertension of the newborn. N Engl J Med 2006; 354: 579–87. [II-2]

47. Chambers CD, Johnson KA, Dick LM, Felix RJ, Jones KL. Birth outcomes in pregnant women taking fluoxetine. N Engl J Med 1996; 335: 1010–15. [II-3]

48. Gentile S. The safety of newer antidepressants in pregnancy and breastfeeding. Drug Safety 2005; 28: 137–52. [review]

49. Weissman AM, Levy BT, Hartz AJ, et al. Pooled analysis of antidepressant levels in lactating mothers, breast milk, and nursing infants. Am J Psychiatry 2004; 161: 1066–78. [review]

50. Halberg P, Sjoblom V. The use of selective serotonin reuptake inhibitors during pregnancy and breast-feeding: a review and clinical aspects. J Clin Psychopharm 2005; 25: 59–73. [review]

51. Gregoire AJ, Kumar R, Everitt B, Henderson AF, Studd JW. Transdermal oestrogen for the treatment of severe postnatal depression. Lancet 1996; 347: 930–3. [RCT, *n* = 61]

52. Dennis CL, Ross LE, Herxheimer A. Oestrogens and progestins for preventing and treating postpartum depression. Cochrane Database Syst Rev 2005; 4. [meta-analysis: 2 RCTs, *n* = 241 – not good, since two studies cannot be combined]

53. Miller LJ. Use of electroconvulsive therapy during pregnancy. Hosp Community Psychiatry 1994; 45: 444–50. [II-3]

22

Respiratory disease

Lauren A Plante

BASIC RESPIRATORY PHYSIOLOGY IN PREGNANCY

See also Chapter 2 of *Obstetric Evidence Based Guidelines*.

- Increase in minute ventilation (30–40%), predominantly by increase in tidal volume.
- Lesser increase in oxygen consumption (15–30%).
- Decrease in expiratory reserve volume and functional residual capacity.
- Reduction in arterial PCO_2 and increase in arterial PO_2.
- Quicker to desaturate with hypoventilation.

RESPIRATORY CONDITIONS

- Common: asthma, pneumonia.
- Less common: tuberculosis.
- Rare: restrictive lung disease, emphysema, cystic fibrosis, interstitial lung disease, sarcoidosis, acute lung injury/adult respiratory distress syndrome (ALI/ARDS).

ASTHMA

KEY POINTS

- Asthma is characterized by airway obstruction, inflammation, and increased responsiveness to stimuli. To reach a diagnosis, once abnormal FEV_1 (forced expiratory volume in 1 second) is found in a patient with historic and physical examination findings consistent with asthma, other differential diagnoses must be excluded.
- Peak expiratory flow rate (PEFR) is essential for management.
- Asthma is classified as mild intermittent, mild persistent, moderate persistent, and severe persistent by symptoms and PEFR.

- Asthma has historically been associated with small increased risks of preterm birth, low birth weight, perinatal mortality, and pre-eclampsia, but these risks are probably just associated with undertreatment of asthma; if asthma is adequately treated, it is not associated with a significant increase in adverse perinatal outcomes.
- Pregnancy has a variable effect on asthma severity, with about two-thirds getting better, and one-third worse. Most exacerbations occur between 24 and 36 weeks.
- The management of asthma in pregnant women should follow the same guidelines as for other non-pregnant patients.
- Management is according to objective measurement of pulmonary function with PEFR by classification (Table 22.1). Other main components are use of environmental control measures, adequate pharmacotherapy, and patient education regarding symptoms, management, and compliance.
- Inhalation therapy is preferred to systemic treatments, with inhaled corticosteroids, not inhaled beta-agonist, the mainstay of therapy.
- Prostaglandin $F_{2\alpha}$ should be avoided.

DIAGNOSIS

Asthma is characterized by episodic symptoms of airway obstruction, which is at least in part reversible, and requires that alternative explanations be excluded. Airway inflammation rather than bronchospasm is the key. Increased airway responsiveness to stimuli is characteristic. Indicators that may suggest a diagnosis of asthma include:

- wheezing
- history of recurrent cough, wheeze, chest tightness, or difficulty in breathing
- worsening of symptoms with exercise, viral infection, exposure to animal fur or feathers, mold, pollen, house

dust mites, tobacco or wood smoke, changes in weather, airborne chemicals or dusts
- preponderance or worsening of symptoms at night, especially if they awaken the patient.

Physical examination is not always reliable, but may include thoracic hyperexpansion or chest deformity, hunching of shoulders or use of accessory muscles, audible wheezing or a prolonged expiratory phase, increased nasal discharge or nasal polyps, or any manifestation of an allergic skin condition. The more indicators present, the more likely the diagnosis; however, the absence of wheezing does not equate with the absence of the diagnosis. If a diagnosis of asthma is being considered, the next step is **spirometry**, to determine whether airflow obstruction is present, and, if so, whether it is reversible. Forced vital capacity (FVC), **forced expiratory volume in 1 second (FEV$_1$)**, and the FEV$_1$/FVC ratio are measured before and after administration of a short-acting bronchodilator.

To reach **a diagnosis, once abnormal FEV$_1$ is found in a patient with historic and physical examination findings consistent with asthma, other differential diagnoses must be excluded,** such as chronic obstructive pulmonary disease (COPD) (bronchitis, emphysema), congestive heart failure (CHF), pulmonary embolus, laryngeal or vocal cord dysfunction, and mechanical airway obstruction (e.g. tumor).

SYMPTOMS

Wheezing, shortness of breath, coughing, chest tightness, difficulty in breathing, dyspnea.

INCIDENCE

Asthma affects approximately **1–4% of pregnant women**.[1] Among US women aged 18–44 years old, 4% reported an asthma attack within the preceding 12 months. However, 11.1% had received a diagnosis of asthma at some point during their lifetimes. Thus, this is a common disease among women of reproductive age. The cause–specific mortality ratio among women aged 18–44 years old averaged 0.8 per 100 000 in the USA in 2000–2002.[2]

ETIOLOGY/BASIC PATHOPHYSIOLOGY

Airway obstruction and inflammation are usually due to an excessive response to stimuli, as described above. Drops in maternal PaO$_2$, especially <60 mmHg, can profoundly reduce the fetal PaO$_2$, because the fetus operates on the steep portion of the oxygen desaturation curve.

CLASSIFICATION

Asthma severity is classified into four stages, as in Table 22.1.[3] The National Heart, Lung, and Blood Institute (NLHBI) classification is as follows:

Mild intermittent asthma

Fewer than two episodes per week and fewer than two nocturnal episodes per month, and peak expiratory flow rate (PEFR) >80% of personal best (or FEV$_1$ >80% of predicted), and less than 20% variation in PEFR in the course of a day.

Mild persistent asthma

Symptoms more than twice a week (but not daily), or nocturnal symptoms more than twice per month, and PEFR >80% of personal best (or FEV$_1$ >80% of predicted), and no more than 20–30% variation in PEFR in the course of a day.

Moderate persistent asthma

Daily symptoms, or nocturnal symptoms more than once per week, or PEFR between 60 and 80% of personal best (FEV$_1$ 60–80% of predicted), or PEFR variation >30%.

Severe persistent asthma

Continual daytime symptoms, or frequent nocturnal symptoms, or PEFR <60% of personal best (FEV$_1$ <60% of predicted). PEFR variation is typically >30%.

COMPLICATIONS

Asthma has historically been associated with small increased risks of **preterm birth** (odds ratio [OR] = 1.6), **low birth weight (OR = 2.0)**, **perinatal mortality (OR = 1.3)**, and **pre-eclampsia (OR = 1.3)**.[4] These risks are probably **associated just with undertreatment of asthma**; if asthma is adequately treated, it is not associated with a significant increase in adverse perinatal outcomes.[5] There are no randomized prospective trials comparing pregnancy outcomes in treated and untreated asthmatics. Women who decrease their asthma medication during pregnancy deliver infants of lower birth weight and slightly shorter gestational age than those who either increase their medication or make no change.[6]

PREGNANCY CONSIDERATIONS

Pregnant women are **less likely than others to receive appropriate asthma care**.[7] Pregnant women are equally

Table 22.1 *NAEPP Asthma Classification*[1,3]

Symptoms	Mild intermittent	Mild persistent	Moderate persistent	Severe persistent
	≤2 times a week Asymptomatic between exacerbations	>2 times a week but <1 time a day	Daily Exacerbations occur ≥2 times a week	Continual Frequent exacerbations
Pulmonary function tests	Normal PEFR between exacerbations FEV_1 or PEFR ≥80% of predicted PEFR variability <20%	FEV_1 or PEFR >80% of predicted PEFR variability 20–30%	FEV_1 or PEFR 60–80% of predicted PEFR variability >30%	FEV_1 or PEFR <60% of predicted PEFR variability >30%
Nocturnal awakening	≤2 times a month	>2 times a month	>1 time a week	Nightly awakenings
Interference with daily activities	None	Mild	Some interference with normal activities but rare severe exacerbation	Limitations of physical activity
Treatment	Inhaled short-acting ß₂-agonist (albuterol)	Inhaled short-acting ß₂-agonist and daily anti-inflammatory (low-dose inhaled corticosteroid or cromolyn)	Inhaled ß₂-agonist and daily medication (medium-dose inhaled corticosteroid *or* low–medium-dose inhaled corticosteroid *and* long-acting bronchodilator)	Inhaled short-acting ß₂-agonist and daily medication (inhaled high-dose corticosteroid *and* long-acting bronchodilator *and* oral corticosteroid)

NAEPP, National Asthma Education and Prevention Program;[3] PEFR, peak expiratory flow rate; FEV_1, forced expiratory volume in 1 second.

likely to be admitted for an asthma attack, but are less likely to receive corticosteroids in the emergency department (ED), and those who are sent home are less likely to be prescribed outpatient steroids. Pregnant women are far more likely than non-pregnant counterparts to report ongoing symptoms 2 weeks after an ED visit, perhaps because of the difference in steroid use.[7]

Pregnancy has a variable effect on asthma severity, which may improve, worsen, or remain unchanged. In general, about **two-thirds of patients get better**, and one-third of patients get worse.[8] **Most exacerbations occur between 24 and 36 weeks**, while the fewest symptoms occur at term. Of patients with mild disease, 2% were hospitalized during pregnancy, 13% were noted to have an exacerbation, and 13% had symptoms at the time of delivery.[9] For patients with moderate asthma, 7% were hospitalized and 26% had an exacerbation during pregnancy, with 21% symptomatic at delivery. Among severe asthmatics, 27% were hospitalized and 52% had an exacerbation during pregnancy, and 46% of severe asthmatics were symptomatic at delivery.[9] Among women with mild disease at the start, 30% were reclassified to a higher degree of severity during the pregnancy; 22% of women with moderate or severe disease initially were reclassified into the mild category. A number of **predictive factors** have been proposed (smoking during pregnancy, carrying a female fetus, and worsening of rhinitis have all been suggested to predict a worsening of symptoms) but studies are inconsistent.[10–12]

MANAGEMENT
Principles

The management of asthma in pregnant women should follow the **same guidelines as for other patients.** The goal is to maintain asthma control during pregnancy. Current recommendations for asthma management and control are available from the National Asthma Education and Prevention Program (NAEPP).[3,13]

Prevention

Eliminate or mitigate asthma triggers. Environmental control measures are shown Table 22.2.

Preconception care

Multidisciplinary care, including at least an obstetrician expert in asthma care, or a maternal–fetal medicine specialist, and a pulmonologist, is recommended for preparation

Table 22.2 *NAEPP summary of control measures for environmental factors that can make asthma worse*

Allergens
Reduce or eliminate exposure to the allergen(s) the patient is sensitive to, including:
- Animal dander: remove animal from house, or, at a minimum keep animal out of patient's bedroom and seal or cover with a filter the air ducts that lead to the bedroom.
- House-dust mites:
  - Essential: encase mattress in an allergen-impermeable cover; encase pillow in an allergan-impermeable cover or wash it weekly; wash sheets and blankets on the patient's bed in hot water weekly (water temperature of >130° F is necessary for killing mites).
  - Desirable: reduce indoor humidity to less than 50%; remove carpets from the bedroom; avoid sleeping or lying on upholstered furniture; remove carpets that are laid on concrete.
- Cockroaches: Use poison bait or traps to control. Do not leave food or garbage exposed.
- Pollens (from trees, grass, or weeds) and outdoor molds: to avoid exposure, adults should stay indoors – especially during the afternoon – with the windows closed during the season in which they have problems with outdoor allergens.
- Indoor mold: fix all leaks and eliminate water sources associated with mold growth; clean moldy surfaces. Consider reducing indoor humidity to <50%.

Tobacco smoke
Advise patients and others in the home who smoke to stop smoking or to smoke outside the home. Discuss ways to reduce exposure to other sources of tobacco smoke, such as from daycare providers and the workplace.

Indoor/outdoor pollutants and irritants:
Discuss ways to reduce exposures to the following:
- Wood-burning stoves or fireplaces.
- Unvented stoves or heaters.
- Other irritates (e.g. perfumes, cleaning agents, sprays).

NAEPP, National Asthma Education and Prevention Program[3]

of pregnancy and during pregnancy. Education regarding prognosis, complications, and management of asthma therapy should be reviewed, with emphasis on the fact that asthma therapy should not change in pregnancy compared with the non-pregnant state, but should still aim for maximal relief of symptoms and best pulmonary function, through attentive patient compliance with suggested management.

Prenatal care

Management is based on four components:
1. **Use** of *objective* measures of lung function such as **PEFR**, both to ascertain severity and to monitor therapy, rather than relying on symptoms.
2. Use of **environmental control** measures to eliminate or mitigate asthma triggers.
3. **Pharmacotherapy** designed to prevent or reverse airway inflammation typical of asthma, as well as drug treatment for exacerbations.
4. Patient **education** regarding symptoms, management, and **compliance**.

Work-up of pulmonary function

Asthma control should be assessed on a regular basis (at least at each prenatal visit) by review of symptoms, medications used, and quality of life over the preceding weeks. The single best measure of pulmonary function is the FEV_1, which is the volume of gas exhaled in 1 second by a forced exhalation after the patient takes a deep breath. This value can only be obtained by spirometry, which limits its clinical value. The **PEFR** can be measured by peak flow meters, which are portable, inexpensive, and disposable. Both FEV_1 and PEFR remain unchanged in pregnancy in the normal state. Predicted PEFR values are based on age, gender, and height. For women, they range from 380 to 550 L/min. Each pregnant woman should establish her personal best during quiescent asthma. PEFR >80% of personal best are normal (green zone); values between 50 and 80% are intermediate (yellow zone); values <50% are associated with severe asthma exacerbation (red zone).[1] **Daily peak flow monitoring** using an inexpensive home meter is advisable in cases of moderate or severe asthma, in order to identify presymptomatic airflow obstruction which may require escalation of therapy. PEFR should be recorded in a log and brought to each prenatal visit.

Therapy

Goals

No limitations at school or work; normal or near-normal pulmonary function assessed by PEFR (or FEV_1); prevent hypoxia in mother and fetus; and minimal-to-none exacerbations, chronic symptoms, use of short-term beta-agonists, or medication side effects. Maternal oxygen saturation must remain >95% to avoid fetal hypoxia.

Suggested medications

These are listed in Table 22.1, according to severity classification. Some of the tables (22.1–22.5) and figures (22.1, 22.2) come from the National Institutes of Health (NIH) National Lung, Heart and Blood Institute (NLHBI) National Asthma Education and Prevention Program (NAEPP).[3] http://www.nhlbi.nih.gov/health/prof/lung/asthma/astpreg/astpreg_full.pdf

Mild intermittent asthma

These patients require **no daily medication**. Quick relief can be provided in the form of **2–4 puffs of a short-acting beta-agonist bronchodilator as needed**. PEFR 50–80% should be treated with an inhaled short-acting beta-mimetic immediately. Values <50% require the same therapy plus an immediate visit to the emergency room. However, the need to use rescue twice a week or more means a step-up in therapy and perhaps a reclassification of severity. These patients can have severe exacerbations interrupting long periods of normal lung function, in which case systemic steroids should be offered.

Mild persistent asthma

These patients should be treated with a **daily inhaled corticosteroid** (low dose); alternative therapies, however, include inhaled cromolyn, leukotriene receptor antagonist, or sustained-release theophylline adjusted to a serum level of 5–12 µg/ml.

Moderate persistent asthma

These patients should be treated either with a **medium-dose inhaled corticosteroid, or a low-dose inhaled corticosteroid plus a long-acting inhaled beta-agonist**. If needed, the long-acting beta-agonist can be combined with a medium-dose corticosteroid.

Alternative therapies include low-dose or medium-dose inhaled corticosteroid in combination with either theophylline or a leukotriene receptor antagonist.

Severe persistent asthma

These patients require **both a high-dose inhaled corticosteroid and a long-acting inhaled beta-agonist**, and may require, in addition, **oral corticosteroids**; when feasible, the oral corticosteroids should be discontinued and control maintained with inhaled agents.

An alternative therapy would be high-dose inhaled corticosteroid plus sustained-release theophylline titrated to therapeutic serum levels, as above.

General

Inhalation therapy is preferred to systemic treatments, because of direct delivery to airway and fewer side effects. Spacer devices can increase delivery to the lungs and minimize oral absorption. Note that for all except the mild intermittent type of asthma, **inhaled corticosteroids**, *not* **inhaled beta-agonist, are the mainstay of therapy.**

Use of one or more canister of beta-agonist per month indicates inadequate asthma control. Gain control as quickly as possible; a short course of oral steroids may be helpful. Review symptoms monthly. Step-down therapy may be attempted if symptoms are well controlled.

An individualized action plan should be generated for an asthmatic patient. This incorporates frequent self-assessment, a daily self-management plan, a long-term self-management plan, and an asthma action plan based on symptoms, peak flow, and medications used. The action plan allows patients to step up therapy at home with exacerbations, and provides criteria for contacting the physician or seeking care in an emergency department. Samples of these plans can be found in the NIH document online at http://www.nhlbi.nih.gov/health/prof/lung/asthma/astpreg/astpreg_full.pdf.

If symptoms are not adequately controlled, review compliance, inhalation technique, and environmental control. If there is no room for improvement in these areas, step up to the next level of therapy. At step 3 or step 4 (moderate or severe persistent disease), consider referral to a specialist in asthma, if not already involved.

Specific management and medications

Enviromental control measures are shown in Table 22.2. Usual dosages for long-term control medications are shown in Table 22.3. Comparative daily dosages of inhaled corticosteroids are shown in Table 22.4. Management of asthma exacerbation at home is shown in Figure 22.1. Management of asthma exacerbation for emergency department management, and criteria for hospitalization are shown in Figure 22.2. Medications for asthma exacerbation are shown in Table 22.5.

Inhaled steroids
Antinflammatory agents decrease edema and secretions in the bronchioles. Indications are shown in Table 22.1. They are used not for acute relief, but for long-term management (4 weeks for maximal benefit). In addition, if a beta-mimetic (e.g. albuterol) is used ≥3 times/week, inhaled steroid therapy should be started. Most of the data

Table 22.3 *NAEPP usual dosages for long-term-control medications during pregnancy and lactation*

Medication	Dosage form	Adult dose
Inhaled corticosteroids (see estimated comparative daily dosages for inhaled corticosteroids (Table 22.4)		
Systematic corticosteroids		**(applies to all three corticosteroids)**
Methylprednisolone	2, 4, 8, 16, 32 mg tablets	• 7.5–60 mg daily in a single dose in a.m. or qod as needed for control
Prednisolone	5 mg tablets, 5 mg/5 ml, 15 mg/5 ml	• Short-course 'burst' to achieve control: 40–60 mg/day as single dose or 2 divided doses for 3–10 days
Prednisone	1, 2.5, 5, 10, 20, 50 mg tablets 5 mg/ml, 5 mg/5 ml	
Long-acting inhaled beta$_2$-agonists (should not be used for symptom relief or for exacerbations. Use with inhaled corticosteroids)		
Salmeterol	MDI 21 µg/puff	2 puffs q 12 hours
	DPI 50 µg/blister	1 blister q 12 hours
Formoterol	DPI 12 µg/single-use capsule	1 capsule q 12 hours
Combined medication		
Fluticasone/Salmeterol	DPI 100, 250, or 500 µg/50 µg	1 inhalation bid; dose depends on severity of asthma
Cromolyn		
Cromolyn	MDI 1 mg/puff	2–4 puffs tid–qid
	Nebulizer 20 mg/ampule	1 ampule tid–qid
Leukotriene receptor antagoenists		
Montelukast	10 mg tablet	10 mg qhs
Zafirlukast	10 or 20 mg tablet	40 mg daily (20 mg tablet bid)
Methylxanthines (serum monitoring is important [serum concentration of 5–12 µg/ml at steady state])		
Theophylline	Liquids, sustained-release tablets, and capsules	Starting dose 10 mg/kg/day up to 300 mg max; usual max 800 mg/day

NAEPP, National Asthma Education and Prevention Program;[3] DPI, dry powder inhaler; MDI, metered-dose inhaler.
Notes:
• The most important determinant of appropriate dosing is the clinician's judgment of the patient's response to therapy.
• Some doses may be outside package labeling, especially in the high-dose range.

Table 22.4 *NAEPP estimated comparative daily dosages for inhaled corticosteroids*

Drug	Adult low daily dose	Adult medium daily dose	Adult high daily dose
Beclomethasone CFC 42 or 84 µg/puff	168–504 µg	504–840 µg	> 840 µg
Beclomethasone HFA 40 or 80 µg/puff	80–240 µg	240–480 µg	>480 µg
Budesonide DPI 200 µg/inhalation	200–600 µg	600–1200 µg	> 1200 µg
Flunisolide 250 µg/puff	500–1000 µg	1000–2000 µg	> 2000 µg
Fluticasone MDI: 44, 110, or 220 µg/puff	88–264 µg	264–660 µg	> 660 µg
DPI: 50, 100, or 250 µg/inhalation	100–300 µg	300–750 µg	>750 µg
Triamcinolone acetonride 100 µg/puff	400–1000 µg	1000–2000 µg	> 2000 µg

NAEPP, National Asthma Education and Prevention Program;[3] DPI, dry powder inhaler; MDI, metered-dose inhaler.

Table 22.5   *NAEPP medications and dosages for asthma exacerbations during pregnancy and lactation*

Medications	Dosages		Comments
	Adult dose	Child dose	
Short-acting inhated beta$_2$-agonists			
Albuterol			
Nebulizer solution (5.0 mg/ml 2.5 mg/3 ml 1.25 mg/3 ml 0.63 mg/3 ml)	2.5–5 mg every 20 minutes for 3 doses, then 2.5–10 mg every 1–4 hours as needed, or 10–15 mg/hour continously	0.15 mg/kg (minimum dose 2.5 mg) every 20 minutes for 3 doses, then 0.15–0.3 mg/kg up to 10 mg every 1–4 hours as needed, or 0.5 mg/kg hour by continuous nebulization	Only selective beta$_2$-agonists are recommended. For optimal delivery, dilute aerosols to minimum of 3 ml at gas flow of 6–8 L/min
MDI (90 μg/puff)	4–8 puffs every 20 minutes up to 4 hours, then every 1–4 hours as needed	4–8 puffs every 20 minutes for 3 doses, then every 1–4 hours inhalation maneuver; use spacer/holding chamber	As effective as nebulized therapy if patient is able to coordinate
Bitolterol			
Nebulizer solution (2 mg/ml)	See albuterol dose	See albuterol dose: thought to be half as potent as albuterol on a mg basis	Has not been studied in severe asthma exacerbations. Do not mix with other drugs
MDI (370 μg/puff)	See albuterol dose	See albuterol dose	Has not been studied in severe asthma exacerbations
Levalbuterol (R-albuterol) Nebulizer solution (0.63 mg/3 ml 1.25 mg/3 ml)	1.25–2.5 mg every 20 minutes for 3 doses, then 1.25–5 mg every 1–4 hours as needed, or 5–7.5 mg/hour continuously	0.075 mg/mg (minimum dose 1.25 mg) every 20 minutes for 3 doses, then 0.075–0.15 mg/kg up to 5 mg every 1–4 hours as needed, or 0.25 mg/kg/hour by continuous nebulization	0.63 mg of levalbuterol is equivalent to 1.25 mg of racemic albuterol for both efficacy and side effects
Pirbuterol MDI (200 μg/puff)	See albuterol dose	See albuterol dose: thought to be half as potent as albuterol on a mg basis	Has not been studied in severe asthma exacerbations
Systemic (injected) beta$_2$-agonists			
Epinephrine 1:1000 (1 mg/ml)	0.3–0.5 mg every 20 minutes for 3 doses sq	0.01 mg/kg up to 0.3–0.5 mg every 20 minutes for 3 doses sq	No proven advantage of systemic therapy over aerosol
Terbutaline (1 mg/ml)	0.25 mg every 20 minutes for 3 doses sq	0.01 mg/kg every 20 minutes for 3 doses, then every 2–6 hours as needed sq	No proven advantage of systemic therapy over aerosol
Anticholinergics			
Ipratropium bromide Nebulizer solution (0.25 mg/ml)	0.5 mg every 30 minutes for 3 doses, then every 2–4 hours as needed	0.25 mg every 20 minutes for 3 doses, then every 2–4 hours	May mix in same nebulizer with albuterol. Should not be used as first-line therapy, should be added to beta$_2$-agonist therapy
MDI (18 μg/puff)	4–8 puffs as needed	4–8 puffs as needed	Dose delivered from MDI is low and has not been studied in asthma exacerbations

(*Continued*)

Table 22.5 *(Continued)*

Medications	Dosages		Comments
	Adult dose	Child dose	
Ipratropium with albuterol			
Nebulizer solution (Each 3 mL vial contains 0.5 mg ipratropium bromide and 2.5 mg albuterol)	3 ml every 30 minutes for 3 doses, then every 2–4 hours as needed	1.5 ml every 20 minutes for 3 doses, then every 2–4 hours	Contains EDTA to prevent discoloration. This additive does not induce bronchospasm
MDI (Each puff contains 18 µg ipratropium bromide and 90 µg albuterol)	4–8 puffs as needed	4–8 puffs as needed	
Systemic corticosteroids (dosages and comments apply to all three corticosteroids)			
Prednisone Methylprednisolone Prednisolone	120–180 mg/day in 3 or 4 divided doses for 48 hours, then 60–80 mg/day until PEFR reaches 70% of predicted or personal best	1 mg/kg every 6 hours for 48 hours, than 1–2 mg/kg/day (maximum – 60 mg/day) in 2 divided doses until PEFR is 70% of predicted or personal best	For outpatient 'burst' use 40–60 mg in single or 2 divided doses for adults (children: 1–2 mg/kg/day, maximum 60 mg/day) for 3–10 days

Notes:
- The most important determinant of appropriate dosing is the clinician's judgment of the patient's response to therapy.
- No advantage has been found for higher-dose corticosteroids in severe asthma exacerbations, nor is there any advantage for intravenous administration over oral therapy provided gastrointestinal transit time or absorption is not impaired. The usual regimen is to continue the frequent multiple daily doses until the patient achieves an FEV_1 or PEFR of 50% of predicted or personal best and then lower the dose to twice daily. This usually occurs within 48 hours. Therapy following a hospitalization or emergency department visit may last from 3 to 10 days. If patients are then started on inhaled corticosteroids, studies indicate there is no need to taper the systemic corticosteroid dose. If the follow-up systemic corticosteroid therapy is to be given once daily, one study indicates that it may be more clinically effective to give the dose in the afternoon at 3 p.m. with no increase in adrenal suppression.

NAEPP, National Asthma Education and Prevention Program.[3]

on inhaled steroids in human pregnancy come from **budesonide** (Pulmicort), which makes it the **preferred drug in this class**.[14] Budesonide and fluticasone propionate (Flovent) are more potent than beclomethasone (Beclovent, Vanceril). Inhaled beclomethasone is associated with improved FEV_1 and less side effects compared with theophylline in moderate asthmatics in the only trial assessing this comparison in pregnancy, consistent with non-pregnant trials.[15] There is **no evidence of increased rates of congenital malformations** with the use of inhaled corticosteroids in pregnancy.[3] They are safe in pregnancy. There is also no effect on fetal growth or preterm birth.[16]

Beta-agonists
Beta-agonists relax the smooth muscle of the bronchioles. There is **no evidence of increased rates of congenital malformations** with the use of beta-agonists in pregnancy.[3]

Short-acting beta-agonists. The most commonly used agent is albuterol. The onset of action is < 5 minutes, with a duration of only 4–6 hours.

Long-acting beta-agonists. Salmeterol (Serevent) and formoterol (Foradil).

Combinations of inhaled corticosteroids and long-acting beta-mimetics
Fluticasone and salmeterol (Advair) combination is more effective than either drug alone in non-pregnant trials.

Cromolyn
Cromolyn sodium is a non-steroidal anti-inflammatory drug (NSAID) used for chronic management of asthma, not acute exacerbations (4 weeks for maximal benefit). There is **no evidence of increased rates of congenital malformations** with the use of cromolyn in pregnancy;[3] this is a safe drug in pregnancy, as is nedocromil.

Theophylline
Theophylline has a long record of use in pregnancy and no teratogenic effects are known; however, the narrow therapeutic window and potential for maternal and fetal toxicity mandates close monitoring of serum levels. The current NAEPP guidelines allow low-dose theophylline as an alternative to a long-acting inhaled beta-agonist when inhaled corticosteroids do not suffice to control symptoms, but clearly state that **this is not a preferred therapy**. Stick then

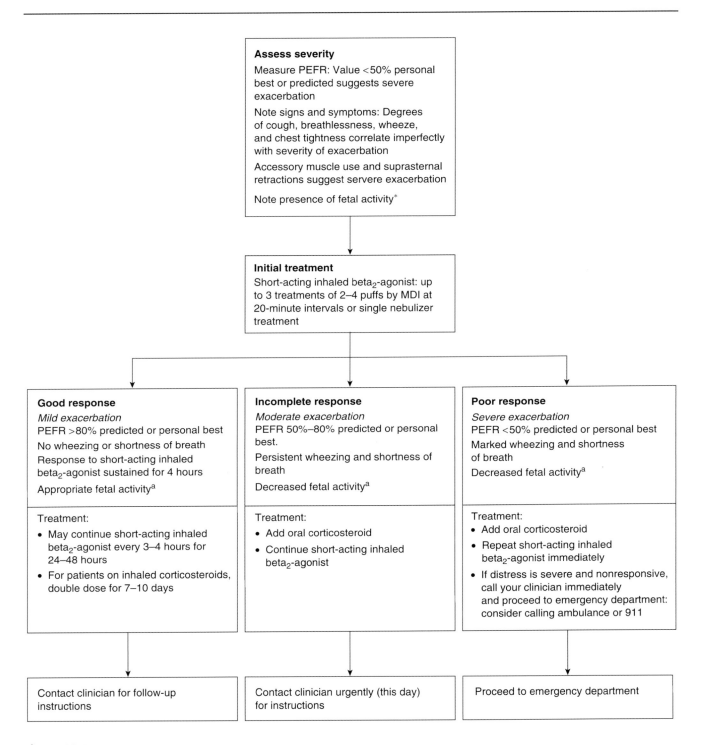

Figure 22.1

Management of asthma exacerbations during pregnancy and lactation: **Home treatment**, as suggested by NAEPP (National Asthma Education and Prevention Program);[3] MDI, metered-dose inhaler; PEFR, peak expiratory flow rate. *Fetal activity is monitored by observing whether fetal kick counts decrease over time.

with inhaled steroids over theophylline. Recommendations for target serum theophylline levels have been changed to 5–12 μg/ml.

Leukotriene modifiers

Limited human data are available on the use of leukotriene modifiers during pregnancy. In non-pregnant individuals, these drugs, while more effective than placebo, are **less**

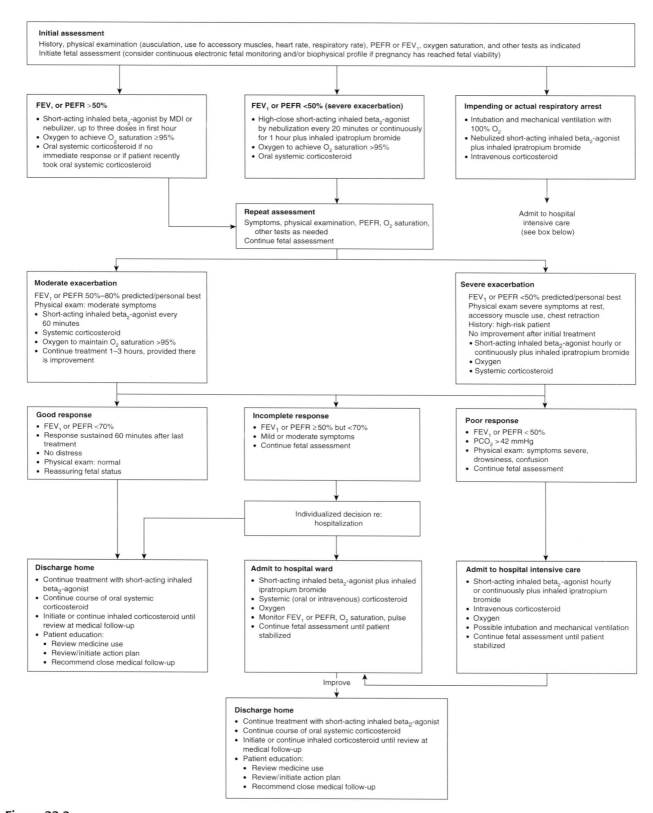

Figure 22.2

Management of asthma exacerbations during pregnancy and lactation: **Emergency department and hospital-based care,** as suggested by NAEPP (National Asthma Educational and Prevention Program).[3] FEV_1, forced expiratory volume in 1 second; MDI, metered-dose inhaler; PCO_2, carbon dioxide partial pressure; PEFR, peak expiratory flow rate; re, regarding.

effective than inhaled corticosteroids, and do not add much benefit to women already on inhaled steroids. They do not reduce the risk of exacerbation requiring systemic steroids, are associated with modest improvement in PEFR, and very modest decrease in use of rescue short-acting beta-2 agonists.[17] These drugs may be considered during pregnancy for women who had a good response to them prior to pregnancy, but they are not a preferred option when initiating therapy. Montelukast and zafirlukast are safe in pregnancy.

Oral corticosteroids

Oral corticosteroids are indicated when any combinations of inhaled steroids, beta-agonists, and cromolyn do not control asthma. Oral steroids use in the first trimester is associated with a possible increased risk of cleft lip (with or without cleft palate) from the background rate of 0.1–0.3%, a small excess risk. The use of oral corticosteroids during pregnancy is associated with an increase in incidence of gestational diabetes, pre-eclampsia, preterm delivery, and low birth weight. These outcomes may be attributed either to the drug or to the severity of the disease process. Available data do not allow for the distinction.

Intravenous corticosteroids may be indicated in severe asthma exacerbation (see Figure 22.2 and Table 22.5). Methyprednisolone 60–80 mg intravenously every 6–8 hours is the usual drug used, with onset of action being several hours.

Criteria for intubation

See Table 22.6.

Antepartum testing

No specific indication.

Delivery

Asthma medications should be continued in labor. Although asthma is typically quiescent during labor and delivery, PEFR should be measured upon admission, and again every 12 hours in labor. Although women who have received systemic steroids are sometimes given stress dose steroids in labor, there is no evidence to support this practice. Women who have received systemic steroids (e.g. ≥ 20 mg of prednisone or its equivalent) for ≥ 3 weeks in pregnancy may receive stress-dose steroids peridelivery, in the form of hydrocortisone 100 mg intravenously every 8 hours (stop ≤ 24 hours postpartum). Addisonian crisis is very rare, especially for short (< 3 weeks) intervals of steroid therapy. Prostaglandins E_1 and E_2 are safe. **Prostaglandin $F_{2\alpha}$ should be avoided**, as it can cause bronchospasm.

Table 22.6 *Criteria for mechanical ventilation of a pregnant asthmatic*

Maternal PaO_2 ≤ 60 mmHg
Maternal $PaCO_2$ ≥ 45 mmHg
Worsening acidosis (pH < 7.35)
Altered mental consciousness
Evidence of maternal exhaustion

Anesthesia

Regional is preferred to general anesthesia in asthmatics. Narcotics which predispose to histamine release (e.g. morphine) are to be avoided because of the potential to provoke bronchospasm. In case of general anethesia, ketamine is preferred to thiopental, preanesthetic use of atropine or glycopyrolate is useful, and even low concentrations of the inhaled halogenated agents may provide bronchodilation.

Postpartum/breastfeeding

Breastfeeding does not protect against asthma in offspring.[18]

PNEUMONIA

KEY POINTS

- The presence of an **infiltrate on chest X-ray** confirms the diagnosis of pneumonia.
- **Complications** of community-acquired pneumonia (CAP) include **mechanical ventilation, maternal mortality, small-for-gestational age** infant, and **perinatal mortality.**
- **Prompt administration of antibiotics** without delay and **appropriate antibiotic** therapy are the most important principles for effective management.
- **Prevention** is effective with **pneumococcal and influenza vaccines.**
- **Hospitalization** is particularly indicated when the pregnant woman with CAP has **coexisting medical conditions** such as malignancy, renal failure, cerebrovascular disease, diabetes, or valvular heart disease, **respiratory rate (RR) ≥ 30 breaths/min, diastolic blood pressure (BP) ≤ 60 mmH/g, systolic BP ≤ 90 mmHg, heart rate (HR) ≥ 125 beats/min, altered mental status, $PaCO_2$ < 60 mmHg on room air, presence of a pleural effusion, hematocrit < 30%, arterial pH < 7.35,** or **multilobe involvement.**
- Most cases of low-risk CAP in pregnancy can be treated with just a **macrolide**, while the more high-risk cases can be treated with a **macrolide** and a **cephalosporin such as ceftriaxone.**
- Antibiotic therapy should not be changed within the first 72 hours unless clinical deterioration is overt or organism sensitivities become available.

DIAGNOSIS

Pneumonia is an infectious process of the lower respiratory tract that should be suspected if a patient presents with new respiratory symptoms of cough, dyspnea, or sputum production, particularly if fever and abnormal breath sounds are also present. The presence of an **infiltrate on chest X-ray** confirms the diagnosis.

ETIOLOGY/BASIC PATHOPHYSIOLOGY

Etiology is usually bacterial, viral, or fungal infection of the lungs. *Streptococcus pneumoniae* (5–30%) and *Mycoplasma pneumoniae* (5–30%) are the most common pathogens, but dozens of different organisms can cause pneumonia.[19] In community-acquired pneumonia, the responsible organism is not identified in 50–90% of cases, depending on how aggressive is the work-up.[20]

CLASSIFICATION

The distinction between community-acquired (CAP) and hospital-acquired pneumonia is made in practice. In the majority of cases, clinical signs and symptoms do not distinguish one pathogen from another. The vast majority of cases of pneumonia in pregnant women in clinical practice and in the literature are cases of CAP. The American Thoracic Society describes four subsets of CAP, stratified by comorbidity and mortality rates.[20] Most pregnant patients with CAP will fall into subset I; this is a group which, non-pregnant, would be appropriately treated as outpatients. There are, however, no reliable data as to stratification of therapy in pregnancy.

SYMPTOMS

Respiratory symptoms of cough, dyspnea, or sputum production, usually fever.

EPIDEMIOLOGY

The attack rate for CAP is no different among pregnant women than among women of reproductive age who are not pregnant, approximately **1.5 per 1000**.[21] Pregnant women hospitalized with CAP have lower severity scores than their non-pregnant counterparts; this may reflect either a tendency for the disease process to be less severe or, more probably, a **lower threshold for hospitalization during pregnancy**. Pneumonia incidence is evenly distributed throughout pregnancy; i.e. there is no specific period of vulnerability.

RISK FACTORS

Smoking and asthma.

COMPLICATIONS

Approximately 2% of pregnant women with pneumonia require tracheal intubation and **mechanical ventilation**.[22] The risk of **maternal mortality** with CAP is 2.9% from the reports from the 1990s.[23] Among women hospitalized for pneumonia during pregnancy, the risk of delivering a **small for gestational age** infant is increased relative to controls, although this may be confounded by different health behaviors in the two groups. There is no statistical difference in prematurity or perinatal mortality in individual studies, but both rates are increased, and **perinatal mortality** was 4.3% in reports from the 1990s.[23]

PREGNANCY CONSIDERATIONS

Women hospitalized for CAP during pregnancy appear to be **less ill** than their non-pregnant counterparts, measured by either severity score or length of stay, but this probably reflects a tendency to hospitalize for less-severe disease because of the pregnancy.

MANAGEMENT
Principles

Prompt administration of antibiotics without delay and **appropriate antibiotic** therapy are the most important principles for effective management.

Prevention

Pneumococcal vaccine prevents 71% of cases of CAP, and 32% of related mortality in non-pregnant adults.[19] **For details on recommended pneumococcal and influenza vaccines**, see Chapter 37.

Work-up

Assess severity of illness by **physical findings** (blood pressure, respiratory rate, mental status, state of hydration) and by **radiographic findings** (e.g. multilobar involvement, pleural effusion). The utility of a sputum Gram stain and culture in guiding initial antibiotic therapy is not supported by sufficient evidence for or against, but may be indicated in the woman with purulent sputum. Sputum culture for pathogens such as *Legionella* spp., fungi, viruses, *Mycobacterium* spp., as well as urinary antigen assays for

Legionella spp. and *S. pneumoniae* and acid-fast stain for mycobacterial infection should be considered in selected cases.

Patients with severe illness or underlying cardiopulmonary disease are candidates for arterial blood gas analysis. Blood culture is positive in 5–11% of cases.

Treatment

Hospitalization

There are no trials to assess if/when hospitalization is beneficial for the pregnant woman with pneumonia. **Hospitalization may be indicated** when there are factors that have been correlated with an increased risk of mortality, or may be indicated when an initial period of close observation is warranted. The PORT prediction model,[24] for prognosticating death or complicated clinical course in non-pregnant adults, included, among others, **coexisting medical conditions** such as malignancy, renal failure, cerebrovascular disease, **respiratory rate (RR) ≥ 30 breaths/min, diastolic blood pressure (BP) ≤ 60 mmHg, systolic BP ≤ 90 mmHg, HR ≥ 125 beats/min, altered mental status, PaCO$_2$ < 60 mmHg on room air, presence of a pleural effusion, hematocrit < 30% and arterial pH < 7.35.** Diabetes, valvular heart disease, and multilobe involvement are other risk factors for a complicated course.[22] The majority of obstetric patients will fail to qualify as high-risk patients by these criteria. Retrospectively applying American Thoracic Society guidelines in place at the time of the study (similar to above), only 25% of pregnant patients with a diagnosis of CAP would have been assigned to outpatient care.[22] A 23-hour observation period might be useful in deciding whether inpatient treatment is warranted in the pregnant patient.

Antibiotics

There are no trials to assess which **antibiotic regimen** is most beneficial for the pregnant woman with pneumonia. There are no published treatment guidelines that alter therapy for pneumonia based on pregnancy. The **fluoroquinolones** are **avoided** in pregnancy because of concerns about interference with cartilage formation in the fetus, and the **tetracyclines** because of concerns about dentition. However, depending on drug allergies and microbiological sensitivities, it may be necessary to alter these preferences. The Infectious Diseases Society of America[25] currently recommends the following treatments for the non-pregnant adult with CAP:

Previously healthy patient, no recent antibiotic therapy

Erythromycin, azithromycin, or clarithromycin. Only 1% of pregnant women with CAP remained febrile with erythromycin 500 mg every 6 hours.[22]

Previously healthy, but antibiotics within the past 3 months for any reason

Azithromycin or clarithromycin **plus** high-dose amoxicillin (1 g po tid), or azithromycin or clarithromycin **plus** high-dose amoxicillin–clavulanic acid (2 g po bid).

Comorbidities (cardiopulmonary, diabetes, renal disease, malignancy), no recent antibiotic therapy

Azithromycin or clarithromycin.

Comorbidity and recent antibiotic therapy

Azithromycin or clarithromycin, **plus** high-dose amoxicillin, high-dose amoxicillin–clavulanate, cefpodoxime, cefprozil, or cefuroxime.

Suspected aspiration with infection

Amoxacillin–clavulanate or clindamycin.

Influenza with bacterial superinfection

High-dose amoxicillin or amoxicillin–clavulanic acid, or cefpodoxime, cefprozil, or cefuroxime.

Inpatient, with or without recent antibiotic therapy

Azithromycin or clarithromycin, **plus** cefotaxime, ceftriaxone, or ampicillin–sulbactam.

Critical illness (ICU), with risk factors for Pseudomonas infection (structural lung disease, recent antibiotic therapy, recent stay in hospital)

Piperacillin, piperacillin–tazobactam, imipenem, meropenem, or cefepime, **plus** aminoglycoside, **plus** azithromycin or clarithromycin.

Critical illness (ICU), no risk factors for Pseudomonas

Piperacillin, piperacillin–tazobactam, imipenem, meropenem, or cefepime, **plus** azithromycin or clarithromycin.

Summary

So in summary, probably most cases of low-risk CAP in pregnancy can be treated with just a **macrolide**, while the more high-risk cases can be treated with a **macrolide and a cephalosporin such as ceftriaxone.**

There are inadequate data to determine the best **duration of antimicrobial treatment** for community-acquired pneumonia. With older agents, a duration of 10–14 days is commonly prescribed, but newer agents have longer half-lives and therefore may be curative over shorter courses of therapy, e.g. 5–7 days; trials are under way.

Typical responses to therapy include defervescence in 2–4 days, with resolution of leukocytosis in the same time period. The chest X-ray may take longer to clear, as may the auscultatory findings.[20] **Antibiotic therapy should not be changed within the first 72 hours unless clinical deterioration is overt or organism sensitivities become available.** There is no evidence in non-pregnant adults that intravenous and oral therapy differ in efficacy. Once the patient has clinically stabilized or improved, she can be switched to oral antibiotics. Criteria for stabilization[20] include:

- improvement in cough and dyspnea
- afebrile (<100° F) on at least two occasions 8 hours apart
- white blood cells (WBCs) decreasing
- adequate oral intake.

If the pathogen and sensitivities are known, the **narrowest spectrum agent should be chosen for oral therapy,** but in most cases this will not be possible, and oral agents should duplicate the spectrum of the parenteral agents used. The American Thoracic Society recommends discharge to home the same day that clinical stability is achieved and the switch to oral agents is made. A follow-up inpatient chest X-ray is not indicated.

Oxygen support should be provided as needed. Criteria for intubation are shown in Table 22.6.

Antepartum testing

No specific indication.

Delivery

No specific changes.

Anesthesia

No specific changes.

Postpartum/breastfeeding

No specific changes.

TUBERCULOSIS
KEY POINTS

- Definite diagnosis of **active** *Mycobacterium tuberculosis* infection is based on **culture** (usually sputum) **for *M. tuberculosis.*** Sputum culture is also required for **drug sensitivity testing.**
- Diagnosis of **latent tuberculosis** is based on a positive tuberculin test in a woman without prior vaccination and no symptoms or positive X-ray/smear/culture for *M. tuberculosis.*
- Pregnancy is not known to influence the progression from latent to active disease.
- The treatment for **latent** tuberculosis infection in pregnancy is **isoniazid 300 mg daily for 6–9 months.**
- Treatment of **active** tuberculosis consists of an initial 2-month phase of therapy, including **isoniazid, rifampin, pyrazinamide,** and **ethambutol.** Directly observed therapy is usually recommended. The following 4 months typically continue isoniazid with either rifampin or ethambutol. **Active tuberculosis treatment is not altered by pregnancy,** as these drugs are **not teratogenic.**

DIAGNOSIS

Definite diagnosis of **active** *M. tuberculosis* infection remains based on **culture** (usually sputum) **for *M. tuberculosis.*** Smear (usually sputum) with acid-fast bacilli is a means of rapid diagnosis.[26] Diagnosis of **latent tuberculosis** is based on a positive tuberculin test in a woman without prior vaccination and no symptoms or positive X-ray/smear/culture.

SYMPTOMS

Symptoms of active disease are cough, lethargy, dyspnea, malaise, fever, sweating, or weight loss. Hemoptysis is a late finding.

EPIDEMIOLOGY/INCIDENCE

Although relatively rare in the developed world, tuberculosis (TB) is an infectious disease killer second only to HIV-AIDS (human immunodeficiency virus/acquired immune deficiency syndrome). The World Health Organization estimates at least 8 million new cases of TB in the world each year, the majority of which occur in people of reproductive age. Two million people worldwide die of tuberculosis every year. The incidence has increased in Africa (highest incidence)

Table 22.7 *Indications for PPD testing in pregnancy (factors which may predispose to progression from latent to active disease)*

Recent conversion
Household contacts of persons with infectious pulmonary TB
Recent immigration from parts of the world with high rates of TB
Homelessness
HIV infection
Living or working in an institutional setting in which TB is common (hospital, jail, homeless shelter)
Injection drug use
Renal failure on hemodialysis
Diabetes
Solid organ transplantation
Certain cancers; certain surgeries such as gastrectomy or jejunal bypass
High-dose corticosteroids for prolonged periods (lower limit not known)
Significantly underweight/poor nutrition

PPD, purified protein derivative (tuberculin); TB, tuberculosis, HIV, human immunodeficiency virus.

secondary to HIV, and in the former Soviet Union secondary to declines in socio-economic conditions and the health system. HIV co-infection (about 11% worldwide) accounts for a significant portion of the growing TB caseload.

ETIOLOGY/BASIC PATHOPHYSIOLOGY

Spread by airborne droplets is facilitated by the ability of these small particles to remain airborne for up to hours after being emitted from an infected respiratory tree. When the mycobacterium is inhaled and taken up by alveolar macrophages, the infection may either be contained by granuloma formation or may progress to active disease.[26] The development of cell-mediated immunity against *M. tuberculosis* occurs in most patients, is associated with the development of a positive tuberculin skin test, and the diagnosis of latent tuberculosis infection. In some patients, especially children <5 years old or immunocompromised adults, the replication of *M. tuberculosis* cannot be contained, and active disease occurs. Latent tuberculosis infection can develop into active tuberculosis, especially in individuals with risk factors (Table 22.7). Pulmonary disease is the most common but not the only form of active tuberculosis, which can also manifest in 20% of cases (extrapulmonary tuberculosis) as meningitis, osteitis, genitourinary involvement, or disseminated disease.

RISK FACTORS/ASSOCIATIONS

HIV is the most important risk factor. Poorly controlled diabetes, renal failure, malignancy, steroids, malnutrition,

and vitamin A or D deficiencies are other risk factors for acquiring active *M. tuberculosis* infection.[26]

PREGNANCY CONSIDERATIONS

Despite varying historical opinions, ranging from the beneficial to the deleterious effect of pregnancy on TB, **no consistent effect can be demonstrated**. TB attack rates appear to be comparable in both the pregnant and non-pregnant states. Presentation is similar among both pregnant and non-pregnant patients, but diagnosis may be delayed in pregnancy because of the ubiquity of constitutional complaints during early pregnancy. **Pregnancy is not known to influence the progression from latent to active disease.** Pregnancy is not associated with higher (or lower) prevalence of anergy compared with other non-pregnant HIV-negative adults.

MANAGEMENT
Principles

Management of *M. tuberculosis* infection in pregnancy should be **multidisciplinary**, with close involvement of obstetrician, maternal–fetal medicine, and infectious diseases specialists.

Screening
Tuberculin skin testing

Tuberculin skin testing is the method usually recommended to **detect both latent and active disease** in countries in

Table 22.8	*Criteria for a positive tuberculin skin test* [27]
Size of reaction	**Persons in whom reaction is considered positive**
≥5 mm	HIV-infected persons Close contacts of persons with infectious tuberculosis Persons with an abnormal chest radiograph consistent with previous tuberculosis[a] Immunosuppressed patients receiving the equivalent of ≥15 mg of prednisone per day for ≥1 month
≥10 mm	Foreign-born persons recently arrived (<5 years earlier) from country with high prevalence of tuberculosis Persons with a medical condition that increases the risk of tuberculosis[b] Injection-drug users Members of medically underserved, low-income populations (e.g. homeless persons) Residents and staff members of long-term care facilities (e.g. nursing homes, correctional institutions, homeless shelters) Healthcare workers Children <4 years of age Persons with conversion on a tuberculin skin test (increase in induration of ≥10 mm within a 2-year period)
≥15 mm	All others

[a]An abnormal chest radiograph consistent with previous tuberculosis reveals fibrotic opacities occupying more than 2 cm² of the upper lobe; radiographs showing pleural thickening or isolated calcified granulomas are not considered to be suggestive of previous tuberculosis.

[b]Medical conditions that increase the risk of development of tuberculosis in the presence of latent tuberculosis infection include silicosis, end-stage renal disease, malnutrition, diabetes mellitus, carcinoma of the head and neck or lung, immunosuppressive therapy, lymphoma, leukemia, loss of more than 10% of ideal body weight, gastrectomy, and jejunoileal bypass.

which BCG (bacille Calmette-Guérin) vaccination is uncommon. The more consistent form of tuberculin, standardized purified protein derivative (**PPD**) is the best available test to diagnose latent *M. tuberculosis* infection: 0.1 ml (5 tuberculin units) of PPD is administered intracutaneously in the volar surface of the forearm. The reaction is read 48–72 hours after the injection, but up to 1 week later, the reading is accurate. Targeted tuberculin testing is recommended in order to identify individuals who are at increased risk for developing *M. tuberculosis* infection and who would benefit by treatment of latent tuberculosis infection. Testing is currently discouraged among persons without these risk factors. Persons at increased risk for development of active disease are those who were recently infected/converted (i.e. converted from a positive to a negative skin test within the preceding 2 years), as well as those who not only have latent infection but also have an increased risk of progression from latent infection to overt disease (see Table 22.7). This is not an exhaustive list but is limited to those conditions which may be found in pregnancy. These represent indications for PPD testing. Interpretation of the PPD results is shown in Table 22.8.[27]

A decision to test is a decision to treat. Therefore, do not perform the first unless prepared to perform the second. With a positive skin test, a **chest X-ray** is indicated to differentiate latent from active infection, as the therapy is different. The screening algorithm is shown in Figure 22.3.

Work-up

Women with a cough lasting for >2 weeks or with symptoms as described above, especially with risk factors and/or from high prevalence areas, should be worked up for *M. tuberculosis* infection. **Radiographic** findings suggesting tuberculosis include upper lobe infiltrate, cavitary lesions, and hilar adenopathy. **Sputum smear** can be negative even in the case of active disease in 15–20% of cases. **Sputum culture** is required both for definite diagnosis and for **drug sensitivity testing**,[26] although both false-positive and false-negative results have been reported. Growth generally occurs in 7–21 days, but may take up to 6 weeks or longer.

Prevention

BCG vaccine has >70% efficacy in preventing *M. tuberculosis* infection in children, but not great efficacy in adults. It is impossible to distinguish induration induced by BCG or *M. tuberculosis* infection. The Center for Disease Control (CDC) recommends that a history of BCG vaccination be

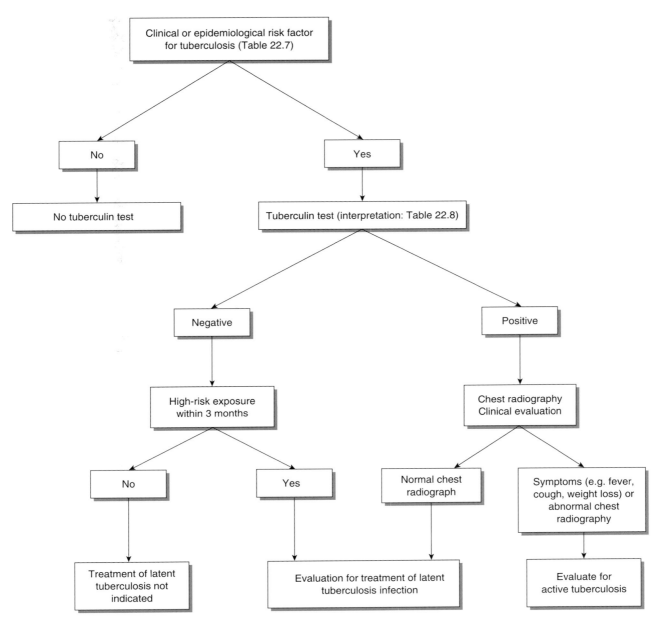

Figure 22.3
Tuberculosis screening algorithm.[27]

ignored when administering and interpreting a tuberculin skin test.

Therapy

Latent tuberculosis infection

The treatment for latent tuberculosis infection in pregnancy is **isoniazid 300 mg daily for 6–9 months.**[28] Alternative rifampin-based regimens have not been evaluated in pregnancy. Because isoniazid can interfere with pyridoxine metabolism and thereby precipitate peripheral neuropathy, coadministration of pyridoxine 25 mg/day is recommended.[29] Isoniazid is 60–90% effective in reducing the risk of progression from tuberculosis latent infection to active disease. The most important but rare (1/1000) side effect of isoniazid is hepatitis. Age >35 years old is no longer considered a contraindication to its use.[27] Advantages of beginning treatment during pregnancy include better compliance and less loss to follow-up.

Table 22.9	WHO-recommended treatment regimens[26]		
		Tuberculosis treatment[a]	
Treatment category	Patients	Initial phase (daily or three times per week)	Continuation phase (daily or three times per week)
I	New cases of smear-positive pulmonary tuberculosis or severe extrapulmonary tuberculosis or severe smear-negative pulmonary tuberculosis or severe concomitant HIV disease	2 months $H_3R_3Z_3E_3$ or 2 months $H_3R_3Z_3S_3$ 2 months HRZE or 2 months HRZS	4 months H_3R_3 4 months HR
II[c]	Previously treated smear-positive pulmonary tuberculosis; relapse; treatment failure; treatment after default	2 months $H_3R_3Z_3E_3S_3$/1 month $H_3R_3Z_3E_3$ 2 months HRZES/1 month HRZE	5 months $H_3R_3E_3$ 5 months HRE
III[d]	New cases of smear-negative pulmonary tuberculosis or with less severe forms of extrapulmonary tuberculosis	2 months $H_3R_3Z_3E_3$ 2 months HRZE	4 months H_3R_3 4 months HR 6 months HE[b]

[a]Subscript after letters refers to the number of doses per week; daily has no subscript. H = isoniazid; R = rifampin; Z = pyrazinamide; S = streptomycin; E = ethambutol.

[b]A continuation phase of 6 months of HE has a higher failure and relapse rate than a continuation phase of 4 months of HR but can be used for mobile patients and those with limited access to health services; the HE regimen can also be used concomitantly with antiretroviral treatment of HIV-infected patients.

[c]CDC/ATS and BTS recommend treatment for such patients based on susceptibility testing, with regimens tailored to the susceptibility profile. WHO recommends susceptibility testing whenever possible for patients with treatment failure.

[d]WHO indicates that ethambutol need not be given in the initial phase of category III treatment if patients have non-cavitary, smear-negative pulmonary tuberculosis, or if patients are known to have a drug-susceptible organism, or for young children with primary tuberculosis.

Recent TB infection or HIV co-infection increase the risk for transplacental spread of tubercle bacilli, and thus for congenital tuberculosis, which implies that treatment for latent infection (i.e. a positive PPD test) in these cases should be especially expeditious and compliant.

Active tuberculosis infection

Multiple drugs for ≥6 months can cure >95% of patients (Tables 22.9 and 22.10).[26] Single-drug therapy is no longer acceptable for active TB. The treatment regimen can be both complicated and long, with an initial period of intensive therapy designed to kill actively growing bacilli and thereby shorten the time the individual is infectious to others, followed by a second phase in which microbiological cure is attempted. The initial 2-month phase of therapy typically includes **isoniazid, rifampin, pyrazinamide,** and **either ethambutol or streptomycin.** Strict adherence to the regimen is important in minimizing drug resistance; for this reason, **directly observed therapy** is usually recommended. The following 4–6 months typically continue isoniazid with either rifampin or ethambutol. Regimens are available from the CDC and the American Thoracic Society[30] as well as from the British Thoracic Society and the International Union Against Tuberculosis and Lung

Disease, and from the World Health Organization (WHO). Advice from a specialist is likely to be helpful. In the case of multidrug-resistant TB, treatment becomes considerably more complex.

Treatment in pregnancy

TB treatment is not altered by pregnancy. Isoniazid, rifampin, pyrazinamide, and ethambutol are **not teratogenic,** and the WHO recommends their use in pregnant women.[26] **Streptomycin** exposure in utero has been associated with infant hearing loss, and so it is **contraindicated** in pregnancy. There are no adequate well-controlled reliable studies in human pregnancy. Pregnant women who are untreated pose an infection risk to the population at large as well as to their own infants. Postponing treatment into the second trimester or later is associated with higher obstetric and neonatal complication rates[29,31] as well as higher rates of prematurity, low birth weight, and perinatal death.

Drug resistance

Data on the second-line agents used in cases of multidrug-resistant tuberculosis in pregnancy are even more limited, but there are case reports as to a number of regimens.[31]

Table 22.10 *Doses, route of administration, and mode of action of primary drugs used in the treatment of tuberculosis*[26]

Drug	Route	Mode of action	Daily dose		Twice weekly dose		Thrice weekly dose	
			Adult	Maximum	Adult	Maximum	Adult	Maximum
Isoniazid	Oral or IM[a]	Bactericidal	5 mg/kg	300 mg	15 mg/kg (range 13–17)	900 mg	10 mg/kg (range 8–12)	900 mg
Rifampin	Oral or IV	Bactericidal	600 mg (range 8–12 mg/kg)	600 mg	600 mg (range 8–12 mg/kg)	600 mg	600 mg (range 8–12 mg/kg)	600 mg
Pyrazinamide[b]	Oral	Bactericidal	1–5 g (<50 kg) 25 g (≥75 kg)	25 g (<50 kg)	20 g (<50 kg) 35 g (≥75 kg)	20 g (<50 kg)	30 g (51–74 kg) 30 g (≥75 kg)	30g (51–74 kg)
Ethambutol[c]	Oral	Bacteriostatic	15–25 mg/kg	25 g	45 mg/kg		30 mg/kg	
Streptomycin	IM, IV	Bactericidal	15 mg/kg	1000 mg	15 mg/kg	1000 mg	15 mg/kg	1000 mg
Thioacetazone	Oral	Bacteriostatic	150 mg		NR	NR	NR	NR

IM = intramuscular; IV = intravenous; NR = not recommended.

[a]Intravenous and suppository forms are available in some countries.

[b]WHO and CDC/ATS recommend dosing of pyrazinamide in adults on a weight basis, but dosing based on weight categories as recommended by BTS and by tuberculosis programs is more useful in practice. Recommendations of dosing for this drug vary widely. Adults weighing < 45 kg can have pediatric doses. The doses given here are based on the New York City Tuberculosis Control Program.

[c]WHO, IUATLD, and BTS recommend 15 mg/kg ethambutol for daily administration in adults and children and 30 mg/kg for thrice-weekly dosing.

Unfortunately, the alternative to treatment of multidrug-resistant tuberculosis is not practical, because of the grave public health implications. Tuberculosis strains which are known to be resistant to one or more of the first-line drugs are treated with alternative agents, which may include amikacin, kanamycin, capreomycin, cycloserine, fluoroquinolones, para-aminosalicylate, thiacetazone, amoxicillin–clavulanic acid, clofazimine, clarithromycin, or ethionamide. Kanamycin, streptomycin, and amikacin, which are ototoxic, have been associated with hearing loss in newborns whose mothers were treated during pregnancy; for all these drugs, well-designed controlled studies in pregnant women are unavailable. Therapy of drug-resistant TB should be driven by microbiological susceptibility patterns either obtained by direct culture or known to be prevalent in the area, rather than by teratogenic concerns. The local, regional, national, or supranational health authority usually plays a role in decisions as to appropriate therapy in cases of drug-resistant TB. The WHO has a tuberculosis gateway which can be easily accessed, and provides links to epidemiology and to treatment of tuberculosis: http://www.who.int/tb/en/.

Infection control issues

Women with active pulmonary tuberculosis are infectious, but if the organism is sensitive, 2 weeks of therapy with multiple agents renders the women non-infectious, so special precautions are not necessary. If the duration of therapy is shorter, or if multidrug-resistant tuberculosis is present or suspected, the mother must be isolated in a negative pressure room for labor, and personal protective equipment should be worn by staff. Measures for the infant may include prophylactic isoniazid, BCG vaccination, or – in cases of multidrug-resistant tuberculosis – potentially, separation from the mother.

Antepartum testing

No specific indications.

Delivery

Cord blood and placenta should be tested for acid-fast bacilli.

Postpartum/breastfeeding

Maternal tuberculosis treatment is not altered by breastfeeding. The neonate should receive PPD, chest X-ray, lumbar puncture, and *M. tuberculosis* smear and culture if the mother had *M. tuberculosis* infection during pregnancy. If tuberculosis is suspected in the offspring, the child should be adequately treated.

REFERENCES

1. Davidson CM, Doyle NM, Ramin SM. Don't undertreat asthma in pregnancy. Contemp Obstet Gynecol 2005; 8: 34–41. [review]

2. National Center for Health Statistics, online at http://209.217.72.34/asthma/ReportFolders/reportFolders.aspx, accessed 3/4/05. [review]

3. National Asthma Education and Prevention Program. NAEPP Working Group Report on Managing Asthma During Pregnancy: Recommendations for Pharmacologic Treatment – Update 2004. NIH Publication 05-3279. [guideline]

4. Kallen B, Rydhstroem H, Aberg A. Asthma during pregnancy – a population based study. Eur J Epidemiol 2000; 16: 671–71. [II-2, $n=37\,000$]

5. Dombrowski MP, Schatz M, Wise R, et al. Asthma during pregnancy. Obstet Gynecol 2004; 103: 5–12. [II-2, $n=2500$]

6. Olesen C, Thrane N, Nielsen GL, Sorensen HT, Olsen J. A population-based prescription study of asthma drugs during pregnancy: changing the intensity of asthma therapy and perinatal outcomes. Respiration 2001; 68: 256–61. [II-2]

7. Cydulka RK, Emerman CL, Schreiber D, et al. Acute asthma among pregnant women presenting to the emergency department. Am J Respir Crit Care Med 1999; 160: 887–92. [II-3]

8. Kwon HL, Belanger K, Bracken MB. Effect of pregnancy and stage of pregnancy on asthma severity: a systematic review. Am J Obstet Gynecol 2004; 190: 1201–10. [review]

9. Schatz M, Dombrowski MP, Wise R, et al. Asthma morbidity during pregnancy can be predicted by severity classification. J Allergy Clin Immunol 2003; 112: 283–8 [II-3, $n = 1700$]

10. Kircher S, Schatz M, Long B. Variables affecting asthma course during pregnancy. Ann Allergy Asthma Immunol 2002; 89: 463–6. [II-3]

11. Gluck JC, Gluck PA. The effect of pregnancy on the course of asthma. Immunol Allergy Clin North Am 2000; 20: 729–43. [II-3]

12. Beecroft N, Cochrane GM, Milburn HF. Effect of sex of fetus on asthma during pregnancy. BMJ 1998; 317: 856–7. [II-3]

13. Busse WW, National Heart, Lung, and Blood Institute, National Asthma Education and Prevention Program Asthma in Pregnancy Working Group. NAEPP expert panel report. Managing asthma during pregnancy: recommendations for pharmacologic treatment – 2004 update. J Allergy Clin Immunol 2005; 115: 34–46. [review]

14. Gluck JC, Gluck PA. Asthma controller therapy during pregnancy. Am J Obstet Gynecol 2005; 192: 369–80. [review]

15. Dombrowski MP, Schatz M, Wise R, et al. Randomized trial of inhaled beclomethasone dipropionate versus theophylline for moderate asthma during pregnancy. Am J Obstet Gynecol 2004; 190: 737–44. [RCT, $n=385$]

16. Namazy J, Schatz M, Long L, et al. Use of inhaled steroids by pregnant asthmatic women does not reduce intrauterine growth. J Allergy Clin Immunol 2004; 113: 427–32. [II-2]

17. Ducharme F, Schwartz Z, Kakuma R. Addition of anti-leukotriene agents to inhaled corticosteroids for chronic asthma. Cochrane Database Syst Rev 2006; 4: [meta-analysis: 27 RCTs, non-pregnant]

18. Rust GS, Thompson CJ, Minor P, et al. Does breastfeeding protect children from asthma? Analysis of NHANES III survey data. J Natl Med Assoc 2001; 93: 139–48. [II-3]

19. File TM. Community-acquired pneumonia. Lancet 2003; 362: 1991–2001. [review]

20. American Thoracic Society. Guidelines for the management of adults with community-acquired pneumonia. Am J Respir Crit Care Med 2001; 163: 1730–54. [review]

21. Jin Y, Carriere KC, Marrie TJ, Predy G, Johnson DH. The effects of community-acquired pneumonia during pregnancy ending with a live birth. Am J Obstet Gynecol 2003; 18: 800–6. [II-3]

22. Yost NP, Bloom SL, Richey SD, Ramin SM, Cunningham FG. An appraisal of treatment guidelines for community-acquired pneumonia. Am J Obstet Gynecol 2000; 183: 131–5. [II-3; $n=119$ pregnant women with pneumonia]

23. Bloom SL, Ramin S, Cunningham FG. A prediction rule for community-acquired pneumonia. N Engl J Med 1997; 336: 1913–14. [meta-analysis in letter to the editor]

24. Fine MJ, Auble TE, Yealy DM, et al. A prediction rule to identify low-risk patients with community-acquired pneumonia. N Engl J Med 1997; 336: 243–50. [II-3]

25. Mandell LA, Bartlett JG, Dowell SF, et al. Update of practice guidelines for the management of community-acquired pneumonia in immuno-competent adults. Clin Infect Dis 2003; 37: 1405–33. [review]

26. Frieden TR, Sterling TR, Munsiff SS, Watt CJ, Dye C. Tuberculosis. Lancet 2003; 362: 887–92. [review]

27. Jasmer RM, Nahid P, Hopewell PC. Latent tuberculosis infection. N Engl J Med 2002; 347: 1860–6. [review]

28. American Thoracic Society. Targeted tuberculin testing and treatment of latent tuberculosis infection. Am J Respir Crit Care Med 2000; 161: S221–47. [review]

29. Figueroa-Damian R, Arredondo-Garcia JL. Pregnancy and tuberculosis: effect of treatment on perinatal outcome. Am J Perinatol 1998; 15: 303–6. [II-3]

30. American Thoracic Society, CDC, and Infectious Diseases Society of America. Treatment of tuberculosis. MMWR Morb Mortal Wkly Rep 2003; 52: 1–77. [review]

31. Figueroa-Damian R, Arredondo-Garcia JL. Neonatal outcome of children born to women with tuberculosis. Arch Med Res 2001; 32: 66–9. [II-3]

23

Antiphospholipid syndrome

James Airoldi

KEY POINTS

- The **diagnosis** of antiphospholipid syndrome (APS) requires the presence of at least **one clinical and one laboratory** criteria.
- **Complications** of APS include venous thromboembolism (VTE), **early-onset pre-eclampsia, pregnancy loss, fetal growth restriction (FGR), fetal death, and preterm birth.**
- Therapy should be:
  - For APS with either ≥3 unexplained consecutive pregnancy losses at <10 weeks, or ≥1 unexplained fetal deaths >10 weeks: **low-dose aspirin (ASA acetylsalicylic acid)** and **prophylactic heparin.**
  - For APS with **VTE** during pregnancy: **therapeutic anticoagulation.**
  - There are no trials to assess therapy for APS with pre-eclampsia and/or FGR.
- All trials on efficacy have used unfractionated heparin as therapy. If on low molecular weight (LMW) heparin, regional anesthesia should be delayed until ≥24 hours after the last dose.

HISTORIC NOTES

Lupus anticoagulant (LA) was first described in the early 1950s as prolonging certain clotting assays. A few years later, LA was found to be associated with the false-positive test for syphilis and, paradoxically, thrombosis.

DIAGNOSIS[1,2]

The diagnosis of antiphospholipid syndrome (APS) requires the presence of at least one clinical and one laboratory criteria. There are no time limits on the interval between the clinical and laboratory events.

Clinical criteria

1. **Pregnancy loss:** ≥3 unexplained consecutive pregnancy losses at <10 weeks, or ≥1 unexplained fetal deaths at >10 weeks (morphologically normal fetus).
2. **Preterm birth (PTB) at <34 weeks for fetal growth restriction (FGR) or pre-eclampsia:** ≥1 preterm births at <34 weeks of a morphologically normal fetus due to severe pre-eclampsia, FGR, oligohydramnios, abnormal Doppler flow or NRFHR testing.
3. **Thrombosis:** one or more clinical venous, arterial, or small vessel venous thromboembolism (VTE) occurring within any tissue or organ. Except for superficial vein thrombosis, thrombosis must be confirmed by imaging or Doppler studies or histopathology.

Laboratory criteria

1. **Anticardiolipin antibodies (ACAs):** Immunoglobulin G (**IgG**) and/or immunoglobulin M (**IgM**) in medium–high titers (≥40 units, or >99th percentile).
2. **LA:** prolonged activated partial thromboplastin time (aPTT), dilute Russel's viper venom time (DRVVT), and kaolin clotting time (Figure 23.1).
3. Anti-β_2 glycoprotein-I IgG or IgM antibody (>99th percentile).

Abnormal laboratory tests must occur in **≥2 occasions, ≥12 weeks apart.**

Antiphospholipid antibody testing

Antiphospholipid antibodies (APAs) are directed against phospholipids, and include ACAs and LA. LA is a double misnomer. LA is seen in many patients without systemic lupus erythematosus (SLE), and is associated with thrombosis, not anticoagulation. ACA is strongly correlated with LA and thrombosis. In the 1990s ACAs were found to require the presence of plasma phospholipid-binding protein B2

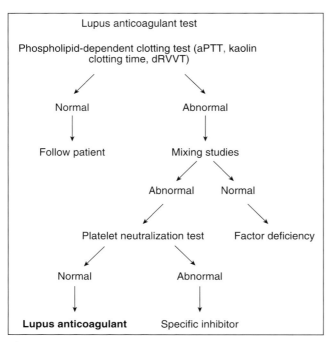

Figure 23.1
Algorithm for interpretation of lupus anticoagulant test:[1,2] aPTT, activated partial thromboplastin time; dRVVT, dilute Russell's viper venom time.

glycoprotein 1 to bind to cardiolipin. In contrast, ACAs from patients with syphilis or other infections are B2 glycoprotein 1 independent. B2 glycoprotein 1 was recently included in the definition. Approximately 80% of patients with LA have ACAs, whereas 20% of patients with ACAs are found positive for LA.[2] Substantial **inter-laboratory variation** when testing the same sera remains a **serious problem**.

SYMPTOMS

Clinical manifestations of APS may involve any organ system, including vascular (arterial or venous), cardiac, cutaneous, endocrine/reproductive, gastrointestinal, hematological, neurological, obstetric, ophthalmological, pulmonary, and renal.

EPIDEMIOLOGY/INCIDENCE

APAs are found in up to 5% of healthy controls. The prospective risks in these are unknown. 25–35% of SLE patients have APS (see Chapter 24). ACAs are present in 15% of women with recurrent miscarriage; LA is found in 8% of patients with recurrent miscarriage. In women with mid-trimester fetal loss, LA is seen in up to 30%, and 70% of definite APS patients have both ACAs and LA.

ETIOLOGY/BASIC PATHOPHYSIOLOGY

APAs may cause pregnancy loss by thrombosis of placental vessels, interference with coagulation factors (reduce levels of annexin V), inhibition of proliferation of trophoblasts, or other yet unknown mechanisms.

CLASSIFICATION

Primary APS refers to patients with APS but no other autoimmune disorders. *Secondary* APS refers to patients with other autoimmune disorders (e.g. SLE).[2]

COMPLICATIONS

Maternal

Venous and arterial thromboembolism (5–12% risk in pregnancy; 0.5–2% of asymptomatic people incidentally found to have APAs have thromboses each year); early-onset **pre-eclampsia** (placental infarction, decidual vasculopathy); **gestational hypertension** (18–48% of women with APS; this rate is not diminished by aspirin, heparin, or glucocorticoids); autoimmune **thrombocytopenia** (40–50%); heparin-induced thrombocytopenia (less with low molecular weight [LMW] heparin); heparin-induced osteoporosis (especially if on glucocorticoids); lupus flare in patients with coexisting SLE.

Fetal

Pregnancy loss; **FGR** (15–30%); **fetal death**; **PTB** (33%, secondary to gestational hypertension or placental insufficiency, either spontaneous or iatrogenic).

PREGNANCY CONSIDERATIONS

Complications are less if pregnancy starts when APS is 'quiescent' without symptoms and negative levels of APAs, whereas complications are more frequent and severe if APS is active with high levels of APAs. As other autoimmune disorders, APS can exacerbate postpartum: fever, pulmonary infiltrates, pleural effusion, occasionally renal, pulmonary, VTE; rarely disseminated intravascular coagulation (DIC) and mortality.

MANAGEMENT

Principles

Multidisciplinary management with a rheumatologist or internal medicine specialist is recommended.

Screening

Women with the following risk factors should be screened for ACA and LA:

- three or more spontaneous unexplained first trimester losses at < 10 weeks
- one or more unexplained fetal loss/death at ≥ 10 weeks
- early-onset (< 34 weeks) pre-eclampsia or FGR leading to PTB
- SLE
- history of vascular thrombosis (VTEs such as deep vein thrombosis [DVT], pulmonary embolus [PE], and stroke).

Work-up

Laboratory tests as described above (ACA, LA, and anti-β_2 glycoprotein-I tests). Testing for antiphospholipid antibodies other than these is not clinically useful in the evaluation of recurrent pregnancy loss.

Prevention

There is no preventive strategy available.

Therapy

There are usually **two ways of dosing heparin:**

1. **Prophylactic anticoagulation** typically implies low dosing (usually without monitoring, Table 26.4). If prophylactic adjusted-dose, this implies anti Xa level of 0.2–0.4 U/ml.
2. **Therapeutic anticoagulation** implies higher dosing (always **adjusted dosing**), meaning usually adjusted to anti Xa levels of 0.5–1.2 U/ml (Table 26.5).

Evidence

- Compared with placebo or usual care, low-dose aspirin (ASA, acetylsalicylic acid) is not associated with any difference in outcome in pregnant women with APS.[3–5] The summary relative risk (RR) for recurrent pregnancy loss is 1.05 (95% CI 0.66–1.68).[6]
- Compared with low dose ASA alone, **unfractionated heparin and low-dose ASA** in APS patients with recurrent pregnancy loss[7–9] are associated with significant reduction in pregnancy loss, with a summary RR of 0.48 (95% CI 0.33–0.68) for the three combined studies.[7–9]
- Compared with low-dose ASA alone or placebo, prednisone and low-dose ASA are not associated with a significant difference in pregnancy loss, with an RR of 0.85 (95% CI 0.53–1.36).[10,11] However, there were significant higher rates of PTB in the prednisone groups in both trials and higher neonatal intensive care unit (NICU)

admissions in one study.[11] There were also lower birth weights in the prednisone group in one of the studies.[10]

- Compared with heparin and low-dose ASA, prednisone and low-dose ASA are associated with no difference in pregnancy loss rates, but again the prednisone group had a significantly higher rate of PTB.[12]
- In women already on heparin and ASA, the addition of intravenous immunoglobulin (IVIG) did not affect pregnancy loss rates in a very small trial, but was associated with a significantly higher PTB rate.[13] This therapy is very expensive, and the only treatment shown to lower anticardiolipin levels.

Actual therapy

APS with pregnancy loss or prior thrombosis: low-dose ASA and prophylactic heparin[2,7–9]

Therapy is usually begun once fetal viability is established, but there is insufficient evidence regarding the best time of initiation of therapy.

- Low-dose ASA dose is usually about 75–100 mg daily.
- For prophylactic unfractionated heparin: 5000–7500 units first trimester; 7500–10 000 units second trimester, 10 000 units third trimester SQ q12h.
- For prophylactic LMW heparin: enoxaparin (Lovenox) 30–40 mg SQ q12h or dalteparin (Fragmin) 5000 u SQ q12h (may adjust prophylaxis in high-risk cases to heparin [antiXa] level range 0.2–0.3).

APS with VTE during pregnancy: therapeutic anticoagulation[2]

- Therapeutic unfractionated heparin: doses need to be adjusted to keep aPTT 2–3 times normal.
- Therapeutic LMW heparin: enoxaparin 1 mg/kg q12h, or dalteparin 200 units/kg q12h.
- Discontinue ASA just before delivery. Must adjust therapeutic LMW heparin to heparin [antiXa] level 0.5–1.2. Consider switching from LMW heparin to unfractionated heparin at 36 weeks (or earlier if high risk for PTB).

APS with PTB secondary to early-onset FGR, other signs of placental insufficiency (see page 175, clinical criteria) or severe pre-eclampsia
- There are no treatment trials to assess any therapy.

Unfractionated heparin is thus the **only** therapy that has shown a statistically significant reduction in pregnancy loss. The optimal dose and the exact population(s) in which this therapy is most effective are difficult to assess precisely given the loose inclusion criteria and small numbers of the trials. It is associated with a 5% decrease in bone mass density (BMD). Supplemental calcium (calcium gluconate/carbonate 1500 mg daily) and vitamin D, as well as weight-bearing exercise, should be encouraged. Idiosyncratic thrombocytopenia, known as heparin-induced thrombocytopenia (HIT), occurs in < 5% of women on heparin therapy, is usually mild, and usually starts 3–15 days after initiation of therapy. There is no evidence to assess warfarin therapy for women with extreme thrombotic histories, including recurrent thromboses or cerebral thrombosis. (See also Chapter 26.)

Antepartum testing

- **Early ultrasound** is essential for accurate dating.
- Prenatal visits can be more frequent, approximately every 2 weeks after 24 weeks. Initiate heparin once viability is confirmed.
- Detailed ultrasound at about 18–20 weeks and follow-up ultrasounds about every 4–6 weeks for growth, fluid volume, and Doppler evaluation of the fetus.
- Fetal surveillance testing at 32 weeks.
- Daily fetal kick counts.

Preparations for delivery

- Delivery by EDC (estimated date of confinement).
- If on LMW heparin, consider switching to unfractionated heparin at 36 weeks to allow regional anesthesia.

Delivery

Send placenta (decreased placental weight, ischemic-hypoxic changes – infarctions, decidual and fetal thrombi, chronic villitis).

Anesthesia

If on unfractionated heparin, regional anesthesia can be administered usually 6–8 hours after the dose, or at least when the aPTT is within normal limits. **If on LMW heparin, regional anesthesia should be delayed until ≥ 24 hours after the last dose,** since there is a risk of spinal hematoma if regional anesthesia is performed within 24 hours. That is why a woman on LMW heparin should be switched off LMW heparin on to unfractionated heparin weeks before any chance of labor or delivery (usually around 36 weeks if no other risk of PTB).

Postpartum/breastfeeding

In women with APS based on recurrent embryonic loss at < 10 weeks, the use of anticoagulation in the postpartum period has never been shown to be helpful.

In women with APS based on fetal loss at ≥ 10 weeks and no thrombotic events, anticoagulation for 6 weeks is usually recommended in the USA[2] (only 3–5 days in the UK).

Women with APS based on prior thrombotic events should be switched to warfarin therapy. Warfarin therapy is safe in breastfeeding women. An international normalized ratio (INR) of 3.0 is desirable.

Estrogen-containing oral contraceptives should be avoided, as they further increase the VTE risk.

It is imperative that women with APS be followed closely by a medical or hematological specialist after pregnancy. About 50% of women with APS develop thromboses in the 3–10 years after delivery, and about 10% develop SLE.[2]

REFERENCES

1. Miyakis S, Lockshin MD, Atsuni T, et al. International consensus statement on an update of the classification criteria for definite antiphospholipid syndrome. J Thromb Haemost 2006; 4: 297–306. [review]
2. American College of Obstetricians and Gynecologists. Antiphospholipid Syndrome. ACOG Practice Bulletin No. 68, 2005. [review]
3. Pattison NS, Chamley LW, Birdsall M, et al. Does aspirin have a role in improving pregnancy outcome for women with the antiphospholipid syndrome? A randomized controlled trial. Am J Obstet Gynecol 2000; 183: 1008–12. [RCT, n=50]
4. Cowchock S, Reece EA. Do low-risk pregnant women with antiphospholipid antibodies need to be treated? Am J Obstet Gynecol 1997; 176: 1099–100. [RCT, n=19]
5. Tulppala M, Marttunen M, Soderstrom-Anttila V, et al. Low-dose aspirin prevention of miscarriage in women with unexplained or autoimmune related recurrent miscarriage: effect on prostacyclin and thromboxane A2 production. Hum Reprod 1997; 12: 1567–72. [RCT, n=66]
6. Empson M, Lassere M, Craig JC, et al. Recurrent pregnancy loss with antiphospholipid antibody: a systematic review of therapeutic trials. Obstet Gynecol 2002; 99: 135–44. [meta-analysis: 10 RCTs; Refs 2, 3, 4, 5, 7–13, n=627]
7. Rai R, Cohen H, Dave M, Regan L. Randomised controlled trial of aspirin and aspirin plus heparin in pregnant women with recurrent miscarriage associated with phospholipids antibodies. BMJ 1997; 314: 253–7. [RCT, n=90]
8. Kutteh WH. Antiphospholipid antibody-associated recurrent pregnancy loss: treatment with heparin and low dose aspirin is superior to low-dose aspirin alone. Am J Obstet Gynecol 1996; 174: 1584–9. [RCT, n=50]
9. Farquharson RG, Quenby S, Greaves M. Antiphospholipid syndrome in pregnancy: a randomized controlled trial of treatment. Lupus 2002; 100: 408–13. [RCT, n=98]
10. Silver RK, MacGregor SN, Sholl JS, et al. Comparative trial of prednisone plus aspirin vs. aspirin alone in the treatment of anticardiolipin antibody positive obstetric patients. Am J Obstet Gynecol 1993; 169: 1411–17. [RCT, n=39]
11. Laskin CA, Bombardier C, Hannah ME, et al. Prednisone and aspirin in women with autoantibodies and unexplained recurrent fetal loss. N Engl J Med 1997; 337: 148–53. [RCT, n=202]
12. Cowchock FS, Reece EA, Balaban D, et al. Repeated fetal losses associated with antiphospholipid antibodies: a collaborative randomized trial comparing prednisone with low-dose heparin treatment. Am J Obstet Gynecol 1992; 166: 1318–23. [RCT, n=45]
13. Branch DW, Peaceman AM, Druzin M, et al. A multicenter, placebo-controlled pilot study of intravenous immune globulin treatment of antiphospholipid syndrome during pregnancy. The Pregnancy Loss Study Group. Am J Obstet Gynecol 2000; 182: 122–7. [RCT, n=16]

24

Systemic lupus erythematosus

Vincenzo Berghella

KEY POINTS

- **Diagnosis:** ≥ 4/11 American College of Rheumatology criteria.
- **Preconception counseling:** feto-neonatal and maternal **complications** are primarily seen in systemic lupus erythematosus (SLE) patients **with active disease periconceptionally or patients with hypertension, or renal, heart, lungs, or brain disease, or antiphospholipid antibodies.** Therefore, it is recommended to screen for all above, and to start pregnancy with SLE in remission. Optimize medical therapy preconceptionally.
- **Laboratories:** complete blood count (CBC) with platelets, transaminases, creatinine, blood urea nitrogen (BUN), anti-SSA/Ro and anti-SSB/La antibodies, anticardiolipin antibodies (ACA), lupus anticoagulant (LA) or dilute Russell's viper venom time (DRVVT), antinuclear antibodies (ANA), anti double-stranded (anti ds) DNA, C3, C4, urine sediment, 24-hour urine for total protein and creatinine clearance.
- **If stable with no recent flares on azathioprine and/or hydroxychloroquine, it is recommended to continue them in pregnancy and postpartum.** Keep at lowest possible efficacious dose of medications, including steroids.
- **For women with antiphospholipid syndrome (APS), see Chapter 23.**
- Women with **anti-SSA/Ro and/or anti-SSB/La antibodies** have a **2–5% risk of congenital heart block (CHB);** preventive screening and therapy for CHB are not evidence based. Women with fetuses with CHB should be managed and delivered at a tertiary care center with the availability of immediate neonatal pacing.

HISTORIC NOTES

- 1950s: systemic lupus erythrematosus (SLE) 5-year survival = 50%.
- 1990s: 10-year survival = 95%.

DIAGNOSIS

The American College of Rheumatology (**ARA**) **criteria** require ≥ 4 out of these 11 criteria to make a diagnosis of SLE – either serially or simultaneously:[1]

1. Malar rash.
2. Discoid rash.
3. Photosensitivity.
4. Oral ulcers – painless.
5. Arthritis (non-erosive, involving two or more peripheral joints).
6. Serositis: pleuritis or pericarditis, conjunctivitis.
7. Renal disorder: persistent proteinuria > 0.5 g/day, or cellular casts.
8. Neurological disorder: seizure or psychosis.
9. Hematological disorder: hemolytic anemia with reticulocytosis, or leukopenia < 4000/mm³, or lymphopenia < 1500/mm³, or thrombocytopenia < 100 000/mm³.
10. Immunological disorder: positive lupus erythematosus cell preparation, or anti double-stranded (ds) DNA, or anti-Smith (SM) antibody, or false-positive serological test for syphilis.
11. Antinuclear antibodies (ANA) in abnormal titers.

SYMPTOMS

See 11 diagnostic criteria. Also, general (fatigue, fever, malaise, weight loss); gastrointestinal (anorexia, ascites, vasculitis); thrombosis, Raynaud's phenomenon, etc.

EPIDEMIOLOGY/INCIDENCE

- 1:700–2000 of the general population (1:200 in African-Americans).
- 90% in women; 1/500 of childbearing age.
- ANA: positive in 95% of SLE patients, but not specific or pathognomonic.

- Anti ds DNA: positive in 70% of SLE patients, associated with clinical activity/flare, renal disease.
- Anti-SSA/Ro antibody: positive in 30% of SLE patients, associated with congenital heart block (CHB) (see below), neonatal lupus, Sjögren's syndrome.
- Anti-SSB/La antibody: positive in 10% of SLE patients; associated with CHB, neonatal lupus, Sjögren's syndrome.
- Anticardiolipin antibodies (ACA): positive in 50% of SLE patients. Associated with antiphospholipid syndrome (APS) (see Chapter 23), thrombosis.
- Lupus anticoagulant (LA): positive in 26% of SLE patients, associated with APS (Chapter 23), fetal growth restriction (FGR), fetal death, and pre-eclampsia.
- 25% of SLE patients meet criteria for APS (see Chapter 23).
- Anti-SM: positive in 30% of SLE patients, specific for SLE.
- Anti-RNP: positive in 40% of SLE patients, associated with neonatal lupus, mixed connective tissue (CT) disease.
- Anti-centromere: 90% in CREST variant of scleroderma.

ETIOLOGY/BASIC PATHOPHYSIOLOGY

Auto-antibody (Ab) to fixed tissue antigen (Ag) in vessel wall, nucleus, cytoplasmic membranes, etc. Ag–Ab complexes in serum.

COMPLICATIONS

Maternal

Hypertension and pre-eclampsia (20–50%), preterm birth (PTB) 30–50% (spontaneous – premature preterm rupture of membranes [PPROM] and preterm labor [PTL] – and indicated), gestational diabetes mellitus.

Fetal/neonatal

Increased incidence of first trimester spontaneous pregnancy loss (10–20%), fetal death (1–30%), FGR (10–20%), CHB (see below), and neonatal lupus (see below).

These adverse outcomes are primarily seen in SLE patients with active disease periconceptionally, or in patients with hypertension, or renal, cardiac, pulmonary, or neurological disease, or antiphospholipid antibodies. APS is associated with most fetal deaths in SLE. Renal disease is present in 50% of SLE patients. The above complications may also be seen more frequently in multiple pregnancies with SLE.

PREGNANCY CONSIDERATIONS
Effect of pregnancy on SLE

Pregnancy usually does not affect long-term prognosis of SLE. Over 90% of women without end-organ disease or antiphospholipid antibodies (APAs) do well, and take home babies. Incidence of flares varies widely, depending on definition of flare, patient selection, and clinical status at conception. Flares can occur in any trimester, but most commonly late and postpartum. Most flares in pregnancy are mild (90%), musculoskeletal, and neurological. Prednisone ≥ 20 mg is usually required for severe flares.

Effect of SLE on pregnancy

Increased incidence of complications (see above). If renal SLE, 50% have hypertension, 10–30% worsening but usually reversible renal disease. If creatinine ≥ 1.3 mg/dl, and/or creatinine clearance < 50 ml/min, and/or proteinuria > 3 g in 24 hours preconceptionally, there is a small risk of irreversible renal deterioration.

MANAGEMENT
Principles

Goal: pregnancy with SLE in remission. **Start pregnancy with SLE in remission. To achieve this, usually need to optimize medical therapy preconceptionally.** Most drugs are safe (see below), and should be continued throughout pregnancy.

Work-up

Baseline prenatal laboratory tests should include the following: complete blood count (CBC) **with platelets, transaminases, creatinine, blood urea nitrogen (BUN), anti-SSA/Ro antibody, anti-SSB/La antibody, ACA, LA, ANA, anti ds DNA, C3, C4, urine sediment, 24-hour urine for total protein, and creatinine clearance.**

Differential diagnosis

Distinguish SLE flare from pre-eclampsia: C3, C4 (decreased in SLE), and anti ds DNA (increased in SLE). Gestational age at onset of symptoms is also helpful, with pre-eclampsia usually occurring after 24 weeks.

Preconception counseling

Review all of the above with the patient and family, especially diagnosis, risks and complications, and management.

Evaluate by history, physical examination, and laboratory tests. Obtain records. Discuss current medications. To insure pregnancy is conceived with SLE quiescent, encourage the patient to wait at least 6 months without flares/active disease before attempting conception. If **stable with no recent flares on azathioprine and/or hydroxychloroquine, it is recommended to continue them in pregnancy and postpartum. Keep at the lowest possible efficacious dose of steroids.** Discuss contraception. Consider multidisciplinary management with a rheumatologist.

Prenatal care

For women with APS, see Chapter 23. Treatment decisions are based on the past obstetric history and any history of prior thromboembolic events. The use of medications to treat or suppress SLE flares will need to be evaluated on an individual basis. If patients have been maintained on medication(s) throughout the pregnancy, these should be continued through the postpartum period. Counsel regarding avoiding excessive sun exposure or fatigue.

Therapy

NSAIDs (non-steroidal anti-inflammatory drugs)

Safe up to 28–30 weeks. Side effects: fetal ductal closure and oligohydramnios, especially after 30 weeks.

Corticosteroids

Mechanism: increase antibody levels. Prednisone: 5–80 mg are usual daily doses. Try to keep maintenance doses ≤ 20 mg/day. For treatment of flares, usually need ≥ 60 mg/day × 3 weeks. Safe in pregnancy (metabolized by placenta, does not cross it). Animal studies report facial clefts. Safe for breastfeeding. High doses: risk of diabetes (perform early glucola test), and of PPROM. Taper if used more than 7 days. Stress steroids in active labor up to one dose post delivery (hydrocortisone 100 mg IV q8h) are indicated only if steroid therapy in pregnancy for ≥ 14 days (to prevent Addisonian collapse [very rare] – general malaise, nausea/vomiting, skin changes). Side effects: increased bone loss, especially together with heparin (give calcium).

Azathioprine (Azasan, Imuran)

A dose of 50–100 mg orally daily or divided bid. Increase after 6–8 weeks. Safe in pregnancy. FGR association is probably due to SLE, not azathioprine. It induces chromosomal breaks, which disappear as the infant grows.

Hydroxychloroquine sulfate (Plaquenil)

Antimalarial drug: 400–600 mg orally daily, then increase to 200–400 mg daily. Probably safe in pregnancy.[2] If stopped, 2.5 times risk of flare compared with placebo.[3] Important not to stop drug periconceptionally.[4] No long-term effects. Safe in breastfeeding.

Other agents

Acetaminophen (paracetamol) is safe throughout pregnancy, but usually not as effective as other therapies. Avoid cyclophosphamide, methotrexate, and penicillamine, which are not safe in pregnancy. Plasmapheresis is a last resort; consult a rheumatologist.

Antepartum testing

Accurate gestational age assessment is important, and therefore a first trimester ultrasound examination is indicated.

Fetal growth can be evaluated throughout pregnancy with ultrasound examinations every 4–6 weeks. For women with anti-SSA/Ro and/or anti-SSB/La antibodies, see CHB below. A fetal echocardiogram is indicated if CHB, an arrhythmia, or hydropic signs are detected.

Patients in whom disease activity is quiescent, and there is no evidence of hypertension, renal disease, FGR, or preeclampsia, can begin weekly fetal testing at 34–36 weeks' gestation. Patients with active disease, APA, renal disease, hypertension, or FGR can begin antepartum testing earlier, e.g. at 30–32 weeks.

Delivery

Stress-dose steroids are indicated only if steroid use ≥ 14 days during pregnancy (see corticosteroids above).

Postpartum/breastfeeding

Flares are more common. Continue, and consider increasing SLE therapies.

CONGENITAL HEAR BLOCK
Incidence

About 2–5% of SSA/SSB-positive women.

Etiology

Anti-SSA/Ro and anti-SSB/La antibodies cause myocarditis and fibrosis in the atrioventricular (AV) node and bundle of His regions.

Counseling

Usually permanent, with pacemaker needed. One-third of untreated CHB infants die within 3 years (sudden death). There is a 15–33% recurrence in future siblings. Complications: congestive heart failure (hydrops).

MANAGEMENT
Prevention

If at high CHB risk given presence of anti-SSA/Ro and/or anti-SSB/La antibodies, consider following with serial echocardiography about every 2 weeks from about 16 to 32 weeks to look for prolonged PR (AV) interval and any dysrrhythmia, especially looking for incomplete (first or second) degree block. The fetal mechanical PR interval is measured from simultaneous mitral and aortic Doppler waveforms.[5] If incomplete block is detected, consider therapy with dexamethasone (4 mg orally) to prevent progression to complete (third) degree block.[6] This screening may not be cost-effective, given CHB is uncommon in prospective series even with positive anti-SSA/Ro and/or anti-SSB/La antibodies, and is not evidence based.[5]

Prenatal care

Fetal echocardiography: 10–20% of CHB have a congenital heart defect (CHD) and not anti-SSA/Ro and/or anti-SSB/La antibodies, but 95% of CHB without CHD have anti-SSA/Ro and/or anti-SSB/La antibodies.

Therapy

A complete (third degree) CHB is considered to be irreversible. The effectiveness of steroids,[6–10] beta-mimetics,[11,12] digoxin, or intravenous immunoglobulin (IVIG) or any other therapy to normalize conduction or improve outcome has not been confirmed in any trial. **Women with fetuses with CHB should be managed and delivered at a tertiary care center with the availability of immediate neonatal pacing.**

Delivery

While trial of labor (TOL) by repeated scalp sampling to assure fetal well-being can be attempted, TOL is often difficult to manage clinically.

NEONATAL LUPUS

Transient neonatal SLE, that results from maternal immunoglobulin G (IgG) passing through the placenta. Usually, neonatal lupus occurs in 10% of anti-SSA-Ro and/or anti-SSB/La positive pregnancies. Thus, prophylaxis is not indicated. Female: male ratio = 14:1. Not always mother has diagnosis of SLE. Most cases are cutaneous (transient rash) and have thrombocytopenia. Can also have other hematological, CHB, etc., complications. Can last for 14–16 weeks. The neonatal death rate is 1–2%.

REFERENCES

1. Tan EM, Cohan AS, Aries JF, et al. The 1982 revised criteria for the classification of systemic lupus erythromatosus. Arthritis Rheum 1982; 25: 1271. [III]
2. Costedoat-Chalumeau N, Amoura Z, Duhaut P, et al. Safety of hydroxychloroquine in pregnant patients with connective tissue diseases: a study of one-hundred thirty-three cases compared with a control group. Arthritis Rheum 2003; 48: 3207–11. [II-1]
3. A randomized study of the effect of withdrawing hydroxychloroquine sulfate in systemic lupus erythematosus. The Canadian Hydroxychloroquine Study Group. N Engl J Med 1991; 324: 150–4. [RCT].
4. Levy RA, Vilela VS, Cataldo MJ, et al. Hydroxychloroquine in lupus pregnancy: double-blind and placebo-controlled study. Lupus 2001; 10: 401–4. [RCT, $n=20$].
5. Van Bergen AH, Cuneo BF, Davis N. Prospective echocardiographic evaluation of atrioventricular conduction in fetuses with maternal Sjögren's antibodies. Am J Obstet Gynecol 2004; 191: 1014–18. [II-3]
6. Copel JA, Buyon JP, Kleinman CS. Successful in utero therapy of fetal heart block. Am J Obstet Gynecol 1995; 173: 1384–90. [II-3]
7. Buyon JP, Waltuck J, Kleinman C, Copel J. In utero identification and therapy of congenital heart block. Lupus 1995; 4: 116–21. [II-3]
8. Saleeb S, Copel J, Friedman D, et al. Comparison of treatment with fluorinated glucocorticoids to the natural history of autoantibody-associated congenital heart block. Arthritis Rheum 1999; 42: 2335–45. [II-3]
9. Shinohara K, Miyagawa S, Fujita T, et al. Neonatal lupus erythromatosus: results of maternal corticosteroid therapy. Obstet Gynecol 1999; 93: 952–7. [II-3]
10. Narne S, Berghella V, Weiner S, et al. Outcome in fetuses with autoantibody associated congenital heart block treated with dexamethasone. Obstet Gynecol 2004; 103: 106s. [II-3]
11. Novi JM, Mulvihill BH. Use of a subcutaneous beta-sympahtomimetic pump for the treatment of fetal congenital complete heart block. A case report. J Reprod Med 2003; 48: 893–5. [II-3]
12. Eronen M, Heikkila P, Teramo K. Congenital complete heart block in the fetus: hemodynamic features, antenatal treatment, and outcome in six cases. Pediatr Cardiol 2001; 5: 385–92. [II-3]

25

Trauma

Lauren A Plante

KEY POINTS

- Trauma during pregnancy is a common complication, and accounts for a significant fraction of maternal deaths as well as perinatal mortality.
- Changes in physiology related to pregnancy must be borne in mind when managing trauma care.
- **There are no evidence based data** to address the initial care of the traumatized pregnant patient, the type and duration of monitoring, the type of testing required, or the follow-up care of ongoing pregnancy after trauma.
- **Initial maternal stabilization takes priority over fetal assessment.**
- **Transfer to a trauma center should be considered for severe cases.** This decision is usually made **at the scene.**
- A **multidisciplinary** approach is important, as obstetrician, maternal–fetal specialist, trauma surgeon, intensivist, anesthesiologist, neonatologist, and others may need to be involved.
- **Maternal stabilization:** 'ABCs' (airway, breathing, circulation).
- **Appropriate studies should not be withheld because of pregnancy.** Necessary radiological procedures should be performed, with abdominal shielding if possible. There is little risk to an ongoing pregnancy. Non-ionizing modalities may be substituted for ionizing radiation if an appropriate alternative exists. The actual fetal (uterine) dose should be estimated wherever possible rather than simply relying on published mean dosimetry.
- **Blunt abdominal trauma:** focused abdominal sonography for trauma (FAST) ultrasound (see **Figures 25.2 and 25.3**) or diagnostic peritoneal lavage.
- **Fetal ultrasound, fetal monitoring, fetal tocodynamometer (toco) monitoring, and Kleihauer– Betke (KB) test can be considered in the management of the pregnant woman with trauma.**
- No clinical trials exist to guide the practitioner as to the duration of electronic fetal monitoring after trauma, use

of ancillary testing (KB test, flow cytometry), or appropriate follow-up care.
- Patients who are stable enough may have fetal monitoring after the gestational age of viability.
- For the stable trauma patient, laboratory testing for fetomaternal hemorrhage (e.g. KB test) may be useful in determining duration of electronic fetal monitoring. If the screening test is negative, the patient may be discharged home; if positive, monitoring may be continued until symptoms appear and are resolved.
- After hospital discharge following trauma, there remains an increased probability of worse perinatal outcome. Ongoing fetal assessment may be indicated, although the exact type of surveillance has not been established.

DEFINITION

Trauma consists of **intentional harm** and **accidents**. Intentional harm includes assault, blunt-force trauma, and penetrating trauma. Accidents include predominantly motor vehicle crashes and falls.

INCIDENCE

The incidence of trauma in pregnancy is unclear. Estimates vary widely from up to 8% (any physical trauma)[1] to 0.2–2% (evaluation for trauma) to 0.4–2 in 10 000 (hospitalization for trauma).[2–4] These ranges may be due to reporting bias, and undercounting of the total number of injuries. Not all cases of maternal trauma are seen at a trauma center, or even referred to a hospital; hospital-acquired data are biased toward more serious injuries. No ongoing national data collection incorporates mention of pregnancy. Among pregnant women involved in a crash, about 25% occur in the first trimester, 39% in the second trimester, and 34% in the third trimester.[5]

ETIOLOGY/BASIC PATHOPHYSIOLOGY

Causes of trauma in pregnancy are shown in Figure 25.1:[2]

- **71% motor vehicle accident** (nearly 3% of all MVAs involve a pregnant woman)[6]
- 12% assault
- 9% fall
- 2% bicycle
- 2% auto vs pedestrian
- < 1% suicide
- 3% other (unintentional).

PROGNOSTIC FACTORS

Factors which predispose injured women to a **worse pregnancy** outcome, defined as delivery, pregnancy loss, or hysterectomy, are ISS [**Injury Severity Score** – http://www.trauma.org/scores/iss.html] > 15, **altered mental status at admission** (Glasgow Coma Score < 8) and **severe head injury** or **injury to thorax, abdomen, lower extremities, or spine**. Drug use and shock at admission are less highly correlated, although an increased risk is noted.[2]

COMPLICATIONS[3,4]

Complications are in general more common if there is severe injury (ISS ≥ 9),[3] or if the woman is delivered at the same hospitalization as when the trauma occurs.[4] Even with no injury or delivery at hospitalization, later complications may occur (estimates below).

Maternal complications

Maternal death

Maternal mortality associated with trauma is about 0.1–1.4%[2,4] (at least a 100-fold increase over the US maternal mortality ratio). The rate of maternal death for women hospitalized for trauma is about 4%.[7–11] Trauma is one of the leading causes of maternal death, as **about 27% of maternal deaths are injury-related.**[12] Of these deaths, the largest fraction is attributed to MVAs (44%), followed by homicide (31%), unintentional injuries (13%), and suicide (10%). Although the majority of pregnancy-associated homicide deaths occur in the postpartum period, in 21% the woman dies undelivered.[12] Trauma and other forms of violence are the leading cause of death in non-pregnant women of reproductive age.

Hospitalization

Women in the third trimester are more likely to be admitted to the hospital than women in the first or second trimester;[5] 3% of all trauma admissions are for pregnant patients.[13]

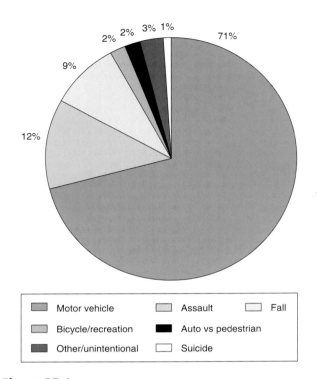

Figure 25.1
Causes of trauma in pregnancy.[2]

Transfusion

Transfusion is required in 0.6–4% of cases.

Hysterectomy

Hysterectomy is required in 0.5–2% of cases.

Fetal/neonatal complications

NRFHR (non-reassuring fetal heart rate) testing
5–20%.

Preterm birth
14–20%.[3]

Abruptio placentae
1–20%, or higher.

Fetal injury
Very few cases have been reported of fetal injury from maternal gunshot or stab wounds and of fetal fractures, visceral ruptures, and intracranial hemorrhage after blunt trauma.

Fetal death
The overall incidence of fetal death is 0.4–1.5%. The rate of fetal death for women hospitalized for trauma is about 11%.[7–11] About 5 in 1000 fetal deaths can be attributed to trauma, or approximately 4 traumatic fetal deaths in 100 000 live births.[14] The majority (> 80%) of these fetal

deaths are associated with MVAs, whereas 6% are related to firearms and another 3% to falls. Less than half, however, include a designation of placental injury (42%), and 20% specify placental abruption. Fetal death is more likely in cases of maternal death, hemorrhagic shock, or no seat belt use. The most significant factors for fetal death after blunt trauma are maternal ejection from a vehicle, maternal tachycardia (heart rate [HR] > 110 beats/min), maternal ISS > 9, fetal bradycardia (fetal heart rate [FHR] < 120 beats/min), and maternal death.[15]

Neonatal death
The incidence of neonatal death is ~1%.

Special considerations for complications from assault[16]

The rate of hospitalization for assault during pregnancy is 0.04%. Of all assaults, 46% were related to an unarmed fight, 12% to firearms or bomb, and 9% to stab injuries. Assaulted women had higher rates of preterm delivery, low birth weight, placental abruption, and uterine rupture compared with women who were never hospitalized for assault during pregnancy. Thirteen percent of women hospitalized after assault delivered during the hospitalization. These women had worse outcomes than either women who were not assaulted or women who were assaulted but discharged undelivered.

Intimate-partner violence accounted for 20% of the assaults in women who were discharged undelivered and for 50% of the assaults in women who delivered during the hospitalization.

PREGNANCY CONSIDERATIONS

Causes of trauma in pregnancy differ from non-pregnant trauma in that **more are attributed to motor vehicles** and fewer to other causes. Pregnancy is generally protective in relation to suicide. Compared with women of the same age who are not pregnant, pregnant women are younger, have **lower ISS, and lower mortality** (1% vs 4%), have shorter length of stay, and lower rates of alcohol and drug use; however, 12% still had been drinking and 20% had been using drugs. A crash rate of 13 per 1000 person-years was calculated for pregnant women aged 15–39 years old,[5] which is half the rate for non-pregnant women in this age group (26 per 1000).[5] The **rate of seat-belt use is higher among pregnant patients** than the comparison group (66 vs 50%). The rate of interpersonal violence is similar among pregnant and non-pregnant women (12 vs 10%).

In 11% of pregnancy trauma cases,[13] the **pregnancy status is unknown** at admission to the receiving trauma team, and in two-thirds of those women the pregnancy was newly diagnosed by serum human chorionic gonadotropin

(hCG) screening – i.e. the status had possibly not been known by the patient either. Of those pregnancies unknown to the trauma team at admission but presumably known to the patient (although she did not or could not communicate the status to the team), **fetal mortality is > 75%**, including both spontaneous and elective abortion. Incidental pregnancies that were news to the trauma team although *not* to the patient carry a 25% probability of fetal mortality.[13] One-third of the non-survivors in the newly diagnosed group were elective abortions, in which the women reported they were fearful of non-specific damage due to either injury or radiation. It must be cautioned, however, that the stated rationale for elective abortion is not always true.

PREGNANCY MANAGEMENT
Prevention/preconception counseling
Seat belts

Full seat belts should be *always* worn by pregnant women, with the shoulder belt over the shoulder, collar bone, and across the chest, between the breasts, and the lap belt as low as possible under the abdomen and the unborn child. Education and written material should be provided to the pregnant woman regarding mandatory seat belt use. Clearly, seat belts save maternal lives – by preventing ejection. Fetal deaths were nearly three times more likely in unrestrained women than in those who had been belted during the crash.[6]

Care of the pregnant trauma patient

There are no trials to assess the effectiveness of the initial care and interventions for the traumatized pregnant patient, including the type and duration of monitoring, the type of testing required, or the follow-up care of ongoing pregnancy after trauma. Therefore, these recommendations are drawn from guidelines in the non-pregnant population (from Eastern Association for the Surgery of Trauma [EAST]).[17]

Work-up and management (Figures 25.2 and 25.3)
Stabilization

General principles from both the American College of Surgeons[18] and the American College of Obstetricians and Gynecologists (ACOG)[1] suggest that **maternal stabilization takes priority over fetal assessment**. The standard algorithm in ATLS (Advanced Trauma Life Support) requires, in order,

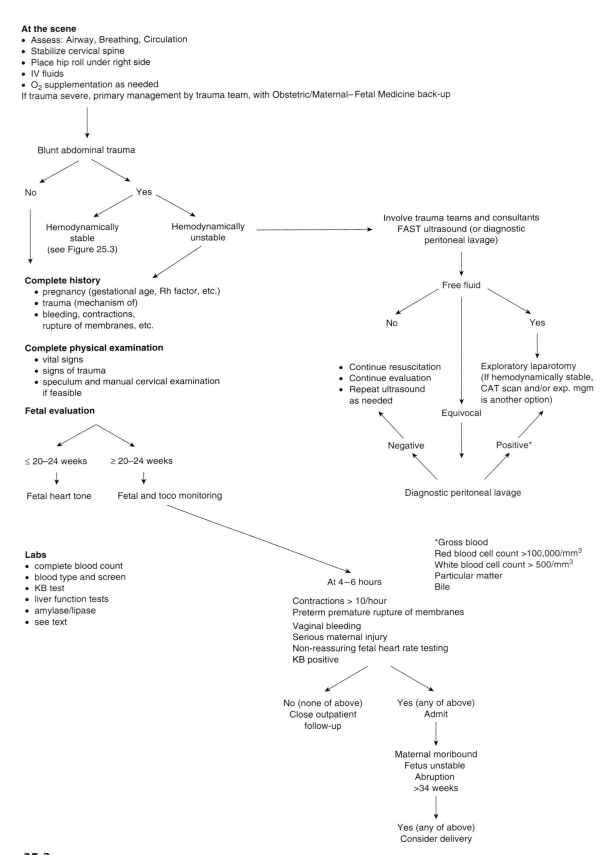

At the scene
- Assess: Airway, Breathing, Circulation
- Stabilize cervical spine
- Place hip roll under right side
- IV fluids
- O$_2$ supplementation as needed

If trauma severe, primary management by trauma team, with Obstetric/Maternal–Fetal Medicine back-up

Blunt abdominal trauma

No   Yes

Hemodynamically stable (see Figure 25.3)

Hemodynamically unstable

Involve trauma teams and consultants
FAST ultrasound (or diagnostic peritoneal lavage)

Free fluid

No   Yes

Complete history
- pregnancy (gestational age, Rh factor, etc.)
- trauma (mechanism of)
- bleeding, contractions, rupture of membranes, etc.

Complete physical examination
- vital signs
- signs of trauma
- speculum and manual cervical examination if feasible

Fetal evaluation

≤ 20–24 weeks   ≥ 20–24 weeks

Fetal heart tone   Fetal and toco monitoring

- Continue resuscitation
- Continue evaluation
- Repeat ultrasound as needed

Exploratory laparotomy
(If hemodynamically stable, CAT scan and/or exp. mgm is another option)

Equivocal

Negative   Positive*

Diagnostic peritoneal lavage

Labs
- complete blood count
- blood type and screen
- KB test
- liver function tests
- amylase/lipase
- see text

At 4–6 hours

*Gross blood
Red blood cell count >100,000/mm^3
White blood cell count > 500/mm^3
Particular matter
Bile

Contractions > 10/hour
Preterm premature rupture of membranes
Vaginal bleeding
Serious maternal injury
Non-reassuring fetal heart rate testing
KB positive

No (none of above)
Close outpatient follow-up

Yes (any of above)
Admit

Maternal moribound
Fetus unstable
Abruption
>34 weeks

Yes (any of above)
Consider delivery

Figure 25.2

Evaluation and management of trauma in pregnancy. FAST, focused abdominal sonography for trauma; KB, Kleihauer-Betke; exp. mgm, expectant management.

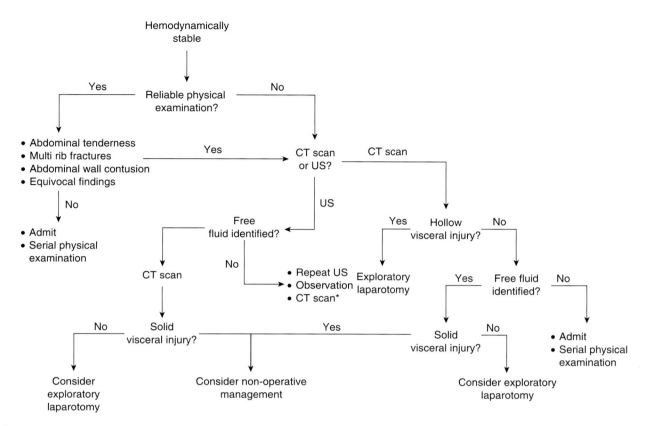

Figure 25.3
Evaluation and management of blunt abdominal trauma in the stable patient. (Adapted from Hoff et al,[17] with permission.)

assessment and stabilization, as shown in Table 25.1. These are now addressed briefly, in regard to pregnant patients.

Airway
Airway edema is more common in pregnant women, so smaller endotracheal tube size is required. Airway reflexes are not changed in pregnancy, but longer gastric emptying times and diminished function of the lower esophageal sphincter leave pregnant women more prone to aspiration of gastric contents.

Breathing
In pregnancy, minute ventilation is increased and functional residual capacity is decreased, so periods of apnea or hypopnea lead more quickly to hypoxemia.

Circulation
Increased cardiac output, expanded plasma volume, and peripheral vasodilation are the signs of hypovolemia seen later in pregnant women because of these compensatory mechanisms. Tachycardia and narrowed pulse pressure are late findings, as pregnant women progress through the stages of hypovolemic shock. Fetal heart rate (FHR) should

Table 25.1 *Maternal stabilization after trauma in pregnancy by Advanced Trauma Life Support principles*
• Airway
• Breathing
• Circulation
• Disability (neurological evaluation)
• Exposure, environmental control (looking everywhere else for injuries, and keeping patients warm)
• Fetus

be evaluated as an additional vital sign. A normal FHR suggests normal uterine perfusion, whereas an abnormal FHR may reflect compromised perfusion and function as an early warning sign of decreased circulatory volume.

Maintenance of left uterine displacement
This procedure is important in maintaining preload and cardiac output after midpregnancy because of the effect of the gravid uterus on compressing the inferior vena cava. If the patient is visibly pregnant to the prehospital provider, the supine position should be avoided.

History and physical examination

After maternal and fetal **stabilization**, a complete **history** (pregnancy and gestational age, trauma, etc.), review of records (ultrasounds, laboratory test – Rh factor), and a more extensive **physical** examination (vital signs, signs of trauma, uterine tenderness, speculum and manual examination) should be performed. In severe trauma, history may be unobtainable as the patient's neurological status is compromised. The mechanism of injury is an important part of the history. Uterine tenderness may be unreliable. A speculum/manual examination is often not feasible because the patient is in cervical spine (C-spine) immobilization or has a pelvic fracture.

Evaluation and diagnostic studies

Appropriate studies should not be withheld because of pregnancy.

Computed tomography

Computed tomography (CT) is recommended for evaluation of hemodynamically stable patients with associated neurological injury, multiple non-abdominal injury, or equivocal physical examination. Patients with a negative CT should nonetheless be admitted for observation[17] (radiation concerns: see below and Tables 25.2–25.4).[19]

Blunt abdominal trauma (see Figures 25.2 and 25.3)

FAST ultrasound.   The maternal abdomen can be evaluated for the presence of intraperitoneal blood either with diagnostic peritoneal lavage (DPL) or with ultrasound; the FAST scan (focused abdominal sonography for trauma – ultrasound of four abdominal quadrants to evaluate for free fluid – signs of blood in abdomen or pelvis) **has recently supplanted DPL in many institutions.**[17] A FAST scan has 80% sensitivity and 100% specificity for intra-abdominal injury in the pregnant patient following blunt abdominal trauma.[20] If DPL is elected, it is typically performed with an open technique in pregnancy. Both of these techniques avoid ionizing radiation altogether.

Exploratory laparotomy.   This procedure is indicated for patients with a positive FAST ultrasound or DPL.[17]

Follow-up CT scan.   In hemodynamically stable patients with positive FAST ultrasound or DPL, a follow-up CT scan should be considered. This may permit non-operative management.

Penetrating abdominal wound

A single preoperative dose of a broad-spectrum **antibiotic** is given (http://www.east.org/tpg/atbpenetra.pdf).[17]

Open fractures

Preoperative prophylactic **antibiotics** with Gram-positive coverage are administered as soon as possible after injury (http://www.east.org/tpg/openfrac.pdf).[17]

Special pregnancy – specific evaluations/studies

Fetal ultrasound.   There is insufficient evidence to assess the effectiveness of performing a fetal ultrasound in the woman with trauma in pregnancy. Assessment of fetus, amniotic fluid volume (AFV), and placenta by ultrasound may be beneficial for management. Ultrasound detects placental abruption when this involves > 50% of the placenta, so that negative ultrasound does not exclude abruption completely, especially since a large abruption may develop many days after the initial trauma.

Fetal monitoring.   There is insufficient evidence to assess fetal monitoring and especially its duration in the woman with trauma in pregnancy. Assessment of fetal status may be beneficial as the fetus is often one of the most sensitive 'organs' to be affected by maternal circulatory compromise. If performed, continuous monitoring is suggested. More than one-third of third trimester women with trauma have ominous findings on monitoring.[9] The fact that maternal and fetal outcomes are worse in women who do not have electronic monitoring in some reports[9] reflects the team priorities (more severely injured mothers require interventions that preclude fetal monitoring, or electronic monitoring is deemed of low priority).

Toco (tocodynamometer) monitoring.   At > 20 weeks' gestation, > 90% of women with trauma presenting for evaluation demonstrate some uterine contractions in the first 4 hours, with uterine activity decreasing over time. Within the first hour, 64% were contracting with a frequency of every ≥ 5 minutes, declining to 29% by hour 4.[21] Patients without contractions or those whose contractions never exceed every 10-minute frequency were discharged at the end of 4 hours, and none had abruption.[21] Those patients who had been contracting at more than every 11-minute frequency were kept for at least 24 hours. There was one placental abruption at 6 hours, resulting in emergent delivery for non-reassuring fetal heart rate (NRFHR) testing, and among the patients hospitalized beyond 24 hours, there was a 40% delivery rate, with one stillborn infant. Total abruption rate was 8%.[21] From these data come the common recommendation for **monitoring at least 4 hours after maternal trauma.** In nearly 5% of trauma in pregnancy cases, fetal compromise or placental abruption becomes evident only after prolonged monitoring of 6–48 hours or more.[22]

The Kleihauer-Betke test.   The KB test assesses for the presence of fetal red blood cells in the maternal circulation. This test is based on the premise that fetal hemoglobin (HbF) is resistant to acid elution. The KB test is particularly helpful with Rh-negative women to assess amount of $Rh_o(D)$ immune globulin needed. Whereas the test is inexpensive and simple to perform, it has been criticized for its subjectivity and lack of reproducibility.[23] Using known admixtures of fetal and maternal blood, KB testing overestimates the volume of fetomaternal hemorrhage and has been demonstrated to vary more than 10-fold with repeat testing of a single sample.[23] Some clinicians have advocated substitution of flow cytometry (using a fluorescence-activated cell sorter) or monoclonal antibodies to HbF as a test for fetomaternal hemorrhage; whereas these are both sensitive and more precise, they are expensive and not widely available. Twenty percent of the patients who had KB test drawn had positive results, although the test proved neither sensitive nor specific for a poor outcome.[22] When control women (i.e. no trauma) in their second and third trimester were evaluated for the presence of fetomaternal hemorrhage using the KB test, a 5.1% positive rate was noted, compared with a 2.6% positive rate among women who underwent maternal evaluation for trauma at the same institution, a difference which is not statistically significant.[24] Ninety-six percent of women with a positive KB test (defined as >0.01 ml of fetal blood in the maternal circulation) had preterm contractions, half of whom met criteria for preterm labor because cervical change was also noted, whereas none of those with a negative test had any contractions during the period of surveillance, which encompassed a minimum of 4 hours. The likelihood ratio of a positive KB test for preterm labor was calculated at >20. In addition, women who required delivery for fetal compromise shortly after admission all had a positive KB test.[25]

Coagulation studies – e.g. fibrinogen, D-dimer, prothrombin time (PT), partial thromboplastin time (PTT). There is no evidence of benefit of coagulation studies, unless massive hemorrhage has occurred or is expected.

Admission. Admission to the hospital for **longer (≥24–48 hours) observation** should be considered for women with evidence of **persistent (>4/hour) contractions, premature preterm rupture of membranes (PPROM), abruption on ultrasound, positive KB test, bleeding, NRFHR testing, or other abnormal fetal testing** with continuous fetal and toco monitoring.

Radiation in the pregnant trauma patient. Recent estimates of **fetal radiation dose** for several examinations are shown in Table 25.2.[19] The gray is the unit of measurement for absorbed dose; it is defined as one joule of energy deposited in 1 kilogram of material. This has replaced the rad or roentgen-absorbed dose, which is defined as the dose delivered to an object of 100 ergs of energy per gram of material. One gray = 100 rads (or, 1 rad = 10 mGy). Teratological effects start usually after 5–10 mGy. Plain radiographs of the spine and chest can be performed in pregnancy with minimal radiation exposure to the fetus, with abdomen and pelvis shielding. Magnetic resonance imaging (MRI) has no ionizing radiation but is less commonly used in the setting of major trauma. With CT scanning, the total radiation dose to the fetus depends on the site imaged, the machine and technique used, and on the distance between cuts.

Table 25.2 *Recent estimates of fetal radiation dose for several examinations*[19]

Examination	Mean fetal dose (mGy)	Maximum fetal dose (mGy)
Skull	<0.01	<0.01
Chest	<0.01	<0.01
Abdomen	1.4	4.2
Thoracic spine	<0.01	<0.01
Lumbar spine	1.7	10
Pelvis	1.1	4
IVP	1.7	10

IVP, intravenous pyelogram.

Table 25.3 *Recent estimates of fetal radiation exposure with computed tomography (CT)*[19]

CT examination	Mean fetal dose (mGy)	Maximum fetal dose (mGy)
Head	<0.005	<0.005
Chest	0.06	0.96
Abdomen	8.0	49
Lumbar spine	2.4	8.6
Pelvis	25	79
Pelvimetry	0.2	0.4

Recent estimates of fetal radiation exposure with CT are shown in Table 25.3.[19]

Since the actual fetal dose given in a procedure may be as much as 10-fold higher than the published mean dose, depending on the patient's size and the technique used, the **actual dose should be estimated** wherever possible **by contacting the institution's radiation physicists for dosimetry.** The proxy for fetal radiation dose is uterine dose.

Concerns about radiation effects on the embryo or fetus include **death, malformation, growth restriction, abnormal development of the brain with severe cognitive sequelae, and cancer.** No data are available for cellular effects per se, only for clinical effects. Threshold doses for the appearance of death or malformation are shown in Table 25.4.[19] Data for **cognitive impairment** (mental retardation), based on survivors of the atomic bomb exposed in utero, suggest no effect with exposure before 10 weeks or after 27 weeks. These data do raise the possibility of a dose–response (rather than threshold) model between 10 and 17 weeks, with a loss of 30 IQ points per Gy (1000 mGy). Diagnostic radiological procedures are orders of magnitude below these limits. Even in the 10–17 week fetus in which a dose–response curve may be postulated for cognitive impairment, an 80 mGy study, such as CT of the pelvis, would have only minimal potential to compromise intellectual function, e.g. 2 IQ points.

Table 25.4	Threshold doses by gestational age for the appearance of embryo/fetus death or congenital malformation[19]	
Weeks from LMP	Embryo/fetus death	Congenital malformation
<---No threshold at conception--->		
4–7	250–500 mGy	200 mGy
7–9	500 mGy	500 mGy
9–23	>500 mGy	Very few observed
23–term	>1000 mGy	Very few observed

LMP, last menstrual period.

Concerns have also been raised about the possibility of **cancer** induction in children exposed to intrauterine radiation. Unlike death or malformation, the induction of cancers is believed to be a dose–response rather than threshold phenomenon. Because childhood cancers are rare events, even a doubling or quadrupling of the risk has little impact on cancer deaths. Excess risk of fatal childhood cancer attributed to fetal exposure with typical diagnostic procedures ranges from 1 in 30 000 to 1 in 1700. The derived risk is estimated at 1 excess case per 33 000 per mGy of exposure. The highest risks, which remain quite small on a population basis, are seen with the highest exposures, e.g. CT of the pelvis.[19] This concern is not a reason to routinely offer termination of pregnancy.[19,26] Recent estimates of conceptus radiation dose with a single anteroposterior chest radiograph (assuming an average maternal size: dose increases with increasing maternal size) range from 0.0021–0.0028 mGy in the first trimester to 0.1–5.9 mGy in the second trimester, and 0.1–1.9 mGy in the third trimester.[27] This corresponds to an excess risk of childhood cancer of approximately 10 per million.

Prenatal care

The indication for **tetanus prophylaxis** does not change during pregnancy (see Chapter 37). If the pregnant patient who had trauma can be discharged undelivered, she should be counseled that **abruption, preterm birth, and other complications** can occur even after discharge (**even > 10 weeks**) of a stable woman after trauma. Even if they have been discharged from the hospital, women who suffered trauma in pregnancy should be aware that a normal baby outcome cannot be guaranteed. Therefore, education and written discharge instructions regarding fetal kick counts, signs of labor, and abruption (vaginal bleeding, uterine tenderness, or persistent abdominal pain) should be given.

Antepartum testing

There is no trial to assess the effectiveness of testing in this population.

Delivery

No specific recommendations.

Anesthesia

Regional or general anesthesia may be appropriate depending on maternal status, injury, and surgical procedure contemplated. Fluid management, airway management, acid aspiration prophylaxis and several other factors, as related to the specific injury and maternal condition, need to be addressed.

Postpartum/breastfeeding

No specific recommendations.

REFERENCES

1. Obstetric aspects of trauma management. ACOG Educational Bulletin No. 251, September 1998. Washington, DC: American College of Obstetricians and Gynecologists; 1998. [The American College of Obstetricians and Gynecologists quotes trauma rates of 1 in 12 pregnancies, but it is unclear how this figure was obtained]
2. Ikossi DG, Lazar AA, Morabito D, Fildes J, Knudson MM. Profile of mothers at risk: an analysis of injury and pregnancy loss in 1,195 trauma patients. J Am Coll Surg 2005; 200: 49–56. [The American College of Surgeons maintains a National Trauma Data Bank (NTDB) – data collected from 130 trauma centers in the USA, including Level I, Level II, and Level III facilities. Review of the NTDB between 1994 and 2001 compared 1195 female admissions that were additionally coded as pregnant to a control group of 76 126 injured women in the same age group. Since during this time there were approximately 27 million live births in the USA (NCHS), that equates to 4 trauma center admissions per 100 000 live births]
3. Schiff MA, Holt VL. Pregnancy outcomes following hospitalization for motor vehicle crashes in Washington State from 1989 to 2001. Am J Epidemiol 2005; 161: 503–10. [State of Washington hospitalizations for MVA in pregnancy from 1989 to 2001, n = 625]
4. El Kady D, Gilbert WM, Anderson J, et al. Trauma during pregnancy: an analysis of maternal and fetal outcomes in a large population. Am J Obstet Gynecol 2004; 1990: 1661–8. [California larger cohort: 10 316 women who sustained trauma during a pregnancy of at least 20 weeks' gestation identified via a statewide hospital discharge database from 1991–1999]
5. Weiss HB, Strotmeyer S. Characteristics of pregnant women in motor vehicle crashes. Injury Prevention 2002; 8: 207–10. [1995–99 National Automotive Sampling System Crashworthiness Data System, drawn from police-reported traffic accidents]
6. Hyde LK, Cook LJ, Olson LM, Weiss HB, Dean JM. Effect of motor vehicle crashes on adverse fetal outcome. Obstet Gynecol 2003; 102: 279–86. [II-3]
7. Corsi PR, Rasslan S, de Oliveira LB, Kronfly FS, Marinho VP. Trauma in pregnant women: analysis of maternal and fetal mortality. Injury 1999; 30: 239–43. [II-3. Fetal death: Corsi's 31%, Shah's 14% if you don't count elective abortion, Rogers was 9%, Warner's–a fairly small study–was 6%, and Theodorou's 18%. Maternal death: Corsi 12%, Shah 9%, Rogers 4%, and Warner 3%]
8. Shah KH, Simons RK, Holbrook T, et al. Trauma in pregnancy: maternal and fetal outcomes. J Trauma 1998; 45: 83–6. [II-3]

9. Rogers FB, Rozycki GS, Osler TM, et al. A multi-institutional study of factors associated with fetal death in injured pregnant patients. Arch Surg 1999; 134: 1274–7. [II-3]

10. Warner MW, Salfinger SG, Rao S, Magann EF, Hall JC. Management of trauma during pregnancy. ANZ J Surg 2004; 74: 125–8. [II-3]

11. Theodorou DA, Velmahos GC, Souter I, et al. Fetal death after trauma in pregnancy. Am Surg 2000; 66: 809–12. [II-3]

12. Chang J, Berg CJ, Saltzmann LE, Herndon J. Homicide: a leading cause of injury deaths among pregnant and postpartum women in the United States, 1991–1999. Am J Public Health 2005; 95: 471–7. [Pregnancy Mortality Surveillance System, established in 1989 by the Centers for Disease Control, identified 7342 deaths among women who were pregnant or within 1 year postpartum]

13. Boccichio GV, Napolitano LM, Hann J, Champion H, Scalea T. Incidental pregnancy in trauma patients. J Am Coll Surg 2001; 192: 566–9. [II-3]

14. Weiss HB, Songer TJ, Fabio A. Fetal deaths related to maternal injury. JAMA 2001; 286: 1863–8. [Fetal death certificates in 16 US states, 1995–97]

15. Curet MJ, Schermer CR, Demarest GB, Bienik EJ, Curet LB. Predictors of outcome in trauma during pregnancy: identification of patients who can safely be monitored for less than 6 hours. J Trauma 2000; 49: 18–24. [8 years' experience at a large Level I trauma center; 271 pregnant women who were admitted after blunt trauma; reviewed delivery outcomes in approximately half]

16. El Kady D, Gilbert WM, Xing G, Smith LH. Maternal and neonatal outcomes of assaults during pregnancy. Obstet Gynecol 2005; 105: 357–63. [II-3, *n* = 2070 pregnant women hospitalized following an assault]

17. Hoff WS, Holevar M, Nagy KK, et al, for the EAST Practice Management Guidelines Work Group. Practice management guidelines for the management of blunt abdominal trauma. 2001. Eastern Association for the Surgery of Trauma, http://www.east.org/tpg/bluntabd.pdf. Accessed 9/10/05 [Eastern Association for the Surgery of Trauma (EAST)] [review]

18. American College of Surgeons. Advanced Trauma Life Support for Doctors Student Manual. Chicago, IL: American College of Surgeons; 1997. [review]

19. National Radiological Protection Board, College of Radiographers and Royal College of Radiologists. Diagnostic medical exposures: advice on exposure to ionizing radiation during pregnancy. 1998. http://www.hpa.org.uk/radiation/publications/misc_publications/advice_during_pregnancy.pdf Downloaded 9/27/05 [National Radiological Protection Board] [review]

20. Brown MA, Sirlin CB, Farahmand N, Hoyt DB, Casola G. Screening sonography in pregnant patients with blunt abdominal trauma. J Ultrasound Med 2005; 24: 175–9. [II-3]

21. Pearlman MD, Tintinalli JE, Lorenz RP. A prospective controlled study of outcome after trauma during pregnancy. Am J Obstet Gynecol 1990; 162: 1502–10. [II-2; *n* = 60. Recommendation for at least 4 hours of monitoring]

22. Dahmus MA, Sibai BM. Blunt abdominal trauma: are there any predictive factors for abruption placentae or maternal-fetal distress? Am J Obstet Gynecol 1993; 169: 1054–9. [II-2; 1988–91; 233 patients > 20 weeks' gestation admitted after non-catastrophic abdominal trauma. Unusually, in this population assaults and falls each outnumbered motor vehicle accidents. Duration of monitoring ranged from 0 to 120 hours, with a mean of 13 hours]

23. Ochsenbein-Imhof N, Ochsenbein AF, Seifert B, et al. Quantification of fetomaternal hemorrhage by fluorescence microscopy is equivalent to flow cytometry. Transfusion 2002; 42: 947–53. [II-3]

24. Dhanraj D, Lambers D. The incidences of positive Kleihauer–Betke test in low-risk pregnancies and maternal trauma patients. Am J Obstet Gynecol 2004; 190: 1461–3. [II-2]

25. Muench MV, Baschat AA, Reddy UM, et al. Kleihauer–Betke testing is important in all cases of maternal trauma. J Trauma 2004; 57: 1094–8. [II-2]

26. Guidelines for diagnostic imaging during pregnancy. ACOG Committee Opinion No. 299, September 2004. Obstet Gynecol 2004; 104: 647–51. [review]

27. Damilakis J, Perisinakis K, Prassopoulos P, et al. Conceptus radiation dose and risk from chest screen-film radiography. Eur Radiol 2003; 13: 406–12. [II-3]

26

Venous thromboembolism and anticoagulation

James Airoldi

KEY POINTS

- Venous thromboembolism (VTE) is the **leading cause of pregnancy-related maternal morbidity and mortality in the developed world.**
- Risk factors include **prior thromboembolism, age of 35 years or more, increased parity, increased maternal weight, instrument-assisted deliveries or cesarean section, prolonged immobilization, smoking, and the presence of an acquired or inherited thrombophilia.**
- **Compressive ultrasonography** is the **primary modality for the diagnosis** of deep vein thrombosis (DVT) in pregnancy.
- The **helical CT scan** is the **primary tool** for the diagnosis of pulmonary embolism (PE) in pregnant patients. A **ventilation–perfusion (V/Q) scan** is an alternative first-line imaging test.
- The three anticoagulants typically used are **unfractionated heparin (UFH), low molecular weight heparin (LMWH),** and **warfarin.**
- **Platelet counts** should be checked 5 days after initiation of UFH, and periodically for the first 2 weeks of **UFH therapy.**
- **LMWH is at least as effective and safe as UFH for the treatment of patients with acute proximal DVT, and for the prevention of DVT. LMWH does not cross the placenta,** and is safe for the fetus. The incidence of bleeding is decreased compared with UFH, while the risk of heparin-induced thrombocytopenia (HIT) and osteoporotic fractures has not been well established for LMWH use in pregnant patients. Pregnant women may require higher doses and these risks could be dose-related. **The dosing of LMWH in pregnancy remains controversial.**
- Warfarin derivatives **cross the placenta** and have the potential to cause both **bleeding in the fetus and teratogenicity.** Warfarin use is believed to be safe in the first 6 weeks of gestation, but has been **associated with warfarin embryopathy in 4–5% of fetuses when maternal exposure occurs between 6 and 9 weeks' gestation.**

- In the pregnant patient with **acute VTE, either adjusted-dose LMWH throughout pregnancy or intravenous UFH** for at least 5 days, followed by adjusted-dose UFH or LMWH for the remainder of the pregnancy, is the recommended approach. Anticoagulants should be administered for at least 6 weeks postpartum.
- There are **three general approaches** to the antepartum management of pregnant patients with **previous VTE: UFH, LMWH, or close surveillance.**
- Among women with a **non-recurring cause for the prior VTE and no thrombophilia,** the risk of recurrent antepartum venous thromboembolism is low, and therefore **routine antepartum low-dose prophylaxis with heparin is not warranted. However postpartum low-dose prophylaxis is still recommended.**
- **If there is a potential recurring cause, low-dose prophylaxis is recommended.**
- In pregnant women with a **prior VTE with** a history of a **low-risk thrombophilia (heterozygous factor V Leiden or prothrombin gene, protein C or S), low-dose prophylactic anticoagulation is recommended.**
- **Adjusted-dose anticoagulation** is recommended for prior VTE and a **high-risk thrombophilia (antithrombin III [AT III] deficiency, homozygous factor V or prothrombin gene or compound heterozygote).**
- **Adjusted-dose anticoagulation** should be used in pregnant women if the woman has had **recurrent VTE episodes, life-threatening thrombosis, or thrombosis while receiving chronic anticoagulation.** Filters in the inferior vena cava should be considered in these situations as well.
- It is recommended that pregnant patients with the **antiphospholipid syndrome** who do not have a history of venous thrombosis receive a low-dose prophylactic regimen of heparin, and that those with previous thrombosis receive an adjusted-dose regimen of heparin (see also Chapter 23).
- The antepartum management of pregnant women with **known thrombophilia** and **no prior VTE** remains controversial because of our limited knowledge of the natural histories of various thrombophilias and a lack of trials of

VTE prophylaxis. Currently, there is **no evidence to suggest benefit of prophylactic low-dose anticoagulation.**

- In pregnant women with **mechanical heart valves**, it appears reasonable to use one of the following four regimens: (1) LMWH or UFH between 6 weeks and 12 weeks and close to term only, and to use vitamin K antagonists (VKAs) at other times; (2) *careful* dose-adjusted UFH throughout pregnancy; (3) *careful* adjusted-dose LMWH throughout pregnancy, or (4) VKAs throughout pregnancy (used in Europe).

See also Chapter 27.

DEFINITION

Venous thromboembolism (VTE) includes any thromboembolic event in a vein, including deep vein thrombosis (DVT) and pulmonary embolism (PE), which are the most common, and others (cerebrovascular event [CVA, or stroke], etc.).

SYMPTOMS

DVT can present with leg swelling, erythema, and calor, with about 25% of patients with these symptoms having DVT. PE is not detected clinically in 70–80% of patients in whom it is detected postmortem. Most patients who die of PE do so within 30 minutes of the event, reinforcing the need for rapid and accurate diagnosis.[1]

EPIDEMIOLOGY/INCIDENCE

VTE is the **leading cause of pregnancy-related maternal morbidity and mortality in the developed world.**[2] Fatal PE remains the leading cause of maternal mortality, accounting for 19.6% of all maternal deaths in the US. Interestingly, hemorrhage is the second leading cause of maternal deaths (about 17%), thus signifying the delicate balance between coagulation and anticoagulation in pregnancy. The incidence of all thromboembolic events averages about **1.3** (range 0.5–3) **per 1000 pregnancies,**[3] and about an equal number are identified antepartum and in the puerperium.[4] There is an equal frequency in all three trimesters. Pulmonary emboli are more frequent postpartum.[4] During pregnancy and postpartum, women in general have a **fivefold increased risk of VTE compared with non-pregnant women.**[4] The risk is increased approximately twofold during pregnancy, and 14-fold in the postpartum period, especially after cesarean delivery. DVT is more common in the left than the right leg. PE occurs in 15% of untreated DVTs, with a mortality rate of 15%. PE occurs in 4.5% of treated DVTs, with a mortality rate of 1%.[5]

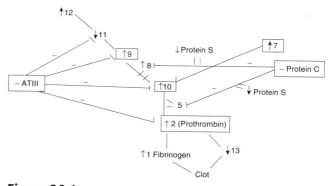

Figure 26.1
Coagulations cascade and some pregnancy changes. ↑↓−, change in pregnancy; ❑, vitamin K dependent; −, negative feedback; ATIII, antithrombin III.

GENETICS

About half of patients with thrombosis have an identifiable underlying genetic disorder.[6] Moreover, approximately 50–60% of patients with a hereditary basis for thrombosis, or a thrombophilia, do not experience a thrombotic event until one other risk factor is present.[4] (see also Chapter 27)

ETIOLOGY/BASIC PATHOPHYSIOLOGY

The coagulation cascade is briefly and schematically shown in Figure 26.1. Pregnancy is associated with marked alterations in the proteins of the coagulation and fibrinolytic systems[7,8] (see Chapter 2 in *Obstetric Evidence Based Guidelines*). A tendency for excessive clotting seems to be an adaptive mechanism to prevent excessive bleeding at delivery. At delivery, about 120 spiral arteries are denuded while carrying about 12% of the woman's cardiac output every minute. Much of the prevention in bleeding is due to myometrial contraction, but there are also increased clotting capacity, impaired fibrinolysis, and decreased anticoagulant activity in pregnancy. The levels of coagulation factors II, VII, VIII, IX, X, and XII increase substantially by the middle of pregnancy. The generation of fibrin also increases markedly. Levels of the anticoagulant protein S appear to decrease about 40% throughout pregnancy, although levels of protein C remain normal. The fibrinolytic system is also inhibited, most substantially in the third trimester.

RISK FACTORS/ASSOCIATIONS

VTE is a multifactorial disease process. Risk factors are shown in Table 26.1, with those more common in pregnancy cases including **prior thromboembolism, age of ≥ 35 years old, increased parity, increased maternal weight,**

Table 26.1	*Conditions associated with increased risk for venous thromboembolism (VTE)[11]*

Advancing age

Obesity

Previous VTE

Surgery

Trauma

Active cancer

Acute medical illnesses – e.g. acute myocardial infarction, heart failure, respiratory failure, infection

Inflammatory bowel disease

Antiphospholipid syndrome

Dyslipoproteinemia

Nephrotic syndrome

Paroxysmal nocturnal hemoglobinuria

Myeloproliferative diseases

Behçet's syndrome

Varicose veins

Superficial vein thrombosis

Congenital venous malformation

Long-distance travel

Prolonged bed rest

Immobilization

Limb paresis

Chronic care facility stay

Pregnancy/puerperium

Oral contraceptives

Hormone replacement therapy

Heparin-induced thrombocytopenia

Other drugs:
   Chemotherapy
   Tamoxifen
   Thalidomide
   Antipsychotics

Central venous catheter

Vena cava filter

Intravenous drug abuse

instrument-assisted deliveries or cesarean section, prolonged immobilization, smoking, and the presence of an acquired or inherited thrombophilia (associated with about 50% of VTE in pregnancy).[9–11]

COMPLICATIONS

- VTE in general: risk of recurrence is about 7–12%.
- DVT: risk of PE, post-thrombotic syndrome.
- PE: risk of death, pulmonary hypertension.

Table 26.2	*Approximate radiation exposures of diagnostic tests for VTE*	
Test		Radiation exposure (rads)
Chest X-ray		0.001
Perfusion scan		0.018
Ventilation scan		0.019
Helical chest CT		0.005
Limited venography		0.050
Pulmonary angiography		0.221
Compression U/S		None
MRI		None

VTE, venous thromboembolism; CT, computed tomography; U/S, ultrasonography; MRI, magnetic resonance imaging.

MANAGEMENT

Principles

Given the paucity of data regarding diagnosis and treatment in pregnancy, most data are derived from the non-pregnant general population.

Diagnosis

To diagnose VTE, clinical suspicion must remain high. Clinical evaluation alone cannot confirm or refute a diagnosis of VTE in the non-pregnant state, and diagnosing VTE in pregnancy is even more challenging. Epidemiological studies have shown that exposure to radiation doses of less than a total of 5 rad has not been associated with significant risk for fetal injury.[12] The diagnostic tests shown in Table 26.2 are all below the safe limit, and most combinations of these tests are also below the 5 rad limit, although they may possibly slightly increase the risks for childhood cancers.[13,14]

Deep vein thrombosis (Figure 26.2)[11]

During pregnancy, thrombosis most frequently begins in the veins of the calf or in the iliofemoral segment of the deep venous system and has a striking predilection for the left leg[15–17] (90%), possibly because of the compressive effects on the left iliac vein by the right iliac artery where they cross.[18] Only about 25% of symptomatic patients have a thrombus.

Compressive ultrasonography

The **primary modality** for the diagnosis of DVT in pregnancy is compressive ultrasonography. It has a sensitivity of 97% and a specificity of 94% for the diagnosis of proximal DVT in the non-pregnant population.[14,19] It is less accurate for symptomatic calf DVTs.[20] It is inadequate for iliac vein

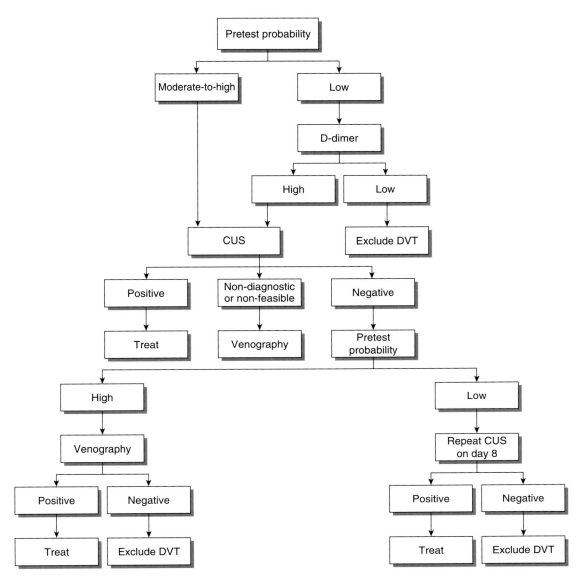

Figure 26.2
Suggested management in patient with symptoms of DVT.[11] CUS, compression ultrasound; DVT, deep vein thrombosis.

thrombosis, for which only magnetic resonance imaging (MRI) has shown a high degree of sensitivity and specificity.[19]

Venography

This technique was widely held to be the standard for establishing a diagnosis of deep vein thrombosis.[21] However, exposure to radiation and the invasive nature of the test have led to its replacement by compressive ultrasound.

D-dimer testing

Noted to have a role in diagnosing VTE in non-pregnant patients and possibly useful during pregnancy, D-dimer testing

is a measurement of the degradation products of cross-linked fibrin. Pregnancy itself may increase D-dimer levels, increasing with gestational age. Preterm labor, pre-eclampsia, and placental abruption can also elevate levels significantly.[22] Sensitivities vary widely, with different assays, ranging from 80–100%,[23] but the main use is derived from a high negative predictive value. The approach using D-dimer is not validated in pregnancy.

Patients who, on clinical evidence, are likely to have thrombosis but whose initial test results are negative, should undergo either venography or serial noninvasive testing. Diagnosis of pelvic vein and internal iliac thrombosis is difficult, and may require MRI.

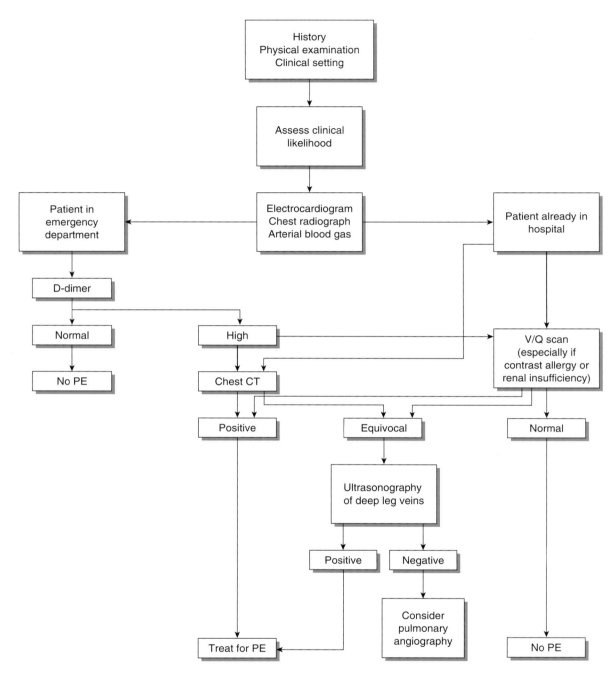

Figure 26.3
Diagnostic algorithm for suspected pulmonary embolism.[24] PE, pulmonary embolism; CT, computed tomography; V/Q, ventilation-perfusion scan.

Pulmonary embolism (Figure 26.3)[24]

Ventilation–perfusion

In the past, the **V/Q scan** has been the **primary tool** for the diagnosis of pulmonary embolism in pregnant patients. If a perfusion defect is seen in a patient with symptoms of PE, this finding can be considered diagnostic. The ventilation portion of the test is useful to distinguish matched defects from unmatched defects if a perfusion defect is not clearly caused by a PE. About 40–60% of V/Q scans are diagnostic (either high probability or normal). For non-diagnostic tests, further studies are necessary.[25]

Helical CT scan

Helical CT scanning has become the first-line imaging test in daily clinical practice, and has become the most widespread imaging test in non-pregnant adults.[24] The sensitivity varies from 57 to 100% and the specificity varies between 64 and

Table 26.3 *Suggested pregnancy management based on VTE and thrombophilia*

Clinical scenario	Pregnancy management
VTE develops during pregnancy	Intravenous UFH for 5–7 days followed by subcutaneous adjusted-dose therapy (UFH or LMWH) for 3–6 months or the remainder of the pregnancy* Adjusted-dose *LMWH* for 3–6 months or the remainder of the pregnancy*
History of a 'low-risk' thrombophilia (heterozygous FVL or PGM, protein C, protein S) *and* No prior VTE Prior VTE	Surveillance only or low-dose prophylatic anticoagulation if strong family history Prophylaxic anticoagulation
History of 'high-risk' thrombophilia (ATIII def, homozygous FVL or PGM, or double heterozygote) No prior VTE Prior VTE	Prophylaxic anticoagulation or surveillance only Adjusted-dose therapeutic anticoagulation*
Prior VTE associated with a non-recurring (transient) risk factor and no known thrombophilia	Surveillance only or prophylactic anticoagulation
Prior VTE related to a recurring factor (pregnancy or OC use) regardless of thrombophilia	Prophylaxic anticoagulation
History of life-threatening thrombosis, recent thrombosis, recurrent thrombosis, or receiving chronic anticoagulation	Adjusted-dose therapeutic anticoagulation˙ Consider IVC filter in certain cases
Antiphospholipid syndrome based on prior thrombosis	Adjusted-dose therapeutic anticoagulation˙
Antiphospholipid syndrome with no prior thrombosis	Prophylaxic anticoagulation
Pregnant women with mechanical heart valves	Warfarin throughout pregnancy except during gestational weeks 6–12 where aggressive adjusted-dose UFH or LMWH should be used. Alternatively, warfarin could be used during entire pregnancy after appropriate counseling˙

VTE, venous thromboembolism; UFH, unfractionated heparin; LMWH, low molecular weight heparin; FVL, factor V Leiden; PGM, prothrombin gene mutation; ATIII, antithrombin III; OC, oral contraceptive; IVC, inferior vena cava; ˙anticoagulation continued for at least 6 weeks postpartum.

100%.[19,23,26] The location of the embolus affects the sensitivity and specificity of helical CT scanning. Helical CT scanning is more sensitive for detecting emboli in the central arteries and is less sensitive for detecting subsegmental emboli.[27] With helical CT, thrombus is directly visualized, and both mediastinal and parenchymal structures are evaluated, which may provide important alternative or additional diagnoses.

Pulmonary angiography
This technique is still the gold standard for ruling out PE. Pulmonary angiography requires expertise for performance and interpretation and is invasive; thus, it is held in reserve for patients in whom the diagnosis cannot be made or excluded based on less-invasive testing.

MANAGEMENT (TABLE 26.3)
Therapy
Agents

Given the paucity of data regarding the efficacy of **anticoagulants** during pregnancy, recommendations about their use during pregnancy are based largely on data from non-pregnant patients. The three anticoagulants typically used are unfractionated heparin (UFH), low molecular weight heparin (LMWH), and warfarin. **Heparin** (UFH or LMWH) is the anticoagulant most often used, given its safety and efficacy during pregnancy.[28–41] Warfarin is also an alternative anticoagulant in certain situations. All three choices are safe during breastfeeding. There are usually **two ways of dosing heparin:**

1. **Prophylactic anticoagulation** typically implies low dosing (usually without monitoring, Table 26.4). If prophylatic adjusted-does, this implies anti Xa level of 0.2–0.4 U/ml.
2. **Therapeutic anticoagulation** implies higher dosing (always **adjusted-dosing**), meaning usually adjusted to anti Xa levels of 0.5–1.2 U/ml (Table 26.5).

Unfractionated heparin
The word heparin derives from the Greek *hepar* for liver, the organ from where it was first isolated. UFH exerts its anticoagulation action by two mechanisms of action:

- stimulation of antithrombin III (ATIII) activity, which is an inhibitor of factors 2, 9, 10 (especially), and 11.
- direct factor 10 inhibition (see Figure 26.1).

Approximately 3% of non-pregnant patients receiving UFH acquire immune-mediated (immunoglobulin G [IgG])

Table 26.4 *Prophylactic low-dose subcutaneous prophylaxic regimens during pregnancy*

- Unfractionated heparin, 5000–7500 U every 12 hours during the first trimester, 7500–10 000 U every 12 hours during the second trimester, 10 000 U every 12 hours during the third trimester, unless the aPTT is elevated
- Unfractionated heparin, 5000–10 000 U every 12 hours throughout pregnancy
- Unfractionated heparin dosed twice daily to target antifactor Xa activity 0.2–0.4 U/ml
- Enoxaparin, 40 mg once or twice daily
- Dalteparin, 5000 U once or twice daily

VTE, venous thromboembolism; aPTT, activated partial thromboplastin time.

Table 26.5 *Therapeutic adjusted-dose subcutaneous regimens during pregnancy*

- Unfractionated heparin (usually ≥ 10 000 U) given 2–3 times per day to achieve aPTT prolongation of 1.5–2.5
- Enoxaparin, 30–80 mg every 12 hours
- Dalteparin, 5000–10 000 U every 12 hours
- Weight-adjusted doses of enoxaparin (1 mg/kg every 12 hours) or dalteparin (200 U/kg every 24 hours)
- Weight-adjusted LMWH with dose sufficient enough to achieve a peak antifactor Xa level of 0.5–1.2 U/ml

VTE, venous thromboembolism; aPTT, activated partial thromboplastin time; LMWH, low molecular weight heparin.

thrombocytopenia (heparin-induced thrombocytopenia, **HIT**), which is frequently complicated by extension of pre-existing VTE or new arterial thrombosis.[42] Antibodies to heparin are detectable. HIT encompasses a range of presentations, from asymptomatic antibodies without thrombocytopenia, to thrombocytopenia, to thrombocytopenia with thrombosis. The mortality rate from untreated HIT and new thrombotic complications is 20–30%.[43] This should be differentiated from an early, benign, transient thrombocytopenia that can occur with initiation of UFH due primarily to platelet clumping. It should be suspected when the platelet count falls to $< 100 \times 10^9$/L or < 50% of the baseline value **5–15 days** after commencing heparin, or sooner with recent heparin exposure.[42] **Platelet counts should be checked 5 days after initiation of UFH, and periodically for the first 2 weeks of UFH therapy.** In pregnant women who acquire HIT and require ongoing anticoagulant therapy, use of the heparinoid **danaparoid sodium** is recommended because it is an effective antithrombotic agent,[38] does not cross the placenta, has much less cross-reactivity with UFH and, therefore, less potential to produce recurrent HIT than LMWH.[44] There was anticipation that LMWH treatment for VTE would decrease the incidence of HIT,[42,45] but this finding has not been demonstrated.[36]

Heparin therapy has been associated with **osteopenia** in pregnant women. Long-term prophylactic UFH therapy during pregnancy is associated with a 2.2% incidence of vertebral fracture.[46] The mean bone loss is about 5%, with unclear reversibility. **LMWHs have a lower risk of osteoporosis than UHF.** Bone mineral density is significantly lower in UFH subjects when compared with both control and dalteparin-treated women in one trial.[47] Multiple logistic regressions found that the type of heparin therapy was the only independent factor associated with reduced bone mass. Cohort studies[48] have also reported no association with osteoporosis and LMWH therapy.

Given that UFH **does not cross the placenta,** there is no risk of teratogenicity.

The rate of **major maternal bleeding** in pregnant patients treated with UFH therapy is about **2%,** which is consistent with the reported rates of bleeding associated with heparin therapy in non-pregnant patients[49] and with warfarin therapy[50] when used for the treatment of DVT. Bleeding at the uteroplacental junction is still possible. The short half-life makes UFH the optimal anticoagulation around the time of delivery or surgery. Protamine sulfate can be used to reverse the effects of UFH. There is insufficient evidence to assess the effectiveness of the pump for heparin therapy in pregnancy.

Low molecular weight heparin

LMWH exerts its anticoagulation action by stimulation of ATIII activity, inhibiting factor 10 (not factor 2) in particular. There is accumulating experience with the use of LMWHs, both in pregnant and non-pregnant patients, for the prevention and treatment of VTE.[34–39] Based on the results of large clinical trials in non-pregnant patients, **LMWH is at least as effective and safe as UFH** for the treatment of patients with acute proximal DVT,[36,38] and for the prevention of DVT in patients who undergo surgery.[39]

LMWH does not cross the placenta, and LMWH is safe for the fetus.[35,48]

Bleeding complications appear to be very uncommon with LMWH. Although it was anticipated that LMWH might have fewer associated risks for bleeding, HIT, and osteoporotic fractures than UFH,[42,45] the incidences of these complications have not been well established for LMWH use in pregnant patients. Pregnant women may require higher doses, and these risks could be dose-related.

The dosing of LMWH remains controversial. Pregnant women may require increases in dalteparin dose of 10–20% compared with doses of non-pregnant women to reach the target anti Xa levels.[51–53] Anticoagulation with LMWH may need to be monitored in pregnant women and the dose adjusted to reach the target Xa level, which decreases the logistical and financial benefits of LMWH. The therapeutic anti Xa level for adjusted-dose therapy is 0.5–1.2 U/ml. The target anti-Xa level for prophylactic dose therapy is 0.2–0.4 U/ml. To achieve these levels, dosing every 12 hours is often necessary.

Warfarin (Coumadin)

Warfarin derivatives are vitamin K antagonists (VKA). Vitamin K gets its initial from the German word *koagulation*. Warfarin inhibits the effects of vitamin K, and hence vitamin K dependent factors (see Figure 26.1). Consequently, warfarin decreases levels of proteins C and S. Warfarin derivatives **cross the placenta** and have the potential to cause both **bleeding in the fetus and teratogenicity.**[54,55] Warfarin use is believed to be safe in the first 6 weeks of gestation, but has been **associated with warfarin embryopathy in 5–15% of fetuses when maternal exposure occurs between 6 and 9 weeks' gestation.** First trimester warfarin embryopathy is mostly skeletal, involving stippled epiphyses, and nasal and limb hypoplasia. Bleeding in the fetus can occur during any trimester. Some clinicians recommend the use of warfarin during pregnancy anyway for specific patients, such as women with mechanical heart valves, those who have a recurrence while receiving adequate heparin, and those with contraindications to heparin therapy. If warfarin is used during pregnancy, patients must be fully informed about the potential adverse effects on the fetus. Warfarin does not induce an anticoagulant effect in the breastfed infant when the drug is given to a nursing mother.[56,57] Therefore, the use of warfarin in breastfeeding women who require postpartum anticoagulant therapy is safe.

Aspirin

Potential complications of aspirin during pregnancy include birth defects and bleeding in the neonate and in the mother. **Low-dose (60–150 mg/day) aspirin** therapy administered during the second and third trimesters of pregnancy in women at risk for gestational hypertension or fetal growth restriction (FGR) is **safe** for the mother and fetus.[58,59] The safety of higher doses of aspirin and/or aspirin ingestion during the first trimester remains uncertain.

Treatment of acute venous thromboembolism in pregnancy

There are now many well-designed randomized trials and meta-analyses comparing intravenous (IV) UFH and subcutaneous (SC) LMWH for the treatment of acute DVT and PE in non-pregnant patients.[36,60] These trials show that LMWH is at least as safe and effective as UFH. However, there are **no trials** comparing UFH to LMWH for the treatment of acute VTE in pregnancy. Therefore, in the pregnant patient with acute VTE, either **adjusted-dose** (adjusted for weight) **LMWH or IV UFH** (80 U/kg bolus followed by a continuous infusion, [at least 1300U/hour], to maintain the activated partial thromboplastin time [aPTT] in the therapeutic range) for at least 5 days, followed by adjusted-dose UFH or LMWH for the remainder of the pregnancy is the recommended approach (see

Table 26.5). The adjusted dose regimen of SC UFH was shown to have equal efficacy in preventing recurrent VTE as compared to warfarin in the first 3 months after an acute VTE.[49] Interestingly, three patients had recurrent VTE during therapy, but all were associated with interruption of anticoagulation.[49] Anticoagulants should be administered **for about 3–6 months in adjusted dose**[11] for the remainder of the pregnancy and at least 6 weeks' postpartum as well. There is insufficient evidence to assess if continuing adjusted-dose anticoagulation after 6 weeks' postpartum is associated with any benefit or detriment. Women with antithrombin deficiency, antiphospholipid antibodies, homozygous or combined thrombophilias, or previous VTE may benefit from indefinite anticoagulation, but this should be decided by an internist after pregnancy.[11] Long-term, low-intensity warfarin therapy is associated with a 50% prevention of recurrent VTE, major hemorrhage, or death in patients with a prior idiopathic VTE.[61]

Filters in the inferior vena cava have been used safely and effectively in pregnant women.[62,63] Suprarenal placement is recommended. No important maternal or fetal morbidity associated with the filters has been reported. **The indications for their use are the same as in non-pregnant patients**: any contraindication to anticoagulant therapy; serious complication of anticoagulation, such as HIT; and the recurrence of PE in patients with adequate anticoagulant therapy.

The **use of thrombolytic agents** during pregnancy has been limited to life-threatening situations because of the risk of substantial maternal bleeding, especially at the time of delivery and immediately postpartum.[64] The risk of placental abruption and fetal death due to these drugs is currently unknown.

Embolectomy, another treatment option when conservative treatment fails, is indicated to prevent death in patients who are hemodynamically unstable despite anticoagulation and treatment with vasopressors.[65] Embolectomy has been associated with a 20–40% incidence of fetal loss,[66] so this treatment must be restricted to cases in which the woman's life is endangered.

Prevention of venous thromboembolism in pregnancy

Avoidance of risk factors shown in Table 26.1 can provide important prevention of VTE and its complications. **Preconception counseling** should review these preventive measures, as well as review in detail any prior history of VTE and risk factors. Risk of VTE should be discussed (see Table 27.2 and Chapter 27).

Women with a history of VTE (with or without thrombophilia) are believed to have a higher **risk of recurrence** in subsequent pregnancies. Estimates of the rate of recurrent venous thrombosis during pregnancy in women with a history of VTE have varied **between < 1% and > 10%.**[67–70] The higher of these estimates has prompted recommendation for anticoagulant prophylaxis during pregnancy and the postpartum period in women with a history of VTE. However, the risk is likely to be lower than has been suggested by some of these studies because they were retrospective, with the possibility of significant bias. The risk is dramatically influenced by risk factors, in particular the presence of thrombophilias (see Table 27.2 in Chapter 27).

There are very few trials for the prevention of VTE in pregnancy (both antepartum and postpartum). The sample sizes of all trials are small and cannot be combined. There is **insufficient evidence** on which to base recommendations for thromboprophylaxis during pregnancy and the early postnatal period, because of limited data, especially regarding rare outcomes such as death and thromboembolic disease and osteoporosis. In general, the studies must be looked at individually one by one.

Antenatal prophylaxis (usually for prior venous thromboembolism) (see Table 26.3)
Compared with UFH, LMWH is associated with a 72% decrease in bleeding episodes; however, all other outcome variables showed no significant differences.[71,72]

Compared with aspirin alone, in pregnant women with recurrent miscarriage associated with antiphospholipid antibodies, **aspirin plus heparin** appears to be associated with a 50% lower risk of fetal loss.[73] (see Chapter 23).

Compared with UFH-only postpartum, UFH antepartum and postpartum is associated with similar results in one very small ($n = 40$) trial, which could not possibly detect differences given its sample size.[74]

In summary, there is **insufficient evidence** on which to base recommendations for VTE prophylaxis during pregnancy and the early postnatal period.[75] In general, in pregnant women with a **prior history of a VTE, low-dose prophylactic anticoagulation** can be used. This may be modified based on the cause of the first VTE and the presence of a thrombophilia. **If the prior VTE was related to a non-recurrent cause** (i.e. broken bone and immobilization) **and the thrombophilia work-up is negative,** the risk of recurrence is very low, and **prophylaxis may be avoided,** especially in women without other risk factors except pregnancy. In fact, the risk of recurrence was 0% in 44 such women followed without anticoagulation.[76] Postpartum prophylaxis may be suggested in all women with a prior VTE. Both antepartum and postpartum prophylaxis may be suggested to the woman with a prior VTE and a thrombophilia, prior unexplained VTE, or a current major risk factor. There are two general therapies for management of pregnant patients with previous VTE who require prophylaxis: UFH or LMWH. For low-dose prophylaxis of VTE during pregnancy, see Table 26.4.

Approximately 50% of gestational VTEs are associated with **heritable thrombophilia** (see Chapter 27). Given that the background rate of VTE during pregnancy is approximately 1:1000, the absolute risk of VTE remains modest for the majority of these thrombophilias, except antithrombin III deficiency, homozygosity for the factor V Leiden mutation and for the prothrombin mutation, and combined defects. The absolute risk of pregnancy-associated VTE has been reported to range from 9% to 16% in homozygotes for the factor V Leiden mutation.[77–80] Compound heterozygosity for the factor V Leiden and prothrombin gene mutations has been reported to have an absolute risk of pregnancy-associated VTE of 4.0% (95% CI 1.4–16.9%).[80] These data suggest that women with antithrombin III deficiency, homozygosity for the factor V Leiden mutation or the prothrombin mutation as well as compound heterozygotes, should be managed more aggressively than those with other low-risk inherited thrombophilias, and thus **adjusted-dose anticoagulation is recommended for prior DVT and a high-risk thrombophilia** (AT III deficiency, homozygous factor V or prothrombin gene mutation or compound heterozygote). Adjusted-dose anticoagulation should also be used in pregnant women if the woman has had recurrent VTE episodes, life-threatening thrombosis, or thrombosis while receiving chronic anticoagulation. Filters in the inferior vena cava should be considered in this situation as well. In pregnant women with a **history of a prior VTE with history of a low-risk thrombophilia** (heterozygous factor V or prothrombin gene, protein C or S), **low-dose prophylactic anticoagulation is recommended.** Persistent antiphospholipid antibodies are associated with an increased risk of VTE during pregnancy and the puerperium.[45] It is recommended that pregnant patients with the antiphospholipid syndrome who do not have a history of venous thrombosis receive a low-dose prophylactic regimen of heparin, and that those with previous thrombosis receive an adjusted-dose regimen of heparin[45] (see also Chapter 23). The antepartum management of pregnant women with known thrombophilia and no prior VTE remains controversial because of our limited knowledge of the natural histories of various thrombophilias and a lack of trials of VTE prophylaxis. We are unaware of prospective data addressing the issue of the incidence of VTE in a large group of pregnant women with thrombophilia and no prior VTE. Currently, there is no evidence to suggest prophylactic low-dose anticoagulation in this group. If there is a very strong family history of VTE (especially at young ages), consideration can be made for low-dose prophylactic anticoagulation.

Postnatal prophylaxis after cesarean delivery
Available data suggest that the risk of VTE is higher after **cesarean section** (especially emergent surgery) than after vaginal delivery.[3] The presence of additional risk factors for pregnancy-associated VTE (e.g. prior VTE, thrombophilia, age > 35 years old, obesity, prolonged bed rest, and concomitant acute medical illness) may exacerbate this risk. Clinical judgment should be used to decide on anticoagulation after cesarean section, taking into account all of the patient's risk factors.

Evidence from small trials reveals that, for post-cesarean delivery VTE prophylaxis:

- Compared with placebo, heparin (either UFH or LMWH) is associated with similar outcomes in two trials.[81,82]
- Compared with UFH, LMWH is associated with similar outcomes in one trial.[83]
- Compared to UFH, hydroxyethyl starch is associated with similar outcomes in one trial.[84]

It has been recommended that **graduated compression stockings** be used during and after cesarean section in patients considered to be at 'moderate risk' of VTE and that **LMWH or UFH prophylaxis** be added in those thought to be at 'high risk.'[85] However, there are **no adequate** randomized controlled trials (**RCTs**) on this subject.

Prophylaxis in women with mechanical heart valves
Women who anticipate ultimately needing valve replacement surgery should be encouraged to complete childbearing before valve replacement. The highest risk for VTE is with first-generation mechanical valves (Starr–Edwards, Bjork–Shiley) in the mitral position, followed by second-generation valves (St Jude) in the aortic position (see also Chapter 2). These women need to be **therapeutically anticoagulated throughout pregnancy and postpartum, with blood levels frequently (usually weekly) checked to ensure therapeutic levels of anticoagulation.** Pregnant women with prosthetic heart valves pose a problem because of the **lack of trials** regarding the efficacy and safety of antithrombotic therapy during pregnancy. There are insufficient data to make definitive recommendations about optimal anticogulation in pregnant patients with mechanical heart valves.

There are in general **four regimens** that can be considered:

1. VKAs throughout pregnancy
2. either LMWH or UFH between 6 weeks and 12 weeks and close to term only, and VKAs at other times
3. careful adjusted-dose UFH throughout pregnancy
4. careful adjusted-dose LMWH throughout pregnancy.

Before any of these approaches is used, it is crucial to explain the risks/benefits carefully to the patient.

In a review, **VKAs throughout pregnancy** was the **regimen associated with the lowest risk of valve thrombosis/systemic embolism** (3.9%); using UFH only between 6 weeks and 12 weeks' gestation was associated with an increased risk of valve thrombosis (9.2%).[86] This analysis suggests that VKAs are more efficacious than UFH for thromboembolic prophylaxis of women with mechanical heart valves in pregnancy; however, coumarins increase the risk of **embryopathy.** In the first trimester coumarin is associated with an overall 5–15% teratogenic risk (nasal hypoplasia, optic atrophy, digital anomalies, mental impairment). European experts have recommended warfarin therapy throughout pregnancy in view of the reports of poor maternal outcomes with heparin and their impression that the risk of embryopathy with coumarin derivatives has been overstated, and may be <5%.[87] If coumarin is used, the dose should be adjusted to attain a target international normalized ratio (INR) of 3.0 (range 2.5–3.5).

A common option utilizes **UFH during the first trimester to minimize teratogenesis, warfarin for the majority of pregnancy (12–36 weeks), and UFH again in the last month to prepare for delivery and allow for epidural anesthesia.** Whereas this regimen may be efficacious, fetal risk is not completely eliminated. **Substituting VKAs with heparin between 6 weeks and 12 weeks** reduces the risk of fetopathic effects but possibly subjects the woman to an increased risk of thromboembolic complications. The reported high rates of thromboembolism with **UFH** might be explained by inadequate dosing and/or the use of an inappropriate target therapeutic range.

The use of **adjusted-dose UFH** warrants careful monitoring and appropriate dose adjustment. A target aPTT ratio of at least twice the control should be attained.[88] If used, SC UFH should be initiated in high doses, usually every 8 hours, and adjusted to prolong a 6-hour postinjection aPTT into the therapeutic range (usually 60–80 seconds); strong efforts should be made to ensure an adequate anticoagulant effect.

LMWH use in pregnant women with prosthetic heart valves[89–95] has been associated with treatment failures,[92–95] and the use of LMWH for this indication has recently become controversial due to a warning from an LMWH manufacturer regarding the drug's safety in this situation.[96] If used, LMWH should be administered twice daily and dosed to achieve antifactor Xa levels of 1.0–1.2 U/ml 4–6 hours (peak) after SC injection, with a trough of 0.6–0.7.

Extrapolating from data in non-pregnant patients with mechanical valves receiving warfarin therapy,[97] for some high-risk women, **the addition of low-dose aspirin, 75–162 mg/day,** can be considered in an attempt to reduce the risk of thrombosis, recognizing that it increases the risk of bleeding.

Antepartum testing

No specific recommendations.

Delivery

In order to avoid an unwanted anticoagulant effect during delivery (especially with neuroaxial anesthesia) in women receiving adjusted-dose SC UFH therapy,[98] it is suggested that heparin be discontinued 24 hours prior to elective induction of labor or cesarean section. If spontaneous labor occurs in women receiving adjusted-dose SC UFH, careful monitoring of the aPTT is required. If it is markedly prolonged near delivery, protamine sulfate may be required to reduce the risk of bleeding. Although bleeding complications appear to be very uncommon with LMWH,[28–37] we suggest the same approach to women receiving adjusted dose of LMWH as in those receiving adjusted-dose UFH: namely, discontinue LMWH 24 hours prior to elective induction of labor or cesarean section.

In women with **mechanical heart valves**, therapeutic anticoagulation can be continued IV (half-life: 90 minutes) until active labor, and then stopped during active labor and for delivery, with therapeutic heparin restarted about 6–12 hours after delivery, and warfarin restarted in an overlapping fashion (to avoid paradoxical thrombosis) 24–36 hours after delivery (the night after delivery). Extensive counseling on all these options and risks is required.

Anesthesia

UFH ≤ 10000 U twice a day does not pose a risk for spinal hematoma. Low-dose UFH and LMWH probably do not cause a risk for spinal hematoma.[1] For precaution, women on low-dose LMWH should not receive regional anesthesia sooner than 12–24 hours after the last dose. Women on therapeutic LMWH should not receive regional anesthesia sooner than 24 hours after the last dose.[99]

Postpartum/breastfeeding

For women who require low-dose anticoagulation, UFH or LMWH can be restarted 12–24 hours postpartum, depending on risk. For women who require therapeutic adjusted-dose anticoagulation, heparin can be restarted (either UFH or LMWH) 6–12 hours postpartum, with warfarin also started about 24–36 hours later, overlapping for the first 5–7 days until warfarin is therapeutic (INR = 2.0–3.0).

REFERENCES

1. American College of Obstetrics and Gynecology Practice Bulletin No. 21. Prevention of deep vein thrombosis and pulmonary embolism. October 2000. [review]
2. Greer IA. Thrombosis in pregnancy: maternal and fetal issues. Lancet 1999; 353: 1258–65. [review]
3. Lindqvist P, Dahlback B, Marsal K. Thrombotic risk during pregnancy: a population study. Obstet Gynecol 1999; 94: 595–9. [II-2]
4. National Institutes of Health Consensus Development Conference. Prevention of venous thrombosis and pulmonary embolism. JAMA 1986; 256: 744–9. [review]
5. Gherman RB, Goodwin TM, Leung B, et al. Incidence, clinical characteristics and timing of objectively diagnosed venous thromboembolism during pregnancy. Obstet Gynecol 1999; 94: 730–4. [II-2]
6. Grandone E, Margaglione M, Colaizzo D, et al. Genetic susceptibility to pregnancy-related venous thromboembolism: roles of factor V Leiden, prothrombin G20210A, and methylenetetrahydrofolate reductase C677T mutations. Am J Obstet Gynecol 1998; 179: 1324–8. [II-2]
7. Lockwood CJ. Heritable coagulopathies in pregnancy. Obstet Gynecol Surv 1999; 54: 754–65. [review]
8. Walker MC, Garner PR, Keely EJ, et al. Changes in activated protein C resistance during normal pregnancy. Am J Obstet Gynecol 1997; 77: 162–9. [II-3]
9. Zotz RB, Gerhardt A, Scharf RE. Inherited thrombophilia and gestational venous thromboembolism. Best Pract Res Clin Haematol 2003; 16: 243–59. [review]
10. Haemostasis and Thrombosis Tack Force, British Committee for Standards in Haematology. Investigation and management of heritable thrombophilia. Br J Haematol 2001; 114: 512–28. [II-2]
11. Kyrle PA, Eichinger S. Deep vein thrombosis. Lancet 2005; 365: 1163–74. [review]
12. Pabinger I, Grafenhofer H. Thrombosis during pregnancy: risk factors, diagnosis and treatment. Pathophysiol Haemost Thromb 2002; 32: 322–4. [review]
13. Ginsberg JS, Hirsh J, Rainbow AJ, Coates G. Risks to the fetus of radiologic procedures used in the diagnosis of maternal venous thromboembolic disease. Thromb Haemost 1989; 61: 189–96. [II-2]
14. Kearon C, Julian JA, Newman TE, Ginsberg JS. Noninvasive diagnosis of deep vein thrombosis. McMaster Diagnostic Imaging Practice Guidelines Initiative. Ann Intern Med 1998; 128: 663–77. [guideline]
15. Bergqvist D, Hedner U. Pregnancy and venous thromboembolism. Acta Obstet Gynecol Scand 1983; 62: 449–53. [review]
16. Bergqvist A, Bergqvist D, Hallbook T. Deep vein thrombosis during pregnancy: a prospective study. Acta Obstet Gynecol Scand 1983; 62: 443–8. [II-1]
17. Hull RD, Raskob GE, Carter CJ. Serial impedance plethysmography in pregnant patients with clinically suspected deep-vein thrombosis: clinical validity of negative findings. Ann Intern Med 1990; 112: 663–7. [II-2]
18. Cockett FB, Thomas ML, Negus D. Iliac vein compression: its relation to iliofemoral thrombosis and the post-thrombotic syndrome. BMJ 1967; 2: 14–16. [II-2]
19. Chan WS, Ginsberg JS. Diagnosis of deep vein thrombosis and pulmonary embolism in pregnancy. Thromb Res 2002; 107: 85–91. [II-2]
20. Heijboer C, Beuller HR, Lensing AW, et al. A comparison of real time diagnosis of deep vein thrombosis in symptomatic outpatients. N Engl J Med 1993; 329: 1365–9. [II-2]
21. Weinmann EE, Salzman EW. Deep-vein thrombosis. N Engl J Med 1994; 331: 1630–41. [review]
22. Nolan TE, Smith RP, Devoe LD. Maternal plasma D-dimer levels in normal and complicated pregnancies. Obstet Gynecol 1993; 81: 235–8. [II-2]
23. Fedullo PF, Tapson VF. Clinical practice. The evaluation of suspected pulmonary embolism. N Engl J Med 2003; 349: 1247–56. [review]
24. Goldhaber SZ. Pulmonary embolism. Lancet 2004; 363: 1295–305. [review]
25. Value of the ventilation/perfusion scan in acute pulmonary embolism. Results of the prospective investigation of pulmonary embolism diagnosis (PIOPED). The PIOPED Investigators. JAMA 1990; 263: 2753–9. [II-2]
26. Rathbun SW, Raskob GE, Whitsett TL. Sensitivity and specificity of helical computed tomography in the diagnosis of pulmonary embolism: a systematic review. Ann Intern Med 2000; 132: 227–32. [II-2]
27. Goodman LR, Curtin JJ, Mewissen MW, et al. Detection of pulmonary embolism in patients with unresolved clinical and scintigraphic diagnosis: helical CT versus angiography. AJR Am J Roentgenol 1995; 164: 1369–74. [II-2]
28. Hunt BJ, Doughty HA, Majumdar G, et al. Thromboprophylaxis with low molecular weight heparin (Fragmin) in high risk pregnancies. Thromb Haemost 1997; 77: 39–43. [II-2]
29. Blomback M, Bremme K, Hellgren M, et al. Thromboprophylaxis with low molecular mass heparin, 'Fragmin' (dalteparin), during pregnancy – a longitudinal safety study. Blood Coagul Fibrinolysis 1998; 9: 1–9. [II-2]

30. Blomback M, Bremme K, Hellgren M, et al. A pharmacokinetic study of dalteparin (Fragmin) during late pregnancy. Blood Coagul Fibrinolysis 1998; 9: 343–50. [II-2]

31. Brennand JE, Walker ID, Greer IA. Anti-activated factor X profiles in pregnant women receiving antenatal thromboprophylaxis with enoxaparin. Acta Haematol 1999; 101: 53–5. [II-3]

32. Dulitzki M, Pauzner R, Langevitz P, et al. Low molecular weight heparin during pregnancy and delivery: preliminary experience with 41 pregnancies. Obstet Gynecol 1996; 87: 380–3. [II-3]

33. Casele HL, Laifer SA, Woelkers DA, et al. Changes in the pharmacokinetics of the low molecular weight heparin enoxaparin sodium during pregnancy. Am J Obstet Gynecol 1999; 181: 1113–17. [II-3]

34. Ellison J, Walker ID, Greer IA. Antifactor Xa profiles in pregnant women receiving antenatal thromboprophylaxis with enoxaparin for prevention and treatment of thromboembolism in pregnancy. Br J Obstet Gynaecol 2000; 107: 1116–21. [II-3]

35. Lepercq J, Conard J, Borel-Derlon A, et al. Venous thromboembolism during pregnancy: a retrospective study of enoxaparin safety in 624 pregnancies. Br J Obstet Gynaecol 2001; 108: 1134–40. [II-2]

36. Dolovich L, Ginsberg JS, Douketis JD, et al. A meta-analysis comparing low molecular weight heparins to unfractionated heparin in the treatment of venous thromboembolism: examining some unanswered questions regarding location of treatment, product type, and dosing frequency. Arch Intern Med 2000; 160: 181–8. [meta-analysis]

37. Gould MK, Dembitzer AD, Doyle RL, et al. Low-molecular-weight heparins compared with unfractionated heparin for treatment of acute deep venous thrombosis: a meta-analysis of randomized, controlled trials. Ann Intern Med 1999; 130: 800–9. [meta-analysis]

38. de Valk HW, Banga JD, Wester JWJ, et al. Comparing subcutaneous danaparoid with intravenous unfractionated heparin for the treatment of venous thromboembolism. A randomized controlled trial. Ann Intern Med 1995; 123: 1–9. [RCT]

39. Nurmohamed MT, Rosendaal FR, Buller HR, et al. Low-molecular-weight heparin versus standard heparin in general and orthopedic surgery: a meta-analysis. Lancet 1992; 340: 152–6. [meta-analysis]

40. Weitz JI. Low-molecular-weight heparins. N Engl J Med 1997; 337: 688–98.

41. Nelson-Piercy C, Letsky EA, de Swiet M. Low-molecular-weight heparin for obstetric thromboprophylaxis: experience of sixty-nine pregnancies in sixty-one women at high risk. Am J Obstet Gynecol 1997; 176: 1062–8. [II-3]

42. Warkentin TE, Levine MN, Hirsh J, et al. Heparin-induced thrombocytopenia in patients treated with low-molecular-weight heparin or unfractionated heparin. N Engl J Med 1995; 332: 1330–5. [II-2]

43. Pravinkumar E, Webster NR. HIT/HITT and alternative anticoagulation: current concepts. Br J Anaesth 2003; 90: 676–85. [review]

44. Magnani HN. Heparin-induced thrombocytopenia (HIT): an overview of 230 patients treated with Orgaran (Org 10172). Thromb Haemost 1993; 70: 554–61. [II-3]

45. Ginsberg JS, Hirsh J. Use of antithrombotic agents during pregnancy. Chest 1995; 108 (Suppl): 305–11S. [review]

46. Dahlman TC. Osteoporotic fractures and the recurrence of thromboembolism during pregnancy and the puerperium in 184 women undergoing thromboprophylaxis with heparin. Am J Obstet Gynecol 1993; 168: 1265–70. [II-3, $n = 184$]

47. Pettila V, Leinonen P, Markkola A, et al. Postpartum bone mineral density in women treated for thromboprophylaxis with unfractionated heparin or LMW heparin. Thromb Haemost 2002; 87: 182–6. [RCT]

48. Sanson BJ, Lensing AWA, Prins MH, et al. Safety of low-molecular-weight heparin in pregnancy: a systematic review. Thromb Haemost 1999; 81: 668–72. [review]

49. Hull RD, Delmore TJ, Carter CJ, et al. Adjusted subcutaneous heparin versus warfarin sodium in the long-term treatment of venous thrombosis. N Engl J Med 1982; 306: 189–94. [RCT]

50. Hull RD, Hirsh J, Jay R, et al. Different intensities of oral anticoagulant therapy in the treatment of proximal-vein thrombosis. N Engl J Med 1982; 307: 1676–81. [RCT]

51. Barbour LA, Oja JL, Schultz LK. A prospective trial that demonstrates that dalteparin requirements increase in pregnancy to maintain therapeutic levels of anticoagulation. Am J Obstet Gynecol 2004; 191: 1024–9. [II-1]

52. Casele HL, Laifer SA, Wolkers DA, Venkataramanan R. Changes in the pharmacokinetics of the low-molecular-weight heparin enoxaparin sodium during pregnancy. Am J Obstet Gynecol 1999; 181: 1113–17. [II-2]

53. Sephton V, Farquharson RG, Topping J, et al. A longitudinal study of maternal dose response to low molecular weight heparin in pregnancy. Obstet Gynecol 2003; 101: 1307–11. [II-2]

54. Ginsberg JS, Hirsh J, Turner CD, et al. Risks to the fetus of anticoagulant therapy during pregnancy. Thromb Haemost 1989; 61: 197–203. [II-3]

55. Hall JAG, Paul RM, Wilson KM. Maternal and fetal sequelae of anticoagulation during pregnancy. Am J Med 1980; 68: 122–40. [II-3]

56. Orme ML, Lewis PJ, de Swiet M, et al. May mothers given warfarin breast-feed their infants? Br Med J 1977; 1: 1564–5. [II-3]

57. McKenna R, Cole ER, Vasan V. Is warfarin sodium contraindicated in the lactating mother? J Pediatr 1983; 103: 325–7. [II-3]

58. Imperiale TF, Petrulis AS. A meta-analysis of low-dose aspirin for prevention of pregnancy-induced hypertensive disease. JAMA 1991; 266: 260–4. [meta-analysis]

59. CLASP Collaborative Group. CLASP: a randomised trial of low dose aspirin for the prevention and treatment of pre-eclampsia among 9,364 pregnant women. Lancet 1994; 343: 619–29. [RCT]

60. Gould MK, Dembitzer AD, Doyle RL, et al. Low-molecular-weight heparins compared with unfractionated heparin for treatment of acute deep venous thrombosis: a meta-analysis of randomized, controlled trials. Ann Intern Med 1999; 130: 800–9. [meta-analysis]

61. Ridker PM, Goldhaber SZ, Danielson E, et al. Long-term, low-intensity warfarin therapy for the prevention of recurrent venous thromboembolism. N Engl J Med 2003; 348: 1425–34. [RCT]

62. Greenfield LJ, Cho KJ, Proctor MC, et al. Late results of suprarenal Greenfield vena cava filter placement. Arch Surg 1992; 127: 969–7. [II-2]

63. Narayan H, Cullimore J, Krarup K, et al. Experience with the Cardial inferior vena cava filter as prophylaxis against pulmonary embolism in pregnant women with extensive deep venous thrombosis. Br J Obstet Gynaecol 1992; 99: 637–40. [II-3]

64. Fagher B, Ahlgren M, Astedt B. Acute massive pulmonary embolism treated with streptokinase during labor and the early puerperium. Acta Obstet Gynecol Scand 1990; 69: 659–61. [II-3]

65. Riedel M. Acute pulmonary embolism 2: treatment. Heart 2001; 85: 351–60. [review]

66. Ahearn GS, Hadjiliadis D, Govert JA, et al. Massive pulmonary embolism during pregnancy successfully treated with recombinant tissue plasminogen activator: a case report and review of treatment options. Arch Intern Med 2002; 162: 1221–7. [II-3]

67. De Swiet M, Floyd E, Letsky E. Low risk of recurrent thromboembolism in pregnancy. Br J Hosp Med 1987; 38: 264. [letter]

68. Howell R, Fidler J, Letsky E, et al. The risk of antenatal subcutaneous heparin prophylaxis: a controlled trial. Br J Obstet Gynecol 1983; 90: 1124–8. [RCT]

69. Badaracco MA, Vessey M. Recurrent venous thromboembolic disease and use of oral contraceptives. Br Med J 1974; 1: 215–17. [II-2]

70. Tengborn L. Recurrent thromboembolism in pregnancy and puerperium: is there a need for thromboprophylaxis? Am J Obstet Gynecol 1989; 160: 90–4. [II-3]

71. Pettila V, Kaaja R, Leinonen P, et al. Thromboprophylaxis with low molecular weight heparin (dalteparin) in pregnancy. Thromb Res 1999; 96: 275–82. [II-2]

72. Hamersley S, Landy H. Low molecular weight heparin is associated with less peripartum blood loss than unfractionated heparin [abstract]. Am J Obstet Gynecol 1998; 178 (1 pt 2): S66. [II-1]

73. Rai R, Cohen H, Dave M, Regan L. Randomised controlled trial of aspirin and aspirin plus heparin in pregnant women with recurrent miscarriage associated with phospholipid antibodies (or antiphospholipid antibodies). BMJ 1997; 314: 253–7. [RCT, n = 90]

74. Howell R, Fidler J, Letsky E, de Swiet M. The risks of antenatal subcutaneous heparin prophylaxis: a controlled trial. Br J Obstet Gynaecol 1983; 90: 1124–8. [RCT]

75. Gates S, Brocklehurst P, Davis LJ. Prophylaxis for venous thromboembolic disease in pregnancy and the early postnatal period. Cochrane Database Syst Rev 2005; 4. [meta-analysis]

76. Brill-Edwards P, Ginsberg JS, Gent M, et al. Safety of withholding heparin in pregnant women with a history of venous thromboembolism. Recurrence of Clot in this Pregnancy Study Group. N Engl J Med 2000; 343: 1439–44. [II-2]

77. Middledorp S, Van der Meer J, Hamulyak K, et al. Counseling women with factor V Leiden homozygosity: use absolute instead of relative risks. Thromb Haemost 2001; 87: 360–1. [review]

78. Middledorp S, Libourel EJ, Hamulyak K, et al. The risk of pregnancy-related venous thromboembolism in women who are homozygous for factor V Leiden. Br J Haematol 2001; 113: 553–5. [II-2]

79. Martinelli I, Legnani C, Bucciarelli P, et al. Risk of pregnancy-related venous thrombosis in carriers of severe inherited thrombophilia. Thromb Haemost 2001; 86: 800–3. [II-2]

80. Pabinger I, Nemes L, Rintelen C, et al. Pregnancy-associated risk for venous thromboembolism and pregnancy outcome in women homozygous for factor V Leiden. Hematol J 2000; 1: 37–41. [II-2]

81. Hill NC, Hill JG, Sargent JM, Taylor CG, Bush PV. Effect of low dose heparin on blood loss at caesarean section. Br Med J (Clin Res Ed) 1988; 296: 505–6. [RCT]

82. Burrows RF, Gan ET, Gallus AS, Wallace EM, Burrows EA. A randomised, double-blind placebo controlled trial of low molecular weight heparin as prophylaxis in preventing venous thromboembolic events after caesarean section: a pilot study. BJOG 2001; 108: 835–9. [RCT, n = 76]

83. Gibson JL, Ekevall K, Walker I, Greer IA. Puerperal thromboprophylaxis: comparison of the anti-Xa activity of enoxaparin and unfractionated heparin. Br J Obstet Gynaecol 1998; 105: 795–7. [RCT, n = 17]

84. Heilman L, Heitz R, Koch FU, Ose C. Perioperative thrombosis prophylaxis at the time of caesarean section: results of a randomised prospective comparative study with 6% hydroxyethyl starch 0.62 and low dose heparin. Geburt Perinatol 1991; 195: 10–15. [RCT] [in German]

85. Report of the RCOG Working Party on Prophylaxis against Thromboembolism in Gynaecology and Obstetrics. London, UK: Royal College of Obstetricians and Gynaecologists; 1995. [review]

86. Chan WS, Anand S, Ginsberg JS. Anticoagulation of pregnant women with mechanical heart valves: a systematic review of the literature. Arch Intern Med 2000; 160: 191–6. [review]

87. Sbarouni E, Oakley CM. Outcome of pregnancy in women with valve prostheses. Br Heart J 1994; 71: 196–201. [II-2]

88. Brill-Edwards P, Ginsberg JS, Johnston M, et al. Establishing a therapeutic range for heparin. Ann Intern Med 1993; 119: 104–9. [II-2]

89. Arnaout MS, Kazma H, Khalil A, et al. Is there a safe anticoagulation protocol for pregnant women with prosthetic valves? Clin Exp Obstet Gynecol 1998; 25:101–4. [II-2]

90. Lee LH, Liauw PC, Ng AS. Low molecular weight heparin for thromboprophylaxis during pregnancy in 2 patients with mechanical mitral valve replacement. Thromb Haemost 1996; 76: 628–30. [letter]

91. Rowan JA, McCowan LM, Raudkivi PJ, et al. Enoxaparin treatment in women with mechanical heart valves during pregnancy. Am J Obstet Gynecol 2001; 185: 633–7. [II-2]

92. Roberts N, Ross D, Flint SK, et al. Thromboembolism in pregnant women with mechanical prosthetic heart valves anticoagulated with low molecular weight heparin. Br J Obstet Gynaecol 2001; 108: 327–9. [II-2]

93. Leyh RG, Fischer S, Ruhparwar A, et al. Anticoagulation for prosthetic heart valves during pregnancy: is low-molecular-weight heparin an alternative. Eur J Cardiothorac Surg 2002; 21: 577–9. [II-2]

94. Mahesh B, Evans S, Bryan AJ. Failure of low molecular-weight heparin in the prevention of prosthetic mitral valve thrombosis during pregnancy: case report and review of options for anticoagulation. J Heart Valve Dis 2002; 11: 745–50. [II-3]

95. Lev-Ran O, Kramer A, Gurevitch J, et al. Low-molecular-weight heparin for prosthetic heart valves: treatment failure. Ann Thorac Surg 2000; 69: 264–5. [II-3]

96. Lovenox Injection (package insert). Bridgewater, NJ: Aventis Pharmaceuticals; 2004. [package insert]

97. Turpie AGG, Gent M, Laupacis A, et al. A comparison of aspirin with placebo in patients treated with warfarin after heart-valve replacement. N Engl J Med 1993; 329: 524–9. [RCT]

98. Anderson DR, Ginsberg JS, Burrows R, et al. Subcutaneous heparin therapy during pregnancy: a need for concern at the time of delivery. Thromb Haemost 1991; 63: 248–50. [II-2]

99. American Society of Regional Anesthesia (ASRA). Recommendations for neuroaxial anesthesia and anticoagulation. Richmond, VA: ASRA; 1998. [guideline]

27

Inherited thrombophilia

James Airoldi

KEY POINTS

- **Inherited thrombophilias** are genetic conditions that **increase the risk of thromboembolic disease.**
- **The risk of thrombotic events is affected by numerous factors,** including thrombophilia, personal history of deep vein thrombosis (DVT), family history of DVT, surgery, age over 35 years old, high parity, high body mass index, smoking, and immobilization.
- The **prevalence** and **thrombogenic potential** of the **inherited thrombophilias** are shown in **Tables 27.1 and 27.2,** respectively. The only significant association in prospective studies is venous thromboembolism (VTE) with factor V Leiden (FVL).
- Meta-analyses of case-control studies show many significant associations between various thrombophilias and adverse pregnancy outcomes. When combining all of the **prospective** cohort studies, there is **no association between thrombophilia and adverse pregnancy outcomes except for late pregnancy loss and pre-eclampsia associated with hyperhomocysteinemia.**
- Fetal carriage of thrombophilic mutations may also have adverse clinical consequences.
- It would be reasonable not to screen universally for inherited thrombophilias, but to screen with a full panel any pregnant women with a **prior personal history of VTE** due to a **non-recurring etiology.**
- Among **women with a non-recurring cause for the prior VTE and no thrombophilia,** the risk of recurrent antepartum VTE is low, and therefore **routine antepartum prophylaxis with heparin may not be warranted.** Anticoagulation can still be given postpartum.
- If protein C (**PC**), protein S (**PS**), heterozygous FVL, or prothrombin G20210A gene mutation (**PGM**) are detected in a woman with **prior VTE, prophylactic anticoagulation is reasonable.**
- If **homozygous FVL or PGM or an antithrombin III (ATIII) deficiency or a compound heterozygote** are detected in a woman with a **prior VTE, full therapeutic anticoagulation** would be indicated.
- In a woman with a **prior personal history of a VTE** and a **recurring etiology, prophylactic anticoagulation is**

recommended. **Screening would be indicated for FVL, PGM, and ATIII.**
- In a woman with a **VTE in the current pregnancy,** screening should be performed for **FVL, PGM, and ATIII.**
- In an otherwise **healthy pregnant woman** with no personal history of VTE or adverse pregnancy outcomes, but whose **first-degree relative has a genetic thrombophilia,** there is **insufficient evidence** to recommend any type of screening. In an otherwise **healthy pregnant woman** with a **prior adverse pregnancy outcome** but no major risk factors for VTE, there is **insufficient evidence** to support screening.
- In women with **one unexplained pregnancy loss** at ≥ 10th week and either heterozygous FVL, PGM, or PS **deficiency,** low molecular weight heparin (**LMWH**) enoxaparin 40 mg starting at 8 weeks is associated with a higher (86 vs 29%) incidence of a **healthy live birth** compared with low-dose aspirin in one trial.

See also Chapter 26.

HISTORIC NOTES

Antithrombin deficiency and dysfibrinogenemia, the first inherited thrombophilias to be described (1965), were found in studies of families in which several members were affected by venous thrombosis.[1,2] Later, heterozygous deficiencies of protein C (PC)[3] and protein S (PS)[4] were identified as causes of inherited thrombophilia. Initially, searches for inherited thrombophilias among patients with idiopathic venous thrombosis were disappointing, since only 5–20% of such patients had inherited thrombophilias.[5] The situation changed remarkably in 1993, after the discovery of resistance to activated PC. This condition is the most common cause of inherited thrombophilia.[6] In most cases it results from a mutation of the factor V gene (G1691A), resulting in a protein called factor V Leiden (FVL).[7] In 1996, the 20210 mutation of the prothrombin gene was found to be another cause of thrombophilia.[8] Homocystinuria, a rare type of thrombophilia, is manifested by both venous and arterial thrombosis.[9] Familial venous thrombosis has also been associated with the occurrence of two or more inherited thrombophilias in the same person.[10]

DEFINITION

Inherited thrombophilias are genetic conditions that increase the risk of venous thromboembolism (VTE), and possibly some other pregnancy-specific complications.[11]

EPIDEMIOLOGY/INCIDENCE

VTE is the leading cause of pregnancy-related maternal morbidity and mortality in the developed world.[12] Estimates for the incidence of thrombotic events occurring during pregnancy and the puerperium vary from 0.2 to 2 per 1000 births.[12] During pregnancy, women have a fivefold increased risk of VTE compared with non-pregnant women,[13] and cesarean delivery carries a fivefold higher risk of thrombosis relative to vaginal delivery.[14,15] The frequency of thrombotic events is equal in the antepartum and postpartum periods. Antepartum risk is equally divided for each trimester.[13] Pulmonary embolism is more common postpartum.[13]

Up to 50% of women who have thrombotic events during pregnancy possess an underlying congenital or acquired thrombophilia.[16] The frequency of the major inherited thrombophilias varies substantially within healthy populations and among patients with previous venous thrombosis (Table 27.1).[17,18] The most common inherited thrombophilias are heterozygosity for the FVL gene mutation, the prothrombin G20210A gene mutation (PGM), and the thermolabile variant of methylenetetrahydrofolate reductase (C677T MTHFR), the most common cause of hyperhomocysteinemia. Lesser thrombophilias include autosomal-dominant deficiencies of antithrombin, PC, and PS. FVL and the G20210A mutation in the prothrombin gene are common among Caucasians but are extremely rare among Asians and Africans.[19] The population prevalence of FVL mutation shows racial differences. In a recent prospective cohort study, the carrier rate was 6.1% in Caucasians, 0.8% in African-Americans, 1.7% in Hispanics, and 1.9% in others[20] (see Table 27.1).

ETIOLOGY/BASIC PATHOPHYSIOLOGY

Changes in the coagulation system, an increase in venous stasis, and vascular injury at delivery substantially increase the risk of developing VTE in pregnancy compared with the non-pregnant state.[12] Coagulation system changes include increases in fibrinogen and factors II, VII, VIII, IX, X, and XII, an increase in the activity of the fibrinolytic inhibitors, a decrease in PS activity (due to estrogen-induced decreases in total PS and increases in the complement 4b binding protein, which binds PS), and an increase in resistance to activated PC

Table 27.1 *Prevalence of different thrombophilias in the general and at-risk population*[17,18]

Thrombophilia	Prevalence in general population (%)	Prevalence in patients with history of thrombosis (%)
Factor V Leiden (heterozygous)	1–15	10–50
Prothrombin gene (heterozygous)	2–5	6–18
ATIII deficiency	0.02	1–3
Protein S deficiency	0.1–1.3	1–5
Protein C deficiency	0.2–0.4	3–5
Hyperhomocysteinemia	5	10
MTHFR (C677T heterozygous)	5–14	N/A

ATIII, antithrombin III; MTHFR, methylenetetrahydrofolate reductase; N/A, not available.

in the second and third trimesters.[21,22] (Figure 26.1) In approximately 50% of patients with a hereditary thrombophilia, the initial thrombotic event occurs in the presence of an additional risk factor such as pregnancy, oral contraceptive use, orthopedic trauma, immobilization, or surgery.[23,24] Histological examination of uteroplacental vessels and intervillous architecture from pathological pregnancies typically displays increased fibrin deposition, thrombosis, and hypoxia-associated endothelial and trophoblast changes.[25] These findings suggest that thrombosis of the uteroplacental circulation may underlie these obstetric conditions. Therefore, in addition to VTE and pulmonary embolism, potential sequelae of the hypercoagulable state may include obstetric complications such as fetal loss, fetal growth restriction (FGR), placental abruption, and pre-eclampsia.

GENETICS/CLASSIFICATION OF EACH THROMBOPHILIA

Congenital (inherited) thrombophilia

Factor V Leiden

The FVL mutation arises from a (G→A) mutation in nucleotide 1691 of the factor V gene's 10th exon, resulting in a substitution of a glutamine for an arginine at position 506 in the factor V polypeptide (factor V Q506). The amino acid substitution impairs the activated PC and PS complex inactivation of factor Va. This defect is termed the FVL mutation and is primarily inherited in an autosomal dominant fashion. It is the most common cause of activated PC resistance. Its prevalence is about 5–10% in Europeans, 3% in Afro–Americans, and rare in Asian and African populations (see Table 27.1). Homozygosity for the mutation, although rare, confers a far higher risk of thromboembolism. Compound heterozygotes should be treated similar to homozygous women.[19]

Prothrombin G20210A

Heterozygosity for a mutation in the promoter of the **prothrombin gene (G20210A)**, i.e. PGM, leads to increased (150–200%) circulating levels of prothrombin and an increased risk of thromboembolism. Homozygosity for the PGM confers a risk of thrombosis equivalent to that of FVL homozygosity. It is inherited in an **autosomal dominant** fashion.[19]

Antithrombin III

Antithrombin III (ATIII) **deficiency** is the **most thrombogenic** of the inherited thrombophilias, with a 70–90% lifetime risk of thromboembolism. Deficiencies in AT result from numerous point mutations, deletions, and insertions, and are usually inherited in an **autosomal dominant** fashion. Because the prevalence of AT deficiency is low, 1:1000 to 1:5000, it is only present in 1% of patients with thromboembolism.[19] The appropriate **cut-off of abnormal activity is < 60%.**

Protein C

Protein C (PC) is a vitamin K dependent polypeptide synthesized primarily in the liver. Activated PC combines with free protein S to inhibit factors V and VIII (Figure 26.1, Chapter 26). PC levels can be decreased by warfarin. Its deficiency can result from numerous mutations. Different mutations have highly variable procoagulant sequelae, making it extremely difficult to predict which patients with PC or PS deficiencies will develop thromboembolism.[19] The inheritance is **autosomal dominant.** PC deficiency is best diagnosed by a **functional assay activity cut-off of < 50%,** which is present in only 0.3% of the population.

Protein S

Protein S (PS) is a vitamin K dependent polypeptide synthesized primarily in the liver. PS is present in plasma in its free (40%) and bound (60%) forms, but it is the free form that is functional. PS specifically functions as a cofactor with protein C (see Figure 26.1, Chapter 26). Its deficiency presents with one of three phenotypes: (1) type I, marked by reduced total and free immunoreactive forms; (2) type II, characterized by normal free immunoreactive levels but reduced APC cofactor activity; and (3) type III, in which there are normal total immunoreactive but reduced free immunoreactive levels. The inheritance is **autosomal dominant. Protein S decreases normally** by about 40% **during pregnancy,** and thus screening during pregnancy is not recommended. **Free PS antigen < 45%** in pregnant and < 55% in non-pregnant women should be detected at least twice to detect true deficiency, and best correlates with genetic deficiency.

MTHFR/homocysteinemia

The most common form of genetic **hyperhomocysteinemia** results from production of a thermolabile variant of **MTHFR** with reduced enzymatic activity (T mutation).[26] The gene encoding for this variant contains an alanine-to-valine substitution at amino acid 677 (C677T).[27] The responsible gene is common, with a population frequency estimated at between 5 and 14%.[28,29] Homozygosity for the thermolabile variant of MTHFR (TT genotype) is a relatively common cause of mildly elevated plasma homocysteine levels in the general population, often occurring in association with low serum folate levels.[30,31] Increased blood levels of homocysteine may reflect deficiency of folate, vitamin B_6, and/or vitamin B_{12}.[32–35] Plasma folate and vitamin B_{12} levels, in particular, are strong determinants of the homocysteine concentration. Homocysteine levels are inversely related to folate consumption, reaching a stable baseline level when folate intake exceeds 400 µg/day.[36,37] Vitamin B_6 is a weaker determinant.[37]

Acquired thrombophilia
Antiphospholipid antibodies

Antiphospholipid antibodies include anticardiolipin antibody (ACA), anti-β_2 glycoprotein-I and lupus anticoagulant (LA). See Chapter 23.

RISK FACTORS/ASSOCIATIONS

The risk of thrombotic events is affected by numerous factors, including **thrombophilia, personal history of** deep vein thrombosis (DVT), **family history of DVT,**[38] **surgery, age over 35 years old, high parity, high body mass index, smoking, and immobilization.**[39]

COMPLICATIONS

To assess the true association between thrombophilias and complications, prospective cohort studies[20,40–42] were preferred over retrospective case-control studies.

Table 27.2   *Risk of VTE with different thrombophilias[17,18,43]*

Thrombophilia	VTE potential (RR of VTE)	VTE risk per pregnancy: no history (%)	VTE risk per pregnancy: prior VTE (%)	Percent of all VTE
FVL heterozygote	5–7	0.25	10	40
FVL homozygote	25	1.5	17	2
Prothrombin gene heterozygote	3–9	0.5	>10	17
Prothrombin gene homozygote	25	2–3	>17	0.5
FVL/prothrombin compound heterozygote	84	4.5–5	>20	1–3
Antithrombin III activity <60%	50–100	0.4–7	40	1
Protein C activity <50%	10–13	0.1–0.8	4–17	14
Protein S free antigen <55%	2–10	0.1	0–22	3
Hyperhomocysteinemia (>16 µm/L)	3–6	0.2	NA	<5%

VTE, venous thromboembolism; RR, relative risk; FVL, factor V Leiden.

Table 27.3   *Thrombophilia and adverse pregnancy outcome[20,40–42]*

Outcome	A True positive	B False positive	C False negative	D True negative	RR	95% CI
FVL ++,+−						
First trimester loss[40]	9	261	54	2156	1.36	0.68–2.68
Second or third trimester loss[40,41]	6	280	40	2742	1.46	0.63–3.31
Any trimester loss[20,40,41]	23	397	358	7175	1.15	0.76–1.72
VTE[20,40,41]	3	417	7	7526	7.68	2.17–27.18
Pre-eclampsia[20,40,41]	10	410	187	7346	0.95	0.52–1.77
Abruption[20,40]	2	402	42	6919	0.82	0.22–3.05
FGR[20,40,41]	19	391	491	6719	0.68	0.44–1.06
Homocysteine						
Second or third trimester loss[42]	2	33	10	704	4.08	1.02–15.62
Pre-eclampsia[42]	2	33	5	709	8.16	1.85–35.21
MTHF ++, +−						
Second or third trimester loss[41]	15	336	9	224	1.11	0.50–2.44
VTE[41]	0	351	0	233	–	–
Pre-eclampsia[41]	6	345	5	228	0.79	0.26–2.44
FGR[41]	5	346	4	229	0.83	0.24–2.83

FVL, factor V Leiden; VTE, venous thromboembolism; RR, relative risk; CI, confidence interval; MTHF, methylenetetrahydrofolate reductase.

Venous thromboembolism

The thrombogenic potential of the inherited thrombophilias and the probability of thrombosis per pregnancy in affected individuals are shown in Table 27.2.[17,18,43] If the woman without history of VTE is a heterozygote for both FVL and PGM, the probability of thrombosis per pregnancy is about 4.6%.[43] Data from older case-control studies show significant associations between thrombophilias and VTE.[16] The largest prospective cohort study showed no association between FVL and VTE,[20] but when combining the three prospective cohort studies that examined FVL,[20,40,41] there was a statistically significant association (Table 27.3).

Adverse pregnancy outcome

Meta-analyses of case-control studies show many significant associations between various thrombophilias and adverse pregnancy outcomes.[44–46] However, the large individual case-control studies fail to support this contention.[47–49] There are four prospective cohort trials in the literature.[20,40–42] The cumulative summary data of these four studies are shown in Table 27.3. Pre-eclampsia included all cases, and FGR was defined as EFW less than the 10th percentile. Chi square and Fisher's exact test were used to construct this table. The **only significant associations** are:

- VTE with FVL
- late pregnancy loss and pre-eclampsia with hyper-homocysteinemia.

FETAL THROMBOPHILIAS

Fetal carriage of thrombophilic mutations may also have adverse clinical consequences. A case-control study evaluated abortuses for the presence of FVL.[50] The mutation was present more frequently among abortuses than in unselected pregnant women. If the placenta showed > 10% infarction, the fetus was 10 times more likely to have the mutation than when the placenta was normal. Carriers of multiple or homozygous thrombophilic defects were at increased risk of having a birth weight in the lowest quartile or lowest decile in a retrospective study.[51] In a prospective study,[20] there was no statistical significance between fetal thrombophilia and any adverse pregnancy outcome. However, fetal FVL mutation carriage was associated with more frequent pre-eclampsia among African-American women and Hispanic women compared with Caucasian women.

MANAGEMENT

These are usually **two ways of dosing heparin:**

1. **Prophylactic anticoagulation** typically implies low dosing (usually without monitoring, Table 26.4). If prophylactic adjusted-dose, this implies anti Xa level of 0.2–0.4 U/ml.
2. **Therapeutic anticoagulation** implies higher dosing (always **adjusted-dosing**), meaning usually adjusted to anti Xa levels of 0.5–1.2 U/ml (Table 26.5).

Screening

The decision to perform screening should clearly be influenced by:

- the prevalence of the risk factor in the studied population
- whether the information gathered would impact on clinical management.

There is **insufficient evidence to support universal screening**, given the overall low prevalence of thrombophilias in the general population, and the low prevalence of VTE and adverse pregnancy outcomes.

Prior VTE and non-recurrent etiology

It would be reasonable to screen with a full panel any pregnant women with a **prior personal history of VTE** due to a **non-recurring etiology** (e.g. immobilization after an accident). Among women with a history of VTE, older case-control studies have demonstrated that recurrent VTE occurs frequently during pregnancy in thrombophilic women.[52] In a prospective study,[41] the frequency of FVL in women with a history of thrombosis was higher than expected (15 vs 2%), but not the frequency of MTHFR. In another prospective study,[53] pregnant women with a single previous episode of VTE without antepartum anticoagulation had a 2.4% antepartum recurrence of VTE. There were **no recurrences in the 44 non-anticoagulated women who had no evidence of thrombophilia and who also had a previous episode of thrombosis that was associated with a non-recurring risk factor.** Among the 51 women with abnormal laboratory results or a previous episode of idiopathic thrombosis, or both, 5.9% had an antepartum recurrence of VTE. Among **women with a non-recurring cause for the prior VTE and no thrombophilia**, the risk of recurrent antepartum VTE is low, and therefore **routine antepartum prophylaxis with heparin may not be warranted.** Anticoagulation can still be given postpartum.[53] If PC, PS, **heterozygous FVL, or PGM are detected, prophylactic anticoagulation would seem reasonable. If homozygous FVL or PGM, or an ATIII deficiency or a compound heterozygote are detected, full therapeutic anticoagulation would be indicated.** An elevated homocysteine and a low folate, vitamin B_6 or vitamin B_{12} level should prompt replacement. Screening for MTHFR is not recommended.

Prior VTE and recurring etiology

In a woman with a **prior personal history of a VTE** and a **recurring etiology** (i.e. oral contraceptives), **prophylactic anticoagulation** is recommended. Being positive for PC or PS would not change clinical management; thus, screening can be avoided. **Screening would be indicated for FVL, PGM, and ATIII** as homozygous FVL, homozygous PGM, compound heterozygote, or an ATIII deficiency would prompt therapeutic anticoagulation. An elevated homocysteine and a low folate, vitamin B_6, or vitamin B_{12} level should prompt replacement. Screening for MTHFR is not recommended.

Current VTE

In a woman with a **VTE in the current pregnancy**, screening can be performed for **FVL, PGM, and ATIII**. A homozygous FVL, a homozygous PGM, compound heterozygote, or an ATIII deficiency might extend the duration of therapeutic anticoagulation, and once switched over to prophylactic doses, again may extend the duration of treatment.

Table 27.4	*Testing characteristics for different thrombophilias*[55]			
Characteristic	Testing method	Can patients be reliably tested during pregnancy?	Is the test reliable during acute thrombosis?	Is the test reliable while on anticoagulation?
Factor V Leiden	APC resistance assay	No	Yes	Yes
	DNA analysis	Yes	Yes	Yes
Prothrombin gene mutation G20210A	DNA analysis	Yes	Yes	Yes
Protein C deficiency	Protein C activity (<50%)	Yes	No	No
Protein S deficiency	Protein S total and free antigen (<45%)	No	No	No
ATIII deficiency	ATIII activity (<60%)	Yes	No	No
Hyperhomocysteinemia	Fasting plasma homocysteine	Yes	Unclear	Yes
	MTHFR	Yes	Yes	Yes

ATIII, antithrombin III; APC, activated protein C; MTHFR, methylenetetrahydrofolate reductase.

Screening for PC or PS and obtaining a positive result would not change the clinical recommendations for anticoagulation greatly (nor would heterozygous FVL or PGM change recommendations), and therefore screening is not recommended in pregnancy. An elevated homocysteine and a low folate, vitamin B_6, or vitamin B_{12} level should prompt replacement. Screening for MTHFR is not recommended.

Multiple risk factors for VTE

In pregnant women with **multiple risk factors for VTE**[54] (e.g. advanced maternal age (AMA), obese, first-degree relative positive for thrombophilia) who is now postpartum (especially if delivered via cesarean section), it may be reasonable to screen for thrombophilias (full panel) at that time (postpartum), as a positive result may influence the decision to use prophylactic anticoagulation for 6 weeks postpartum.

Family with thrombophilia

In an otherwise **healthy pregnant woman** with no personal history of VTE or adverse pregnancy outcomes, but whose **first-degree relative has a genetic thrombophilia**, there is **insufficient evidence** to recommend any type of screening. Postpartum screening may be reasonable if delivered via cesarean section. If such information has already been screened for and is positive, therapeutic anticoagulation should be offered for homozygous FVL, homozygous PGM, compound heterozygote, or ATIII deficiency. However there is insufficient evidence that prophylactic anticoagulation for PC, PS, heterozygous FVL, or heterozygous PGM will benefit outcome. An elevated

homocysteine and a low folate, vitamin B_6, or vitamin B_{12} level should prompt replacement. Screening for MTHFR is not recommended.

Prior adverse pregnancy outcome

In an otherwise **healthy pregnant woman** with a **prior adverse pregnancy outcome** but no major risk factors for VTE, there is **insufficient evidence** to support screening either antepartum or postpartum. If such information has already been screened for and is positive, therapeutic anticoagulation should be offered for homozygous FVL, homozygous PGM, compound heterozygote or ATIII deficiency. However, there is no convincing evidence that prophylactic anticoagulation for PC, PS, heterozygous FVL, or heterozygous PGM will benefit outcome. An elevated homocysteine and a low folate, vitamin B_6, or vitamin B_{12} level should prompt replacement.

Diagnosis

Table 27.4 describes testing of thrombophilias. Potential causes of false-positive results when testing for thrombophilias include:[55]

- Hyperhomocysteinemia – deficiencies of folic acid, vitamin B_{12}, or vitamin B_6; older age, renal failure, smoking.
- Protein C activity – liver disease, childhood, use of oral anticoagulants, vitamin K deficiency, disseminated intravascular coagulation (DIC), the presence of antibodies against protein C.
- Protein S total and free antigen – pregnancy, liver disease, childhood, use of oral anticoagulants, vitamin K

deficiency, DIC, use of oral contraceptives, nephrotic syndrome, the presence of antibodies to protein S.

- Antithrombin III activity – liver disease, use of heparin therapy, nephrotic syndrome, DIC.

Therapy

There are only two trials on inherited thrombophilias and pregnancy complications, so, in effect, there is **insufficient evidence** to make any recommendation in this area.

Pregnancy loss ≥ 10 weeks and thrombophilia

A prospective randomized, non-blinded, non-placebo-controlled trial evaluated the effect of thromboprophylaxis in women with **one unexplained pregnancy loss** at ≥ 10th week of amenorrhea and either heterozygous **factor V Leiden** mutation, **prothrombin G20210A** gene mutation, or **protein S deficiency** (free antigen < 55%).[56] Women were given 5 mg of folic acid daily before conception, to be continued during pregnancy, and either **low-dose aspirin** 100 mg daily **or** low molecular weight heparin (LMWH) enoxaparin 40 mg starting at 8 weeks. LMWH was associated with a higher (86 vs 29%) incidence of a **healthy live birth**, and lower incidence of low birth weight (LBW) (10 vs 30%). No significant side effects of the treatments could be evidenced in patients or newborns. This was not a blinded trial. As there is no argument to prove that low-dose aspirin may have been deleterious, these results support enoxaparin use during such at-risk pregnancies.

Recurrent pregnancy losses and thrombophilia

See also Chapter 14 of *Obstetric Evidence Based Guidelines*.

A recent cohort study showed that in women with a **thrombophilia** (heterozygous factor V, activated protein C resistance, MTHFR 677 TT genotype, protein S deficiency, heterozygous prothrombin G20210A, ATIII deficiency, hyperhomocysteinemia, and/or protein C deficiency) and a **history of ≥ 3 first trimester losses, ≥ 2 second trimester losses, or a fetal death in the third trimester**, enoxaparin 40 mg/day was associated with an approximate 80% rate of **live births**, similar to enoxaparin 80 mg/day.[57]

Hyperhomocysteinemia

There are no trials to assess interventions for the pregnant woman with hyperhomocysteinemia. It might be reasonable to suggest safe therapy aimed at normalizing the homocysteine level, with folic acid 4 mg once a day, in addition to vitamin B_6 25 mg three to four times a day, and vitamin B_{12} 100 mg once a day, but counseling should emphasize that this therapy has not been tested in trials.

For **antepartum testing, delivery, anesthesia,** and **postpartum/breastfeeding,** see Chapter 26.

REFERENCES

1. Egeberg O. Inherited antithrombin III deficiency causing thrombophilia. Thromb Diath Haemorrh 1965; 13: 516–30. [II-3]
2. Beck EA, Charache P, Jackson DP. A new inherited coagulation disorder caused by an abnormal fibrinogen ('fibrinogen Baltimore'). Nature 1965; 208: 143–5. [II-3]
3. Griffin JH, Evatt B, Zimmerman TS, Kleiss AJ, Wideman C. Deficiency of protein C in congenital thrombotic disease. J Clin Invest 1981; 68: 1370–3. [II-3]
4. Comp PC, Esmon CT. Recurrent venous thromboembolism in patients with a partial deficiency of protein S. N Engl J Med 1984; 311: 1525–8. [II-2]
5. Koeleman BP, Reitsma PH, Bertina RM. Familial thrombophilia: a complex genetic disorder. Semin Hematol 1997; 34: 256–64. [II-2]
6. Dahlback B, Carlsson M, Svensson PJ. Familial thrombophilia due to a previously unrecognized mechanism characterized by poor anticoagulant response to activated protein C: prediction of a cofactor to activated protein C. Proc Natl Acad Sci USA 1993; 90: 1004–8. [II-3]
7. Bertina RM, Koeleman BP, Koster T, et al. Mutation in blood coagulation factor V associated with resistance to activated protein C. Nature 1994; 369: 64–7. [II-2]
8. Poort SR, Rosendaal FR, Reitsma PH, Bertina RM. A common genetic variation in the 3′-untranslated region of the prothrombin gene is associated with elevated plasma prothrombin levels and an increase in venous thrombosis. Blood 1996; 88: 3698–703. [II-2]
9. Mudd SH, Skovby F, Levy HL, et al. The natural history of homocystinuria due to cystathionine beta-synthase deficiency. Am J Hum Genet 1985; 37: 1–31. [II-3]
10. Seligsohn U, Zivelin A. Thrombophilia as a multigenic disorder. Thromb Haemost 1997; 78: 297–301. [II-2]
11. Lockwood CJ. Inherited thrombophilias in pregnant patients. Prenat Neonat Med 2001; 6: 3–14. [review]
12. Greer IA. Thrombosis in pregnancy: maternal and fetal issues. Lancet 1999; 353: 1258–65. [review]
13. Thromboembolism in pregnancy. ACOG Practice Bulletin, No. 19, August 2000. [review]
14. Lindqvist P, Dahlback B, Marsal K. Thrombotic risk during pregnancy: a population study. Obstet Gynecol 1999; 94: 595–9. [II-2]
15. Macklon NS, Greer IA. Venous thromboembolic disease in obstetrics and gynaecology: the Scottish experience. Scott Med J 1996; 41: 83–6. [II-2]
16. Grandone E, Margaglione M, Colaizzo D, et al. Genetic susceptibility to pregnancy-related venous thromboembolism: roles of factor V Leiden, prothrombin G20210A, and methylenetetrahydrofolate reductase C677T mutations. Am J Obstet Gynecol 1998; 179: 1324–8. [II-2]
17. Franco RF, Reitsma PH. Genetic risk factors of venous thrombosis. Hum Genet 2001; 109: 369–84. [II-2]
18. Haverkate F, Samama M. Familial dysfibrinogenaemia and thrombophilia. Report on a study of the SSC Subcommittee on Fibrinogen. Thromb Haemost 1995; 73: 151–61. [II-2]
19. Lockwood C. Inherited thrombophilias in pregnant patients: detection and treatment paradigm. Obstet Gynecol 2002; 99: 333–41. [review]
20. Dizon-Townsend D, Miller C, Sibai B, et al. The relationship of the factor V Leiden mutation and pregnancy outcomes for mother and fetus. Obstet Gynecol 2005; 106: 517–24. [II-1]

21. Lockwood CJ. Heritable coagulopathies in pregnancy. Obstet Gynecol Surv 1999; 54: 754. [review]

22. Walker MC, Garner PR, Keely EJ, et al. Changes in activated protein C resistance during normal pregnancy. Am J Obstet Gynecol 1997; 77: 162. [II-3]

23. De Stefano V, Leone G, Mastrangelo S, et al. Clinical manifestations and management of inherited thrombophilia: retrospective analysis and follow-up after diagnosis of 238 patients with congenital deficiency of antithrombin III, protein C, protein S. Thromb Haemost 1994; 72: 352–8. [II-3]

24. Middledorp S, Henkens CM, Koopman MM, et al. The incidence of venous thromboembolism in family members of patients with factor V Leiden mutation and venous thrombosis. Ann Intern Med 1998; 128: 15–20. [II-2]

25. Kingdom JC, Kaufmann P. Oxygen and placental villous development: Origins of fetal hypoxia. Placenta 1997; 18: 613–21. [II-3]

26. Kang SS, Wong PW, Susmano A, et al. Thermolabile methylenetetrahydrofolate reductase: an inherited risk factor for coronary artery disease. Am J Hum Genet 1991; 48: 536–45. [II-3]

27. Frosst P, Blom HJ, Milos R, et al. A candidate genetic risk factor for vascular disease: a common mutation in methylenetetrahydrofolate reductase. Nat Genet 1995; 10: 111–13. [II-3]

28. Gallagher PM, Meleady R, Shields DC, et al. Homocysteine and risk of premature coronary heart disease. Evidence for a common gene mutation. Circulation 1996; 94: 2154–8. [II-3]

29. Guttormsen AB, Ueland PM, Nesthus I, et al. Determinants and vitamin responsiveness of intermediate hyperhomocysteinemia (> or =40 micromol/liter). The Hordaland Homocysteine Study. J Clin Invest 1996; 98: 2174–83. [II-3]

30. Harmon DL, Woodside JV, Yarnell JW, et al. The common 'thermolabile' variant of methylenetetrahydrofolate reductase is a major determinant of mild hyperhomocysteinemia. QJM 1996; 89: 571–7. [II-3]

31. Kluijtmans LA, Young IS, Boreham CA, et al. Genetic and nutritional factors contributing to hyperhomocysteinemia in young adults. Blood 2003; 101: 2483–8. [II-3]

32. Robinson K, Arheart K, Refsum H, et al. Low circulating folate and vitamin B_6 concentrations: risk factors for stroke, peripheral vascular disease, and coronary artery disease. European COMCAC Group. Circulation 1998; 97: 437–43. [II-2]

33. Rimm EB, Willett WC, Hu FB, et al. Folate and vitamin B_6 from diet and supplements in relation to risk of coronary heart disease among women. JAMA 1998; 279: 359–64. [II-2]

34. Voutilainen S, Rissanen TH, Virtanen J, Lakka TA, Salonen JT. Low dietary folate intake is associated with an excess incidence of acute coronary events: The Kuopio Ischemic Heart Disease Risk Factor Study. Circulation 2001; 103: 2674–80. [II-1]

35. Vermeulen EG, Stehouwer CD, Twisk JW, et al. Effect of homocysteine-lowering treatment with folic acid plus vitamin B_6 on progression of subclinical atherosclerosis: a randomised, placebo-controlled trial. Lancet 2000; 355: 517–22. [RCT]

36. Selhub J, Jacques PF, Wilson PW, Rush D, Rosenberg IH. Vitamin status and intake as primary determinants of homocysteinemia in an elderly population. JAMA 1993; 270: 2693–8. [II-1]

37. Ubbink JR, Vermaak WJ, van der Merwe A, Becker PJ. Vitamin B-12, vitamin B-6, and folate nutritional status in men with hyperhomocysteinemia. Am J Clin Nutr 1993; 57: 47–53. [II-2]

38. Zotz RB, Gerhardt A, Scharf RE. Inherited thrombophilia and gestational venous thromboembolism. Best Pract Res Clin Haematol 2003; 16: 243–59. [review]

39. Haemostasis and Thrombosis Task Force, British Committee for Standards in Haematology. Investigation and management of heritable thrombophilia. Br J Haematol 2001; 114: 512–28. [review]

40. Lindqvist PG, Svensson PJ, Marsal K, et al. Activated protein C resistance (FVQ506) and pregnancy. Thromb Haemost 1999; 81: 532–7. [II-1]

41. Murphy RP, Donoghue R, Nallen R. Prospective evaluation of the risk conferred by factor V Leiden and thermolabile methylenetetrahydrofolate reductase polymorphisms in pregnancy. Arterioscler Thromb Vasc Biol 2000; 20: 266–70. [II-1]

42. Murakamis S, Matsubara N, Miyakaw S, et al. The relation between homocysteine concentration and methylenetetrahydrofolate reductase genetic polymorphism in pregnant women. J Obstet Gynaecol Res 2001; 27: 349–52. [II-1]

43. Gerhardt A, Scharf RE, Beckmann MW, et al. Prothrombin and factor V mutations in women with a history of thrombosis during pregnancy and the puerperium. N Engl J Med 2000; 342: 374–80. [II-2]

44. Rey E, Kahn SR, David M, Shrier, I. Thrombophilic disorders and fetal loss: a meta-analysis. Lancet 2003; 361: 901–8. [II-2]

45. Howley HE, Walker M, Rodger MA. A systematic review of the association between factor V Leiden or prothrombin gene variant and intrauterine growth restriction. Am J Obstet Gynecol 2005; 192: 694–708. [II-2]

46. Lin J, August P. Genetic thrombophilias and preeclampsia: a meta-analysis. Obstet Gynecol 2005; 105: 182–92. [II-2]

47. Roque H, Paidas MJ, Funai EF, Kuczynski E, Lockwood CJ. Maternal thrombophilias are not associated with early pregnancy loss. Thromb Haemost 2004; 91: 290–5. [II-2]

48. Infante-Rivard C, Rivard GE, Yotov WV, et al. Absence of association of thrombophilia polymorphisms with intrauterine growth restriction. N Engl J Med 2002; 347: 19–25. [II-2]

49. Prochazka M, Happach C, Marsal K, et al. Factor V Leiden in pregnancies complicated by placental abruption. BJOG 2003; 110: 462–6. [II-2]

50. Dizon-Townson DS, Meline L, Nelson LM, Varner M, Ward K. Fetal carriers of the factor V Leiden mutation are prone to miscarriage and placental infarction. Am J Obstet Gynecol 1997; 177: 402–5. [II-2]

51. von Kries R, Junker R, Oberle D, Kosch A, Nowak-Gottl U. Foetal growth restriction in children with prothrombotic risk factors. Thromb Haemost 2001; 86: 1012–16. [II-2]

52. Simioni P, Tormene D, Prandoni P, Girolami A. Pregnancy-related recurrent events in thrombophilic women with previous venous thromboembolism. Thromb Haemost 2001; 86: 929. [II-2]

53. Brill-Edwards P, Ginsberg JS, Gent M, et al. Safety of withholding heparin in pregnant women with a history of venous thromboembolism. Recurrence of Clot in This Pregnancy Study Group. N Engl J Med 2000; 343: 1439–44. [II-1, $n=125$]

54. Lindqvist PG, Olofsson P, Dahlback B. Use of selective factor V Leiden screening in pregnancy to identify candidates for anticoagulation. Obstet Gynecol 2002; 100: 332–6. [II-3]

55. Seligsohn U, Lubetsky A. Medical progress: genetic susceptibility to venous thrombosis. N Engl J Med 2001; 344: 1222–31. [review]

56. Gris JC, Mercier E, Quere I, et al. Low-molecular-weight heparin versus low-dose aspirin in women with one fetal loss and a constitutional thrombophilic disorder. Blood 2004; 103: 3695–9. [RCT, $n=160$]

57. Brenner B, Hoffman R, Carp H, Dulitsky M, Younis J; LIVE-ENOX Investigators. Efficacy and safety of two doses of enoxaparin in women with thrombophilia and recurrent pregnancy loss: the LIVE-ENOX study. J Thromb Haemost 2005; 3: 227–9. [II-1]

28

Hepatitis A

James Airoldi

KEY POINTS

- The vast majority of hepatitis A virus (HAV) infections are **self-limited**.
- There is **no perinatal transmission of HAV.**
- The inactived live HAV **vaccines** can be **safely used for prevention**, including during pregnancy, if a patient is at risk for HAV exposure.
- **Exposed pregnant women** can receive **HAIg (hepatitis A immunoglobulin) injections**, which are > 85% effective in preventing HAV infection if given within 2 weeks of exposure.
- Therapy of acute HAV infection in pregnancy is supportive.

DIAGNOSIS

Anti-HAV IgM (immunoglobulin M [IgM] antibody to hepatitis A) is the diagnostic criterion for acute hepatitis A virus (HAV) infection.

SYMPTOMS

Fever, malaise, decreased appetite, nausea, abdominal discomfort, dark urine, jaundice.

EPIDEMIOLOGY/INCIDENCE

Incidence is ≤ 1/1000 pregnancies.[1] About 17 000 cases in the USA in 1999 (down almost 50% since 1995).[2] About 40% of population is HAV IgG+ (usually immune from old infection).

GENETICS

RNA picornavirus (family of enteroviruses).

ETIOLOGY/BASIC PATHOPHYSIOLOGY

Fecal/oral contact with infected person or contaminated food/water; rarely from blood transmission. Most US cases are from person-to-person or sexual contact transmission during outbreaks. The average incubation period is 28 (15–49) days; then abrupt onset. HAV infection can be symptomatic (adults) but also asymptomatic (mostly children < 6 years old). Symptoms last usually < 2 months (up to 6 months in 10–15% of patients). **The vast majority of cases are self-limited.**

RISK FACTORS/ASSOCIATIONS

Increased risk of acquiring HAV infection in:

- travelers to developing/high prevalence countries
- homosexuals and other men who have sex with men
- intravenous drug abusers
- people who work with non-human primates
- people with chronic liver disease.

COMPLICATIONS

Mortality is < 0.3%. A chronic carrier state does not exist.

PREGNANCY CONSIDERATIONS

No perinatal transmission.

PREGNANCY MANAGEMENT
Work-up

HAV IgM and IgG (consider rest of hepatitis work-up – see Chapters 29 and 30). Check AST/ALT (aspartate aminotransferase/alanine aminotransferase), bilirubin.

Prevention/preconception counseling

Havrix (Smith Kline Beecham) and VAQTA (Merck) are inactivated live virus vaccines. Two intramuscular (IM) doses (Havrix 1 ml [50 U] or VAQTA 1 g [1440 U]), given 6–12 months apart, are needed to confer immunity. They can be safely used during pregnancy if a patient is at risk for HAV exposure. Immunity after vaccination lasts > 10 years.

Therapy

Acute infection

No anti-HAV drug is available at present. Supportive therapies can be offered to outpatients. Consider hospitalization only in rare cases of severe dehydration, encephalopathy, or coagulopathy.

Exposure

Exposed pregnant women can receive HAIg (hepatitis A immunoglobulin) injections (0.02 mg/kg IM), which are > 85% effective in preventing HAV infection if given within 2 weeks of exposure (close house or sexual contact).

Antepartum testing

Not indicated.

Delivery

Follow obstetric indications.

Anesthesia

No particular precautions necessary.

Postpartum/breastfeeding

Breastfeeding is not contraindicated.

REFERENCES

1. Viral hepatitis in pregnancy. ACOG Educational Bulletin No. 248, July 1998. [review]
2. APGO Educational Series on Women's Health Issues. Hepatitis B and C: the Ob/Gyn's role. APGO, Maryland, 2002. [good pregnancy review]

29

Hepatitis B

James Airoldi

KEY POINTS

- All women should be **screened for hepatitis B virus (HBV) by HBsAg during pregnancy.**
- **Vertical transmission** of HBV occurs in **90% of women with HBeAg+, and 90% of women with acute hepatitis in the third trimester.**
- **Vertical transmission** can occur in **10–20% of women with HBsAg + without the above conditions.**
- **90% of newborns infected with HBV develop chronic hepatitis B without intervention,** with 25% of chronic hepatitis B carriers eventually dying of complications (cirrhosis, hepatocellular cancer) of HBV infection.
- **All neonates born to women with HBsAg + should receive HBIg and hepatitis B vaccine within 12 hours of birth. This prevents 85–95% of neonatal HBV infection.**

DIAGNOSIS/DEFINITION (TABLE 29.1)

- Acute: HBsAg +, HBcAb +, HBcIgM +, HBsAb –.
- Chronic: HBsAg + >6 months, HBsAb–.[1,2]

The virus can be found by polymerase chain reaction (PCR) in blood, urine, feces, seminal fluid, saliva, and the gastrointestinal (GI) tract. The initial differential diagnosis of hepatitis includes hepatitis A, B or C viruses (HAV, HBV, HCV), cytomegalovirus (CMV), Epstein–Barr virus, varicella zoster virus (VZV), coxsackie B virus, herpes simplex virus (HSV), rubella virus, and autoimmune viruses.

SYMPTOMS

Only 30–50% of patients acutely infected have symptoms such as loss of appetite, malaise, nausea and vomiting, etc. About 10% have jaundice. The onset is usually insidious.

EPIDEMIOLOGY/INCIDENCE

More than 400 million people worldwide have chronic HBV infection. Over 300 000 liver cancers per year are due to HBV (>50% of 530 000 total liver cancer cases – 118 000 cases due to HCV – so hepatitis is responsible for 82% of all liver cancers). One-third of the word's population (2 billion people) have been infected with HBV: 5% overall develop **chronic HBV infection, but 90% in children < 1 year old,** and only 2% in persons > 5 years old. **About 25% of HBV chronic infection** patients **die** of liver disease (> 1 million per year worldwide – 0.5% mortality).[3]

The vaccine is about 95% effective against HBV. More than 90 countries implement universal vaccination: the worldwide eradication of HBV is a distinct possibility, but far away at present. More than 75% of chronic HBV infection patients are Chinese, second is subSaharan Africa (10–20% incidence in these countries). Incidence is 0.2–0.5% in North America, Europe, and Australia. The incidence of HBV infection has decreased >60% in the USA from 1985 to 1995.

GENETICS

Small partially double-stranded DNA virus ('Dane particle'). There are seven major HBV genotypes.

ETIOLOGY/BASIC PATHOPHYSIOLOGY

HB virus exposure, then incubation of about 60–90 days (depends on amount of viral exposure), then laboratory changes (see Table 29.1).
Antigens:

's' surface – infected. If present > 6 months, chronic HBV infection.
'c' core
'e' – infectious.

Antibodies:

's' – immune
'c' – covers 'window' period, and usually precedes HBsAb conversion.

About 5% of HBV infections become chronic. This can lead to cirrhosis, hepatocellular carcinoma, and death.

Test	Results	Interpretation	Vertical transmission
HBsAg anti-HBc anti-HBs	Negative Negative Negative	Susceptible	0%
HBsAg anti-HBc anti-HBs	Negative Positive Positive	Immune due to natural infection	0%
HBsAg anti-HBc anti-HBs	Negative Negative Positive	Immune due to hepatitis B vaccination	0%
HBsAg anti-HBc anti-HBc IgM anti-HBs	Positive Positive Positive Negative	Acutely infected	First trimester: 10% Third trimester: 80–90% HBeAg −: 10–20% HBeAg +: 90%
HBsAg anti-HBc anti-HBc IgM anti-HBs	Positive Positive Negative Negative	Chronically infected	First trimester: 10% Third trimester: 80–90% HBeAg −: 10–20% HBeAg +: 90%
HBsAg anti-HBc anti-HBs	Negative Positive Negative	Four interpretations possible: 1. May be recovering from acute HBV infection 2. May be distantly immune and test is not sensitive enough to detect very low level of anti-HBs in serum 3. May be susceptible with false-positive anti-HBc 4. May be an undetectable level of HBsAg present in the serum and the person is actually a carrier	0%

Table 29.1   *Interpretation of the hepatitis B panel*

CLASSIFICATION

See Table 29.1.

RISK FACTORS/ASSOCIATIONS

Transmission is parenteral (percutaneous) and sexual (permucosal). The highest risk of chronic HBV infection is perinatal transmission from HBV-infected mothers. Twenty-five percent of sexual contacts become positive. Intravenous drug abuse (IVDA), sexually transmitted diseases (STDs), multiple sex partners, house contacts, mental institution/prison, and acupuncture are other risk factors, as is the rare HBV-infected blood transfusion. HBV-infected patients are at higher risk of HIV (human immunodeficiency virus) and HCV infections.

COMPLICATIONS

Over 90% of patients resolve the infection (clear the s and e Ag), and develop HBsAb. About 5% develop chronic hepatitis B (maintain HBsAg). Of these, most are asymptomatic with normal liver function tests (LFTs) and no HBV detectable by PCR. The other 15–30% of chronic hepatitis B has persistent viral replication: these patients can develop cirrhosis and hepatocellular cancer. Mortality is 0.5–1%.

PREGNANCY CONSIDERATIONS

Vertical transmission occurs in about **10–20% of HbsAg+ mothers**, if no immunoprophylaxis. **If HBsAg+ and HBeAg+, vertical transmission is 80–90%; about 90% of neonates will become chronic carriers.** Vertical transmission is lowest (< 10%) if HbeAb+. **Vertical transmission** is also **trimester dependent: first trimester 10%, third trimester 80–90%**, of which 90% occurs because of intrapartum exposure to blood and secretions. Only about 10% of all transmission is transplacental hematogenous or from breastfeeding. Pregnancy course is otherwise not altered by HBV (same incidences of pregnancy loss, congenital anomalies, etc.), except for higher preterm birth rates for acute third trimester HBV infection.

MANAGEMENT

Principles

The main goal is prevention of vertical transmission.

Work-up

HBsAg, HBsAb, HBcAb, HBcIgM, HBeAg. It is important to specifically request the HBcIgM as this helps to differentiate between an acute or chronic infection. See Table 29.1 for interpretation of diagnosis, and disease stage.

Other tests rarely necessary in pregnancy:

- HBV DNA by quantitative PCR (to monitor the progression of disease and the effectiveness of treatment).
- Liver biopsy (for initial assessment of severity of disease for chronic HBV).

Prevention/preconception counseling

Vaccinate preconceptionally or early in pregnancy every reproductive-age woman who is susceptible. **Universal maternal screening with HBsAg is recommended at first visit or preconceptionally.**

If HBsAg+, test for HBsAb, eAg, eAb, and cAb. **All HBsAg+ women should have their neonate receive HBIg and HB vaccine within 12 hours of birth.** This combination prevents >90% of vertical transmission.

If HBsAg−, consider vaccine in pregnancy for high-risk groups such as STDs, HIV+, HepC+, IVDA, etc.

Prenatal care

Universal maternal screening with HBsAg at first visit or preconceptionally. If HBsAg+, send work-up as above. If HBsAg−, no further work-up. Consider repeating in early third trimester in high-risk groups (sex with acutely or chronically hepatitis B-infected person, sex workers, multiple/new partner, multiple STDs, HIV, IVDA, occupational contact with blood, receivers of unscreened blood, hemodialysis patients, household contacts of infected patients, persons in prisons, institutions or countries with high rates of HBV infections).

Therapy

Main intervention therapies

HB vaccine

Series of three intramuscular (IM) injections over 6 months of recombinant DNA. 95% seroconversion (HBsAb+ and immune) rate. It is safe in pregnancy and for neonate.

Recombivax HB (Merck): adults >20 years old = 10 mg (1 ml); 11–19 years old = 5 (0.5); <11 years old = 2.5 (0.25); within 12 hours of delivery and maternal HBeAg+ = 5; within 12 hours of delivery and maternal HBeAg− = 2.5. Engerix-B (Smith Kline Beecham): adults >20 years old = 20 mg (1 ml); 11–19 years old = 20 (1); <11 years old = 10 (0.5); within 12 hours of delivery and maternal HBeAg+ = 10; within 12 hours of delivery and maternal HBeAg−= 10.

HBIg

Immunoglobulins specific for HB (0.5 ml/kg IM for adult; 0.13 ml/kg IM for neonate). It is safe in pregnancy and for neonate.

Conditions

Acute hepatitis B in pregnancy

Diagnosis: document conversion of HBsAg− to +. Check all labs as above. Outpatient supportive therapy. Consider hospitalization for severe anemia, diabetes mellitus, severe dehydration, coagulopathy, bilirubin >15 mg/dl. Consider **interferon** (see Chapter 30 and below). Vitamin K 10 mg IM (or po) every 8 hours × 3 can be given to pregnant women with coagulopathy.

Exposure to HB in pregnancy

Check all labs as above. If HBsAg− and sAb−, give HBIg and HB vaccine: this combination will prevent 75% of transmission. Must give HBIg within 14 days of sexual contact. Repeat HBIg within 1 month if blood or mucous membrane exposure.

Vertical transmission prevention

All newborns born to women with HBsAg+ should receive HBIg and HB vaccine within 12 hours of birth.[1,2] This combination is about 95% effective in preventing neonatal HBV infection.

Maternal chronic hepatitis B

No maternal treatment aimed at interfering with disease progression is usually implemented in pregnancy because of safety issues with standard therapy for the non-pregnant adult. This may be reconsidered in the near future, especially as more reassuring data become available for interferon. Therapy for non-pregnant adults is indicated if ALT (alanine transaminase) >1.5 upper limit of normal, *and* HBV DNA >about 150 000 (exact cut-off controversial). HBV DNA <150 000 and undetectable HbeAg are the goals of treatment.[4] Before therapy, liver biopsy may be considered as baseline.

Drugs

Interferon α – immunomodulator

Safety: see Chapter 30. Efficacy: 35% interferon α vs 15% placebo for achieving above goals.

Lamivudine – nucleoside analog

Safety: not safe in pregnancy. Efficacy: >95% achieve < 150 000 HBV DNA copies; can reverse cirrhosis of the liver.

Others

Adefovir dipivoxil and other new nucleoside analogs have no pregnancy data yet.

All the above therapies can reduce HBV replication and histological activity. The future of HBV medical therapy is probably combination therapy.[4] Liver transplantation is for patients not responding to medical therapy.

Antepartum testing

Antepartum testing is not indicated.

Delivery

Delivery follows obstetric indications.

Anesthesia

No particular precautions are necessary.

Postpartum/breastfeeding

Breastfeeding is not contraindicated, as long as the neonate receives HBIg and HB vaccine as above.

RARE/RELATED

Hepatitis D virus is an incomplete RNA virus that can superinfect 20–25% of chronic HBV-infected patients. HDV infection worsens chronic HBV infection, so that 25% of patients may die from disease. If HBV is prevented, HDV infection is prevented, too. HDV has no effect on pregnancy or the fetus/neonate.

REFERENCES

1. Viral hepatitis in pregnancy. ACOG Educational Bulletin No. 248, July 1998. [review]
2. APGO Educational Series on Women's Health Issues. Hepatitis B and C: the Ob/Gyn's role. APGO, Maryland, 2002. [good pregnancy review]
3. Lai CL, Ratziu V, Yuen MF, Poynard T. Viral hepatitis B. Lancet 2003; 362: 2089–94. [general review, non-pregnant]
4. Lok ASF. The maze of treatments for hepatitis B. N Engl J Med 2005; 352: 2743–6 [review, non-pregnant]

30

Hepatitis C

James Airoldi

KEY POINTS

- Chronic hepatitis C (HCV) infection is defined by HCV IgG + with detectable HCV RNA. Chronic active HCV infection is defined as **chronic HCV infection with abnormal liver function tests**.
- HCV is **acquired** via infected blood, sexual contact, or mother-to-infant (vertical transmission).
- Complications of chronic HCV infection include **cirrhosis** and **hepatocellular carcinoma**.
- **Mother-to-infant transmission** is diagnosed by **positive serum HCV RNA on two occasions 3–4 months apart after the infant is 2 months old and/or anti-HCV detected after the infant is 18 months old**. Co-infection **with HIV and high maternal viral load** are associated with a higher risk of transmission.
- **Risk factors** for HCV should be avoided to prevent HCV infection, and used for screening.
- HCV-positive pregnant women should be worked up with **HCV RNA viral load; hepatitis B surface antigen (HBsAg); liver function testing; human immunodeficiency virus (HIV) screening; gastroenterology referral; and sexually transmitted diseases (STD) screening**.
- **Treatment** for HCV chronic infection with efficacious therapy (pegylated interferon-α and ribavirin) for non-pregnant adults **cannot be used during or immediately prior to pregnancy**, because of teratogenicity of ribavirin.
- In **HCV-positive but HIV-negative women, cesarean delivery should be reserved for obstetric indications**.
- **Breastfeeding** is generally not considered to be a risk factor for vertical transmission of HCV in non-HIV infected women. Breastfeeding is instead contraindicated in women with both HCV and HIV infections.
- **Therapy** with ribavirin and alpha interferon should be **started postpartum** for the same indications as in other non-pregnant adults.

DIAGNOSIS/DEFINITION (TABLE 30.1)

- Acute: HCV IgM +.
- **Chronic: HCV IgG + with detectable HCV DNA.**
- **Chronic active disease: HCV IgG + with detectable HCV DNA and abnormal liver function tests (LFTs).**

The virus can be found by polymerase chain reaction (PCR) in blood, urine, feces, seminal fluid, saliva, and the gastrointestinal (GI) tract. The initial differential diagnosis of hepatitis includes hepatitis A, B or C viruses (HAV, HBV, HCV), cytomegalovirus (CMV), Epstein–Barr virus, varicella-zoster virus (VZV), coxsackie B virus, herpes simplex virus (HSV), rubella virus, and autoimmune viruses.

SYMPTOMS

Most HCV infections are asymptomatic (75%). Symptomatic patients present with malaise, fever, abdominal pains, and jaundice.

EPIDEMIOLOGY/INCIDENCE

It is found that 0.6–4.5% of pregnant US women have HCV antibodies, with considerable worldwide geographic

Table 30.1	Definitions of various types of HCV infections
HCV	HCV Ab positive
Chronic HCV	HCV Ab positive, and HCV RNA positive
Chronic active HCV	HCV Ab positive, and HCV RNA positive, and elevated LFTs

HCV, hepatitis C virus (infection); Ab, antibody; LFTs, liver function tests.

variation. HCV is the most common chronic bloodborne infection in the USA, and is responsible for 20–40% of all cases of acute hepatitis. **Worldwide, over 170 million people are chronically infected with HCV.** It is found that 1.8% (3.9 million) of non-institutionalized US citizens carry antibodies; 74% of these individuals (2.7 million) have detectable viral RNA in their serum (chronic disease). The prevalence is projected to decrease from the current 1.8% to about 1% by the year 2030. On the contrary, the prevalence of liver disease caused by HCV is on the rise. This is because of the significant lag time, often 20 years or longer between the onset of infection and clinical manifestations of liver disease.

GENETICS

Single-stranded RNA virus; striking genetic heterogeneity, including six major genotypes, with rapid accumulation of mutations.

ETIOLOGY/BASIC PATHOPHYSIOLOGY

HCV is acquired via infected blood, sexual contact, or mother-to-infant (vertical transmission). The incubation time is usually 30–60 days. Chronic HCV (the presence of serum RNA) develops in 75–85% of adult and pediatric patients. The course of chronic HCV infection is usually insidious. Chronic active disease (elevation in LFTs) develops in 60–70% of chronic HCV infection.

CLASSIFICATION

Genotype 1 (subtypes 1a and 1b) is most common in the USA, and is associated with lower response to antiviral therapy.

RISK FACTORS/ASSOCIATIONS (TABLE 30.2)

Up to 40% of HCV-infected women have no risk factors. HCV can be found in semen[1] and acquired through artificial insemination.[2]

COMPLICATIONS

Complications of chronic infection include **cirrhosis** (10–20%) and **hepatocellular carcinoma** (1–5%).

Table 30.2   *Risk factors for HCV infection*

- History of blood transfusion or exposure to blood products
- History of intravenous drug abuse
- History of multiple sexually transmitted diseases
- HIV infection
- Hepatitis B viral infection
- Sexual partner who abuses intravenous drugs or has HIV, HBV, or HCV infection
- Three or more lifetime sexual partners
- Incarceration
- History of body piercing and tattooing
- Recipient of organ transplants before 1992
- Unexplained elevated transaminases
- Patient or staff members involved in chronic dialysis programs
- Participant in in-vitro fertilization programs from anonymous donors

HCV, hepatitis C virus; HBV, hepatitis B virus; HIV, human immunodeficiency virus.

Table 30.3   *Rate of vertical transmission of hepatitis C[3]*

	Weighted rate[a] (%)
Anti-HCV only	1.7
Viremic (HCV RNA positive)	4.3
HIV positive	19.4
HIV negative	3.5
Injection drug use	8.6

HCV, hepatitis C virus; HIV, human immunodeficiency virus.

[a]Weighted rate adjusts for sample size of study and variance.

PREGNANCY CONSIDERATIONS
Mother-to-infant transmission

Diagnostic confirmation of vertical transmission is obtained with **positive serum HCV RNA on two occasions 3–4 months apart after the infant is 2 months old and/or anti-HCV detected after the infant is 18 months old.** Table 30.3 summarizes transmission rates compiled from 77 studies and 383 cases of mother-to-infant transmission.[3] **Co-infection with HIV greatly increases** vertical transmission.[4] Chronic HCV infection and HIV co-infection are consistently associated with increased transmission. Highly-active antiretroviral therapy (HAART) has been shown to decrease HCV transmission in HCV-HIV co-infected women.[5] Vertical transmission correlates with **high maternal HCV viral load,**[3,5,6,7] but a specific cut-off that predicts transmission has not been identified. Vertical transmission **does not correlate with mode of delivery** in non-HIV women. HIV co-infected women delivered by cesarean section were 60% less likely to have an HCV-infected child than those delivered vaginally.[8] It is controversial whether prolonged rupture of the membranes (i.e. for more than 6 hours) increases risk. Two recent cohort studies showed an increase in HCV transmission with rupture of membranes greater than 6 hours.[5,7] The use of a **scalp electrode is discouraged**. There is no association between gestational age and risk of transmission. Amniocentesis does not appear to significantly increase the risk,[9] but very few studies have addressed this subject. If amniocentesis is requested, try to avoid a transplacental route.

MANAGEMENT
Prevention

There is no HCV vaccine available. **Risk factors** for HCV (see Table 30.2) should be **avoided**. Prevention of complication of liver disease includes avoidance of alcohol and hepatotoxic medicines (including alternative and herbal remedies) and foods.

Principles
Effect of pregnancy on hepatitis C

Pregnancy does not affect the clinical course of acute or chronic hepatitis C. There is an improvement in biochemical markers of liver damage in HCV-positive women during pregnancy.[10] There is a linear increase in HCV viremia throughout pregnancy,[1] 50% above baseline.[10]

Effect of hepatitis C on pregnancy

HCV vertical transmission and its consequences can affect the neonate. Chronic active hepatitis C is associated with an increased incidence of preterm delivery and intrauterine growth restriction.[11,12] Long-term complications of HCV infection for either the mother or the baby can lead to cirrhosis, cancer, and mortality.

Screening

It is not cost-effective to screen universally for HCV in pregnancy. Screening is recommended in women with risk factors for HCV infection (see Table 30.2). Screening is performed with anti-HCV (HCV IgG) antibody. Universal screening may become recommended when therapy for HCV in pregnancy is deemed safe and effective.

Work-up

Any woman with anti-HCV (HCV IgG) antibody should have **HCV RNA viral load, hepatitis B surface antigen** (HBsAg), LFTs, human immunodeficiency virus (HIV) screening, gastroenterology referral, and sexually transmitted diseases (STD) screening.

Preconception/pregnancy counseling

The effect of pregnancy on HCV infection and vice versa should be reviewed. Counseling of the pregnant woman with HCV infection should include review of risk factors known to increase mother-to-infant transmission (HIV co-infection; HCV viremia, especially with high viral loads; vaginal delivery in HIV co-infected women; scalp electrode; and breastfeeding in HIV co-infected women) and reassurance for factors known not to increase transmission (vaginal delivery in HIV-negative women, gestational age at time of infection, chorioamnionitis, and breastfeeding in HIV-negative women). Amniocentesis, especially non-transplacental, is associated with a minimal risk of HCV vertical transmission, and duration of ruptured membranes with unknown risk. Counseling should also include other possible complications, management, and postpartum follow-up.

Therapy

Currently, there is no approved treatment of HCV infection during pregnancy. Pegylated interferon-α and ribavirin can eradicate the virus in >50% of non-pregnant patients, reduce liver fibrosis progression, and reverse cirrhosis. **Treatment with this efficacious therapy for non-pregnant adults cannot be used during or immediately prior to pregnancy, because of teratogenicity of ribavirin.** Interferon-α is relatively contraindicated in pregnancy due to potential fetal neurotoxicity, but no teratogenic effect has been reported in 35 cases of fetal exposure.[13] There is no HCV vaccine or immune globulin available.

Antepartum testing

Antepartum testing is not indicated just for HCV.

Delivery

In HCV-positive but HIV-negative women, mode of delivery does not affect vertical transmission, so that **cesarean delivery should be reserved for obstetric indications**. In HCV- and HIV-positive women, mode of delivery should be cesarean delivery if the HIV viral load is ≥ 1000 copies/ml.[8]

Anesthesia

No particular precautions are necessary.

Postpartum/breastfeeding

Breastfeeding is generally not considered to be a risk factor for vertical transmission of HCV in non-HIV infected women. The safety of breastfeeding operates on the assumption that traumatized, cracked, or bleeding nipples are not present. However, with HIV co-infection, those who breastfed were four times more likely to infect their children than those who bottle-fed.[8] Breastfeeding is therefore contraindicated in women with both HCV and HIV infections. Therapy with ribavirin and interferon should be started postpartum for the same indications as in other non-pregnant adults.[14]

REFERENCES

1. Leurez-Ville M, Kunstmann JM, De Almeida M, et al. Detection of hepatitis C virus in the semen of infected men. Lancet 2000; 356: 42–3. [II-2]

2. Lesourd F, Izopet J, Mervan C, et al. Transmission of hepatitis C during the ancillary procedures for assisted conception: case report. Hum Reprod 2000; 15: 1083–5. [II-3]

3. Yeung LT, King SM, Roberts EA. Mother-to-infant transmission of hepatitis C virus. Hepatology 2001; 34: 223–9. [II-2]

4. Zanetti AR, Tanzi E, Paccagnini S, et al. Mother-to-infant transmission of hepatitis C virus. Lombard Study Group on Vertical HCV Transmission. Lancet 1995; 345: 289–91. [II-2]

5. European Pediatric Hepatitis C Virus Network. A significant sex - but not elective cesarean section – effect on mother-to-child transmission of hepatitis C virus infection. Infect Dis 2005; 192: 1872–9. [II-1]

6. Ohto H, Terazawa S, Sasaki N, et al. Transmission of hepatitis C virus from mothers to infants. N Engl J Med 1994; 330: 744–50. [II-2]

7. Mast EE, Huang L, Seto DS. Risk factors for perinatal transmission of hepatitis C virus and the natural history of HCV infection acquired in infancy. Infect Dis 2005; 192: 1880–9. [II-1]

8. European Paediatric Hepatitis C Virus Network. Effects of mode of delivery and infant feeding on the risk of mother-to-child transmission of hepatitis C virus. BJOG 2001; 108: 371–7. [II-2]

9. Delamare C, Carbonne B, Heim N, et al. Detection of hepatitis C virus RNA (HCV RNA) in amniotic fluid: a prospective study. J Hepatol 1999; 31: 416–20. [II-2]

10. Conte D, Fraquelli M, Prati D, et al. Prevalence and clinical course of chronic hepatitis C virus (HCV) infection and the rate of vertical transmission in a cohort of 15,250 women. Hepatology 2000; 31: 751–5. [II-2]

11. Simms J, Duff P. Viral hepatitis in pregnancy. Semin Perinatol 1993; 17: 384–93. [review]

12. Zanetti AR, Tanzi E, Newell ML. Mother-to-infant transmission of hepatitis C virus. J Hepatol 1999; 3 (Suppl 1): S96–100. [II-2]

13. Pelham J, Berghella V. Alpha interferon use in pregnancy. Obstet Gynecol 2004; 103: 77s. [II-3]

14. Poynard T, Yuen MF, Ratziu V, Lai CL. Viral hepatitis C. Lancet 2003; 362: 2095–100. [review]

31

HIV

Amanda M Cotter and A Marie O'Neill

KEY POINTS

- **Identification** of HIV (human immunodeficiency virus) infection in pregnancy is **essential for the prevention of perinatal transmission.** An opt-out approach has been shown to increase acceptance rates for HIV testing in pregnant women and is the recommended approach to universal prenatal screening.
- The **goal** of HIV treatment in pregnancy is to **prevent vertical transmission,** primarily by reducing maternal viral load to **< 1000 copies/ml or below the limit of detection of the assay.**
- The **rate of perinatal transmission is correlated to maternal viral load but other factors also appear to play a role.**
- All HIV-positive women should be offered **combination antiretroviral therapy, including AZT** (azidothymidine; zidovudine), regardless of clinical or immunological diagnosis, to maximally suppress viral replication, reduce the risk of perinatal transmission, and minimize the risk of development of resistant virus.
- Plasma **HIV-1 RNA levels** should be **monitored each trimester.**
- Women with a **viral load > 1000 copies/ml** should be counseled regarding the **benefit of elective cesarean delivery at 38 weeks** to reduce the risk of transmission.
- With effective antiretroviral therapy leading to undetectable viral load, elective cesarean delivery for viral load ≥ 1000 copies/ml, and formula feeding, the risk of perinatal transmission is reduced to < 2%.

HISTORIC NOTES

The first cases of what would soon thereafter be called AIDS (acquired immune deficiency syndrome) were reported in homosexual males on June 5th, 1981. In 1994, the PACTG-076 regimen of antepartum and intrapartum AZT (azidothymidine; zidovudine) administered to the mother and then to the newborn for 6 weeks resulted in a reduction of maternal–infant transmission of human immunodeficiency virus-1 (HIV-1) from 25.5% to 8%.[1]

DIAGNOSIS

Diagnosis is made when a screening **ELISA** (enzyme-linked immunosorbent assay) is **positive** and is followed by a **confirmatory positive Western blot.** Regarding **rapid testing,** the sensitivity and specificity of each of the available rapid testing assays ranges from 95 to 100%, while the positive predictive value depends on the prevalence of disease in the population. In a population with low prevalence of disease, the positive predictive value is low while the false-positive rate is high. For example, with a prevalence of disease of ~1% in the population, the positive predictive value of the test may be as low as 60%.

EPIDEMIOLOGY

Over 25 million people worldwide have died of the consequences of HIV infection. The total number of cases of HIV/AIDS in adolescents and adults worldwide is currently estimated to be over 42 million, with approximately 47% of those cases occurring in women.[2] There is great variation in distribution and prevalence from region to region, as shown in Table 31.1. More than 90% of all infected persons live in the developing world. Nigeria, Ethiopia, Russia, India, and China together make up 40% of the world's population, and all have early- to middle-stage HIV epidemics. Transmission of HIV in all five of these countries is projected to increase steeply and outside of high-risk populations, such as commercial sex workers and injection drug users, to the general population through unsafe heterosexual contact and the movement of migrant or displaced populations.[3] The projected increase will have significant implications for women, infants, and children in these populations. A second human immunodeficiency virus, HIV-2, is found primarily in West Africa and rarely in Angola and Mozambique. In the USA, AIDS in women has risen from 7% early in the epidemic to 24% of adult cases today. African-American and Hispanic women have been disproportionately affected.

Worldwide, heterosexual contact is the predominant mode of transmission in women, followed by intravenous

Table 31.1   *Prevalence of HIV infection in various regions of the world*

Region	No. of cases	Prevalence (%)	Percent of cases in women
Sub-Saharan Africa	26 million	7.4	57
Caribbean	0.5 million	2.3	49
Eastern Europe/Central Asia	1.75 million	0.8	34
South/Southeast Asia	8 million	0.6	30
Latin America	2 million	0.6	36
North America	1 million	0.6	25
West/Central Europe	0.75 million	0.3	25
North Africa/Middle East	0.6 million	0.3	48
East Asia	1.2 million	0.1	22

Adapted from AIDS Epidemic Update 2004, UNAIDS/WHO.

(IV) drug use with sharing of needles. Over 90% of pediatric HIV/AIDS cases result from perinatal transmission/breastfeeding. In developed countries, continued perinatal transmission is due to lack of awareness among pregnant women about their HIV status and lack of prenatal care. An estimated 40% of women in the US who delivered HIV-infected infants in 2000 had not been diagnosed prior to delivery.[4] In undeveloped countries the lack of access to prophylactic treatment in women who are aware of their status presents an additional risk for perinatal transmission.

PATHOPHYSIOLOGY

HIV primarily infects T lymphocytes that express the CD4 antigen, resulting in a progressive loss of these cells and impairment of cellular immunity. When CD4 lymphocytes are sufficiently depleted, there is the progression to AIDS, characterized by opportunistic infections and malignancies.

CLASSIFICATION

The CDC (Centers for Disease Control and Prevention) classification is based on clinical and laboratory evaluations. (Table 31.2) There are three clinical categories: asymptomatic (A), symptomatic (B), or an AIDS-defining condition (C), with three ranges of CD4 count of ≥ 500 (1), 200–499 (2), and < 200 cells/mm^3 (3). Regardless of symptoms, a CD4 < 200 cells/mm^3 or the presence of an AIDS-defining illness in an HIV-positive person is an AIDS diagnosis.[5]

RISK FACTORS

Risk of perinatal transmission is closely related to viral load (VL) at the time of delivery.[6–8] Other risk factors include low CD4+ T-lymphocyte count, lack of antiretroviral (ARV) therapy, biological phenotype of the virus, substance abuse, duration of membrane rupture > 4 hours, hepatitis C virus (HCV) co-infection, sexually transmitted infections (STIs), preterm delivery, and chorioamnionitis.[9–11] Risk factors for maternal infection include unprotected sexual contact, including oral, with an infected person; sharing drug needles or syringes; sexual contact with someone whose HIV status is unknown; and transfusions of contaminated blood or blood components. The presence of ulcerating or non-ulcerating STIs, including syphilis, genital herpes, chlamydial infection, gonorrhea, or bacterial vaginosis, increases susceptibility to HIV infection during sex with infected partners. There is no evidence that HIV is spread through sweat, tears, urine, feces, or by insect bites such as mosquito bites.

COMPLICATIONS
Maternal

Increased risks of chorioamnionitis, postpartum endometritis, and wound infection have been reported. The risk of peripartum infection is inversely proportional to the CD4+ count at the time of delivery.

Fetal

Possible increased risk of preterm delivery if on a protease inhibitor (PI)-containing regimen, but no increased risk of fetal growth restriction (FGR), stillbirth, or low Apgar scores.[12–14]

PREGNANCY CONSIDERATIONS
Effect of pregnancy on disease

Pregnancy has no clear effect on HIV progression. A transient but clinically insignificant decrease in the CD4+ T-lymphocyte count has been described.

Table 31.2 *Classification for HIV infection*

CD4 count (cells/mm³)	Clinical categories		
	A Asymptomatic, acute (primary) HIV, or PGL	B Symptomatic, not A or C conditions	C AIDS-indicator conditions
1. ≥ 500	A1	B1	Cl
2. 200–499	A2	B2	C2
3. < 200 AIDS-indicator T-cell count	A3	B3	C3

PGL, persistent generalized lymphadenopathy.

From Centers for Disease Control and Prevention. 1993 Revised classification system for HIV infection and expanded surveillance case definition for AIDS among adolescents and adults. MMWR Morb Mortal Wkly Rep 1992: 41:1–19.

Effect of disease on pregnancy

Perinatal transmission can occur antepartum (25–40%), intrapartum (60–75%), or postpartum with breastfeeding (14%). **Perinatal transmission appears closely related to viral load.** There is a strong correlation between high maternal VL at delivery and risk of transmission, but transmission has occurred at all levels of VL.[15] Transmission rates are about 1.2% on highly active antiretroviral therapy (HAART), 10.4% on AZT monotherapy, and 25% on no ARV.[6]

PREGNANCY MANAGEMENT

Screening

Regulations and policies about HIV screening in pregnancy vary from state to state. Given the effectiveness of intervention, **standard serological testing with counseling is recommended for all pregnant women at the initiation of prenatal care** with a screening ELISA, which if positive is followed by a confirmatory Western blot. An **opt-out approach** in which the patient is informed that she will be tested for HIV along with other standard prenatal labs unless she declines has been shown in several studies to significantly increase testing rates from < 40% to 85–98%.[16–19] Screening should be **repeated at 28–32 weeks'** gestation **if high-risk behavior, high prevalence area, or previously declined testing.**[20] **Rapid testing** is recommended for previously untested women presenting in labor, or those expected to be delivered for maternal or fetal indications before results of conventional testing can be obtained.[21] If a rapid HIV test result is positive, ARV prophylaxis should be offered without waiting for the results of the confirmatory conventional tests.

Principles

The **goal** of HIV therapy is to achieve an HIV-1 RNA level < 1000 copies/ml or below the limit of detection of the assay.

The **risk of perinatal transmission can be < 2%** with effective ARV therapy, elective cesarean delivery (CD) as appropriate, and formula feeding. ARV therapy is recommended in pregnancy predominantly to decrease maternal viral load and thereby decrease the risk of perinatal transmission and to improve maternal health. **Combination ARV therapy is indicated in pregnancy regardless of clinical or immunological status and should always include AZT.** When combination ARV therapy is not available, or the patient chooses not to undertake this therapy, several short-course peripartum drug regimens have been shown to significantly decrease the risk of vertical transmission to ~10%.

Preconception counseling

Many HIV-positive women enter pregnancy aware of their diagnosis, and more than half of these women enter the first trimester on ARV therapy. Preconception counseling should include:

- initiate or modify ARV therapy, avoiding potentially teratogenic agents (Table 31.3)
- opportunistic infection prophylaxis as indicated by CD4 count (Table 31.4)
- appropriate immunizations
- optimize maternal nutritional status, initiating folic acid supplementation
- screen for and treat STIs
- screen for psychological and substance abuse disorders
- advise how to optimize the chance of conception while minimizing the risk of sexual transmission.

Prenatal care

Care in pregnancy should be **multidisciplinary**, with close collaboration between the obstetrician, maternal–fetal medicine, and infectious disease specialists. A specialist with experience in the treatment of pregnant women with HIV-1 infection should be involved in the prenatal care.

Initial prenatal visit

History

- Complete medical and obstetric/gynecological history at first prenatal visit.
- Document history of prior or current ARV use.
- Evaluation for symptoms of AIDS should include fever; night sweats; weight loss; a new persistent dry cough; diarrhea; refractory vaginal candidiasis; oral candidiasis; and new outbreaks of herpes.

Physical examination

Complete physical examination at initial visit. During subsequent visits, screen for HIV disease progression. With CD4 < 200 cells/mm^3, specifically evaluate for thrush; HSV; lymphadenopathy or a rash.

Labs

Baseline laboratory investigations: hepatitis B surface antigen, hepatitis B core antibody, hepatitis C core antibody, HIV RNA viral load, T-lymphocyte profile (CD4, CD8, CD4:CD8), complete blood count (CBC) with differential, toxoplasmosis immunoglobulin G (IgG), cytomegalovirus (CMV) IgG, liver profile, venereal disease research laboratory (VDRL), gonorrhea and chlamydia testing, purified protein derivative (PPD), diabetes screening of patients on a PI at first contact, Papanicolaou (Pap) smear (all abnormal Pap smears require colposcopy). Resistance testing should be performed for the same indications as for non-pregnant patients: acute HIV-1 infection, virological failure, suboptimal viral suppression after initiation of ARV therapy, high likelihood of exposure to resistant virus based on community prevalence or source characteristics.

Counseling

- Discuss risks of transmission and factors that modify those risks.
- Discuss risks and benefits of ART for both the patient and the fetus.
- Educate on safe sex practices with condoms.

Continuing prenatal care

- Monitor CD4 count and HIV-1 RNA levels every trimester to determine the need to alter therapy or initiate prophylaxis against opportunistic infections.
- VL should decrease by 1–2 logs within 4 weeks of starting ARV therapy. If, despite good adherence, an adequate response is not seen, or there is re-emergence of

detectable levels of virus, resistance testing should be performed on the failing regimen.
- Repeat VL at 34–36 weeks to allow discussion of options for mode of delivery.
- Repeat liver profile and CBC every trimester for those patients on ARV therapy.
- If CD4+ count < 200 cells/mm^3, Pap smear every trimester with colposcopy for all abnormal Pap smears.

Antiretroviral therapy (Figures 31.1 and 31.2 and Table 31.3)

If the patient is newly diagnosed in the first trimester of pregnancy and is not severely immunocompromised, then treatment is deferred until 14 weeks to eliminate the potential for embryopathy related to medications. Women who would not require HIV treatment outside of pregnancy are offered ARV therapy for the duration of the pregnancy to prevent perinatal transmission. ARV therapy should be started by 28 weeks to achieve undetectable viral load in the mother prior to delivery for optimal benefit (lowest chance of transmission). Treatment protocols must be individualized for each patient. Resistance to therapeutic agents and regimen failure are commonly related to patient compliance. Therefore, regimens are tailored to maximize compliance.[22]

AZT[1] should be part of the regimen in all pregnant women unless contraindicated: antepartum AZT orally 300 mg bid from week 14 until delivery; intrapartum infusion of AZT IV 2 mg/kg over the first hour followed by a continuous infusion of 1 mg/kg/h until delivery. The newborn should receive AZT for at least the first 6 weeks of life (dose = 2 mg/kg qid). AZT can cause anemia and neutropenia, so monitor CBC.

Regimens for second and third trimester

In women that meet criteria for ARV therapy outside of pregnancy, use optimal ARVs for the woman's health but consider the potential impact on the fetus. **Standard ARV regimens as in non-pregnant women, but include AZT.**

Medications/combinations to avoid

Efavirenz, hydroxyurea, amprenavir solution, combinations of AZT with stavudine (d4T) or d4T with didanosine (ddI).

Support decision-making by the woman after discussion of risks and benefits of ARV: see Table 31.3.[14,22]

Regimens for untreated women and their infants

See Figure 31.1.

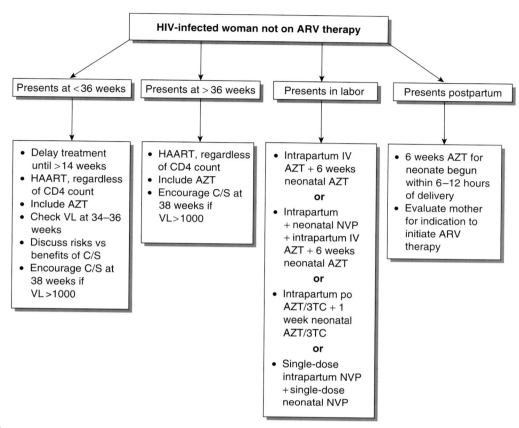

Figure 31.1
Regimens for untreated women and their infants. ARV, antiretroviral; HAART, highly active antiretroviral therapy; AZT, azidothymidine (zidovudine); 3TC, lamuvidine; VL, viral load; IV, intravenous; NVP, nevirapine; C/S, cesarean delivery. (Adapted from Reference 22.)

Monitor for side effects[14,22]

Nucleoside reverse transcriptase inhibitor (NRTI) – AZT

Indications of toxicity that require interrupting or stopping AZT include hemoglobin < 8 g/dl; absolute neutrophil count < 750 cells/mm³; aspartate aminotransferase (AST) or alanine aminotransferase (ALT) > 5 × upper limit of normal. Potential toxicities that may affect the neonate must be considered. Animal data have noted an association between AZT use and squamous tumors in rats in later life.

NRTI use has rarely been linked to mitochondrial toxicity in neonates.

Protease inhibitors

New-onset diabetes mellitus (DM) or exacerbation of existing DM, hyperglycemia, and diabetic ketoacidosis have been reported in patients taking PIs. There are no studies that report an increased risk of pregnancy-associated hyperglycemia in women on a PI-containing regimen. One large prospective cohort of non-pregnant women demonstrated a threefold increased risk for developing DM while on PI therapy.[23] Pregnant women taking PIs should be screened for diabetes each trimester. Amprenavir solutions should be avoided because of potential propylene glycol toxicity.

Nucleoside analog drugs

Mitochondrial toxicity and clinical disorders include neuropathy, cardiomyopathy, myopathy, pancreatitis, hepatic steatosis, and lactic acidosis, which could be confused with HELLP (Hemolysis, Elevated Liver enzymes, and Low Platelet count) syndrome or acute fatty liver of pregnancy. Monitor liver enzymes and electrolytes in the third trimester. Fatalities due to lactic acidosis during pregnancy or in the early postpartum period have been reported in women on ART regimens that included the combination of d4T and ddI (Table 31.3).

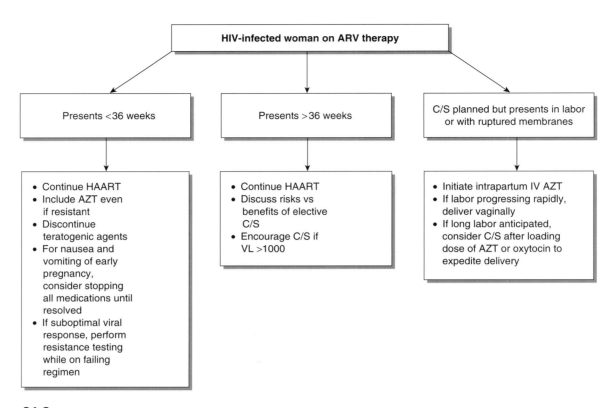

Figure 31.2
Management of women on ARV therapy. ARV, antiretroviral; HAART, highly active antiretroviral therapy; AZT, azidothymidine (zidovudine); VL, viral load; IV, intravenous; C/S, cesarean delivery. (Adapted from Reference 22.)

Non-nucleoside reverse transcriptase inhibitor (NNRTI) – Nevirapine (NVP)

Side effects are rash and hepatotoxicity: the risk is higher in women, especially if CD4 > 250 cells/mm³. Women entering pregnancy on an effective NVP-containing regimen may continue NVP. Pregnant women on NVP should have transaminase levels monitored, especially in the first 18 weeks of treatment. If the patient is symptomatic with even mildly elevated transaminase levels, or asymptomatic with severely elevated levels, NVP should be stopped and avoided in the future. In animal teratology studies with **efavirenz,** an increased incidence of neural tube defects was demonstrated.

Prophylaxis for opportunistic infections

See Table 31.4.

Immunizations

Although HIV infection is primarily a disease of cell-mediated immunity, humoral immunity is also impaired in HIV-positive individuals. Serological response to vaccination may be suboptimal, especially in advanced disease. Live virus vaccines have historically been withheld from HIV-positive individuals because of the risk of contracting the disease from the vaccine. Vaccines should be administered early in the course of HIV infection if possible to increase the likelihood of adequate responses and to minimize the risk of disseminated infection from live vaccines in immunocompromised patients.

All patients should receive **pneumovax, hepatitis B** vaccine series, and **influenza** vaccine. Patients who are HCV positive should be offered the **hepatitis A** vaccine series. **Tetanus and diphtheria** immunization should be updated.[24–26]

Inactivated polio vaccine as a primary series or booster should be administered to those at risk of exposure.

If risk of exposure to yellow fever is high and the CD4 count is > 200 cells/mm³, yellow fever vaccine may be administered; however, serological response may be as low as 35%.[27]

Patients who are rubella non-immune and have a CD4 count > 200 cells/mm³ should be offered vaccination in the postpartum period.[28]

Varicella vaccine is currently being evaluated in HIV-positive adults, and as of this writing, is **not** recommended in the postpartum period for varicella non-immune women. BCG (bacille Calmette-Guérin) vaccine should **not** be

Table 31.3 *Antiretroviral therapy in pregnancy* [14]

	NRTI		NNRTI		PI	
Recommended agents	Zidovudine (AZT) Lamivudine (3TC)	• Efficacy studies and extensive experience • AZT + 3TC is the recommended dual NRTI backbone	Nevirapine	• No evidence of teratogenicity • Increased risk of liver toxicity in women who start nevirapine with CD4 >250 cells/mm³ • In women with CD4 < 250 cells/mm³, nevirapine is acceptable • Monitor closely, especially in first 18 weeks of therapy • No liver toxicity seen with single dose in labor	Nelfinavir Saquinavir	• PK studies and extensive experience • Preferred PI for combination therapy • PK studies and moderate experience • Unboosted saquinavir→ inadequate drug levels in pregnant women
Alternate agents	Didanosine (ddI) Emtricitabine Stavudine (d4T) Abacavir	• Cases of fatal lactic acidosis have occurred with ddI + d4T. Use ONLY if no other alternative			Indinavir Lopinavir/ ritonavir Ritonavir	• Lower drug levels in pregnancy • Unboosted Indinavir NOT recommended • Requires boosting with ritonavir, but optimal dosing in pregnancy is not known • Possibly elevated bilirubin in neonate • Limited experience; study is in progress • Dosing in pregnancy is not established • Lower drug levels in pregnancy • Minimal experience
Insufficient data to recommend	Tenofovir	• No studies in human pregnancies. Bone toxicity in monkey studies			Amprenavir	• No studies in human pregnancy • Oral solution contains ethylene glycol and is contraindicated

Table 31.3 (Continued)		NRTI		NNRTI		PI	
						Atazanavir	• No studies in human pregnancy • Possible elevated bilirubin in neonate
						Fosamprenavir	• No studies in human pregnancy
Not recommended	Zalcitabine	• Teratogenic in animals	Efavirenz	• Teratogenic in monkeys • Cases of CNS defects in humans • Pregnancy category D • Avoid in first trimester • Avoid in women who may become pregnant • Consider after first trimester only if no alternative			
			Delavirdine	• Teratogenic in rodent studies			

NRTI, nucleoside reverse transcriptase inhibitor; NNRTI, non-nucleoside reverse transcriptase inhibitor; PI, protease inhibitor; PK, pharmacokinetic.

administered to HIV-infected women or their newborns – even if the risk of acquiring tuberculosis is high. Disseminated BCG has been reported after immunization.[28,29]

Antepartum testing

Ultrasound evaluation should be performed for the usual obstetric indications. Invasive procedures such as amniocentesis, chorionic villus sampling (CVS), and cordocentesis indicated for diagnostic or therapeutic purposes may place the fetus at increased risk of transmission of the HIV virus, and appropriate counseling with review of indication for these interventions is recommended.[30] The risk of perinatal transmission associated with these invasive procedures may be proportional to maternal viral load. In women not receiving ARV therapy, the risk of transmission in a pregnancy that undergoes amniocentesis has been reported to be 35–40%.[30] In several case series and case-control reports, women on ARV therapy had a 0–3.3% rate of vertical transmission after early invasive testing – which included CVS, amniocentesis, and cordocentesis.[30–32]

If such a procedure is necessary, aim to perform it with maximum suppression of viral load on ARV therapy.

Preterm premature rupture of membranes

The risks of prematurity-related morbidity/mortality must be balanced against the risk of vertical transmission with prolonged rupture of membranes. If premature preterm rupture of membranes (PPROM) occurs prior to 32 weeks, expectant management with administration of corticosteroids for fetal lung maturity and antibiotics for latency is recommended. At a gestational age ≥32 weeks, delivery without the benefit of corticosteroids should be considered if appropriate support is immediately available to care for the premature infant. Consultation with a neonatologist should be sought if considering delivery prior to 32 weeks without the benefit of steroids, as prognosis is dependent on resources available for care of the preterm infant.[9,10]

Delivery

Maintain universal body fluid precautions for all deliveries. Inform pediatrician of mother's status. Bulb suction baby at delivery and wash off maternal secretions as soon as possible after birth are suggested.

Table 31.4 *Prophylaxis for opportunistic infections*

Infection	Indication	First-line treatment	Alternate treatment
Pneumocystis jiroveci pneumonia[a]	• CD4 count <200 cells/mm^3 • History of oropharyngeal candidiasis • History of *Pneumocystis jiroveci* pneumonia (secondary prophylaxis)	Trimethoprim–sulfamethoxazole (TMP–SMZ) one DS tablet daily	TMP–SMZ one SS tablet daily *or* one DS tablet 3x/week Dapsone 50 mg bid or 100 mg daily Aerosolized pentamidine 300 mg monthly
Toxoplasmic encephalitis[b]	CD4 <100 cells/mm^3 and seropositive for *Toxoplasma gondii* IgG	Trimethoprim–sulfamethoxazole (TMP–SMZ) one DS tablet daily	TMP–SMZ one SS tablet daily Dapsone 200 mg po + leucovorin 25 mg po weekly
Disseminated *Mycobacterium avium* complex[c]	CD4 count <50 cells/mm^3	Azithromycin 1200 mg po/week	Rifabutin 300 mg po daily or Rifabutin 300 mg po daily + azithromycin 1200 mg po weekly

Mycobacterium tuberculosis	PPD $\geq$5 mm
	or
	Prior positive PPD without adequate treatment
	or
	Contact with person with active tuberculosis regardless of PPD status
		INH sensitive:
		  INH 300 mg po + pyridoxine 50 mg po daily for 9 months
		  or
		  INH 900 mg po + pyridoxine 100 mg po twice weekly for 9 months
		INH resistant:
		  Rifampin 600 mg po daily *or* rifabutin 300 mg po daily for 4 months
			Rifampin 600 mg po daily *or* rifabutin 300 mg po daily for 4 months

Varicella zoster virus	Varicella non-immune and exposed to chickenpox or shingles	Varicella zoster immune globulin – 5 vials (1.25 ml each) within 48–96 hours of exposure	

[a]SS, single strength; DS, double strength; po, orally; bid, twice a day; PPD, purified protein derivative; INH, isoniazid; HAART, highly active antiretroviral therapy.
[a]Primary prophylaxis should be discontinued after sustained response to HAART with a CD4 count >200 cells/mm^3 for >3 months. Secondary prophylaxis should be discontinued if CD4 count increases from <200 cells/mm^3 to >200 cells/mm^3 for >3 months.
[b]Discontinue primary prophylaxis after sustained response to HAART with CD4 count >200 cells/mm^3 for >3 months. Discontinue secondary prophylaxis when initial therapy completed and asymptomatic with sustained CD4 count >200 cells/mm^3 for >6 months.
[c]Discontinue primary prophylaxis after sustained response to HAART with CD4 count >100 cells/mm^3 for >3 months.

Use the most recent VL level to counsel regarding **mode of delivery**. Risk of perinatal transmission with persistently undetectable VL on ARV therapy is <2%, regardless of mode of delivery. Honor the woman's decision regarding mode of delivery. **Women with a VL >1000 copies/ml should be counseled regarding the potential benefit of scheduled CD to reduce the risk of transmission.**[33] Some clinicians recommend that the absence of ARV therapy or AZT monotherapy only are indications for CD.[34] Schedule CD at 38 weeks using best LMP (last menstrual period) and ultrasound estimate of gestational age without assessing fetal lung maturity by amniocentesis; this entails a small but substantially increased risk of respiratory distress syndrome (RDS).[35] Continue HAART therapy as usual and initiate **AZT infusion for 3 hours prior to CD** and continue until cord clamped. Women with a low CD4 count may

be at increased risk of complications after CD. All women should receive prophylactic antibiotics after cord clamping to reduce risk of postpartum infection.[36] Women with a recent VL <1000 copies/ml can be counseled that trial of labor and vaginal delivery does not significantly increase the very low (<2%) risk of perinatal transmission. There is no evidence of benefit of CD to reduce transmission after labor or rupture of membranes have occurred; the delivery plan in these situations should be individualized.

Intrapartum care

Avoid induction of labor and only consider it at 41 weeks with a favorable cervix. Admit in early labor and augment labor to expedite delivery. Continue HAART regimen in labor;

administer intravenous AZT in labor with loading and maintenance dosing continuously until the umbilical cord is clamped. Delay amniotomy; however, it is not contraindicated and may be used to facilitate labor later in the active phase. Avoid invasive fetal monitoring, intrauterine pressure catheter (IUPC), fetal scalp electrode (FSE), fetal blood sampling (FBS), episiotomy, and forceps or vacuum delivery.[10,37]

Breastfeeding

Women with HIV infection who have access to an adequate supply of infant formula or other suitable source of nutrition should not breastfeed.[38] If access to an alternate nutrition source is not sufficient to completely replace breastfeeding, then exclusive breastfeeding is preferable to alternating breastfeeding/formula feeding regimens. Any woman considering breastfeeding should be aware of her HIV status. A decision not to breastfeed may raise issues regarding confidentiality of a mother's HIV diagnosis and requires sensitivity and supportive interventions.[39,40]

Maternal postpartum care

Establish ongoing primary care for the HIV disease. Long-term planning is essential to ensure that the woman does not fall out of the healthcare system. Continue ARV therapy if needed for maternal health indications; otherwise, discontinue. Prevent nosocomial infection. Rubella vaccines should be administered postpartum to those women with a CD4 count > 200 cells/mm³.[28]

Family planning is critical to the prevention of perinatal transmission. Condom use should be strongly encouraged. Monitor for gynecological manifestations associated with disease progression. Pap smear every 6 months, with colposcopy for any abnormal Pap smear are suggested.

FOLLOW-UP OF INFANTS

Baby should be bathed soon after delivery to remove potentially infectious maternal secretions. Baseline CBC followed by AZT prophylaxis, referral to an HIV specialist. HIV diagnostic testing to establish or rule out HIV infection as early as possible is suggested. Initiate PCP (P*neumocystis carinii* pneumonia) prophylaxis at 6 weeks (until there are two consecutive negative HIV results). Long-term follow-up of HIV and ARV-exposed infants.

DIAGNOSIS OF HIV INFECTION IN THE INFANT

Establishing the diagnosis of HIV infection in the neonate is complicated by the presence of transplacentally acquired maternal antibodies, which makes serological testing unreliable. The mean time to clear maternal antibodies is 10.3 months, but it can take up to 18 months.[41] For this reason, a qualitative HIV-1 DNA PCR assay that detects HIV proviral DNA in peripheral blood mononuclear cells is the primary test used for the diagnosis of HIV-1 perinatally acquired infection in developed countries. Testing should be performed at birth, at 4–6 weeks of age, and approximately 2 months after the second test, at which time the infant has been off ARV prophylaxis for at least 2 weeks. Babies who test negative on all three virological tests should undergo HIV antibody testing at 12 months of age. If this test is positive, it should be repeated at 18 months of age. A positive HIV antibody test after 18 months indicates HIV infection.[42] HIV clade B is the predominant viral strain in the USA. Non-clade B strains are more prevalent in other parts of the world. Some HIV DNA PCR assays may be less sensitive in detecting non-B clades. Assays for HIV-1 RNA detection are available and have comparable sensitivity and specificity for detection of neonatal infection to those of DNA-based assays; however, these assays may be less reliable in infants exposed to ARV with an undetectable viral load.[43]

REFERENCES

1. Connor EM, Sperling RS, Gelber R, et al. Reduction of maternal–infant transmission of human immunodeficiency virus type 1 with zidovudine treatment. Pediatric AIDS Clinical Trials Group Protocol 076 Study Group. N Engl J Med 1994; 331(18): 1173–80. [RCT, *n* = 363]
2. Zarocostas J. Number of people infected with HIV worldwide reaches 40m. BMJ 2005; 331(7527): 1224. [epidemiology report]
3. National Intelligence Council. The Next Wave of HIV/AIDS: Nigeria, Ethiopia, Russia, India, and China. Washington, DC: NIC; 2002. [epidemiology report]
4. Centers for Disease Control & Prevention. Rapid HIV Testing of Women in Labor and Delivery <http://www.cdc.gov/hiv/pubs/rt-women.htm>. Accessed 11/17/2005. Centers for Disease Control & Prevention, 2003. [guideline]
5. Castro KG, Ward JW, Slutsker L, et al. 1993 revised classification system for HIV infection and expanded surveillance case definition for AIDS among adolescents and adults. MMWR Recomm Rep 1992; 41(RR–17): 1–19. [guideline]
6. Cooper ER, Charurat M, Mofenson L, et al; Women and Infant's Transmission Study Group. Combination antiretroviral strategies for the treatment of pregnant HIV-1-infected women and prevention of perinatal HIV-1 transmission. J Acquir Immune Defic Syndr 2002; 29(5): 484–94. [review]
7. Garcia PM, Kalish LA, Pitt J, et al. Maternal levels of plasma human immunodeficiency virus type 1 RNA and the risk of perinatal transmission. Women and Infants Transmission Study Group. N Engl J Med 1999; 341(6): 394–402. [II-2]
8. Mofenson LM, Lambert JS, Stiehm ER, et al. Risk factors for perinatal transmission of human immunodeficiency virus type 1 in women treated with zidovudine. Pediatric AIDS Clinical Trials Group Study 185 team. N Engl J Med 1999; 341(6): 385–93. [II-2]
9. Landesman SH, Kalish LA, Burns DN, et al. Obstetrical factors and the transmission of human immunodeficiency virus type 1 from mother to child. The Women and Infants Transmission Study. N Engl J Med 1996; 334(25): 1617–23. [II-2]

10. International Perinatal HIV Group. Duration of ruptured membranes and vertical transmission of HIV-1: a meta-analysis from 15 prospective cohort studies. AIDS 2001; 15(3): 357–68. [meta-analysis: 15 studies]

11. Minkoff H, Burns DN, Landesman S, et al. The relationship of the duration of ruptured membranes to vertical transmission of human immunodeficiency virus. Am J Obstet Gynecol 1995; 173(2): 585–9. [II-2]

12. European Collaborative Study, Swiss Mother and Child HIV Cohort Study. Combination antiretroviral therapy and duration of pregnancy. AIDS 2000; 14(18): 2913–20. [II-3]

13. Cotter AM, Garcia AG, Duthely ML, Luke B, O'Sullivan MJ. Is antiretroviral therapy associated with an increased risk of preterm delivery, low birth weight, or stillbirth? J Infect Dis 2006; 193: 1195–201. [II-2]

14. Tuomala RE, Shapiro DE, Mofenson LM, et al. Antiretroviral therapy during pregnancy and the risk of an adverse outcome. N Engl J Med 2002; 346(24): 1863–70. [II-2]

15. Ioannidis JP, Abrams EJ, Ammann A, et al. Perinatal transmission of human immunodeficiency virus type 1 by pregnant women with RNA virus loads < 1000 copies/ml. J Infect Dis 2001; 183(4): 539–45. [II-2]

16. Stanley B, Fraser J, Cox NH. Uptake of HIV screening in genitourinary medicine after change to "opt-out" consent. BMJ 2003; 326(7400): 1174. [II-2]

17. Mossman CL, Ratnam S. Opt-out prenatal HIV testing in Newfoundland and Labrador. CMAJ 2002; 167(6): 630; author reply 630–1. [II-2]

18. Jayaraman GC, Preiksaitis JK, Larke B. Mandatory reporting of HIV infection and opt-out prenatal screening for HIV infection: effect on testing rates. CMAJ 2003; 168(6): 679–82. [II-2]

19. Centers For Disease Control And Prevention (CDC). HIV testing among pregnant women – United States and Canada, 1998–2001. MMWR Morb Mortal Wkly Rep 2002; 51: 1013–16. [epidemiology report]

20. ACOG Committee on Obstetric Practice. ACOG Committee Opinion No. 304, November 2004. Prenatal and perinatal human immunodeficiency virus testing: Expanded recommendations. Obstet Gynecol 2004; 104(5 Pt 1): 1119–24. [review]

21. Bulterys M, Jamieson DJ, O'Sullivan MJ, et al. Rapid HIV-1 testing during labor: a multicenter study. JAMA 2004; 292(2): 219–23. [II-2]

22. United States Public Health Service Task Force. Perinatal HIV Guidelines Working Group Members. Public health service task force recommendations for use of antiretroviral drugs in pregnant HIV-1-infected women for maternal health and interventions to reduce perinatal HIV-1 transmission in the United States (revised February, 2005). HIV Clin Trials 2001; 2(1): 56–91. [guideline]

23. Justman JE, Benning L, Danoff A, et al. Protease inhibitor use and the incidence of diabetes mellitus in a large cohort of HIV-infected women. J Acquir Immune Defic Syndr 2003; 32(3): 298–302. [II-2]

24. Laurence JC. Hepatitis A and B immunizations of individuals infected with human immunodeficiency virus. Am J Med 2005; 118 (Suppl 10A): 75–83S. [II-3]

25. McDonald P, Lighton L, Anderson R. Pneumococcal vaccine for HIV patients. Patients with HIV infection should be immunised. BMJ 1995; 311(7001): 387–8. [II-3]

26. Poland GA, Love KR, Hughes CE. Routine immunization of the HIV-positive asymptomatic patient. J Gen Intern Med 1990; 5(2): 147–52. [II-3]

27. Cetron MS, Martin AA, Julian KG, et al. Yellow fever vaccine. Recommendations of the Advisory Committee on Immunization Practices. MMWR Morb Mortal Wkly Rep 2002; 51(RR-17): 1–11. [guideline]

28. Centers for Disease Control and Prevention, Division of Tuberculosis Elimination. Fact Sheet – BCG Vaccine. Centers for Disease Control and Prevention, 2005. [guideline]

29. Hussey G, Hawkridge T, Eley B, et al. Adverse effects of Bacille Calmette-Guérin vaccination in HIV-positive infants. Clin Infect Dis 2004; 38(9): 1333–4; author reply 1334–5. [II-2]

30. Bucceri AM, Somigliana E, Vignali M. Early invasive diagnostic techniques during pregnancy in HIV-infected women. Acta Obstet Gynecol Scand 2001; 80(1): 82–3. [II-3]

31. Maiques V, Garcia-Tejedor A, Perales A, Cordoba J, Esteban RJ. HIV detection in amniotic fluid samples. Amniocentesis can be performed in HIV pregnant women? Eur J Obstet Gynecol Reprod Biol 2003; 108(2): 137–41. [II-3]

32. Somigliana E, Bucceri AM, Tibaldi C, et al. Early invasive diagnostic techniques in pregnant women who are infected with the HIV: a multicenter case series. Am J Obstet Gynecol 2005; 193(2): 437–42. [II-3]

33. The International Perinatal HIV Group. The mode of delivery and the risk of vertical transmission of human immunodeficiency virus type 1 – a meta-analysis of 15 prospective cohort studies. The international Perinatal HIV Group. N Engl J Med 1999; 340(13): 977–87. [II-2]

34. Management of HIV in pregnancy. Royal College of Obstetricians and Gynecologists. Guideline No. 39, April 2004. [guideline]

35. Committee on Obstetric Practice. ACOG Committee Opinion. Scheduled cesarean delivery and the prevention of vertical transmission of HIV infection, No. 234, May 2000. Obstet Gynecol 2001; 73(3): 279–81. [guideline]

36. American College of Obstetricians and Gynecologists. ACOG Practice Bulletin No. 47, October 2003. Prophylactic antibiotics in labor and delivery. Obstet Gynecol 2003; 102(4): 875–82. [review]

37. Mandelbrot L, Mayaux MJ, Bongain A, et al. Obstetric factors and mother-to-child transmission of human immunodeficiency virus type 1: the French perinatal cohorts. SEROGEST French Pediatric HIV Infection Study Group. Am J Obstet Gynecol 1996; 175(3 Pt 1): 661–7. [II-2]

38. Coutsoudis A. Breastfeeding and the HIV positive mother: the debate continues. Early Hum Dev 2005; 81(1): 87–93. [review]

39. Dunn DT, Newell ML, Ades AE, Peckham CS. Risk of human immunodeficiency virus type 1 transmission through breastfeeding. Lancet 1992; 340(8819): 585–8. [II-2]

40. Tess BH, Rodrigues LC, Newell ML, Dunn DT, Lago TD. Infant feeding and risk of mother-to-child transmission of HIV-1 in Sao Paulo State, Brazil. Sao Paulo Collaborative Study for Vertical Transmission of HIV-1. J Acquir Immune Defic Syndr Hum Retrovirol 1998; 19(2): 189–94. [II-2]

41. Louisirirotchanakul S, Kanoksinsombat C, Likanonsakul S, et al. Patterns of anti-HIV IgG3, IgA and p24Ag in perinatally HIV-1 infected infants. Asian Pac J Allergy Immunol 2002; 20(2): 99–104. [II-3]

42. King SM, American Academy of Pediatrics Committee on Pediatric AIDS. American Academy of Pediatrics Infectious Diseases and Immunization Committee. Evaluation and treatment of the human immunodeficiency virus-1 – exposed infant. Pediatrics 2004; 114(2): 497–505. [review]

43. Nesheim S, Palumbo P, Sullivan K, et al. Quantitative RNA testing for diagnosis of HIV-infected infants. J Acquir Immune Defic Syndr 2003; 32(2): 192–5. [II-3]

32

Gonorrhea

A Marie O'Neill

KEY POINTS

- Gonorrhea has been associated with an increased risk of spontaneous abortion, premature labor, early rupture of fetal membranes, chorioamnionitis, and perinatal mortality, as well as neonatal conjunctivitis leading to blindness, increased HIV transmission, and postpartum infection.
- Prevention strategies shown to be effective include use of **condoms, screening high-risk populations, early diagnosis and treatment**, and **partner notification and treatment without clinical assessment.**
- There is insufficient evidence to recommend screening of low-risk pregnant women.
- Pregnant women at **high risk** for gonorrhea are those aged **<25 years old, with prior sexually transmitted infection (STI), multiple sexual partners, a partner with a past history of any STD, sex work, drug use, or inconsistent condom use.** These women should be **screened** in pregnancy **for gonorrhea.**
- Definitive **diagnosis** requires isolation by **culture** *and* confirmation by **nucleic acid amplification tests.**
- First-line treatment for gonorrhea in pregnancy is **ceftriaxone** or **cefixime.**
- If chlamydial infection has not been ruled out, co-treatment with azithromycin single dose or amoxicillin should be provided.
- Patients presenting with preterm premature rupture of membranes (PPROM) who have active gonorrheal infection can be managed expectantly as long as prompt treatment for gonorrhea is instituted.
- Because of the potential for concomitant infection, **testing for *Chlamydia trachomatis*, syphilis, HIV, and hepatitis B is recommended.**

EPIDEMIOLOGY/INCIDENCE

Worldwide, it is estimated that 62 million new cases of gonorrhea occur annually.[1] The highest incidences of gonorrhea and its complications occur in developing countries.

As a result of a national gonorrhea control program implemented in the USA in the 1970s, the national rate of gonorrheal infection has decreased more than 75% over the last three decades. In 2004, there were 330 132 cases of gonorrhea reported to the CDC (Centers for Disease Control and Prevention), with approximately 40 000 of these infections occurring in pregnant women. The CDC estimated that only about half of all infections are reported.[2] The incidence is substantially lower in all countries of western Europe than in the USA, but high and rising rates have been documented in eastern Europe. Gonorrhea disproportionately affects African-Americans, with the reported rate of infection in this population being 19 times greater than that in whites.[2,3] The median prevalence of gonorrhea in unselected populations of pregnant women has been estimated to be 10% in Africa, 5% in Latin America, and 4% in Asia.[4]

ETIOLOGY

Neisseria gonorrhoeae is a Gram-negative diplococcus that primarily infects non-ciliated, columnar, or cuboidal epithelium of the endocervix, urethra, rectum, or pharynx. Gonococci are obligate human pathogens and can survive only briefly outside of the human reservoir.

PATHOPHYSIOLOGY/ TRANSMISSION

N. gonorrhoeae is easily transmitted during oral, vaginal, or anal sex.

The transmission rate from male to female during vaginal intercourse is approximately 50% per contact, rising to 90% after three exposures.[5] The incubation period for *N. gonorrhoeae* is on average 2–7 days, but may vary between 1 and 14 days. **Vertical transmission to the infant occurs in 30–47% of cases if cervical infection is present at the time of delivery.** The eye is the most common site of neonatal infection, but disseminated gonococcal infection or gonococcal arthritis may also occur in the newborn.[6,7] The vast majority of vertical transmission occurs **during vaginal delivery**; however, transmission has been reported after cesarean delivery in patients with ruptured membranes.

SYMPTOMS

The clinical manifestations of gonorrhea are unchanged in pregnant women, except that pelvic inflammatory disease (PID) and perihepatitis are uncommon after the first trimester. Cervical infection is **asymptomatic in up to 80% of women.**[8] When symptoms are present, they include a purulent or mucopurulent cervical exudate, edema, and easily induced cervical or endocervical bleeding. Urethral infection is present in 70–90% of women who have gonococcal cervicitis – most will present with dysuria.[9] *N. gonorrhoeae* does not cause vaginitis; however, co-infection with bacterial vaginosis, trichomonas, or *Chlamydia trachomatis* is common and often causes abnormal vaginal discharge. Pharyngeal infection is typically asymptomatic, but may cause exudative pharyngitis and cervical lymphadenopathy: it occurs in 10–20% of women with cervical gonorrhea.[10,11] Rectal infection is typically asymptomatic, but may cause anal pruritus, mucopurulent discharge, and sometimes pain, tenesmus, and bleeding: it occurs in about 40% of women with cervical gonorrhea.[8] Disseminated gonococcal infection occurs in 0.5–3% of infected individuals, and usually causes septic arthritis accompanied by a rash of hemorrhagic papules and pustules.[12] There are conflicting reports as to whether pregnancy is a risk factor for disseminated infection; however, a recent publication reports an incidence of 0.04–0.09% in pregnancy.[13]

COMPLICATIONS

- Gonorrhea has been associated with an increased risk of **spontaneous abortion, premature labor, early rupture of fetal membranes, chorioamnionitis, and perinatal mortality.** It is not clear if these complications are a direct result of gonococcal infection, or if infection is a marker for other high-risk factors.[14–16]
- Vertical transmission to the infant can cause conjunctivitis, which if left untreated may result in **blindness.** Prior to routine prophylaxis of all infants at the time of birth, approximately 25% of congenital blindness in the USA was caused by gonorrheal conjunctivitis, and it remains a major cause of congenital blindness in underdeveloped countries.[7,17]
- Epidemiological and biological studies provide strong evidence that gonococcal infections **facilitate the transmission of HIV infection,** which has major implications for the pregnancy.[18]
- Women with active cervical infection at the time of delivery are at increased risk for **postpartum infection.**[19]

MANAGEMENT

Prevention

Condoms, when used correctly and consistently, provide a high degree of protection from gonorrheal infection, as well as from other sexually transmitted diseases (STDs).[20] Other important practices for prevention of gonorrhea are **screening to identify asymptomatic cases in high-risk populations, early diagnosis and treatment, and partner notification and treatment.** Several recent randomized trials reported a reduction in the rate of reinfection using an expedited approach to partner therapy whereby **partners are treated without a clinical assessment.** In this approach, the patient delivers either medication or prescriptions to her partner.[21,22] The legal status of such an approach is uncertain in some states.

Screening (Table 32.1)[23–25]

There is no evidence that screening low-risk pregnant women is beneficial.

Screening pregnant women at high risk for gonorrhea may prevent other complications associated with gonococcal infection during pregnancy. **Risk factors** include **age <25 years old, prior sexually transmitted infection (STI), multiple sexual partners, having a partner with a past history of any STD, sex work, drug use, and inconsistent condom use.** Because *N. gonorrhoeae* can cause infection at a variety of body sites, the decision of which sites to test should be guided by sexual history and physical examination findings.

Diagnosis (see Table 32.1)[23–25]

Isolation of *N. gonorrhoeae* by culture is the historic mainstay of gonorrhea diagnosis. A **definitive diagnosis requires isolation by culture *and* confirmation** of isolates by biochemical, enzymatic, serological, or nucleic acid testing. In many laboratories, culture is rapidly being replaced by **nucleic acid amplification tests** (NAATs), including ligase chain reaction (LCR), polymerase chain reaction (PCR), transcription-mediated amplification (TMA), and strand displacement amplification (SDA), or by unamplified DNA probe tests (non-NAATs). A **presumptive** diagnosis of gonorrhea is made with these tests. Clinicians who perform STD screening tests should be aware of the prevalence of STDs in the population being screened and have a conceptual understanding of positive predictive value and of the impact of screening low-risk individuals with a test that has limited specificity. The positive predictive value of nucleic acid based tests is less than 60% when the prevalence of infection in the population is less than 1%. Some assays can detect *C. trachomatis* or *N. gonorrhoeae* in a single specimen. Several of these combined assays do not differentiate

Table 32.1 *Screening and diagnostic tests for gonorrhea*[23–25]

Test	Sensitivity	Specificity	Advantages	Disadvantages
Culture	80–90%	100%	• Can obtain specimen from any potentially infected site • Preserve isolate for antimicrobial sensitivity testing and forensics	• Organism is especially fastidious – can be difficult to grow in culture • Overgrowth of contaminating microorganisms can give a false-negative result • Organism can be rendered non-viable during transport if incorrect media used or delay in transport • 48–72 hours to complete
Gram stain	40–60% compared with culture	70–90%	• Rapid results • Negative predictive value is 99–100% • In setting of limited resources can be used for screening with follow-up testing of screen positives	• Least sensitive/specific • Higher false-negative rate results in more failure to treat
NAAT	96.7% compared with culture	98%	• High sensitivity • Approved for testing on voided urine • Approved for testing on liquid based Pap medium • Rapid results • Specimen less affected by handling and transport	• Most expensive option • No isolate preserved for forensics or sensitivity testing • Highest false-positive rate when persons at low risk are tested • Limited to cervical or urine specimens • Non-viable organisms or contaminants will give false-positive result
Non-NAAT	92.1% compared with culture	99%	• Inexpensive • Rapid results • Specimen less affected by handling and transport	• Non-viable organisms or contaminants will give false-positive result • Limited to cervical specimens

NAAT, nucleic acid amplification test.

between the two organisms, so a positive result should be followed by tests for each organism to obtain an organism-specific result.

Treatment

Antimicrobial resistance is an important consideration in the treatment of gonorrhea. The Gonococcal Isolate Surveillance Project (GISP) of the CDC has reported resistance to penicillins and tetracyclines, and more recently to fluoroquinolones. To date, cephalosporin resistance has not been identified; however, some isolates have demonstrated decreased susceptibility to ceftriaxone or cefixime. **Current CDC recommendations for treatment are presented in Table 32.2,**[26–28] but as resistance patterns change so too may treatment recommendations. **Ceftriaxone IM (intramuscular) or cefixime po (orally) are currently the preferred first-line regimens for genital infection.** Updates can be found at http://www.cdc.gov/STD/treatment/. The only outcome reported in the two available trials was the incidence of 'cure' assessed by bacterial culture.[29] Failure to achieve 'microbiological cure' was similar for each antibiotic regimen: amoxicillin+probenecid compared with spectinomycin; amoxicillin+probenecid compared with ceftriaxone; and ceftriaxone compared with cefixime. Side effects were uncommon for all the tested regimens. Although no differences were detected between the different antibiotic regimens, the trials were limited by their small sample size in their ability to detect important but modest differences. For women who are allergic to penicillin, treatment with ceftriaxone or spectinomycin appears to have similar effectiveness in producing microbiological cure.[29]

Table 32.2 *Current CDC recommendations for treatment of gonorrhea infection* [26–28]

Site of infection	Recommended treatment	Alternate treatment
Cervix/urethra/rectum	Ceftriaxone 125 mg IM single dose (99.1% efficacy), *or* Cefixime 400 mg po single dose (97.4% efficacy)	Spectinomycin 2 g IM single dose if allergic to cephalosporins (98.2% efficacy)
Pharynx	Ceftriaxone 125 mg IM single dose (99% efficacy), *or* Cefixime 400 mg po single dose (95% efficacy)	Spectinomycin 2 g IM single dose[a]
Conjunctiva	Ceftriaxone 1 g IM in a single dose	

[a]Spectinomycin 2 g IM single dose (only 50% efficacy).

For uncomplicated gonococcal infection treated with one of the recommended regimens, a test of cure is *not* necessary. However, if other treatment regimens are used, consider performing a test of cure 4–6 weeks after completing treatment. **35–50% of women who have endocervical gonorrhea are co-infected with *C. trachomatis*. If chlamydial infection has not been ruled out, co-treatment with azithromycin 1 gram orally single dose, or amoxicillin 500 mg po tid × 7 days should be provided.**

If a patient fails one of the recommended treatment regimens, a culture should be obtained for antimicrobial susceptibility testing. Treatment is considered to have failed if the patient reports compliance with medication regimen, simultaneous treatment of her partner, and no sexual activity without barrier protection after completing treatment. It is difficult to exclude reinfection as the cause of a positive result on repeat testing. In the USA, clinicians should contact their local or state health department or the CDC for guidance and assistance in follow-up of these patients as part of the ongoing GISP.

Patients presenting with preterm premature rupture of membranes (PPROM) who are found to have active gonorrheal infection can be managed expectantly as long as treatment for gonorrhea is initiated promptly.[30]

Azithromycin 2 g, as a single oral dose, has demonstrated an efficacy of 99.2% for urogenital and rectal infections, and treatment efficacy of 100% for pharyngeal infection in non-pregnant adults.

Concomitant infections

Because of the potential for concomitant infection, testing for *C. trachomatis*, syphilis, HIV, and hepatitis B is recommended.

REFERENCES

1. World Health Organization. World Health Report 1998. Geneva, Switzerland: WHO; 1998. [epidemiological data]
2. Centers for Disease Control and Prevention. Sexually Transmitted Disease Surveillance, 2004. Atlanta, GA: U.S. Department of Health and Human Services; 2005. [epidemiological data]
3. Centers for Disease Control and Prevention. STDs and Pregnancy Fact Sheet. Atlanta, GA: Department of Health and Human Services; 2004. [review]
4. Handsfield HH, Sparling FP. Neisseria gonorrhoeae. In: Mandell GL, Bennett JE, Dolin R, eds. Principles and Practices of Infectious Diseases, 6th edn. Philadelphia: Churchill Livingstone; 2005: 2514–27. [review]
5. Lin JS, Donegan SP, Heeren TC, et al. Transmission of *Chlamydia trachomatis* and *Neisseria gonorrhoeae* among men with urethritis and their female sex partners. J Infect Dis 1998; 178(6): 1707–12. [II-2]
6. Fransen L, Nsanze H, Klauss V, et al. Ophthalmia neonatorum in Nairobi, Kenya: the roles of *Neisseria gonorrhoeae* and *Chlamydia trachomatis*. J Infect Dis 1986; 153(5): 862–9. [II-3]
7. Galega FP, Heymann DL, Nasah BT. Gonococcal ophthalmia neonatorum: the case for prophylaxis in tropical Africa. Bull World Health Organ 1984; 62(1): 95–8. [review]
8. McCormack WM, Stumacher RJ, Johnson K, Donner A. Clinical spectrum of gonococcal infection in women. Lancet 1977; 1(8023): 1182–5. [review]
9. Brunham RC, Paavonen J, Stevens CE, et al. Mucopurulent cervicitis – the ignored counterpart in women of urethritis in men. N Engl J Med 1984; 311(1): 1–6. [II-2]
10. Wiesner PJ. Gonococcal pharyngeal infection. Clin Obstet Gynecol 1975; 18(1): 121–9. [II-2]
11. Wiesner PJ, Tronca E, Bonin P, Pedersen AH, Holmes KK. Clinical spectrum of pharyngeal gonococcal infection. N Engl J Med 1973; 288(4): 181–5. [II-3]
12. Holmes KK, Counts GW, Beaty HN. Disseminated gonococcal infection. Ann Intern Med 1971; 74(6): 979–93. [II-3]
13. Phupong V, Sittisomwong T, Wisawasukmongchol W. Disseminated gonococcal infection during pregnancy. Arch Gynecol Obstet 2005; 273(3): 185–6. [II-3]
14. Edwards LE, Barrada MI, Hamann AA, Hakanson EY. Gonorrhea in pregnancy. Am J Obstet Gynecol 1978; 132(6): 637–41. [II-3]

15. Schulz KF, Cates W Jr, O'Mara PR. Pregnancy loss, infant death, and suffering: legacy of syphilis and gonorrhoea in Africa. Genitourin Med 1987; 63(5): 320–5. [II-3]

16. McGregor JA, French JI, Richter R, et al. Antenatal microbiologic and maternal risk factors associated with prematurity. Am J Obstet Gynecol 1990; 163(5 Pt 1): 1465–73. [II-2]

17. Fox KK, Whittington WL, Levine WC, et al. Gonorrhea in the United States, 1981–1996. Demographic and geographic trends. Sex Transm Dis 1998; 25(7): 386–93. [epidemiological data]

18. Cohen MS, Hoffman IF, Royce RA, et al. Reduction of concentration of HIV-1 in semen after treatment of urethritis: implications for prevention of sexual transmission of HIV-1. AIDSCAP Malawi Research Group. Lancet 1997; 349(9069): 1868–73. [II-2]

19. Alger LS, Lovchik JC, Hebel JR, Blackmon LR, Crenshaw MC. The association of Chlamydia trachomatis, Neisseria gonorrhoeae, and group B streptococci with preterm rupture of the membranes and pregnancy outcome. Am J Obstet Gynecol 1988; 159(2): 397–404. [II-2]

20. Paz-Bailey G, Koumans EH, Sternberg M, et al. The effect of correct and consistent condom use on chlamydial and gonococcal infection among urban adolescents. Arch Pediatr Adolesc Med 2005; 159(6): 536–42. [II-2]

21. Golden MR, Whittington WL, Handsfield HH, et al. Effect of expedited treatment of sex partners on recurrent or persistent gonorrhea or chlamydial infection. N Engl J Med 2005; 352(7): 676–85. [II-2]

22. Kissinger P, Mohammed H, Richardson-Alston G, et al. Patient-delivered partner treatment for male urethritis: a randomized, controlled trial. Clin Infect Dis. 2005; 41(5): 623–9. [RCT]

23. Crotchfelt KA, Welsh LE, DeBonville D, Rosenstraus M, Quinn TC. Detection of Neisseria gonorrhoeae and Chlamydia trachomatis in genitourinary specimens from men and women by a coamplification PCR assay. J Clin Microbiol 1997; 35(6): 1536–40. [II-2]

24. Koumans EH, Black CM, Markowitz LE, et al. Comparison of methods for detection of Chlamydia trachomatis and Neisseria gonorrhoeae using commercially available nucleic acid amplification tests and a liquid Pap smear medium. J Clin Microbiol 2003; 41(4): 1507–11. [II-2]

25. Martin DH, Cammarata C, Van Der Pol B, et al. Multicenter evaluation of AMPLICOR and automated COBAS AMPLICOR CT/NG tests for Neisseria gonorrhoeae. J Clin Microbiol 2000; 38(10): 3544–9. [II-2]

26. Ramus RM, Sheffield JS, Mayfield JA, Wendel GD, Jr. A randomized trial that compared oral cefixime and intramuscular ceftriaxone for the treatment of gonorrhea in pregnancy. Am J Obstet Gynecol 2001; 185(3): 629–32. [RCT]

27. Sexually transmitted diseases treatment guidelines 2006. Centers for Disease Control and Prevention. MMWR 2006; 55 (No. RR–11): 1–100. [Guideline]

28. Cavenee MR, Farris JR, Spalding TR, et al. Treatment of gonorrhea in pregnancy. Obstet Gynecol 1993; 81(1): 33–8. [review]

29. Brocklehurst P. Antibiotics for gonorrhoea in pregnancy. Cochrane Database Syst Rev 2006; 1. [meta-analysis: 2 RCTs, n=346]

30. Maxwell GL, Watson WJ. Preterm premature rupture of membranes: results of expectant management in patients with cervical cultures positive for group B streptococcus or Neisseria gonorrhoeae. Am J Obstet Gynecol 1992; 166(3): 945–9. [II-3]

33

Chlamydia

A Marie O'Neill

KEY POINTS

- Untreated maternal genital *Chlamydia trachomatis* has been associated with increased incidences of **preterm premature rupture of membranes (PPROM), preterm birth, low birth weight, and decreased perinatal survival.**
- **Neonatal infection** is associated with neonatal **conjunctivitis and pneumonitis.**
- Prevention strategies shown to be effective include **condoms, screening to identify asymptomatic cases in high-risk populations, early diagnosis and treatment, and partner notification and treatment without a clinical assessment.**
- Screening and treatment of women at risk for chlamydial infection improves pregnancy outcome.
- **Pregnant women with risk factors should undergo screening: age < 25 years old (strongest risk factor), multiple sex partners, new partner within past 3 months, single marital status, inconsistent use of barrier contraception, previous or concurrent sexually transmitted infection (STI), vaginal discharge, mucopurulent cervicitis, friable cervix, or signs of cervicitis on physical examination.**
- Women who test positive and/or who have on-going risk factors should be retested in the third trimester.
- There is insufficient evidence to recommend for or against routine screening of asymptomatic, low-risk pregnant women aged ≥ 26 years old for chlamydial infection.
- A **nucleic acid amplification test (NAAT)** – e.g. ligase chain reaction (LCR) or polymerase chain reaction (PCR) – **screening test, confirmed by another NAAT test**, achieves the highest predictive accuracy for the **diagnosis of maternal genital chlamydial infection.**
- Azithromycin, amoxicillin, and **erythromycin** (in order of preference) are all accepted treatments of maternal genital chlamydial infection. A **test of cure** and **repeat testing in the third trimester**, as well as **testing for** *Neisseria gonorrhoeae*, syphilis, HIV, and hepatitis B are recommended for those women with positive testing earlier in pregnancy.

BACKGROUND

The major sexually transmitted diseases caused by *Chlamydia trachomatis* are cervicitis, urethritis, proctitis, and lymphogranuloma venereum (LGV). *C. trachomatis* is also a significant pathogen causing conjunctivitis in both the newborn and in sexually active adolescents and adults.

EPIDEMIOLOGY/INCIDENCE

Worldwide it is estimated that over 92 million chlamydial infections occur annually, with just less than half occuring in women.[1] The incidence of chlamydial infections in the USA and worldwide continues to rise annually. The CDC (Centers for Disease Control and Prevention) estimates that there are approximately 4 million new chlamydial infections annually in the USA, and approximately 200 000 of these occur in pregnant women.[2] The age-specific rate for chlamydial infection is highest in the 15–24-year-old age category. The rate of chlamydial infection in African-American females in the USA is more than 7.5 times higher than the rate among white females.[2] The prevalence of chlamydia varies significantly across the world. Selected rates of genital *C. trachomatis* infection in pregnant women are shown in Table 33.1.

Ocular trachoma is rare in the developed world, but worldwide it is estimated that 7–9 million people are blind as a result of this condition.[3]

LGV occurs sporadically in developed countries but is endemic in Africa, India, Southeast Asia, South America, and the Caribbean. The World Health Organization (WHO) and several partner organizations have initiated a program for global elimination of ocular trachoma as a disease of public health importance by the year 2020. Infection with *C. trachomatis* confers little protection against reinfection, and the limited protection that is conferred is short lived.

Table 33.1	*Rates of chlamydial infection in pregnant women* [1]			
Papua New Guinea	26%	Thailand	5.7%
		USA	5%
India	17%	Italy	2.7%
Cape Verde	13%	Brazil	2.1%
Iceland	8%		
Tanzania	6%		

CLASSIFICATION

C. trachomatis infections can be divided into **four clinical categories:**

- classic ocular trachoma
- other ocular and genital diseases in adults
- LGV
- perinatal infection – conjunctivitis and pneumonia primarily.

In pregnant women, genital infections including LGV, and conjunctivitis are the most clinically significant of these.

SYMPTOMS
Maternal genital infections

The clinical manifestations of *C. trachomatis* are unchanged in pregnant women, except that pelvic inflammatory disease (PID) and perihepatitis are uncommon after the first trimester; 70–90% of women with cervical or urethral *C. trachomatis* infection are asymptomatic.

Cervicitis/urethritis

Mucopurulent cervicitis that may be perceived as vaginal discharge, cervical edema, and friability, dysuria if urethritis present, and low abdominal pain if upper genital tract infection is present.

Lymphogranuloma venereum (LGV)

LGV is often a difficult diagnosis to make because it is not thought of in the differential.

- The first stage is formation of a primary lesion – a small papule or herpetiform ulcer – usually on the genital mucosa or adjacent skin that causes few or no symptoms.
- The secondary stage occurs days to weeks later and is characterized by painful inguinal lymphadenopathy and systemic symptoms.
- The third stage manifests as hypertrophic chronic granulomatous enlargement with ulceration of the external genitalia. Lymphatic obstruction may also lead to elephantiasis of the genitalia.

Proctitis/proctocolitis

These conditions result from anal intercourse or secondary spread of secretions from the cervix:

- Serovars D through K – anal pruritus and a mucous rectal discharge that may become mucopurulent. The infection remains superficial, is limited to the rectum, and closely resembles gonococcal proctitis. Infection is often asymptomatic.
- LGV strains – rectal pain, tenesmus, rectal bleeding, and fever. The disease extends into the colon. The rectal and colonic mucosa become ulcerated, and a granulomatous inflammatory process occurs in the bowel wall, with both non-caseating granulomas and crypt abscesses. Sinus tract formation can lead to rectovaginal fistulas in women.

Chlamydial conjunctivitis

Chlamydial conjunctivits is the most common cause of chronic follicular conjunctivitis. Common manifestations are a unilateral or bilateral asymmetric conjunctivitis associated with moderate hyperemia and mucopurulent discharge.

ETIOLOGY/BASIC PATHOPHYSIOLOGY

C. trachomatis is an **obligate intracellular** pathogen that exhibits morphological and structural similarities to Gram-negative bacteria. The organism has a unique life cycle that includes an extracellular infectious form and an intracellular replicative form. The target cells of *C. trachomatis* are the squamocolumnar epithelial cells of the endocervix and upper genital tract, the conjunctiva, urethra, and rectum.

The LGV biovar of *C. trachomatis* penetrates the skin or infects epithelial cells of the mucous membranes of the genital tract or rectum. It is then carried by lymphatic drainage to the regional lymph nodes, where it multiplies inside mononuclear phagocytes. *C. trachomatis* serovars D through K cause conjunctivitis in neonates as well as in adults. The incubation for *C. trachomatis* is variable, depending on the type of infection, but in general is 7–21 days.

TRANSMISSION

- *C. trachomatis* is readily transmitted during vaginal, oral, or anal sex, and mother-to-infant transmission commonly occurs at delivery.
- The risk of acquisition of *C. trachomatis* with a single episode of sexual intercourse with an infected partner is not known. However, it appears to be substantially less than that for *Neisseria gonorrhoeae*.[4] (Chapter 32)

- Between 22% and 44% of infants born to infected women develop neonatal conjunctivitis.[5]
- Between 11% and 20% of infants born to infected mothers develop pneumonia caused by *C. trachomatis.* [6]

COMPLICATIONS/RISKS

Untreated maternal genital *C. trachomatis* has been found to be an independent risk factor for a statistically significant increase in **preterm premature rupture of membranes (PPROM), preterm birth, low birth weight, and decreased perinatal survival** when compared with either treated women or controls without the infection.[7] Successful treatment is associated therefore with prevention of PPROM and small-for-gestational-age infants.[8]

Neonatal infection acquired from an infected maternal genital tract at the time of delivery is associated with neonatal **conjunctivitis** and **pneumonitis**.

MANAGEMENT

Prevention

Condoms, when used correctly and consistently, provide a high degree of protection from this and other sexually transmitted infections (STIs).[9] Other important practices for prevention of chlamydia are **screening to identify asymptomatic cases in high-risk populations, early diagnosis and treatment,** and **partner notification and treatment.** The rate of reinfection is reduced using an expedited approach to partner therapy, whereby **partners are treated without a clinical assessment.** In this approach, the patient delivers either medication or prescriptions to her partner. The legal status of such an approach is uncertain in some states.[10,11]

Screening

There is no trial to assess the efficacy of universal or risk-based screening for chlamydial genital infection in pregnancy. The Canadian Task Force and the CDC recommend that all pregnant women be screened for chlamydial infection.[12,13] The American College of Obstetricians and Gynecologists (ACOG) and the American Academy of Pediatrics (AAP) recommend **screening pregnant women with risk factors or signs of cervicitis on physical examination** rather than routinely screening all women.[14] Risk factors for acquiring chlamydial infection (extrapolated mainly from non-pregnant studies) are **young age <25 years old** (strongest risk factor), **multiple sex partners, new partner within past 3 months, single marital status, inconsistent use of barrier contraception, previous or concurrent STI, vaginal discharge, mucopurulent cervicitis, friable cervix, and cervical ectopy.**

Diagnosis

A **nucleic acid amplification test (NAAT) – ligase chain reaction (LCR) or polymerase chain reaction (PCR) – screening test, confirmed by another NAAT test**, achieves the highest predictive accuracy for the **diagnosis of maternal genital chlamydial infection** (Table 33.2).[15–17]

- Anti-*Chlamydia* immunoglobulin M (IgM) is uncommon in adults with genital tract infection. The prevalence of anti-*Chlamydia* immunoglobulin G (IgG) is high in sexually active adults (30–60%), even in those who do not have an active infection, and is probably due to past infection. The sensitivity, specificity, and predictive values of serologies are not high enough to make them clinically useful in the diagnosis of active disease. Thus, **chlamydial serologies are not recommended for diagnosis** of active disease, except in suspected cases of LGV.
- Two prospective studies compared an LCR NAAT performed on voided urine to endocervical culture in pregnant women, and found LCR to be more sensitive.[18,19]
- A prospective study comparing endocervical culture with endocervical direct fluorescent antibody (DFA), enzyme immunoassay (EIA), and polymerase chain reaction (PCR) found that **non-culture tests have a higher sensitivity,** even in a population with a prevalence rate as low as 4.3%.[20]
- Clinicians who perform STI screening tests should be aware of the prevalence of STIs in the population being screened and have a conceptual understanding of positive predictive value and the implications of screening low-risk individuals with a test that has limited specificity. In low-prevalence populations (<5% infected), a significant proportion of positive test results are false positives. For example, with a prevalence of 3%, out of 1000 patients 30 are infected. A test with a sensitivity of 80% and a specificity of 99% detects 24 of the infected people but falsely identifies 10 uninfected individuals as infected. The positive predictive value in this example is 70%.
- **A positive result on a non-culture test should be considered presumptive evidence of infection. Consideration should be given to performing an additional test after a positive screening test and requiring that both the screening test and the additional test be positive to make a diagnosis of *C. trachomatis* infection.**
- Using a blocking antibody format to verify a positive EIA screening test and a competitive probe format to verify a positive nucleic acid probe screening test have been the additional tests most widely used. These follow-up tests are usually performed on the original screening specimen.
- Because of the greater sensitivity of NAATs, a NAAT is the only recommended additional test to verify a result from another NAAT and is, potentially, a superior additional test to verify a non-NAAT result.

Table 33.2   *Tests for diagnosis of maternal genital chlamydial infection*[15–17]

Test	Sensitivity	Specificity	Advantages	Disadvantages
Culture	40–80%[16]	99.9%	High specificity	• Handling requirements limit utility – temperature for storage must be 4°C and time to inoculation < 24 hours • Limited availability • Long incubation in tissue culture (48–72 hours)
DFA	50–80%	99.8%	Relatively quick results	• Requires a highly skilled microscopist for proper interpretation • Some assays can cross-react with other bacteria, including other species of *Chlamydia*
EIA	40–60%	99.5%	• Not technically demanding to perform • Less expensive than nucleic acid based tests • Relatively quick results	Relatively low sensitivity
NAAT	Cervix 81–100% Urine 80–96%	99.7%	• Highest sensitivity and specificity comparable to culture • Can be used on voided urine specimen • Faster results than culture • Relatively quick results	Expensive
Non-NAAT	40–65%	99%	• Relatively easy to perform and interpret • Relatively quick results	Relatively low sensitivity

DFA, direct fluorescent antibody; EIA, enzyme immunoassay; NAAT, nucleic acid amplification test.

• Except for using culture to obtain an isolate, a non-NAAT should not be used as an additional test after a NAAT because of the lower sensitivity of the non-NAAT.

Treatment

Azithromycin, amoxicillin, and **erythromycin** (in order of preference) are all accepted treatments of maternal genital chlamydial infection. Compared with erythromycin, azithromycin is associated with a similar efficacy (test of cure rates = 93% for erythromycin and 100% for azithromycin) but higher compliance and fewer reported side effects in pregnant women.[21–24] Compared with erythromycin, amoxicillin is associated with a similar efficacy in achieving a negative test of cure, and is better tolerated by pregnant women.[25–28] That is why **azithromycin is the first choice** (Table 33.3).[13] Clindamycin and erythromycin may be

considered if azithromycin and amoxicillin are contraindicated or not tolerated.[29]

Doxycycline is the treatment of choice in non-pregnant women, but is not recommended in pregnancy because it may cause permanent discoloration in developing fetal teeth. Results of clinical trials in non-pregnant populations indicate that azithromycin and doxycycline are equally efficacious, with 97% and 99% negative test of cure rates, respectively.[30] In-vitro studies suggest that *C. trachomatis* is not sufficiently sensitive to amoxicillin to consider it as an appropriate treatment; however, several randomized trials have demonstrated that amoxicillin does eradicate chlamydial infection in pregnancy. Treatments for LGV and conjunctivitis caused by *C. trachomatis* have not been studied in pregnancy. Recommendations are based on treatment recommendations in non-pregnant populations.

A follow-up test of cure is recommended in pregnant women treated for *Chlamydia*. If a nucleic acid based test is used, follow-up testing should be performed at least 3 weeks

Table 33.3 *Treatment of chlamydial infection in pregnancy* [13]

Infection	Recommended treatment	Alternate treatment
Cervicitis/urethritis/proctitis	**Azithromycin 1 g orally single dose** *or* Amoxicillin 500 mg orally three times a day for 7 days	Erythromycin base 500 mg orally four times a day for 7 days *or* Erythromycin base 250 mg orally four times a day for 14 days *or* Erythromycin ethylsuccinate 800 mg orally four times a day for 7 days *or* Erythromycin ethylsuccinate 400 mg orally four times a day for 14 days
Conjunctivitis	Azithromycin 1 g orally single dose	Erythromycin base 250 mg orally four times a day for 21 days
Lymphogranuloma venereum	Erythromycin base 500 mg orally four times a day for 21 days	

post-treatment because non-viable organisms may remain present for some days after successful treatment and can give a false-positive test result.

Concurrent treatment for gonorrhea is not indicated unless a positive test for this organism is obtained. **Because of the potential for concomitant infection, testing for *N. gonorrhoeae*, syphilis, HIV, and hepatitis B is recommended.**

One prospective study of cervical chlamydial infection in women presenting with preterm premature rupture of membranes who were conservatively managed and not treated for *Chlamydia* showed no effect on duration of latency and no increase in the incidence of chorioamnionitis or early endometritis.[31]

Repeat testing in the third trimester of pregnancy is recommended for women who test positive earlier in pregnancy to reduce transmission to the neonate at birth.[19]

REFERENCES

1. World Health Organization Department of HIV/AIDS. Global Prevalence and Incidence of Selected Curable Sexually Transmitted Infections. Geneva: World Health Organization; 2001. [epidemiological data]
2. Centers for Disease Control and Prevention. Sexually Transmitted Disease Surveillance, 2004. Atlanta, GA: US Department of Health and Human Services; 2005. [epidemiological data]
3. Chidambaram JD, Melese M, Alemayehu W, et al. Mass antibiotic treatment and community protection in trachoma control programs. Clin Infect Dis 2004; 39(9): e95–7. [II-2]
4. Lycke E, Lowhagen GB, Hallhagen G, Johannisson G, Ramstedt K. The risk of transmission of genital *Chlamydia trachomatis* infection is less than that of genital *Neisseria gonorrhoeae* infection. Sex Transm Dis 1980; 7(1): 6–10. [II-2]
5. Hammerschlag MR, Roblin PM, Gelling M, et al. Use of polymerase chain reaction for the detection of *Chlamydia trachomatis* in ocular and nasopharyngeal specimens from infants with conjunctivitis. Pediatr Infect Dis J 1997; 16(3): 293–7. [II-2]
6. Schachter J, Grossman M, Sweet RL, et al. Prospective study of perinatal transmission of *Chlamydia trachomatis*. JAMA 1986; 255(24): 3374–7. [II-2]
7. Ryan GM, Jr, Abdella TN, McNeeley SG, Baselski VS, Drummond DE. *Chlamydia trachomatis* infection in pregnancy and effect of treatment on outcome. Am J Obstet Gynecol 1990; 162(1): 34–9. [II-2]
8. Cohen I, Veille JC, Calkins BM. Improved pregnancy outcome following successful treatment of chlamydial infection. JAMA 1990; 263(23): 3160–3. [II-2, *n*=325]
9. Paz-Bailey G, Koumans EH, Sternberg M, et al. The effect of correct and consistent condom use on chlamydial and gonococcal infection among urban adolescents. Arch Pediatr Adolesc Med 2005; 159(6): 536–42. [II-2]
10. Golden MR, Whittington WL, Handsfield HH, et al. Effect of expedited treatment of sex partners on recurrent or persistent gonorrhea or chlamydial infection. N Engl J Med 2005; 352(7): 676–85. [II-2]
11. Kissinger P, Mohammed H, Richardson-Alston G, et al. Patient-delivered partner treatment for male urethritis: a randomized, controlled trial. Clin Infect Dis 2005; 41(5): 623–9. [RCT]
12. Davies HD, Wang EE. Periodic health examination, 1996 update: 2. Screening for chlamydial infections. Canadian Task Force on the Periodic Health Examination. CMAJ 1996; 154(11): 1631–44. [review and guideline]
13. Sexually transmitted diseases treatment guidelines 2006. Centers for Disease Control and Prevention. MMWR 2006; 55 (No. RR-11): 1–100. [guideline]
14. American Academy of Pediatrics and American College of Obstetricians and Gynecologists. Guidelines for Perinatal Care, 4th edn. Washington, DC: American College of Obstetricians and Gynecologists; 1997. [guideline]
15. Dille BJ, Butzen CC, Birkenmeyer LG. Amplification of *Chlamydia trachomatis* DNA by ligase chain reaction. J Clin Microbiol 1993; 31(3): 729–31. [II-3]
16. Mahony JB, Luinstra KE, Waner J, et al. Interlaboratory agreement study of a double set of PCR plasmid primers for detection of

Chlamydia trachomatis in a variety of genitourinary specimens. J Clin Microbiol 1994; 32(1): 87–91. [II-3]

17. Ossewaarde JM, Rieffe M, Rozenberg-Arska M, et al. Development and clinical evaluation of a polymerase chain reaction test for detection of *Chlamydia trachomatis*. J Clin Microbiol 1992; 30(8): 2122–8. [II-3]

18. Andrews WW, Lee HH, Roden WJ, Mott CW. Detection of genitourinary tract *Chlamydia trachomatis* infection in pregnant women by ligase chain reaction assay. Obstet Gynecol 1997; 89(4): 556–60. [II-3]

19. Gaydos CA, Howell MR, Quinn TC, Gaydos JC, McKee KT Jr. Use of ligase chain reaction with urine versus cervical culture for detection of *Chlamydia trachomatis* in an asymptomatic military population of pregnant and nonpregnant females attending Papanicolaou smear clinics. J Clin Microbiol 1998; 36(5): 1300–4. [II-2]

20. Thejls H, Gnarpe J, Gnarpe H, et al. Expanded gold standard in the diagnosis of *Chlamydia trachomatis* in a low prevalence population: diagnostic efficacy of tissue culture, direct immunofluorescence, enzyme immunoassay, PCR and serology. Genitourin Med 1994; 70(5): 300–3. [II-2]

21. Adair CD, Gunter M, Stovall TG, et al. Chlamydia in pregnancy: a randomized trial of azithromycin and erythromycin. Obstet Gynecol 1998; 91(2): 165–8. [RCT, *n* = 106]

22. Bush MR, Rosa C. Azithromycin and erythromycin in the treatment of cervical chlamydial infection during pregnancy. Obstet Gynecol 1994; 84(1): 61–3. [II-2]

23. Edwards MS, Newman RB, Carter SG, et al. Randomized clinical trial of azithromycin for the treatment of chlamydia cervicitis in pregnancy. Infect Dis Obstet Gynecol 1996; 4: 333–7. [RCT]

24. Rosenn MF, Macones GA, Silverman NS. Randomized trial of erythromycin and azithromycin for treatment of chlamydial infection in pregnancy. Inf Dis Obstet Gynecol 1995; 3: 241–4. [RCT]

25. Alary M, Joly JR, Moutquin JM, et al. Randomized comparison of amoxycillin and erythromycin in treatment of genital chlamydial infection in pregnancy. Lancet 1994; 344(8935): 1461–5. [RCT]

26. Silverman NS, Sullivan M, Hochman M, Womack M, Jungkind DL. A randomized, prospective trial comparing amoxicillin and erythromycin for the treatment of *Chlamydia trachomatis* in pregnancy. Am J Obstet Gynecol 1994; 170(3): 829–32. [RCT]

27. Magat AH, Alger LS, Nagey DA, Hatch V, Lovchik JC. Double-blind randomized study comparing amoxicillin and erythromycin for the treatment of *Chlamydia trachomatis* in pregnancy. Obstet Gynecol 1993; 81(5(Pt 1)): 745–9. [RCT]

28. Turrentine MA, Troyer L, Gonik B. Randomized prospective study comparing erythromycin, amoxicillin, and clindamycin for the treatment of *Chlamydia trachomatis* in pregnancy. Inf Dis Obstet Gynecol 1995; 2: 205–9. [RCT]

29. Brocklehurst P, Rooney G. Interventions for treating genital *Chlamydia trachomatis* infection in pregnancy. Cochrane Database Syst Rev 2006; 1. [meta-analysis: 11 RCTs, *n* = > 300]

30. Thorpe EM Jr, Stamm WE, Hook EW 3rd, et al. Chlamydial cervicitis and urethritis: single dose treatment compared with doxycycline for seven days in community based practises. Genitourin Med 1996; 72(2): 93–7. [RCT]

31. Ismail MA, Pridjian G, Hibbard JU, Harth C, Moawad AA. Significance of positive cervical cultures for *Chlamydia trachomatis* in patients with preterm premature rupture of membranes. Am J Perinatol 1992; 9(5–6): 368–70. [II-2]

34

Syphilis

A Marie O'Neill

KEY POINTS

- **Prenatal screening** and treatment of pregnant women for syphilis is **cost-effective, even in areas of low prevalence of disease** ($< 0.1\%$).
- **Penicillin** remains the only recommended **treatment** for syphilis in pregnancy.
- Pregnant women with a **penicillin allergy** should be **desensitized** and then treated with penicillin.
- Staging of disease and penicillin dosing are not altered by pregnancy.
- Current treatment regimens are based on over 50 years of clinical experience with penicillin, expert opinion, and observational clinical studies rather than on randomized clinical trials.

DEFINITION

Treponema pallidum is the causative agent of syphilis.

INCIDENCE/EPIDEMIOLOGY

- Worldwide, it is estimated that over 12 million new cases of syphilis occur annually.[1]
- **Each year at least half a million infants are born with congenital syphilis worldwide, and another half a million stillbirths and spontaneous abortions occur as a result of maternal infection.**
- Over 90% of new cases occur in developing countries. These cases are more likely to remain untreated and result in significant morbidity and mortality. In sub-Saharan Africa an estimated 2 million pregnant women are infected with syphilis annually, and 80% of these infections remain undiagnosed.[2] Syphilis is responsible for 21% of perinatal deaths in Zimbabwe, making it the leading cause of perinatal mortality.[3] In Latin America the overall prevalence of syphilis in pregnant women is 3.1%. The prevalence in pregnant women in Paraguay is 6.2%, and in Honduras 1.2% of all live births are affected with congenital syphilis.[4] Since 1989 the newly independent states of the former Soviet Union have experienced a 43-fold increase in reported cases, with rises proportionally larger among reproductive-aged women.[5] In South and Southeast Asia over 2 million reproductive-aged women are infected with syphilis annually.[1]

- The number of cases of primary and secondary syphilis in the USA has been increasing since 2000, with 7980 new cases reported to the CDC (Centers for Disease Control and Prevention) in 2004. Approximately 40% of these infections occur in reproductive-aged women.[6] Despite the recent increasing trend in the number of cases of primary and secondary syphilis in the USA, the number of cases of congenital syphilis continues to decrease, with 353 cases reported in 2004.[6] Syphilis disproportionately affects African-Americans, with the reported rate of infection in this population being 5.6 times greater than that in whites.[6,7] The Syphilis Elimination Effort (SEE) is a national initiative launched by the CDC in 1999 to reduce or eliminate syphilis in the USA. Updates on the progress of this project can be found at http://www.cdc.gov/stopsyphilis/

PATHOPHYSIOLOGY AND TRANSMISSION

Treponema pallidum is a Gram-negative spirochete unable to survive outside the human host, and therefore has never been grown in culture. Unlike most other infectious diseases, it is rarely if ever diagnosed by isolation and characterization of the causative organism. *T. pallidum* can survive in the human host for several decades.

T. pallidum is easily transmitted by sexual contact, and the overwhelming majority of cases are transmitted by **sexual intercourse**. Endemic syphilis is transmitted non-venerally by close contact with an active lesion and occurs in communities living under poor hygiene conditions. Syphilis is rarely transmitted during transfusion of blood or blood products or through needle sharing by intravenous

(IV) drug abusers. The organism generally enters the body through small breaches in epithelial surfaces of genital, anorectal, oropharyngeal, or other cutaneous sites; however, penetration of intact mucous membranes can occur. Once inside the body, it rapidly disseminates. The **incubation period** for *T. pallidum* averages 3 weeks, but can range from 10 to 90 days. During the incubation period, infected patients have, by definition, neither clinical nor serological evidence of disease but are potentially infectious. The period of greatest infectivity is early in the disease when a chancre, mucous patch, or condyloma latum is present. Infectivity decreases over time, and after 4 years it is very unlikely that an untreated individual will spread syphilis, even by sexual contact. The risk of infection during a single sexual encounter with an infected individual is up to 60%, depending on the stage of disease, and approaches 100% after five sexual encounters.[8]

Fetal syphilis occurs as a result of transplacental passage of the spirochete, which enters fetal circulation and causes infection. **Neonates** may acquire syphilis at the time of delivery by contact with infectious maternal secretions, blood, or genital lesions. Perinatal transmission may occur during any stage of maternal disease; however, it is most common in cases of maternal primary, secondary, or early latent syphilis, with up to 83% of fetuses and newborns affected.[9]

SYMPTOMS AND CLASSIFICATION

Syphilis has been called 'the great pretender' because of the **myriad of clinical manifestations** it can produce. It is a chronic, systemic infection characterized by several stages. The immune response to *T. pallidum* plays a significant role in the manifestations of all stages of syphilis. Much of the pathology observed in the disease is attributable to **vascular abnormalities caused by proliferative endarteritis** that occurs in all stages of syphilis. The pathophysiology of the endarteritis is not known, although the scarcity of treponemes and the intense inflammatory infiltrate suggest that the immune response plays a role in the development of these lesions. **Manifestations of syphilis are not altered by pregnancy.**

Incubation period

- Asymptomatic with no serological evidence of disease. Transmission can occur during this period.

Primary syphilis[8,10–12]

- Symptoms develop at the site of the initial treponemal invasion as a result of local replication of the organism.
- Treponemes also spread throughout the body by hematological and lymphatic dissemination, even before the appearance of the chancre.

- Regional **adenopathy** often develops within the first week and usually consists of several discrete non-tender, rubbery nodes. Inguinal adenopathy is often bilateral.
- Primary lesions are papular, but rapidly ulcerate to form a chancre.
- The classic **chancre** is a solitary, painless lesion with raised, firm, everted edges, central ulceration, and a granular base. However, up to 40% of individuals have multiple chancres.
- The most common site is the labia or cervix in females, but primary lesions may also occur on the lips, breasts, mouth, and anus.
- Without treatment the local lesion **spontaneously resolves within 3–6 weeks.**
- Approximately 25% of individuals will have an adequate immune response and spontaneously clear the infection.

Secondary syphilis[8,10–12]

- If the primary infection is untreated, **secondary syphilis develops 2–8 weeks later in approximately 75% of untreated individuals.**
- Secondary infection demonstrates a wide diversity in physical features involving virtually any organ and is often not thought of early in the diagnostic process.
- Secondary syphilis generally begins with a **non-specific constitutional illness** that commonly includes a sore throat, low-grade fever, myalgias, and generalized lymphadenopathy.
- **Skin rashes** are the classic and most commonly recognized lesions, but the appearance is highly variable, and differential diagnosis is often challenging.
- The rash is often initially macular and non-pruritic, and becomes papular by 3 months.
- The rash frequently involves the **palms of the hands** and **soles of the feet**, and may be accompanied by mucous patches in the mouth, pharynx, or cervix and condyloma lata in the anogenital region or axilla. **Condyloma lata** are hypertrophic lesions resembling flat warts that occur in moist areas.
- Individuals are highly contagious during this stage, especially upon contact with mucous patches or condyloma lata.
- Secondary disease **lasts for an average of 3.6 months** and spontaneously resolves. Approximately 25% of individuals experience a relapse of secondary disease during the first year of infection.

Latent syphilis[8,10–12]

- In latent syphilis, by definition, there are **no clinical stigmata of active disease**, although disease remains detectable by **positive specific treponemal serological tests** (FTA-ABS or MHA-TP; see later). Latent syphilis is further subdivided into stages based on the duration of infection: early latent, late latent, and latent of unknown duration.

Early latent syphilis

- Early latency is defined as the time period within 1 year of initial infection.
- Ninety percent of relapse occurs during this time period; mucocutaneous lesions are most common. The patient *is* infectious while lesions are present.
- Patients are believed to be potentially infectious in the absence of lesions.
- Vertical transmission of infection may occur.

Late latent syphilis

- Initial infection has occurred > 1 year previously.
- This stage is associated with host resistance to reinfection.
- Sexual transmission is unlikely.
- Transplacental infection of the fetus can occur, but is less likely than with earlier stages of disease.
- Infection via blood transfusion is possible.

Latent syphilis of unknown duration

- The date of initial infection cannot be established as having occurred within the previous year *and* the patient is aged 13–35 years old *and* has a non-treponemal titer ≥ 1:32.

Late benign syphilis (tertiary syphilis)[8,10–12]

- Without treatment at earlier stages of disease, tertiary syphilis eventually develops in 30–40% of infected patients.
- Tertiary syphilis usually becomes clinically manifest **after a period of 15–30 years** of untreated infection.
- Characteristic manifestations of tertiary disease include cardiovascular and gummatous lesions.
- **Cardiovascular** syphilis typically presents as inflammatory lesions of the cardiovascular system – especially aortitis.
- **Gummas** are granulomatous, nodular lesions that can occur in a variety of organs, most commonly skin, and bone.
- In patients with untreated syphilis, about 10% develop cardiovascular syphilis, 16% develop gummatous syphilis, and 6.5% develop symptomatic neurosyphilis.[10]
- The diagnosis of late syphilis is confounded by the lack of sensitivity of the non-treponemal tests in these conditions.

- If a patient suspected of having late syphilis has a non-reactive non-treponemal test, a confirmatory treponemal test should be performed.
- Approximately one-third of patients will remain seroreactive for decades, but will *not* develop clinical manifestations of tertiary syphilis.
- Treatment of tertiary syphilis achieves a microbiological cure, but many of the clinical manifestations will be irreversible.

Neurosyphilis[8,10–12]

- The diagnosis of neurosyphilis is made at **any** stage of disease when *both* clinical and laboratory criteria are met.
- *T. pallidum* disseminates widely after initial infection. Examination of **cerebrospinal fluid (CSF)** will reveal evidence of infection (elevated lymphocytes and protein, **positive VDRL** [venereal disease research laboratory]) in approximately 15% of patients with primary syphilis, and as many as 40% of patients with secondary syphilis.
- Many patients with CSF evidence of infection will be asymptomatic in the early stages of disease.
- Persistence of CSF abnormalities for over 5 years in the untreated patient is highly predictive of the development of clinical neurosyphilis.
- Clinical evidence of central nervous system (CNS) infection with *T. pallidum* includes:
  - acute syphilitic meningitis
  - meningovascular syphilis/seizures/stroke syndrome
  - general paresis/dementia/depression/memory loss/ change in personality
  - Argyll Robertson pupils – small fixed pupils that do not react to light but do react to convergence-accommodation
  - tabes dorsalis – paresthesias, abnormal gait, shooting pains in the extremities or trunk, diminished peripheral reflexes, loss of position and vibration senses.
- Laboratory evidence of neurosyphilis includes a reactive serological test for syphilis and a reactive VDRL in the CSF.
- The CSF-VDRL is a highly specific test, but has a **sensitivity of only about 30%**.
- Treponemal specific **testing of CSF is helpful only when negative** – this rules out neurosyphilis. Immunoglobulin G (IgG) antibodies cross the blood–brain barrier and can give a positive result in the absence of neurosyphilis; therefore, **a positive treponemal specific test is not helpful in making the diagnosis**.
- A CSF examination is essential in patients with signs or symptoms of neurological involvement at any stage of *T. pallidum* infection, and is also recommended in **all**

Table 34.1 *Screening tests for syphilis*[15, 16]

Test	Sensitivity	Specificity	Advantages	Disadvantages
Serology	85.5%	97.1%	• Relatively inexpensive • Rapid • Technically simple	• Not useful in primary disease • RPR and VDRL detect antigens not specific to treponemes
Dark-field microscopy	80%	100*	• Useful in evaluating lesions of primary disease • Immediate diagnosis if positive findings	• Not widely available – requires special equipment and an experienced operator
ICS	84.1–95.3%	92%	• Point of care testing • Inexpensive • Can use in the most resource-poor settings	• Slightly lower sensitivity than other methods
PCR	95.8%	95.7%	• In trials PCR does differentiate syphilis from other treponematoses • May be useful in primary disease	• Expensive • Not yet available for clinical use

RPR, rapid plasma reagin; VDRL, venereal disease research laboratory; ICS, immunochromatographic strip; PCR, polymerase chain reaction.
*If infection with other pathogenic treponemes can be excluded.

patients with untreated syphilis of unknown duration or of duration greater than 1 year.

- A CSF evaluation should include a cell count, protein level, and VDRL. Elevated lymphocytes and protein, and positive VDRL are typical findings.
- Treatment of neurosyphilis achieves a microbiological cure, but many of the neurological manifestations will be irreversible.

RISK FACTORS

Risk factors for maternal infection include multiple sexual partners, unprotected sex, sex in exchange for money or drugs, presence of other sexually transmitted infections (STIs), African-American race, and spending time in a correctional facility.

The **single most significant risk factor for congenital syphilis infection is maternal stage of disease.** With early-stage disease (primary, secondary, and early latent), up to 83% of fetuses and newborns are affected.[9]

COMPLICATIONS

- Untreated syphilis can profoundly affect pregnancy outcome, resulting in **spontaneous abortion, stillbirth, non-immune hydrops fetalis, preterm birth, or**

perinatal morbidity and mortality. Fetal syphilis has similar complications and manifestations to those seen in neonatal syphilis: hepatomegaly, ascites, elevated transaminases, anemia, and thrombocytopenia are common.[9]

- The longer the interval between infection and pregnancy, the more benign the outcome for the infant.[13]
- In general, infection during early gestation ends in spontaneous abortion or stillbirth; infection in late gestation results in full-term delivery of an infant with congenital syphilis; while infection in the distant past often results in an unaffected infant.[13]
- The greatest risk of stillbirth caused by congenital syphilis occurs at 24–32 weeks' gestation.[14]
- Rates of **vertical transmission** in untreated women based on stage of disease:[14]
  - 70–100% in primary syphilis
  - 40% in early latent syphilis
  - 10% in late latent disease.

MANAGEMENT
Prevention

Important practices for prevention of syphilis are early diagnosis and treatment, partner notification and treatment, and screening to identify asymptomatic cases in high-risk populations.

Screening (Table 34.1)[15,16]

- Most pregnant women with syphilis are asymptomatic and can only be identified through serological screening.
- Prenatal screening and treatment programs are limited or non-existent in many developing countries where the incidence and burden of disease is greatest.
- **Screening all pregnant women for syphilis and appropriately treating those found to be reactive effectively reduces complications associated with infection during pregnancy.**[17]
- In the USA, serological screening during pregnancy has been legislated since the 1930s; however, only 90% of states currently have statutes requiring antepartum syphilis screening.[18] Of those states with mandatory screening, 76% require one prenatal test early in pregnancy, and 26% require repeat screening in the third trimester. The most cost-effective approach is to screen all pregnant women at their initial prenatal visit, and to repeat screening in the third trimester in those women with significant risk factors.[19]
- The genus *Treponema* includes *Treponema carateum*, the causative agent of pinta, and *Treponema pallidum*. The latter species is subdivided into 3 subspecies: *T. pallidum* subsp. *pallidum*, which causes syphilis; *T. pallidum* subsp. *pertenue*, which causes yaws; and *T. pallidum* subsp. *endemicum*, which causes bejel. The subspecies causing pinta, yaws, and bejel are morphologically and serologically indistinguishable from *T. pallidum pallidum* (syphilis), so there is no test in current clinical use that can differentiate one of these treponemal infections from another. The transmission of yaws, pinta, or bejel is not via sexual contact and the clinical course of each disease is significantly different, which differentiates them from syphilis.
- **Serological testing** remains the mainstay for screening and laboratory diagnosis of secondary, latent, and tertiary syphilis. These tests include non-treponemal and treponemal antibody detection.
- Non-treponemal tests are useful for screening. These include the rapid plasma reagin (**RPR**) card test and the venereal disease research laboratory (**VDRL**) test.
- Non-treponemal tests are also useful for monitoring treatment as titers drop over time, and often revert to negative; however, with repeated infection, complete seroreversion may not occur.

Diagnosis

- Treponemal tests are used to confirm the diagnosis. These include the serum fluorescent treponemal antibody absorption test (**FTA-ABS**) and the microhemagglutination (**MHA**) test for *T. pallidum*.

- Treponemal tests remain reactive for many years in over 85% of persons adequately treated, and they give a false-positive result in about 1% of the general population; therefore, they should not be used for screening.[20]
- Serological tests are generally not reactive until several weeks after the appearance of the primary lesion, and therefore are not useful in diagnosing primary syphilis.
- Dark-field microscopy and direct fluorescent-antibody testing for *T. pallidum* (DFA-TP) are diagnostic options for primary syphilis.
- **Dark-field microscopy** is the most specific technique for diagnosing syphilis when an active chancre or condyloma latum is present. Its sensitivity is limited by the experience of the operator performing the test, the number of live treponemes in the lesion, and the presence of non-pathological treponemes in oral or anal lesions. Given the inherent difficulties of dark-field microscopy, negative examinations on three different days are necessary before a lesion may be considered negative for *T. pallidum*.[21]
- A new screening test, consisting of an immunochromatographic strip (ICS) impregnated with treponemal antigen that tests blood obtained by fingerprick and offers immediate results, is available.[15] It has been found to be cost-effective, and has the potential to have a significant impact on the epidemiology of this disease in undeveloped, resource-poor countries.
- The complete genome of *T. pallidum* has been sequenced, and specific polymerase chain reaction (PCR) primers have been developed; however, PCR is not yet available for routine clinical use.[22,23]

Work-up

- **Lumbar puncture** is indicated with:
  - neurological/ophthalmological signs
  - aortitis/gummas
  - treatment failure/treatment with agent other than penicillin
  - HIV infection
  - titer > 1:32.
- CSF with a positive VDRL is diagnostic for neurosyphilis.

Treatment (Table 34.2)[24]

- The efficacy of penicillin for the treatment of syphilis was well established through clinical experience before the value of randomized controlled clinical trials was recognized. Therefore, almost all the recommendations for the treatment of syphilis are based on the opinions of persons knowledgeable about sexually transmitted diseases (STDs) and are reinforced by case series, clinical trials, and > 50 years of clinical experience.

Table 34.2   *Treatment of syphilis[24]*

Primary syphilis	Benzathine penicillin G 2.4 million units IM in a single dose
Secondary syphilis	Benzathine penicillin G 2.4 million units IM in a single dose
Early latent syphilis	Benzathine penicillin G 2.4 million units IM in a single dose
Late latent syphilis or Syphilis of unknown duration	Benzathine penicillin G 2.4 million units IM each at 1-week intervals × 3 weeks (7.2 million units total)
Tertiary syphilis	Benzathine penicillin G 2.4 million units IM each at 1-week intervals × 3 weeks (7.2 million units total)
Neurosyphilis	Aqueous crystalline penicillin G 18–24 million units per day, administered as 3–4 million units IV every 4 hours or continuous infusion, for 10–14 days or Procaine penicillin 2.4 million units IM once daily + Probenecid 500 mg orally four times a day, both for 10–14 days

Table 34.3   *Oral desensitization protocol for patients with a positive skin test*

Penicillin V suspension dose number	Units	Cumulative dose (units)
1	100	100
2	200	300
3	400	700
4	800	1,500
5	1,600	3,100
6	3,200	6,300
7	6,400	12,700
8	12,000	24,700
9	24,000	48,700
10	48,000	96,700
11	80,000	176,700
12	160,000	336,700
13	320,000	656,700
14	640,000	1,296,700

Note: Observation period: 30 minutes before parenteral administration of penicillin. Interval between doses, 15 minutes; elapsed time, 3 hours and 45 minutes; cumulative dose, 1.3 million units. Adapted from Wendel et al.[27]

- **Parenteral penicillin G** is the only therapy with documented efficacy for syphilis during pregnancy. The success of therapy is > 98%.[25]
- The highest risk of fetal treatment failure exists with maternal secondary syphilis.[25]
- High VDRL titers at treatment and delivery, earlier maternal stage of syphilis, shorter interval from treatment to delivery, and delivery of an infant at ≤ 36 weeks' gestation are associated with the delivery of a congenitally infected neonate after adequate treatment for maternal syphilis.[26]
- Pregnant women with syphilis in any stage who report **penicillin allergy** should be evaluated to determine the need for **desensitization, and treated with penicillin** (Table 34.3).[27]
- Women with a penicillin reaction other than anaphylaxis should undergo skin testing. Those with a history of anaphylaxis or a positive skin test to one of the penicillin determinants should be desensitized and treated with penicillin.
- Desensitization is a straightforward, relatively safe procedure that can be done orally or intravenously. Oral desensitization is regarded as safer, and is easier to perform. Patients should be desensitized in a hospital setting because serious IgE-mediated allergic reaction can rarely occur. Desensitization is typically completed in approximately 4 hours, after which the first treatment dose of penicillin is administered. After desensitization, patients must be maintained on a penicillin regimen for the duration of therapy if multiple weekly doses are indicated by stage of disease.
- The **Jarisch–Herxheimer** reaction is an acute febrile reaction frequently accompanied by headache, myalgias, and other symptoms that usually occurs within the first 24 hours after any therapy for syphilis. It occurs most often in early disease – especially primary – and is thought to represent massive lysis of treponemes. The reaction begins within 1–2 hours of treatment, peaks at 8 hours, and typically resolves within 24–48 hours. It **occurs in up to 45%** of pregnant women treated for syphilis. The

Jarisch–Herxheimer reaction may induce labor or cause fetal compromise in pregnant women; however, these concerns should **not** prevent or delay therapy.

- Ultrasonography provides a non-invasive means to evaluate the fetus for signs of syphilis. Abnormal findings indicate a risk for obstetric complications and fetal treatment failure.[28]
- **Sexual contacts must be elicited, tracked, and treated** (by law in the USA).

Follow-up after treatment

- Non-treponemal antibody serological titers should be checked at 1, 3, 6, 12, and 24 months following treatment.[13]
- Among patients with primary and secondary syphilis, **a fourfold decline** (2 dilutions) **by 6 months and an eightfold decline** (4 dilutions) **by 12 months are expected.**
- Among patients with early latent syphilis, a fourfold decline by 12 months is expected.
- Titers that show a fourfold rise or do not decrease appropriately suggest either treatment failure or reinfection. The treatment regimen should be repeated in these cases.
- It is important that the same testing method (RPR or VDRL) be used for all follow-up examinations, since titers may vary by 1–2 dilutions if different tests are used.
- Patients with neurosyphilis should have repeat CSF evaluation every 6 months for the first 2 years, or until the CSF shows no evidence of disease.[13]
- Treponemal tests usually stay positive for life.

NEONATAL

Neonatal congenital syphilis is characterized by macropapular rash, hepatosplenomegaly, osteochondritis/periostosis (perform an X-ray of long bones: 95% of these infants will have osteochondritis), jaundice, ascites/hydrops, petechiae/purpura, lymphadenopathy, chorioretinitis, anemia, thrombocytopenia, hyperbilirubinemia, elevated liver enzymes, and reactive syphilis serological tests in blood/CSF. Babies can be asymptomatic. Fifty percent of congenitally affected babies are born to mothers without prenatal care. **Infants of mothers with** untreated syphilis, relapse/reinfection, treated with erythromycin, treated < 1 month before delivery, without good history of treatment, without fourfold decrease in titers, or without enough serological follow-up **should be treated. Lumbar puncture** should be carried out on any infant suspected of having congenital syphilis.

REFERENCES

1. World Health Organization Department of HIV/AIDS. Global Prevalence and Incidence of Selected Curable Sexually Transmitted Infections. Geneva: World Health Organization; 2001. [epidemiological data]

2. Deperthes BD, Meheus A, O'Reilly K, Brouet N. Maternal and congenital syphilis programmes: case studies in Bolivia, Kenya, and South Africa. Bull World Health Organ 2004; 82: 410–16. [epidemiological data]

3. Aiken CG. The causes of perinatal mortality in Bulawayo, Zimbabwe. Cent Afr J Medi 1992; 38: 263–81. [II-3]

4. Valderrama J, Zacarias F, Mazin R. [Maternal syphilis and congenital syphilis in Latin America: big problem, simple solution]. Rev Panam Salud Publica 2004; 16(3): 211–17. [review] [in Spanish]

5. Borisenko KK, Tichonova LI, Renton AM. Syphilis and other sexually transmitted infections in the Russian Federation. Int J STD AIDS 1999; 10(10): 665–8. [epidemiological data]

6. Centers for Disease Control and Prevention. Sexually Transmitted Disease Surveillance, 2004. Atlanta, GA: US Department of Health and Human Services; 2005. [review]

7. Centers for Disease Control and Prevention. STD's and Pregnancy Fact Sheet. Atlanta, GA: US Department of Health and Human Services; 2004. [review]

8. Garnett GP, Aral SO, Hoyle DV, Cates W Jr, Anderson RM. The natural history of syphilis. Implications for the transmission dynamics and control of infection. Sex Transm Dis 1997; 24(4): 185–200. [review]

9. Hollier LM, Harstad TW, Sanchez PJ, Twickler DM, Wendel GD Jr. Fetal syphilis: clinical and laboratory characteristics. Obstet Gynecol 2001; 97(6): 947–53. [II-2]

10. Clark EG, Danbolt N. The Oslo study of the natural history of untreated syphilis; an epidemiologic investigation based on a restudy of the Boeck–Bruusgaard material; a review and appraisal. J Chronic Dis 1955; 2(3): 311–44. [II-2]

11. Danbolt N, Clark EG, Gjestland T. The Oslo study of untreated syphilis; a re-study of the Boeck–Bruusgaard material concerning the fate of syphilitics who receive no specific treatment; a preliminary report. Acta Derm Venereol 1954; 34(1–2): 34–8. [II-2]

12. Rockwell DH, Yobs AR, Moore MB Jr. The Tuskegee study of untreated syphilis; the 30th year of observation. Arch Intern Med 1964; 114: 792–8. [II-2]

13. Singh AE, Romanowski B. Syphilis: review with emphasis on clinical, epidemiologic, and some biologic features. Clin Microbiol Rev 1999; 12(2): 187–209. [review]

14. Fiumara NJ. Review of congenital syphilis. Sex Transm Dis 1984; 11(1): 49–50. [review]

15. Montoya PJ, Lukehart SA, Brentlinger PE, et al. Comparison of the diagnostic accuracy of a rapid immunochromatographic test and the rapid plasma reagin test for antenatal syphilis screening in Mozambique. Bull World Health Organ 2006; 84(2): 97–104. [II-3]

16. Young H. Syphilis serology. Dermatol Clin 1998; 16(4): 691–8. [II-3]

17. United States Preventive Services Task Force. Screening for syphilis infection: recommendation statement. Rockville, MD: Agency for Healthcare Research and Quality; 2004. [guideline]

18. Hollier LM, Hill J, Sheffield JS, Wendel GD Jr. State laws regarding prenatal syphilis screening in the United States. Am J Obstet Gynecol 2003; 189(4): 1178–83. [review]

19. Turrentine MA, Troyer L, Gonik B. Randomized prospective study comparing erythromycin, amoxicillin, and clindamycin for the treatment of *Chlamydia trachomatis* in pregnancy. Inf Dis Obstet Gynecol 1995; 2: 205–9. [RCT]

20. Larsen SA, Steiner BM, Rudolph AH. Laboratory diagnosis and interpretation of tests for syphilis. Clin Microbiol Rev 1995; 8(1): 1–21. [II-3]

21. Cummings MC, Lukehart SA, Marra C, et al. Comparison of methods for the detection of *Treponema pallidum* in lesions of early syphilis. Sex Transm Dis 1996; 23(5): 366–9. [II-1]

22. Liu H, Rodes B, Chen CY, Steiner B. New tests for syphilis: rational design of a PCR method for detection of *Treponema pallidum* in clinical specimens using unique regions of the DNA polymerase I gene. J Clin Microbiol 2001; 39(5): 1941–6. [II-2]

23. Serwin AB, Kohl PK, Chodynicka B. The centenary of Wassermann reaction – the future of serological diagnosis of syphilis, up-to-date studies. Przegl Epidemiol 2005; 59(3): 633–40. [review]

24. Sexually transmitted diseases treatment guidelines 2006. Centers for Disease Control and Prevention. MMWR 2006; 55(No. RR–11): 1–100. [guidelines]

25. Alexander JM, Sheffield JS, Sanchez PJ, Mayfield J, Wendel GD Jr. Efficacy of treatment for syphilis in pregnancy. Obstet Gynecol 1999; 93(1): 5–8. [II-2]

26. Sheffield JS, Sanchez PJ, Morris G, et al. Congenital syphilis after maternal treatment for syphilis during pregnancy. Am J Obstet Gynecol 2002; 186(3): 569–73. [II-2]

27. Wendel GD Jr, Stark BJ, Jamison RB, Molina RD, Sullivan TJ. Penicillin allergy and desensitization in serious infections during pregnancy. N Engl J Med 1985; 312(19): 1229–32. [II-2]

28. Wendel GD Jr, Sheffield JS, Hollier LM, et al. Treatment of syphilis in pregnancy and prevention of congenital syphilis. Clin Infect Dis 2002; 35(Suppl 2): S200–9. [II-2]

35

Trichomonas

A Marie O'Neill

KEY POINTS

- Pregnant women colonized with *Trichomonas vaginalis* in the second trimester have a **higher risk of delivering an infant with low birth weight** *or* **delivering before term**, but metronidazole treatment, unfortunately, has been **associated with an 80% increase of preterm birth.**
- *T. vaginalis* infection is a **risk factor for sexual transmission of human immunodeficiency virus-1 (HIV-1), with a twofold increase reported.**
- **Condoms,** when used correctly and consistently, provide a high degree of **protection from many sexually transmitted infections (STIs), including** *T. vaginalis.*
- There is no evidence that identifying asymptomatic *T. vaginalis* is beneficial in reducing the associated risk of preterm delivery or delivery of a low birth weight infant; therefore, **there is insufficient evidence to recommend screening of asymptomatic pregnant women, and some evidence that treatment of these patients may in fact be harmful.**
- **Metronidazole as a single 2 g oral dose, or 500 mg twice a day for 7 days, at any gestational age,** is the treatment of choice for *symptomatic T. vaginalis* infection.
- **Concurrent treatment of sexual partners** is recommended to prevent reinfection.

EPIDEMIOLOGY/INCIDENCE

Worldwide, it is estimated that 180 million new cases of trichomoniasis occur annually.[1] Undeveloped countries account for a disproportionate number of cases. Trichomoniasis affects 2–3 million women and approximately 80 000 pregnant women in the USA annually. The frequency of infection in European women is similar. The World Health Organization (WHO) estimates 30 million new infections annually in Africa.[2] In contrast to bacterial sexually transmitted infections (STIs) such as *Neisseria gonorrhoeae* and *Chlamydia trachomatis*, *T. vaginalis* infection rates are as high or higher in middle-aged women when compared with adolescents. Incidence is highest among women with multiple sexual partners, and in populations with high rates of other STIs.

SYMPTOMS/SIGNS

The clinical manifestations of trichomoniasis are unchanged in pregnant women. Infection is **asymptomatic in up to 50% of women.** The most common symptoms include vulvovaginal pruritus (23–82%), vaginal discharge (50–75%), dysuria (30–50%), and dyspareunia (10–50%). The most common signs are copious vaginal discharge (50–75%), yellow/green in 5–20%, frothy in 10–50%; inflammation of vaginal mucosa (40–75%); and vulvar erythema (10–20%).

ETIOLOGY/BASIC PATHOPHYSIOLOGY

Trichomoniasis is caused by the protozoan *Trichomonas vaginalis*, which had been previously thought to be a harmless commensal. *T. vaginalis* can infect the vagina and the Skene's glands of the urethra. The incubation period for *T. vaginalis* is 4–7 days on average, but ranges from 2 to 28 days.

TRANSMISSION

T. vaginalis is easily transmitted during **vaginal intercourse.** The organism will survive for several hours in a moist environment outside the host and is rarely transmitted nonvenerally. The transmission rate from male to female during vaginal intercourse has been reported to be 66–100%.[3] Vertical transmission to a female infant occurs in 2–17% if vaginal infection is present at the time of delivery.[4] Urinary and respiratory infections occur in <5% of cases.

COMPLICATIONS/RISKS

Pregnant women colonized with *T. vaginalis* in the second trimester have a 30% **higher risk of delivering an infant with low birth weight** *or* **delivering before term**, and a 40% higher risk of giving birth to an infant who is both preterm *and* of low birth weight.[5] In pregnant women with *T. vaginalis*, **metronidazole treatment,** unfortunately, has been **associated**

Table 35.1   *Screening/diagnostic tests for T. vaginalis[15–17]*

Test	Sensitivity	Specificity	Advantages	Disadvantages
Wet mount	62–80%	>99%	• Rapid results • Inexpensive • High specificity	• Low sensitivity compared with culture • Sensitivity and specificity are strongly dependent on the skills and experience of the microscopist and also on the quality of the sample
Culture	95%	100%	• High sensitivity and specificity	• Organism can be rendered non-viable if incorrect media used or delay in transport • 3–7 days to complete • Not available in most clinical labs
PCR	95%	98%	• Results available more quickly than with culture	• Most expensive option • Limited availability

PCR, polymerase chain reaction.

with an **80% increase of preterm birth** compared with no treatment, with the majority of the increase in preterm delivery attributed to spontaneous preterm labor.[6–8] The proposed mechanism for treatment with metronidazole causing preterm labor is that lysis of dying trichomonads elicits an inflammatory response that triggers labor. (see also Chapter 15 of *Obstetric Evidence Based Guidelines*).

T. vaginalis infection is a **risk factor for sexual transmission of human immunodeficiency virus-1 (HIV-1)** in women. Studies from Africa have suggested that *T. vaginalis* infection approximately doubles the rate of HIV transmission.[9] The proposed mechanism for this increased risk is twofold:

• local infiltration of large number of leukocytes, including CD4+ lymphocytes – the primary target of HIV infection
• disruption in the integrity of the vaginal mucosa.

MANAGEMENT

Prevention

Condoms, when used correctly and consistently, provide a high degree of protection from many STIs.[10]

Screening

There is no evidence that identifying asymptomatic *T. vaginalis* is beneficial in reducing the associated risk of preterm delivery or delivery of a low birth weight infant.[6–8]

Diagnosis

Wet mount preparation of vaginal secretions suspended in normal saline with microscopic observation of motile trichomonads is the most **commonly utilized** method of diagnosing trichomoniasis in women; however, the **sensitivity** of this method is **low**.

Isolation of *T. vaginalis* by **culture is the gold standard**, but the greater cost and longer time to diagnosis make this an underutilized diagnostic option. Commonly used culture media include:[11,12]

• modified Diamond's broth media, sensitivity 95%
• InPouch transport and test system, sensitivity 87%
• modified Columbia agar, sensitivity 98%.

To increase the detection rate in a high-risk population without substantially increasing cost, culture could be performed on those symptomatic patients with a negative wet mount. Although nucleic acid based tests are available, they are not yet widely used. Conventional Papanicolaou (Pap) smear is not considered accurate for the identification of *T. vaginalis*. Confirmatory testing is necessary for those cases reported by Pap: sensitivity = 60–70%, specificity = 88%. Liquid-based Pap smear is accurate for the identification of *T. vaginalis* and warrants treatment without further testing; however, the sensitivity is low (61.4%).[13] Clinicians who perform STD (sexually transmitted disease) screening tests should be aware of the prevalence of STDs in the population being screened and have a conceptual understanding of positive predictive value and the impact of screening low-risk individuals with a test that has limited specificity (Table 35.1).[14–16]

Treatment

The nitroimidazoles are the only class of drugs useful for the oral or parenteral treatment of trichomoniasis. In randomized clinical trials, oral nitroimadazoles have resulted in parasitological cure rates of 90–95%. Metronidazole and tinidazole are most commonly used. **Metronidazole can be given as a single 2 g oral dose, or 500 mg twice a day for 7** days, and can be given to symptomatic women **at any gestational age**. Multiple studies and meta-analyses have not demonstrated a definitive association between metronidazole use during pregnancy and teratogenic or mutagenic effects in infants.[17,18] Tinidazole is given as a single 2 g oral dose. Its use is contraindicated in the first trimester of pregnancy. Metronidazole resistance is increasingly common. The CDC (Centers for Disease Control and Prevention) estimated that **5% of clinical isolates of *T. vaginalis* exhibit** some degree of **metronidazole resistance**. An escalated dosing regimen of metronidazole 2 g daily for 3–5 days has been successful in some cases of resistant infection. Tinidazole is effective in treating up to 60% of metronidazole-resistant *T. vaginalis* infections. **Concurrent treatment of sexual partners** is recommended to prevent reinfection.

REFERENCES

1. World Health Organization. World Health Report 1998. Geneva, Switzerland: WHO; 1998. [epidemiological data]
2. Gerbase AC, Mertens TE. Sexually transmitted diseases in Africa: time for action. Afr Health 1998; 20(3): 10–12. [review]
3. Krieger JN. Trichomoniasis in men: old issues and new data. Sex Transm Dis 1995; 22(2): 83–96. [II-3]
4. Danesh IS, Stephen JM, Gorbach J. Neonatal *Trichomonas vaginalis* infection. J Emerg Med 1995; 13(1): 51–4. [II-3]
5. Cotch MF, Pastorek JG 2nd, Nugent RP, et al. *Trichomonas vaginalis* associated with low birth weight and preterm delivery. The vaginal infections and prematurity study group. Sex Transm Dis 1997; 24(6): 353–60. [II-2]
6. Klebanoff MA, Carey JC, Hauth JC, et al. Failure of metronidazole to prevent preterm delivery among pregnant women with asymptomatic *Trichomonas vaginalis* infection. N Engl J Med 2001; 345(7): 487–93. [RCT, n = 617. 2 g metronidazole q48h × 2 doses]
7. Gulmezoglu AM. Interventions for trichomoniasis in pregnancy. Cochrane Database Syst Rev 2007; 1. [meta-analysis: 2 RCTs, *n* = 842]
8. Ross SM, Van Middelkoop A. Trichomonas infection in pregnancy: does it affect outcome? S Afr Med J 1983; 63: 566–7. [RCT, *n* = 225. 2 g metronidazole × 1 to women and their partners]
9. Laga M, Manoka A, Kivuvu M, et al. Non-ulcerative sexually transmitted diseases as risk factors for HIV-1 transmission in women: results from a cohort study. AIDS 1993; 7(1): 95–102. [II-2]
10. Paz-Bailey G, Koumans EH, Sternberg M, et al. The effect of correct and consistent condom use on chlamydial and gonococcal infection among urban adolescents. Arch Pediatr Adolesc Med 2005; 159(6): 536–42. [II-3]
11. Borchardt KA, Zhang MZ, Shing H, Flink K. A comparison of the sensitivity of the InPouch TV, Diamond's and Trichosel media for detection of *Trichomonas vaginalis*. Genitourin Med 1997; 73(4): 297–8. [II-2]
12. Stary A, Kuchinka-Koch A, Teodorowicz L. Detection of *Trichomonas vaginalis* on modified Columbia agar in the routine laboratory. J Clin Microbiol 2002; 40(9): 3277–80. [II-2]
13. Lara-Torre E, Pinkerton JS. Accuracy of detection of *Trichomonas vaginalis* organisms on a liquid-based Papanicolaou smear. Am J Obstet Gynecol 2003; 188(2): 354–6. [II-2]
14. Radonjic IV, Dzamic AM, Mitrovic SM, et al. Diagnosis of *Trichomonas vaginalis* infection: the sensitivities and specificities of microscopy, culture and PCR assay. Eur J Obstet Gynecol Reprod Biol 2005; 126(8): 116–20. [II-2]
15. Aslan DL, Gulbahce HE, Stelow EB, et al. The diagnosis of *Trichomonas vaginalis* in liquid-based Pap tests: correlation with PCR. Diagn Cytopathol 2005; 32(6): 341–4. [II-3]
16. Patel SR, Wiese W, Patel SC, et al. Systematic review of diagnostic tests for vaginal trichomoniasis. Infect Dis Obstet Gynecol 2000; 8(5–6): 248–57. [review]
17. Burtin P, Taddio A, Ariburnu O, Einarson TR, Koren G. Safety of metronidazole in pregnancy: a meta-analysis. Am J Obstet Gynecol 1995; 172(2 Pt 1): 525–9. [meta-analysis]
18. Sorensen HT, Larsen H, Jensen ES, et al. Safety of metronidazole during pregnancy: a cohort study of risk of congenital abnormalities, preterm delivery and low birth weight in 124 women. J Antimicrob Chemother 1999; 44(6): 854–6. [II-2]

36

Group B streptococcus

Marianne Vendola

KEY POINTS

- Asymptomatic group B streptococcus (GBS) colonization in the mother is associated with an incidence of neonatal GBS disease of ~1–2% without intervention. **Neonatal disease** is divided into **early-onset** or **late-onset** disease, with possible complications being **sepsis, pneumonia, meningitis**, and, less frequently, **focal infections** and death.
- Major **risk factors** for neonatal GBS sepsis are **prolonged rupture of membranes** (≥ 18 hours), **preterm delivery**, and maternal **temperature $\geq 100.4°F$ ($\geq 38°C$).**
- **Universal prenatal maternal screening and intrapartum antibiotic treatment** are the most efficacious of the current strategies for prevention of early-onset disease, and >50% more effective than a risk factor-based strategy. There is no known prevention of late-onset GBS sepsis.
- **Women with GBS bacteriuria** in the current pregnancy or who had a **prior infant with GBS sepsis** are candidates for **intrapartum antibiotics prophylaxis**, and should be the only two groups **not screened**. **Asymptomatic women with even low** (<100) **CFU (colony-forming units) of GBS in the urine culture should be treated both antepartum and intrapartum.**
- **Screening** involves collecting an **anovaginal specimen at 35–37 weeks** (labeled penicillin-allergic if appropriate). Women who are GBS positive are treated with **penicillin in labor**. Ampicillin is a reasonable alternative. If the patient is penicillin-allergic but not at high risk for anaphylaxis, cefazolin is the agent of choice.
- **Intrapartum treatment for chorioamnionitis is recommended, regardless of GBS maternal status.**

DIAGNOSIS/DEFINITION

Streptococcus agalactiae, or Lancefield group B streptococcal (GBS) disease is a bacterial infection involving the pregnant woman and her newborn infant.

SYMPTOMS

In the **mother**, GBS is usually **asymptomatic**. It can cause urinary tract infection, chorioamnionitis, endometritis, bacteremia, and stillbirth. Two forms of infection occur in **newborns: early-onset** and **late-onset disease**. Early-onset GBS disease usually causes illness within the first 24 hours of life. However, illness can occur up to 6 days after birth. Late-onset disease usually occurs at 3–4 weeks of age; it can occur any time from 7 days to 3 months of age. Symptoms of both kinds of neonatal GBS include breathing problems, not eating well, irritability, extreme drowsiness, unstable temperature (low or high), and weakness or listlessness (in late-onset disease).

EPIDEMIOLOGY/INCIDENCE (FIGURE 36.1)

GBS is a major cause of invasive disease at all ages and can cause serious bacterial sepsis, including neonatal meningitis. The prevalence of asymptomatic GBS anovaginal colonization in pregnant women is **about 20%**, with a range of 1.6–30.4%.[1–3] Usually 40–75% of neonates born to colonized mothers are colonized themselves (about 15% of all neonates). The prevalence of **early-onset GBS sepsis** fell in the USA from 2.0/1000 in 1990 to **0.4/1000** in 2004, attributable to the increasing use of intrapartum antibiotics.[4] The screening-based approach to GBS infection brought a dramatic decrease in the overall rate of neonatal early-onset GBS even **among VLBW (very low birth weight) infants (3.3 cases $\times$ 1000 VLBW births).**[4]

ETIOLOGY/BASIC PATHOPHYSIOLOGY

GBS is now best known as a cause of postpartum infection and as one of the most common causes of neonatal sepsis.

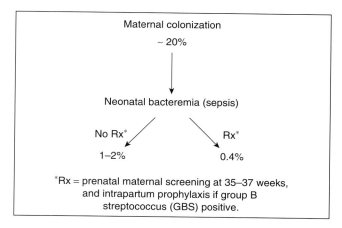

Figure 36.1
Natural history of GBS infection.

There are several serotypes. Group B streptococci colonize the vaginal and gastrointestinal tract (reservoir) in healthy women. Neonates acquire the organism as a result of **vertical transmission from the maternal genital tract** to the infant in utero or **usually at delivery**.

CLASSIFICATION

Disease in the neonate is divided into early and late disease. **Early neonatal sepsis** with GBS is often observed within 24 hours of delivery, but it can become apparent as late as 7 days after birth. Early-onset disease presents within the first 6 days of life, with breathing difficulty, shock, pneumonia, and occasionally infection of the spinal fluid and brain (meningitis). Nothing specific regarding the clinical presentation in early disease differentiates group B streptococci as

the etiology from other pathogens. Pneumonia with bacteremia is common and meningitis less likely. **Late GBS disease** is defined as infection after 1 week and before 3 months after birth. Late disease is commonly serotype III, characterized by bacteremia and meningitis. Infections in the infant can be localized, or may involve the entire body.

RISK FACTORS/ASSOCIATIONS

For early-onset GBS disease, **prolonged rupture of membranes (≥18 hours), preterm delivery (but >80% GBS neonates are term), temperature ≥100.4°F (≥38°C)**, maternal GBS colonization between 35 and 37 weeks, birth of a previous infant with invasive GBS disease, maternal chorioamnionitis, young maternal age, African-American race, Hispanic ethnicity, and GBS bacteriuria during pregnancy. Diabetes or maternal GBS colonization in a previous pregnancy are not risk factors for early-onset GBS disease.

COMPLICATIONS (TABLE 36.1)

In newborns GBS can cause **sepsis, pneumonia, meningitis**, and, less frequently, **focal infections** such as osteomyelitis, septic arthritis, or cellulites. Early-onset GBS sepsis is defined as occurring within the first week of life, usually around 48 hours and within 72 hours. Late-onset disease occurs after the first week.[5] **Neonatal death** due to GBS infection occurs in 1 in 10 000 neonates.

Rarely, intrauterine fetal GBS infection can occur, even with intact membranes, from ascending colonization. Growth restriction, microcephaly, hydranencephaly, cerebellar necrosis, chorioretinitis, cataract, microphthalmia,

Table 36.1	*Early- versus late-onset GBS characteristics*	
Characteristic	Early-onset disease	Late-onset disease
Definition	Occurs <1 week	≥1 week
Usual timing of manifestation after birth	48 hours	≥1 week
Incidence (of all neonatal GBS sepsis)	80% (natural); 50% (screen and treat)[5]	20% (natural); 50% (screen and treat)[5]
Most common/predominant clinical signs/symptoms	Rapid RDS, pneumonia (meningitis 10–30%)	Meningitis, localized infections (ears, eyes, breasts, bone, joints, skin, etc.)
Serotype		III (95%)
Mortality	5%	<2%
Long-term morbidity		If meningitis – 15–50% can have neurological sequelae

GBS, group B streptococcus; RDS, respiratory distress syndrome.

and hepatosplenomegaly can be present. Some of these findings are easily ascertained by ultrasound.

MANAGEMENT
Principles/prevention

Several approaches to the prevention of **early-onset** GBS neonatal infection have been studied or devised.[6] There are **no trials** to assess the effectiveness of any of these approaches, probably because they would have to include about > 100 000 screened pregnancies to show a difference in early-onset GBS sepsis given the current incidence of the disease (< 0.5%).

Maternal vaccination

Vaccination against GBS is potentially the most effective method of preventing the morbidity and mortality caused by infection.

Active vaccination
Active vaccination needs to be polyvalent to cover all serotypes. It has the potential to prevent about twice as many cases of death in the neonate as microbiological screening, and three times as many as risk factor-based screening, but a large randomized trial should be carried out.[7] The first capsular polysaccharide vaccines were poorly immunogenic, so a trial of protein conjugate vaccines followed, using tetanus toxoid as the conjugate. They were shown to be safe, well tolerated, and the antibody response was persistent for over a year in the mother and the passive protection in the neonate protected him/her against late-onset disease.[8] But there is need for a large, randomized trial recording neonatal disease events (phase 3).[9] Vaccination is the only strategy that would protect against late-onset disease, which current strategies do not cover.

Passive vaccination
Passive vaccination with 'specific' GBS immunoglobulin G (IgG) is not available.

Universal maternal treatment

There are insufficient data to evaluate universal treatment of all women during birth.

Prenatal maternal screening and prelabor maternal treatment

Antibiotic therapy (with erythromycin) does not prevent preterm birth (PTB) or affect stillbirths in women with GBS colonization. Subanalysis by heavy colonization did not change results.[10] **Antibiotics should not be used before the antepartum period to treat asymptomatic maternal GBS** colonization, except if GBS is present in the urine (2–4% of pregnancies). **Asymptomatic women with even low** (< 100) **CFU** (colony-forming units) of **GBS in the urine culture at 27–31 weeks have decreased PTB < 37 weeks when treated with penicillin 1 million IU three times per day for 6 days** compared with placebo.[11] Therefore, GBS bacteriuria should be always adequately treated at diagnosis. In fact, every urine specimen sent in pregnancy should be labeled 'pregnant', so as to alert the laboratory to report any isolation of GBS. GBS identified in urine is a marker for heavy maternal colonization, is also associated with a higher risk for early-onset GBS sepsis, and is therefore also an indication for intrapartum antibiotic prophylaxis.

No prenatal maternal screening and intrapartum treatment based on risk factors

Risk factors are described above; the ones used for this strategy are delivering < 37 weeks, intrapartum temperature ≥ 100.4°F (≥ 38°C), or rupture of membranes ≥ 18 hours.[7] Over 20% of neonates with early-onset GBS sepsis are born to women without risk factors. As shown below, while this was a popular strategy in the past, it is less effective than a screening-based strategy.[12,13] A risk factor-based strategy is still common in the UK and other European countries. **Intrapartum treatment for chorioamnionitis is recommended, regardless of GBS maternal status.**[4]

Universal prenatal maternal screening and intrapartum treatment (Figure 36.2)

A screening-based strategy is > 50% more effective than a risk factor-based strategy.[13] This is the protocol with the most evidence for efficacy.[14] After the Center for Disease Control (CDC) recommended this screening strategy compared to either this or a risk factor-based strategy in 2002,[7] the incidence of early-onset GBS sepsis declined from 0.47 in 1000 live births (1999–2001) to 0.32–0.34 in 1000 (2003–2004).[5] A screening-based strategy involves an incidence of intrapartum antibiotic prophylaxis similar (24%) to that of the risk factor approach;[13] therefore, the treatment risks should be similar. Even this approach of screening for GBS colonization and intrapartum treatment **does not affect the incidence of late-onset GBS sepsis.** A screening-based strategy is recommended in the USA and Australia (see Screening section below for more details).

Neonatal (screening and) treatment only

Screening and/or treatment of just the neonate without some form of in-utero prophylaxis is a much inferior approach than the maternal screening approaches just

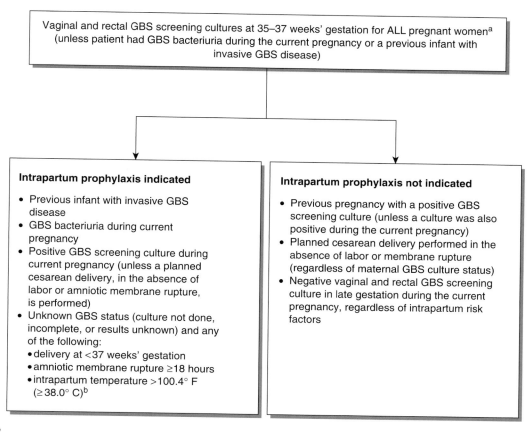

Figure 36.2

Indications for intrapartum antibiotic prophylaxis to prevent perinatal GBS disease under a universal prenatal screening strategy based on combined vaginal and rectal cultures collected at 35–37 weeks' gestation from all pregnant women. (Reproduced from Schrag et al.[7])

[a]If onset of labor or rupture of amniotic membranes occurs at <37 weeks' gestation and there is a significant risk for preterm delivery (as assessed by the clinician), a suggested algorithm for group B streptococcus (GBS) prophylaxis management is provided (Figure 36.3).
[b]If amnionitis is suspected, broad-spectrum antibiotic therapy that includes an agent known to be active against GBS should replace GBS prophylaxis.

described (screening or risk-factor based). Neonatal treatment is only 'too little too late', as 40% of neonates with GBS are already bacteremic at birth. Evaluation of neonates born to GBS-positive mothers who were not treated or to mothers with risk factors is imperative.[4]

Screening/diagnosis (see Figure 36.2)

Detection

Detecting vaginal GBS colonization of pregnant women is a way of detecting women at high risk for early-onset GBS infection. Because colonization is intermittent, the earlier in pregnancy a swab is done the less it is predictive. Taking a swab at 35–37 weeks is the generally recommended time, but it misses late colonization. The positive and negative predictive values of GBS carriage at 35–37 weeks (prevalence about 20%) for carriage at time of parturition are > 79

and > 93%, respectively.[4] **Women with GBS bacteriuria in the current pregnancy or who had a prior infant with GBS sepsis** are candidates for **intrapartum antibiotics prophylaxis** and **should not be screened.**[7]

Collection of screening specimen

An anovaginal swab is collected at 35–37 weeks. At 35–37 weeks, swab first the lower vagina, then the anal area. The anogenital specimen obtains the highest yield for GBS. Vaginal–rectal swabs, during which > 70% of women report at least mild pain, do not increase GBS detection rates compared with vaginal–perianal swabs.[15] When women collect the specimens themselves as outpatients, GBS yield is similar to when the specimens are collected by a healthcare worker.[16] Swab is transported in a special medium (e.g. Amies or Stuart's without charcoal), which maintains GBS viability for ≤4 days, and **labeled 'penicillin allergy' if**

Table 36.2 *Recommended regimens for intrapartum antimicrobial prophylaxis for perinatal GBS disease prevention*[a]	
Recommended	Penicillin G, 5 million units IV initial dose, then 2.5 million units IV every 4 hours until delivery
Alternative	Ampicillin, 2 g IV initial dose, then 1 g IV every 4 hours until delivery
If penicillin allergic[b] Patients not at high risk for anaphylaxis	Cefazolin, 2 g IV initial dose, then 1 g IV every 8 hours until delivery
Patients at high risk for anaphylaxis[c] GBS susceptible to clindamycin and erythromycin[d]	Clindamycin, 900 mg IV every 8 hours until delivery or Erythromycin, 500 mg IV every 6 hours until delivery
GBS resistant to clindamycin or erythromycin or susceptibility unknown	Vancomycin,[e] 1 g IV every 12 hours until delivery

[a] Broader-spectrum agents, including an agent against group B streptococcus (GBS), may be necessary for treatment of chorioamnionitis.

[b] History of penicillin allergy should be assessed to determine whether a high risk for anaphylaxis is present. Penicillin-allergic patients at high risk for anaphylaxis are those who have experienced immediate hypersensitivity to penicillin, including a history of penicillin-related anaphylaxis; other high-risk patients are those with asthma or other diseases that would make anaphylaxis more dangerous or difficult to treat, such as persons being treated with beta-adrenergic-blocking agents.

[c] If laboratory facilities are adequate, clindamycin and erythromycin susceptibility testing should be performed on prenatal GBS isolates from penicillin-allergic women at high risk for anaphylaxis.

[d] Resistance to erythromycin is often but not always associated with clindamycin resistance. If a strain is resistant to erythromycin, but appears susceptible to clindamycin, it may still have inducible resistance to clindamycin.

[e] Cefazolin is preferred over vancomycin for women with a history of penicillin allergy other than immediate hypersensitivity reactions, and pharmacological data suggest it achieves effective intra-amniotic concentrations. Vancomycin should be reserved for penicillin-allergic women at high risk for anaphylaxis.

Reproduced from Schrag et al.[7]

appropriate. The swabs are cultured using a selective enrichment broth media (e.g. Todd-Hewitt broth with antibiotics) over 18–24 hours. For penicillin-allergic patients, clindamycin and erythromycin disk susceptibility is carried out.[7]

Identification

Definitive microbiological identification is performed by serological detection of group B antigen or a polymerase chain reaction (PCR).[12] A **PCR test** has a sensitivity of 97%, a specificity of 100%, and a positive predictive value of 100% compared with conventional anovaginal cultures, but is not widely available, and PCR universal screening has not been sufficiently tested in clinical studies.[12]

Rapid screening

The availability of a sensitive rapid screening test to detect accurately women in labor who are colonized with GBS would make prevention strategies more efficient, but the available **rapid tests still lack acceptable performance characteristics**. A rapid and sensitive test with appropriate therapy would further decrease the incidence of GBS sepsis.

Intrapartum antibiotic prophylaxis (Table 36.2)

Intrapartum antibiotic prophylaxis in women colonized with GBS is associated with a 90% **decreased incidence of infant colonization** and 83% decreased **early-onset neonatal infection with group B streptococcus**.[17] Intrapartum antibiotic treatment is also associated with a **strong trend for an 88% decreased incidence of neonatal mortality**.[17] The rate of infant GBS sepsis in the control groups of the studies where this outcome was reported ranged from 2 to 9%. This is higher than the overall infection rates of 1–2% that are reported in babies whose mothers are colonized with GBS, raising questions as to how representative the populations studied were.

Penicillin is the first-line agent for intrapartum GBS prophylaxis (see Table 36.2). When antibiotics are given ≥ 2 hours before delivery, early-onset sepsis is minimized.[18] For women with penicillin allergy, see Table 36.2.[7] Clindamycin for penicillin-allergic women with GBS colonization has also been suggested,[19] but the rate of resistance can be as high as 15%.[7,12] If the culture results are unknown, the risk-based approach can be used (see Figure 36.2). Women with negative GBS cultures ≤ 5 weeks do not require intrapartum prophylaxis even if the above risk factors develop.[7] If intrauterine infection is diagnosed, broad-spectrum antibiotic therapy (e.g. ampicillin and gentamicin) is recommended.[19]

Adverse consequences of prophylaxis are anaphylaxis to penicillin (4–40 in 100 000), drug resistance, and neonatal infection from agents different than GBS. Regarding drug resistance, penicillin is the preferred antibiotic to decrease resistance. If the patient is penicillin-allergic but not at high risk for anaphylaxis, cefazolin is the agent of choice (see Table 36.2). Early-onset sepsis from pathogens other than GBS requires continuous surveillance.

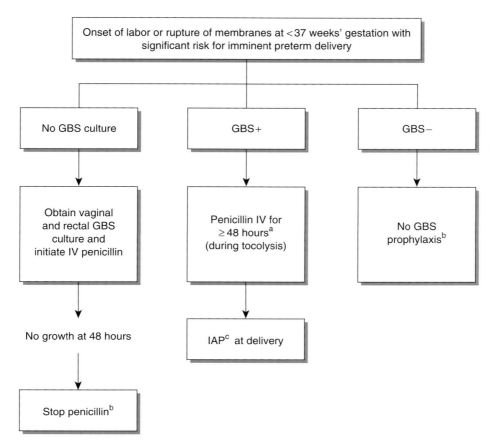

Figure 36.3
Sample algorithm for GBS prophylaxis for women with threatened preterm delivery. This algorithm is not an exclusive course of management. Variations that incorporate individual circumstances or institutional preferences may be appropriate. (Reproduced from Schrag et al.[7])

[a] Penicillin should be continued for a total of at least 48 hours, unless delivery occurs sooner. At the physician's discretion, antibiotic prophylaxis may be continued beyond 48 hours in a group B streptococcus (GBS) culture-positive woman if delivery has not yet occurred. For women who are GBS culture positive, antibiotic prophylaxis should be reinitiated when labor likely to proceed to delivery occurs or recurs.
[b] If delivery has not occurred within 4 weeks, a vaginal and rectal GBS screening culture should be repeated and the patient should be managed as described, based on the result of the repeat culture.
[c] Intrapartum antibiotic prophylaxis.

Women undergoing **cesarean delivery** before labor or rupture of membranes (ROM) do not benefit from intrapartum GBS prophylaxis. But women planning to be delivered by cesarean should still undergo screening for GBS at 35–37 weeks, in case they present in labor or with ROM.

For women with **threatened preterm delivery**, see Figure 36.3.

Vaginal chlorhexidine is associated with a statistically significant (28%) reduction in GBS colonization of 7-day-old neonates, but is not associated with reductions in other outcomes, including neonatal early-onset GBS infection, pneumonia, sepsis, or mortality.[20] The lack of efficacy may be due to insufficient data (type II error).

Antepartum testing

No specific indication for GBS carriers.

Delivery

Intrapartum antibiotic prophylaxis is as described (see Figure 36.2). There is insufficient evidence to assess if digital vaginal examinations or intrauterine fetal monitoring affect the incidence of GBS sepsis.[7] There seems to be no increase in GBS sepsis in pregnancies undergoing stripping of membranes,[21] but none of the studies reported screening or results for GBS.

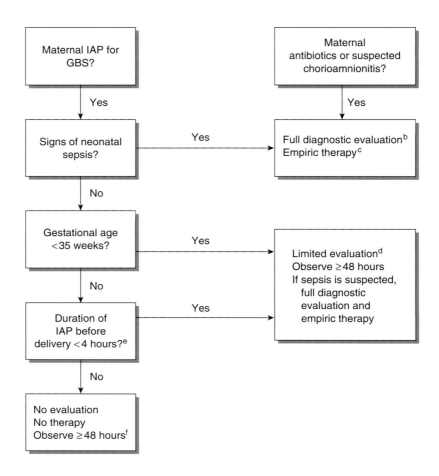

Figure 36.4

Sample algorithm for management of a newborn whose mother received intrapartum antimicrobial agents for prevention of early-onset group B streptococcal disease[a] or suspected chorioamnionitis. This algorithm is not an exclusive course of management. Variations that incorporate individual circumstances or institutional preferences may be appropriate. (Reproduced from Schrag et al.[7])

[a] If no maternal intrapartum prophylaxis (IAP) for group B streptococcus (GBS) was administered despite an indication being present, data are insufficient on which to recommend a single management strategy.

[b] Includes complete blood cell count and differential, blood culture, and chest radiograph if respiratory abnormalities are present. When signs of sepsis are present, a lumbar puncture, if feasible, should be performed.

[c] Duration of therapy varies, depending on results of blood culture, cerebrospinal fluid findings, if obtained, and the clinical course of the infant. If laboratory results and clinical course do not indicate bacterial infection, duration may be as short as 48 hours.

[d] Complete blood count (CBC) with differential and blood culture.

[e] Applies only to penicillin, ampicillin, or cefazolin and assumes recommended dosing regimens (Table 36.2).

[f] A healthy-appearing infant who was ≥38 weeks' gestation at delivery and whose mother received ≥4 hours of IAP before delivery may be discharged home after 24 hours if other discharge criteria have been met and a person able to comply fully with instructions for home observation will be present. If any one of these conditions is not met, the infant should be observed in the hospital for at least 48 hours and until criteria for discharge are achieved.

Neonatal management

See Figure 36.4.[7]

REFERENCES

1. Valkenburg-van den Berg AW, Sprij AJ, Oostvogel PM, et al. Prevalence of colonization with GBS in pregnant women of a multi-ethnic population in the Netherlands. Eur J Obstet Gynecol Reprod Biol 2006; 124: 178–83. [II-2]

2. Adriaanse AH, Kollee LA, Muytjens HL, et al. Randomized study of vaginal chlorhexidine disinfection during labor to prevent vertical transmission of GBS. Eur J Obstet Gynecol Reprod Biol 1995; 61(2): 135–41. [RCT]

3. Regan JA, Klebanoff MA, Nugent RP. The epidemiology of GBS colonization in pregnancy. Vaginal infections and prematurity study group. Obstet Gynecol 1991; 77(4): 604–10. [II-2]

4. Puopolo KM, Madoff LC, Eichenwald EC. Early-onset group B streptococcal disease in the era of maternal screening. Pediatrics 2005; 115(5): 1240–6. [II-2]

5. Centers for Disease Control and Prevention (CDC). Early-onset and late-onset neonatal group B streptococcal disease – United States,

1996–2004. MMWR Morb Mortal Wkly Rep 2005; 54: 1205–8. [epidemiological report]

6. Rouse DJ, Goldenberg RL, Cliver SP, et al. Strategies for the prevention of early-onset neonatal group B streptococcal sepsis: a decision analysis. Obstet Gynecol 1994; 83: 483–94. [decision analysis]

7. Schrag S, Gorwitz R, Fultz-Butts K, Schuchat A. Prevention of perinatal group B streptococcal disease. Revised guidelines from CDC. MMWR Recomm Rep 2002; 51(RR-11): 1–24 [review/guideline; www.cdc.gov/groupbstrep]

8. Lin FY, Philips JB III, Azimi PH, et al. Level of maternal antibody required to protect neonates against early-onset disease caused by group B Streptococcus type Ia: a multicenter, seroepidemiology study. J Infect Dis 2001; 184: 1022–8. [II-2]

9. Law MR, Palomaki G, Alfiveric Z, et al. The prevention of neonatal group B streptococcal disease: a report by a working group of the Medical Screening Society. J Med Screen 2005; 12: 60–8. [III]

10. Klebanoff MA, Regan JA, Rao AV, et al. Outcome of the Vaginal Infections and Prematurity Study: results of a clinical trial of erythromycin among pregnant women colonized with group B streptococci. Am J Obstet Gynecol 1995; 172: 1540–5. [RCT, $n = 938$; vaginal-cervical GBS at 23–26 weeks: erythromycin 333 mg tid or placebo for 10 weeks or up to 35 6/7 weeks, whichever came first]

11. Thomsen AC, Morup L, Hansen KB. Antibiotic elimination of group-B streptococci in urine in prevention of preterm labour. Lancet 1987; 1(8533): 591–3. [RCT, $n = 69$]

12. Gibbs RS, Schrag S, Schuchat A. Perinatal infections due to Group B streptococci. Obstet Gynecol 2004; 104: 1062–76. [review]

13. Schrag SJ, Zell ER, Lyndfield R, et al. A population-based comparison of strategies to prevent early-onset group B streptococcal disease in neonates. N Engl J Med 2002; 347: 233–9. [II-1]

14. Locksmith GJ, Clark P, Duff P. Maternal and neonatal infection rates with three different protocols for prevention of group B streptococcal disease. Am J Obstet Gynecol 1999; 180: 416–22. [II-1]

15. Jamie WE, Edwards RK, Duff P. Vaginal–perianal compared with vaginal–rectal cultures for identification of group B streptococcus. Obstet Gynecol 2004; 104: 1058–61. [II-2]

16. Mercer BM, Taylor MC, Fricke JL, Baselski VS, Sibai BM. The accuracy and patient preference for self-collected group B streptococcus cultures. Am J Obstet Gynecol 1995; 173: 1325–8. [II-2]

17. Smaill F. Intrapartum antibiotics for Group B streptococcal colonisation. Cochrane Database Syst Rev 2005; 4. [5 RCTs, $n => 751$. Overall poor quality RCTs]

18. De Cueto M, Sanchez MJ, Sampedro A, et al. Timing of intrapartum ampicillin and prevention of vertical transmission of group B streptococcus. Obstet Gynecol 1998; 91: 112–14. [II-2]

19. Royal College of Obstetricians and Gynaecologists. Prevention of early onset neonatal group B streptococcal disease. Guideline No. 36, 2003. [guideline]

20. Stade B, Shah V, Ohlsson A. Vaginal chlorhexidine during labour to prevent early-onset neonatal group B streptococcal infection. Cochrane Database Sys Rev 2007; 1: CD003520. [meta-analysis: 5 RCTs, $n = 3081$]

21. Boulvain M, Stan C, Irion O. Membranes stripping for induction of labor. Cochrane Database Syst Rev 2007; 1. [meta-analysis]

37

Vaccination

A Marie O'Neill

KEY POINTS

- **Preconception immunization** is preferred to vaccination during pregnancy.
- If not administered preconceptionally, **inactivated influenza and tetanus/diphtheria vaccines should be given in pregnancy to all pregnant women as appropriate.**
- In most cases, vaccines should be administered **to pregnant women believed to be at high risk for acquiring a vaccine-preventable illness.**
- MMR (measles–mumps–rubella), **varicella and pertussis vaccines** should be administered to all **postpartum** women who are non-immune, and have no contraindications to vaccination.
- No vaccine is 100% safe and 100% effective in non-pregnant or pregnant adults.
- There is **no vaccine** that is **more dangerous to a pregnant woman or her fetus than the disease it is designed to prevent.**

GOALS OF VACCINATION IN PREGNANCY

- To prevent maternal infection that poses a risk to the mother and/or the fetus.
- To provide passive immunity against vaccine-preventable illness to the neonate. Maternal antibodies transferred across the placenta during pregnancy confer protection against viral and bacterial diseases that are often serious in the first months of life.[1]

GENERAL GUIDELINES FOR VACCINATION IN PREGNANCY

Preconception

Preconception immunization is preferred to vaccination of pregnant women. If not administered preconceptionally,

Table 37.1 *Vaccines recommended for all pregnant women*		
Vaccine	Dosing regimen	Indications
Influenza (inactivated)[5,6]	Annually	Pregnancy at any gestation during the influenza season Do not administer live vaccine (LAIV/FluMist)
Tetanus/diphtheria (Td) (toxoids)[7,8]	Booster every 10 years after primary series completed	Uncertain history or incomplete primary series, administer 3 dose primary series: • first 2 doses at least 4 weeks apart • third dose 6–12 months later

Influenza vaccine has been administered to pregnant women since the 1950s. A population-based study of >2000 pregnant women who were vaccinated in 1959–1965 found no association with fetal malformations or pregnancy loss.[9]

Maternal tetanus toxoid vaccination has been shown to be up to 98% effective in preventing neonatal tetanus.[7] The WHO estimates that 1.5 million cases of neonatal tetanus have been prevented since a 1989 initiative to eliminate maternal and neonatal tetanus. When a tetanus vaccine product which also contains diphtheria toxoid is available, it is preferable choice to provide immunity to this disease also without any increased risk to the mother or fetus.

Table 37.2 *Vaccines recommended for pregnant women at significant risk for exposure*

Vaccine	Dosing regimen	Indications
Hepatitis A (inactivated)[1,10]	2 dose series: • second dose 6–18 months after the first Post-exposure prophylaxis: • 2 dose vaccination series + immunoglobulin	Chronic liver disease, illicit drug use, travel/live/work in endemic area[a]
Hepatitis B (recombinant)[11,12]	3 dose series: • second dose 1–2 months after the first • third dose 3–4 months later	Exposure to blood in workplace, dialysis patient, injection drug use, multiple sex partners, other sexually transmitted infections, hepatitis C, household contact of person with chronic hepatitis B, travel to area of high prevalence for >6 months[a]
Pneumococcal (polysaccharide)[13]	Single dose	Chronic pulmonary disease excluding asthma, chronic liver disease, chronic renal failure, nephrotic syndrome, functional or anatomic asplenia, sickle cell disease, diabetes mellitus, immunosuppressive conditions (e.g. HIV), Native American or Alaskan Native
	One-time revaccination after 5 years	Chronic renal failure or nephrotic syndrome, functional or anatomic asplenia, sickle cell disease, chronic high-dose steroids, immunosuppressive conditions
Rabies[14,15]	Pre-exposure prophylaxis: • Given on days 0, 7, and 21 or 28 • Serological testing every 6 months for continuous exposure or every 2 years for frequent intermittent exposure Post-exposure prophylaxis: • If previously vaccinated, IM doses of vaccine immediately, and repeat dose 3 days later. Rabies immunoglobulins not indicated for appropriately vaccinated persons • Not previously vaccinated: Single dose of rabies immunoglobulin (RIG) or equine rabies immunoglobulin (ERIG) 5 doses of IM vaccine given on days 0, 3, 7, 14, and 28	Veterinary workers, other persons having frequent contact with animal species at risk for rabies, travelers to areas where dog rabies is enzootic and rapid access to medical care may not be available Immediately wash and thoroughly irrigate all bite/scratch/puncture wounds caused by animal contact Post-exposure prophylaxis is an urgent rather than an emergent situation. In many cases it is administered when not truly indicated. Consultation with an infectious disease expert should be obtained if feasible
Meningococcal (polysaccharide)[16,17]	Single dose, revaccination after 5 years recommended if continued high risk for infection	Anatomic or functional asplenia, terminal complement component deficiency, military recruits, boarding school or college students, travel or reside in endemic or epidemic area[a]
Polio: inactivated polio vaccine (IPV)	3 dose primary series if not previously completed : • second dose 1–2 months after first • third dose 6–12 months later	Travel to or live in areas where polio is common, lab worker who might handle poliovirus, healthcare worker who might care for polio-infected persons

(Continued)

Table 37.2	*Vaccines recommended for pregnant women at significant risk for exposure (continued)*	
Vaccine	Dosing regimen	Indications
Polio: oral polio vaccine (OPV)	Booster – if risk of exposure and primary series completed more than 10 years previously: • single dose of IPV If less than 4 weeks available to immunize, a single dose of OPV may be given[1] 3 dose primary series and booster recommendations are same as above	Because of superior immunogenicity and no risk of vaccine-related polio infection, the USA and many industrialized nations have adopted IPV for routine immunization.[18] In developing nations where rates of exposure to wild-type poliovirus are high, the superior secretory immunity in the gastrointestinal tract induced by OPV is considered an advantage. OPV is also less expensive than IPV. For these reasons OPV is the only product available in many developing nations and should be used in pregnancy as indicated
Anthrax[a] (inactivated bacteria)	6 dose series: • first 3 doses at 3-week intervals • then 6, 12, and 18 months after first dose [a]Exposure to aerosolized *Bacillus anthracis* spores also requires a 60-day course of appropriate antibiotics	Persons exposed to anthrax in a lab setting, work with imported animal hides or furs considered to be potentially infectious, military personnel deployed to high-risk areas, and victims of acts of bioterrorism
Japanese encephalitis (inactivated virus)[19]	3 dose series: • 0, 7, and 30 days	Travel to areas where Japanese encephalitis is prevalent[a]

Typhoid
  Oral TY21a (live attenuated)
 	
  Injectable Vi (polysaccharide)
 	
  Inactivated whole-cell vaccine
	Oral: 3 dose series
	• one dose every 2 days
	
	Injection Vi:
	• single dose
	Inactivated injection:
	• 2 doses 4 weeks apart
		Travel to or live in area where typhoid is endemic, close contact of typhoid carrier, lab exposure to *Salmonella typhi* bacteria

Yellow fever[20, 21] (live virus)[22]	Single dose Booster every 10 years for continued risk/exposure	Live in or travel to area where yellow fever is endemic, lab exposure to the virus

[a]List of high-risk areas at http://www.cdc.gov/travel/diseases.htm#hepa

Influenza and polio vaccines were the first to be recommended and routinely administered during pregnancy in the period 1957–1966. More than 50 000 women were vaccinated and no association with adverse pregnancy or postnatal outcomes was found.[6]

OPV can cause rare cases of vaccine-associated paralytic poliomyelitis (VAPP) – approximately 1 case per 2.6 million OPV doses administered.[18] The spread of OPV virus to unimmunized children is considered to be advantageous, especially in areas in which vaccine acceptance levels are low.

There has been no documentation of risk to the fetus from maternal vaccination for typhoid.[6]

It is unknown if vaccinating a pregnant woman against Japanese encephalitis poses a risk to the fetus. In general, inactivated virus exposure is believed to pose minimal or no risk.[6]

Clinical studies indicate that yellow fever vaccination during pregnancy is not associated with increased risk of congenital anomalies or spontaneous abortion.[20–22]

inactivated influenza and tetanus/diphtheria vaccines should be given in pregnancy to all pregnant women as appropriate, and several other vaccines should be administered to women with certain risk factors. No vaccine is 100% safe and 100% effective in non-pregnant or pregnant adults.

Live attenuated vaccines

• Pregnancy is a contraindication to live vaccines because of a *theoretical* risk of transmission of the infectious agent to the fetus. These vaccines should not routinely be administered during pregnancy or within 4 weeks of conception.

Table 37.3 *Vaccines not recommended in pregnancy*

Vaccine	Dosing regimen	Comments
MMR (measles–mumps–rubella) (live virus)	Single dose	Not given to pregnant women or women planning to become pregnant within 4 weeks **Administer this MMR vaccine in the immediate postpartum period to those women determined to be rubella non-immune** on prenatal evaluation
Varicella (live virus)	2 dose series: <ul><li>second dose 4–8 weeks after first</li></ul> Post-exposure prophylaxis: <ul><li>Varicella zoster immune globulin (VZIG) within 96 hours of exposure to varicella or herpes zoster</li><li>If VZIG is not available: – IVIG can be used at a dose of 400 mg/kg given IV as a single dose or – closely monitor for development of disease and treat with acyclovir if disease develops</li></ul>	Not given to pregnant women or women planning to become pregnant within 4 weeks **Initiate series in the immediate postpartum period to those women determined to be varicella non-immune** on prenatal evaluation VZIG and IVIG are safe in pregnancy and breastfeeding. Acyclovir in Pregnancy Registry was completed in 1999. Data on 1246 exposures in pregnancy did not find an association with any adverse pregnancy outcome[23]
T$_{DAP}$ (Toxoid/Acellular)[32]	Single dose to replace one Td booster	Women in whom > 2 years have elapsed since last Td vaccine should be offered T$_{DAP}$ postpartum or prior to conception.
BCG (bacille Calmette-Guérin)	Single dose	No harmful fetal effects have been associated with BCG, but its use is not recommended in pregnancy[24]
Smallpox[25] – (live vaccinia virus)	Single inoculation Immunity decreases 3–5 years after vaccination Post-exposure prophylaxis: <ul><li>Vaccination within 3 days of exposure will completely prevent or significantly modify smallpox in the vast majority of persons</li><li>Vaccination 4–7 days after exposure likely offers some protection from disease or decreases severity</li></ul>	Pregnant women, or women planning to become pregnant within 4 weeks should not be vaccinated in the absence of exposure to active disease Close contacts of pregnant women or women planning to become pregnant within 4 weeks should not be vaccinated unless exposed to active disease – exposure to the resulting lesion can cause vaccinia viral infection in the pregnant woman and/or fetus

The first live attenuated rubella vaccines were introduced in 1969 – the Cendehill and HPV-77 vaccine virus strains. In 1971 the Centers for Disease Control (CDC) established the Vaccine in Pregnancy (VIP) Registry of women who had received either of these two rubella vaccines within 3 months before or after conception.[26,27] None of the 290 infants born to the 538 women entered into this Registry through April 1979 had defects indicative of congenital rubella syndrome (CRS); this included 94 liveborn infants of women who were known to be non-immune before receiving the vaccine.[27, 28]

In January 1979, the RA 27/3 rubella vaccine was licensed for use in the USA. Concerns were raised that this new live attenuated-virus vaccine might have greater fetotropic and teratogenic potential than the earlier vaccines. 272 women known to be susceptible to rubella who received the RA 27/3 vaccine within 3 months of their estimated date of conception were enrolled in the VIP Registry between 1979 and 1988. Data collected by CDC in the VIP Registry since 1979 show no evidence that the RA 27/3 rubella vaccine administered in pregnancy can cause defects indicative of CRS. Therefore, the observed **risk for CRS following rubella vaccination continues to be zero.** These results are consistent with the experiences in the Federal Republic of Germany and the United Kingdom,[29,30] where rubella vaccine has not been associated with CRS among infants born to susceptible mothers who were vaccinated around the time of conception.

Varicella: vaccination while pregnant or within 3 months of conception is not an indication for recommending termination of pregnancy. Data from the first 5 years of Varicella Vaccine in Pregnancy Registry (March 1995 to March 2000) identified no cases of congenital varicella syndrome or other birth defects related to vaccine exposure during pregnancy.[31]

BCG: 'Although no harmful effects to the fetus have been associated with BCG vaccine, **its use is not recommended during pregnancy.**'[24]

Smallpox: the last case of smallpox in the USA was in 1949. The last naturally occurring case in the world was in Somalia in 1977.

Risk of vaccinia – 14–52 people per 1 million vaccinated experienced potentially life-threatening reactions, including eczema vaccinatum, vaccinia necrosum, or postvaccinal encephalitis, and 1–2 deaths occurred. The vaccine can cause a very rare but serious complication in the fetus called fetal vaccinia – less than 50 cases of fetal vaccinia have ever been reported in the world, and only three of these cases were reported in the USA. In the period 1967–1971 when smallpox vaccine was routinely given in the USA, only one case of fetal vaccinia occurred among an estimated 90 000 to 280 000 pregnant women who received the vaccine. Fetal vaccinia can lead to preterm birth, skin rash with scarring, stillbirth, or neonatal death. Because fetal vaccinia is so rare, smallpox vaccination during pregnancy should not be a reason to consider termination of pregnancy.[25, 33]

CDC's Advisory Committee on Immunization Practices does not recommend preventive use of Vaccinia Immune Globulin (VIG) for pregnant women. However, if a woman has a complication from smallpox vaccine that could be treated with VIG, she should recieve it while pregnant.[25]

- Exposure to a live attenuated vaccination within 28 days of conception or during gestation is *not* an indication for termination of pregnancy.
- Some pregnant women are at high risk for acquiring a vaccine-preventable infection because of their occupation, habits, travel plans, or where they live. The **real** risk of exposure to a vaccine-preventable illness associated with serious morbidity or mortality for the mother or fetus outweighs the *theoretical* risk of fetal infection after vaccination. These women should be immunized if an appropriate vaccine is available.
- **There is no vaccine that is more dangerous to a pregnant woman or her fetus than the disease it is designed to prevent.**
- Breastfeeding is not a contraindication to live vaccine.[2]
- Live vaccines include LAIV (live attenuated influenza vaccine), MMR (mumps, measles, and rubella), BCG (bacille Calmette-Guérin), varicella, vaccinia (smallpox), yellow fever, and TY21a (typhoid).

Inactivated or killed vaccines, toxoids, immune globulins, antisera

- There is no evidence that exposure to an inactivated vaccine, toxoid, immune globulin, or antisera poses any risk to a pregnant woman or her fetus.[3,4]
- It is not necessary to delay conception after exposure to one of these products.
- With the exception of the inactivated flu vaccine, however, it is preferable to delay administration of these medications until the second trimester whenever prompt administration is not medically indicated. Waiting until the second trimester helps to avoid false associations in the patient's mind between the vaccine and adverse first trimester events such as spontaneous abortion and structural anomalies.
- There is no contraindication to administration of these products to breastfeeding women.

CONTRAINDICATIONS TO VACCINATION

The only true contraindication applicable to all vaccines is a history of a *severe* allergic reaction after a prior dose of vaccine or to a vaccine component, unless the recipient has been desensitized. An extensive listing of vaccine components, their use, and the vaccines that contain each component is available from CDC's National Immunization Program website at http://www.cdc.gov/nip

REFERENCES

1. Gall SA. Maternal immunization. Obstet Gynecol Clin North Am 2003; 30(4): 623–36. [review]
2. Pickering LK, Granoff DM, Erickson JR, et al. Modulation of the immune system by human milk and infant formula containing nucleotides. Pediatrics 1998; 101(2): 242–9. [review]
3. Grabenstein JD. Pregnancy and lactation in relation to vaccines and antibodies. Pharm Pract Manag Q 2001; 20(3): 1–10. [review]
4. Koren G, Pastuszak A, Ito S. Drugs in pregnancy. N Engl J Med 1998; 338(16): 1128–37. [review]
5. Harper SA, Fukuda K, Uyeki TM, Cox NJ, Bridges CB; Advisory Committee on Immunization Practices (ACIP); Centers for Disease Control and Prevention (CDC). Prevention and control of influenza. Recommendations of the Advisory Committee on Immunization Practices (ACIP). MMWR Recomm Rep 2004; 53(RR-6): 1–40. [guideline]
6. Munoz FM, Greisinger AJ, Wehmanen OA, et al. Safety of influenza vaccination during pregnancy. Am J Obstet Gynecol 2005; 192(4): 1098–106. [review]
7. Demicheli V, Barale A, Rivetti A, Demicheli V. Vaccines for women to prevent neonatal tetanus. Cochrane Database Syst Rev 2007; 1 [meta-analysis: 2 RCTs, $n = 10\,560$]
8. Sheffield JS, Ramin SM. Tetanus in pregnancy. Am J Perinatol 2004; 21(4): 173–82. [review]
9. Heinonen OP, Slone D, Shapiro S. Immunizing agents. In: Kaufman DW, ed. Birth Defects and Drugs in Pregnancy. Littleton, MA: Publishing Sciences Group; 1977: 314–21. [review]
10. Duff B, Duff P. Hepatitis A vaccine: ready for prime time. Obstet Gynecol 1998; 91(3): 468–71. [review]
11. Ayoola EA, Johnson AO. Hepatitis B vaccine in pregnancy: immunogenicity, safety and transfer of antibodies to infants. Int J Gynaecol Obstet 1987; 25(4): 297–301. [review]
12. Levy M, Koren G. Hepatitis B vaccine in pregnancy: maternal and fetal safety. Am J Perinatol 1991; 8(3): 227–32. [review]
13. Chaithongwongwatthana S, Yamasmit W, Limpongsanurak S, et al. Pneumococcal vaccination during pregnancy for preventing infant infection. Cochrane Database Syst Rev 2006; 1. [meta-analysis: 3 RCTs, $n = 280$]
14. Chabala S, Williams M, Amenta R, Ognjan AF. Confirmed rabies exposure during pregnancy: treatment with human rabies immune globulin and human diploid cell vaccine. Am J Med. 1991; 91(4): 423–4. [II-3]
15. Sudarshan MK, Madhusudana SN, Mahendra BJ. Post-exposure prophylaxis with purified vero cell rabies vaccine during pregnancy – safety and immunogenicity. J Commun Dis 1999; 31(4): 229–36. [review]
16. Adam I, Abdalla MA. Is meningococcal polysaccharide vaccine safe during pregnancy? Ann Trop Med Parasitol 2005; 99(6): 627–8. [review]
17. McCormick JB, Gusmao HH, Nakamura S, et al. Antibody response to serogroup A and C meningococcal polysaccharide vaccines in infants born of mothers vaccinated during pregnancy. J Clin Invest 1980; 65(5): 1141–4. [II-3]
18. Prevots DR, Burr RK, Sutter RW, Murphy TV; Advisory Committee on Immunization Practices. Poliomyelitis prevention in the United States. Updated recommendations of the Advisory Committee on Immunization Practices (ACIP). MMWR Recomm Rep 2000; 49 (RR-5): 1–22; quiz CE1–7. [guideline]
19. Inactivated Japanese encephalitis virus vaccine. Recommendations of the Advisory Committee on Immunization Practices (ACIP). MMWR Recomm Rep 1993; 42(RR-1): 1–15. [guideline]
20. Tsai TF, Paul R, Lynberg MC, Letson GW. Congenital yellow fever virus infection after immunization in pregnancy. J Infect Dis 1993; 168(6): 1520–3. [II-3]

21. Nasidi A, Monath TP, Vandenberg J, et al. Yellow fever vaccination and pregnancy: a four-year prospective study. Trans R Soc Trop Med Hyg 1993; 87(3): 337–9. [II-2]
22. Nishioka Sde A, Nunes-Araujo FR, Pires WP, Silva FA, Costa HL. Yellow fever vaccination during pregnancy and spontaneous abortion: a case-control study. Trop Med Int Health 1998; 3(1): 29–33. [II-2]
23. Stone KM, Reiff-Eldridge R, White AD, et al. Pregnancy outcomes following systemic prenatal acyclovir exposure: conclusions from the international acyclovir pregnancy registry, 1984–1999. Birth Defects Res A Clin Mol Teratol 2004; 70(4): 201–7. [II-2]
24. The role of BCG vaccine in the prevention and control of tuberculosis in the United States. A joint statement by the Advisory Council for the Elimination of Tuberculosis and the Advisory Committee on Immunization Practices. MMWR Recomm Rep 1996; 45(RR-4): 1–18. [guideline]
25. Centers for Disease Control and Prevention. Smallpox vaccination information for women who are pregnant or breastfeeding. 2003; 5. [review]
26. Centers for Disease Control and Prevention. Revised ACIP recommendation for avoiding pregnancy after receiving a rubella-containing vaccine. JAMA 2002; 287(3): 311–12. [guideline]
27. Bart SW, Stetler HC, Preblud SR, et al. Fetal risk associated with rubella vaccine: an update. Rev Infect Dis 1985; 7 (Suppl 1): S95–102. [review]
28. Centers for Disease Control (CDC). Rubella vaccination during pregnancy – United States, 1971–1988. MMWR Morb Mortal Wkly Rep 1989; 38(17): 289–93. [review]
29. Enders G. Rubella antibody titers in vaccinated and nonvaccinated women and results of vaccination during pregnancy. Rev Infect Dis 1985; 7 (Suppl 1): S103–7. [II-3]
30. Sheppard S, Smithells RW, Dickson A, Holzel H. Rubella vaccination and pregnancy: preliminary report of a national survey. Br Med J (Clin Res Ed) 1986; 292(6522): 727. [survey]
31. Shields KE, Galil K, Seward J, et al. Varicella vaccine exposure during pregnancy: data from the first 5 years of the pregnancy registry. Obstet Gynecol 2001; 98(1): 14–19. [II-3]
32. Center for Disease Control and Prevention. Preventing tetanus, diptheria and pertussis among adults: use of tetanus toxoid reduced diptheria toxoid and accellular pertussis vaccine. MMWR 2006; 55(RR–17): 1–33 [Guideline].
33. Centers for Disease Control and Prevention (CDC). Women with smallpox vaccine exposure during pregnancy reported to the National Smallpox Vaccine in Pregnancy Registry – United States, 2003. MMWR Morb Mortal Wkly Rep 2003; 52(17): 386–8. [II-3]

Part II

Fetus

A **Multiple gestations**
38. Multiple gestations

B **Growth disorders**
39. Fetal growth restriction
40. Fetal macrosomia

C **Fetal infections**
41. CMV
42. Toxoplasmosis
43. Parvovirus
44. Herpes
45. Varicella

D **Fetal death**
46. Fetal death

E **Immune disorders**
47. Hemolytic disease of the fetus/neonate
48 Neonatal alloimmune thrombocytopenia

F **Non-immune hydrops fetalis**
49. Non-immune hydrops fetalis

G **Amniotic fluid disorders**
50. Sonographic assessment of amniotic fluid: oligohydramnios and polyhydramnios

H **Antenatal testing**
51. Antepartum testing
52. Fetal lung maturity

38

Multiple gestations

Edward J Hayes

KEY POINTS

- **Preterm birth** is the largest reason for the **increased morbidity and mortality associated with multiples.**
- To date **no preterm birth prevention strategy has been shown to be effective in multiple gestations,** and although multiple tests have been developed to determine one's risk for early delivery, since there is no proven intervention, screening cannot be recommended.
- **Multifetal pregnancy reduction** is implemented in higher-order gestations **to decrease the likelihood of a very premature delivery, with the benefits of reduction from quadruplets or higher felt to outweigh the risks.**
- Discordant growth between multiples may be a marker for genetic or structural anomalies, infection, twin–twin transfusion, or placental issues; however, evidence of **fetal growth restriction (FGR), not discordance, predicts adverse neonatal outcome.**
- Nuchal translucency (NT) for aneuploidy screening is accurate in multiple gestations.
- Multiples have a **higher rate of pre-eclampsia,** which tends to occur in an atypical fashion.
- A **single fetal death in multiple gestations** should **not mandate immediate delivery,** for the risk of disseminated intravascular coagulation (DIC) is theoretical. If the twins are monochorionic, adverse effects on the remaining fetus from the co-twin death occur immediately, before prompt delivery can prevent them.
- Routine antepartum testing has not been proven to be advantageous in multiple gestations without coexisting morbidity.
- **Monoamniotic twins** have a high rate of mortality that increases as gestational age increases; consequently, **delivery should be considered at 32 weeks.**
- **Twin–twin transfusion syndrome** has significant mortality if left untreated, particularly if diagnosed in the second trimester. Although laser coagulation of vascular anastomoses has recently been proposed as possibly an effective treatment, it still results in a 66% chance of one of the twins dying or suffering significant neurological injury.

DEFINITION

Multiple gestation is a gestation carrying >1 fetus. The vast majority involve twins. There are two types of twins:

- Monozygotic (MZ) twins are formed when a single fertilized ovum splits into two individuals who are almost always genetically identical, unless after their division a spontaneous mutation causes a genetic difference between the twins.
- Dizygotic (DZ) twins are formed when two separate ova are fertilized by two different sperm, resulting in genetically different individuals.

EPIDEMIOLOGY/INCIDENCE

It is important to differentiate the natural from the actual incidence of multiple gestations.

Natural incidence of multiple gestations (Figure 38.1)

- MZ twinning occurs at a constant rate of about 4 per 1000 (1/250).
- DZ twinning rates vary with the individual's characteristics, such as race (low in Asians, high in blacks), age (increases with advanced maternal age), parity (increases with parity), and family history (especially on maternal side). The 'natural' incidence of twins and triplets in the USA as reported in 1973 was 1 in 80 and 1 in 800, respectively.[1]

Actual incidence of multiple gestations

The actual incidence of multiple gestations has been heavily influenced by use of **assisted reproductive technologies**

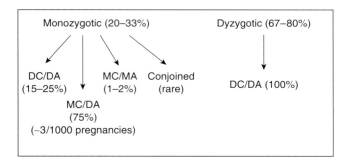

Figure 38.1
Natural incidence of multiple gestations. DC/DA, dichorionic
diamniotic; MC/DA, monochorionic, diamniotic; MC/MA,
monochorionic monoamniotic.

(ART) since the 1980s. Currently, >50% of multiple gestations in developed countries are from ART. The proportion of live births that are multiple gestations in the USA has increased significantly over the last two decades, with a 65%

increase in twins and a 500% increase in triplets and higher-order births.[2] This rise is associated with the increased use of ART treatments and the increasing maternal age at the time of pregnancy. The rate of multiple gestations, as recorded in 2002, was 3.3% of total births, with 3.1% twins and 0.2% triplets or higher-orders multiples.[3] The vast majority of these pregnancies are DZ. MZ twin rates increase with ART to 3–5%.[4] ART multiple pregnancies are associated with a higher incidence of fetal/neonatal and maternal complications.

ETIOLOGY (TABLE 38.1)

- DZ twins are formed by two distinct fertilized ova and always have separate chorion and amnion (dichorionic/diamniotic, DC/DA).
- MZ twins are formed from the division of one fertilized egg. The type is determined by the timing of the fertilized ovum division.

Table 38.1 *Timing of zygote division and types of twins*			
Timing of division	Type of twins	Characteristics	Picture
Day 1–3	Dichorionic diamniotic (DC/DA)	Two placentas with two chorions and two amnions	Dichorionic diamniotic (fused placentae) Dichorionic diamniotic (separate placentae)
Day 3–8	Monochorionic diamniotic (MC/DA)	Monochorionic placenta with two amnions	Monochorionic diamniotic
Day 8–13	Monochorionic monoamniotic (MC/MA)	Monochorionic placenta with a single amniotic sac	Monochorionic monoamniotic
Day 13–15	Conjoined twins	Fused twins	

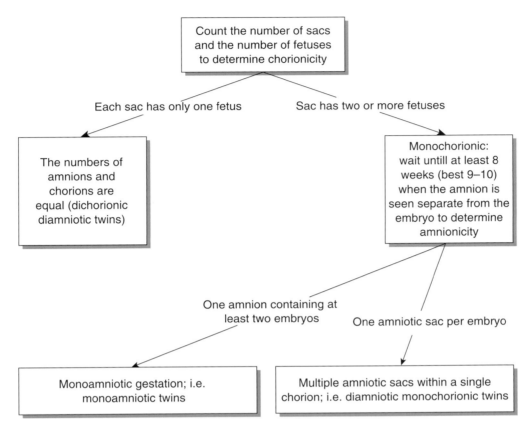

Figure 38.2
Determination of chorionicity and amnionicity in the first trimester.

DIAGNOSIS

The clinical signs for suspecting multiple gestations are a uterus larger than dates, and now pregnancy that has resulted from ART. The accuracy of diagnosing twins on clinical criteria is poor, as 37% of women who do not undergo routine ultrasound screening will not have their twins diagnosed by 26 weeks, and 13% of multiples will only be diagnosed at the time of admission for delivery.[5]

Ultrasound is 100% accurate in diagnosing multiple gestations.[5] The best time for accurate diagnosis is the **first trimester**, as this is the **optimum time to determine** not only fetal number but also **chorionicity and amnionicity** in particular. Determination of chorionicity and zygocity is paramount for correct risk assessment, counseling, and management of complications: e.g. twin–twin transfusion syndrome (TTTS), fetal growth restriction (FGR), and single fetal death. In addition, this determination will help future medical care of the babies for genetic component of diseases and organ transplantation compatibility.

DETERMINATION OF CHORIO-AMNIONICITY

Determination of chorionicity and amnionicity in the first trimester is shown in Figure 38.2.

Determination of chorionicity and amnionicity after the first trimester is shown in Figures 38.3 and 38.4.

In the 30–40% of cases in which there are clearly two placentas, or differing fetal sex, the pregnancy is DC/DA, and dizygotic. In the majority of cases, the best ultrasound characteristic to distinguish chorionicity and amnionicity is the **twin peak sign**. The twin peak sign (also called the lambda or delta sign) is a triangular projection of tissue with the same echogenicity as the placenta, extending beyond the chorionic surface of the placenta[6] (see Figure 38.4).

DNA fingerprinting through polymorphisms or other means can also determine zygocity, but it is invasive and therefore associated with complications.

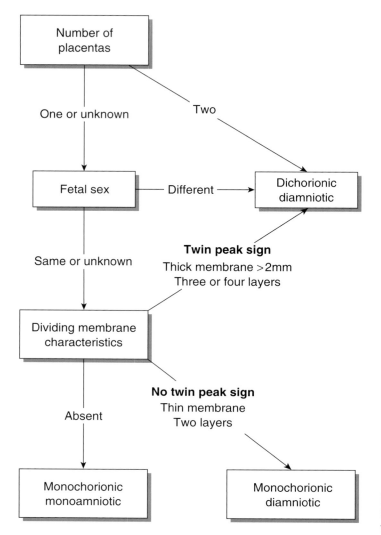

Figure 38.3
Determination of chorionicity and amnionicity after the first trimester.

COMPLICATIONS

The incidence and severity of complications is related to chorionicity and amnionicity. Complications are more common in all types of multiple gestations than in singleton gestations and can be classified as follows.

Fetal

Spontaneous reduction

A significant number of multiple gestations diagnosed in the first trimester undergo spontaneous reduction of one sac in the first trimester, referred to as the 'vanishing twin'. The rates of wastage of at least one gestation directly correlate with the initial number of gestational sacs, i.e. about 20–50% of twins, 53% of triplets, and 65% of quadruplets.[7] Since the maternal serum alpha fetoprotein (MSAFP) is elevated in pregnancies

with vanishing twins, this test is not accurate for screening in this situation, and therefore should not be performed.

Spontaneous loss

The risk of miscarriage, especially in the first but also in the second trimester, is increased.

Higher rates of chromosomal and congenital anomalies

Owing to the increased number of fetuses, particularly dizygotic, the risk of having one fetus affected by a trisomy is increased above the baseline risk of a singleton.[8] Therefore, the Down syndrome risk of a 35-year-old singleton mother is obtained in twins of a 31–33 year old mother,[9] and for triplets this risk is obtained for a 28 year old mother.[10] Structural defects occur two to three times more commonly

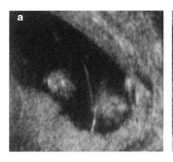
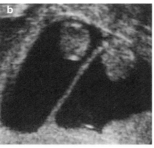

Figure 38.4
T sign and twin peak sign. (a) T sign (MC/DA gestation); always monozygotic. (b) Twin peak sign (DC/DA gestation)

Table 38.2 *Mean gestational age (GA) at birth according to number of fetuses*	
No. of fetuses	Mean GA at birth (weeks)
1	~40
2	~36
3	~33
4	~29–30
5	~24
≥6	~<20

in liveborn MZ twins than in DZ twins or singletons.[11] Only in 5–20% are both MZ twins affected.

Intrauterine growth restriction and discordant growth

Discordant growth of multiples is usually defined as a 20–25% reduction in estimated fetal weight (EFW) of the smaller compared with the larger fetus (larger minus smaller EFW, divided by larger EFW). Discordance may be a marker for structural or genetic anomalies, infection, TTTS, or placental issues. However, it is not the discordance per se, even >30%, but evidence of intrauterine growth restriction (**IUGR**) **of one fetus** that **predicts adverse neonatal outcome.** The risk of mortality or neonatal morbidity is higher among neonates in small for gestational age (SGA)-discordant twins than in adequate for gestational age (AGA)-discordant twins (20 vs 6%).[12]

Single fetal demise in multiple gestations

Up to 5% of twins and 17% of triplets in the second or third trimester undergo spontaneous loss of one or more fetuses.[13] This has been associated with a slight increase in risks of preterm birth (PTB) and growth restriction in the remaining fetuses. Other impacts on the remaining fetuses are dependent on chorionicity:

- Dichorionic twins: no significant neurological morbidity in the remaining fetus after the death of one twin.[10]
- Monochorionic twins: due to vascular anastomoses, the remaining fetus is at significant risk of morbidity (about 25% neurological) and mortality (about 10% perinatal) as a result of significant hypotension that occurs at the time of the demise.

Preterm birth

Human uteri are designed to carry to term one fetus. Increasing the number of fetuses is inversely associated with gestational age at birth, so that about 50% of twins deliver preterm, most pregnancies with three or four fetuses have significant perinatal morbidity and mortality, and most pregnancies carrying more than four fetuses do not even reach viability (Table 38.2). PTB is mostly spontaneous from preterm labor (PTL) or preterm premature rupture of membranes (PPROM), but also iatrogenic due to complications. **PTB is the main reason for the increased morbidity and mortality associated with multiples.** In-vitro fertilization (IVF) twins have higher rates of PTB (68 vs 41%) and a significantly lower gestational age at delivery (35 weeks) compared with spontaneously conceived twins.[14] Multiples account for 30% of very low birth weight (VLBW) infants, nearly 20% of infant mortality,[15] and significant morbidity evidenced by the rate of **cerebral palsy,** which is correlated to number of fetuses, varying from 1.6 per 1000 in singletons to 7.3 and 28 for twins and triplets, respectively.[16]

Immaturity

Twins may have a higher rate of respiratory distress syndrome (RDS) when matched with gestational-age-matched singletons.[17]

Intrapartum complications

These complications are more common, especially in multiple gestations with first fetus non-vertex and trial of labor.

Perinatal neurological damage

These complications are related to complications described above.

Perinatal mortality

Twins have a higher rate (5 vs 1%) of perinatal mortality than singletons. This risk comes mostly from MZ twins, since MZ twins have a higher (2.5–5 times) risk compared with DZ twins.

Maternal

Heartburn; hemorrhoids; tiredness; anxiety; hyperemesis gravidarum; maternal anemia; as well as:

Pre-eclampsia

Multiples have a higher rate of pre-eclampsia, whose incidence is inversely proportional to the total fetal number. Increasing incidence with twins (8%), triplets (10%), and quadruplets (12%) have been reported.[18] Multiples, besides having a higher rate of pre-eclampsia, are more likely to manifest this disease in an atypical fashion.[19]

Abruptio placentae

Abruptio placentae is more common in multiples and exhibits a correlation to the number of fetuses (1.2% of twins; 1.6% of triplets).[18]

Thrombocytopenia

Up to one-third of triplets' gestations can be complicated by thrombocytopenia, and unlike singletons where the number one cause of thrombocytopenia is gestational, severe pre-eclampsia is the most common cause in triplets.[20]

Acute fatty liver

In contrast to singleton gestations where the rate of fatty liver is 1 in 10 000, the rate in triplets is up to 7%.[21]

Gestational diabetes

There is a mild correlation between twins and gestational diabetes when compared with singletons, although insulin requirements between these two groups are not significantly different.[22] A significant association is demonstrated with triplets with a gestational diabetes rate of 22%.[23]

Other maternal complications are postpartum hemorrhage, peripartum hysterectomy, with a significantly increased risk of emergent peripartum hysterectomy compared with singletons,[24] **postpartum depression, and maternal death.**

Table 38.3	*Staging for TTTS*[25]
Stage 1	MC/DA gestation with oligohydramnios (MVP < 2 cm) and polyhydramnios (MVP > 8 cm)
Stage 2	Absent (empty) bladder (in donor)
Stage 3	Abnormal Doppler[a]
Stage 4	Hydrops
Stage 5	Death of one twin

[a]Defined as either umbilical artery absent or reversed diastolic flow; ductus venosus absent or reversed diastolic flow; or umbilical vein pulsatile flow.[25]

TTTS, twin–twin transfusion syndrome; MC/DA, monochorionic diamniotic; MVP, maximum vertical pocket.

Complications specific to monochorionic gestations

Twin–twin transfusion syndrome

Incidence
Occurs in 10–15% of monochorionic diamniotic (MC/DA) pregnancies, and therefore in about 1/2 500 pregnancies. Rare cases have been reported in monochorionic monoamniotic (MC/MA) pregnancies.

Etiology
All monochorionic pregnancies have one placenta only, with anastomoses of artery-to-artery (AA), vein-to-vein (VV), and artery-to-vein (AV) of the two twins. TTTS may not occur in MC/MA gestations because of more AA, and less AV anastomoses than in MC/DA gestations. An imbalance of arterial circulation of one twin (donor) to the venous circulation of another (recipient) probably through an AV anastomosis can lead to TTTS. Over 50% of TTTS placentas have ≥ 1 velamentous cord insertion, possibly associated with this imbalance. The donor twin develops anemia and resultant effects (e.g. IUGR, oligohydramnios), while the recipient twin has polyhydramnios, becomes polycythemic, and can develop heart failure.

Diagnosis
The antepartum diagnosis requires ultrasound. The criteria are **MC/DA gestation** (see above) with **oligohydramnios** (maximum vertical pocket [MVP] <2 cm) in one sac, and **polyhydramnios** (MVP >8 cm) in the other. Supporting criteria can be the presence of same-sex twins with a single placenta, and significant discordance in fetal growth. It is important to rule out other etiologies for similar findings, such as FGR of just one twin with normal other twin, chromosomal or structural abnormalities, infection, etc.

Staging
Staging for TTTS is described in Table 38.3.[25]

Prognosis
Prognosis is poor, and depends mostly on gestational age at diagnosis and stage of disease. About 5% of TTTS, especially in early stages, can regress. Survival with diagnosis at < 26 weeks without treatment is 30%.[26] Survival can often be with severe morbidity, including neurological, cardiac, ischemia/necrosis of extremities, renal cortical necrosis, etc. Given this poor prognosis, support is important (e.g. ww.tttsfoundation.org).

Monoamniotic twins

Incidence is 1 in 10 000 pregnancies, but more common with IVF using zona manipulation affecting up to 17% of multiples after this technique.[27] Diagnosis is by ultrasound: prior to 8 weeks, one yolk sac and two fetal poles are diagnostic;[28] after 8 weeks, same sex, single placenta, and single amniotic sac with no dividing amniotic membrane allow diagnosis. Fetuses must be of the same sex. Demonstration of umbilical cord entanglement is also diagnostic of monoamniotic twins.

The rate of loss, especially from cord accidents in utero, but also from congenital anomalies, and very PTB in pregnancies > 22 weeks, is up to 32% despite intensive care and monitoring at tertiary care centers.[29] Perinatal mortality with aggressive inpatient monitoring (see below) and delivery at 32 weeks has recently been reported to be as low as 10%, with later delivery probably associated with continuing risk of mortality.[30]

Acardiac twin (also called twin reversal arterial perfusion [TRAP] syndrome) is an MZ/MC pregnancy characterized by a fetus lacking a normally developed heart and usually a head ('acardiac twin'). It occurs in 1% of MC twins, or about 1 in 35 000 pregnancies. This acardiac fetus survives in utero due to placental anastomoses shunting blood flow from the 'pump twin'. Diagnosis needs ultrasound Doppler confirmation of blood being pumped in from the 'pump' twin. The 'pump twin' can develop a high cardiac output state and subsequent failure, resulting in intrauterine or neonatal death of this normal twin in about 35–50% of cases.[31]

Conjoined twins are an anomaly linked to MZ twinning with an incidence of 1 in 50 000 to 1 in 10 000 births.[32] Classification is based on the site of connection with the suffix *pagus* added. Of those diagnosed in utero, 28% will die prior to delivery, 54% die immediately after birth, with only an 18% survival rate.[33] Diagnosis of shared anatomy is imperative to management and prognosis.[31]

PREGNANCY CONSIDERATIONS

Compared with singleton gestations, physiological changes in twins include a 50–60% increase in maternal blood volume (40–50% in singletons), leading to higher incidence of anemia, higher increase in cardiac output, slightly lower diastolic blood pressure, and more discomfort such as pressure, difficulty in ambulation, etc.

PREGNANCY MANAGEMENT
Nutrition

The recommended weight gain for twin pregnancies starting with normal body mass index (BMI) is about 35–40 lbs. Diet should include an increase in caloric intake by 300 kcal above singletons (600 kcal above non-pregnant state); folic acid ≥ 1 mg/day; and iron 60 mg/day.

Prenatal diagnosis
First trimester

Nuchal translucency (NT) alone in multiple gestations has been shown to be as sensitive as in singletons, and has an 88% detection rate for trisomy 21, with a 7.3% screen positive rate.[34] Serum-based screening in multiples is not as sensitive as in singletons. Chorionic villus sampling can be performed between 10 and 12 weeks. It has the same risks as amniocentesis in multiples,[35] and has a 4–6% rate of twin–twin contamination.[36] (See also Chapter 4 in *Obstetric Evidence Based Guidelines*.)

Second trimester

Serum screening for neural tube defects with MSAFP using a cut-off of 4.5 MoM has a detection rate of 50–85% with a 5% false-positive rate. Serum screening for Down syndrome is not considered clinically helpful in multiples, given the poor detection rates and high rates of false positives and negatives.[37] Genetic amniocentesis has been reported to have a loss rate with multiples similar to singletons.[39] At sampling of the first sac, indigo carmine or Evan's blue can be injected; a clear sample obtained from the second sac insures that two different sacs have been sampled. Methylene blue dye should not be used because of the risks of fetal hemolytic anemia, small intestinal atresia, and fetal demise. If gestation is MC, sampling of one sac is suggested for karyotype.

Prediction of preterm birth

Women with twin gestations are at low risk (5%) to deliver prior to 32 weeks if at 24 weeks the transvaginal ultrasound (TVU) cervical length is ≥ 3 cm, or the fetal fibronectin (fFN) level is negative.[39] Clinical findings associated with delivery prior to 32 weeks are a TVU cervical length < 25 mm at 16–24 weeks and a positive fFN at 24–28 weeks.[40] Since there is currently no beneficial intervention if these screening tests are positive, routine screening of multiples at risk for preterm delivery cannot be recommended.

Prevention and management of complications

Selective termination of an anomalous fetus

Selective termination of an anomalous fetus is usually performed in the second trimester due to the time of diagnosis of the fetal anomaly.

In DC pregnancies, the procedure consists of injection of potassium chloride into the fetal heart transabdominally. The loss rate of the entire pregnancy is about 4% of those performed prior to 24 weeks, with a difference if twins were reduced vs higher-order multiples (2.4% vs 11.1%) and if more than one fetus is terminated (2.6% loss if one fetus vs 42.9% if two).[41]

In MC pregnancies, potassium chloride should not be used, as it crosses to the other fetus through the placental anastomoses and therefore causes fetal death of both fetuses. Cord ligation, or occlusion with clips, diathermy, or other means have been used, with insufficient data for effective comparison.

Preterm birth

(See also Chapters 15 and 16 of *Obstetric Evidence Based Guidelines*.)

Prevention of multiple gestations
The incidence of multiple gestation is increased with both ovulation induction, which represents the majority of ART multiples, and IVF. Unfortunately, it is difficult to prevent multiple gestations with ovarian stimulation. Excessive stimulation and insemination in the presence of an excessive number of ripe follicles should be avoided. Transfer of one embryo almost guarantees avoidance of multiple gestation, and is associated with rates of successful pregnancy similar to transfer of more than one embryo with modern techniques. Many developed countries have laws which allow the transfer of only one, or maximum of two embryos. No more than three embryos should ever be transferred, even in the woman with poor prognosis (i.e. > 40 years old). The successful outcome of ART should be based on the rate of healthy term singleton babies per cycle.

Multifetal pregnancy reduction in dichorionic gestations
The goal of first trimester fetal reduction is to decrease the number of fetuses in higher-order gestations, thereby lessening the likelihood of a premature delivery and the associated morbidity and mortality. Although there has been no randomized controlled trial, several retrospective studies of higher-order gestations reduced to twins or singletons have shown significant prolongation of gestation when compared with those who did not undergo reduction.[42] Based on these findings, The American College of Obstetricians and Gynecologists (ACOG) states that '… the risks associated with a quadruplet or higher pregnancy clearly outweigh the risks associated with fetal reduction.'[43] There seems to be an increasing risk of IUGR with increasing fetal number. Compared with triplets, triplets reduced to twins have a higher (about 6–9%) incidence of loss < 24 weeks, but lower incidences of PTB < 32 weeks, maternal hospitalization, cesarean delivery (CD), and better neonatal outcome of the remaining twins after reduction compared with triplets. As reduction involves termination of one triplet fetus, overall perinatal survival is not different, and might actually be slightly decreased, but improvement in morbidity and mortality is seen in the 'remaining' twin fetuses compared with non-reduced triplets and yields a higher rate of 'intact' normal babies in the reduced-to-twins compared with the non-reduced triplets. Over 90% of women who underwent pregnancy reduction would opt for the procedure again.

Bed rest
Bed rest, either prophylactic (before symptoms) or therapeutic (with symptoms of PTL), does not prevent PTB in multiple gestations.[44] Compared with normal activity, **prophylactic bed rest in the hospital increases the rate of delivery before 34 weeks by 84%**[44,45] in uncomplicated twin pregnancies. **There is no reduction in LBW or perinatal mortality** (see also Chapter 15 of *Obstetric Evidence Based Guidelines*).

Cerclage
Cerclage, either history-indicated[46] or ultrasound-indicated,[47] does not prevent PTB in twin and triplet[48] gestations.

Other prophylactic interventions such as education and support, home uterine activity monitoring,[49] progesterone,[50] and infection screening have either been shown to be ineffective or insufficiently studied for prevention of PTB in multiple gestations.

Tocolytics
Prophylactic tocolysis has no proven effect on the incidence of PTB, LBW, or neonatal mortality (all similar incidences with placebo) in twin gestations, and therefore this practice should be avoided.[51]

Preterm labor
No tocolysis is indicated if any of the following are present: ≥ 34 weeks' gestation, fetal lung maturity, PPROM, chorioamnionitis, or non-reassuring testing.

If < 34 weeks and none of the above criteria are present, evaluation of multiples presenting < 34 weeks in threatened PTL may be based on cervical length (CL), for this directly correlates with delivery within 7 days in women with regular painful contractions at 24–36 weeks:

- >25 mm, 0%
- 21–25 mm, 7%
- 16–20 mm, 21%
- 11–15 mm, 29%
- 6–10 mm, 46%
- 1–5 mm, 80%.[52]

Corticosteroids (one course: betamethasone 12 mg q24h × 2 doses) should be administered to all patients who are between 24 and 33 6/7 weeks and at high risk (e.g. CL < 20 mm) of delivery within 7 days.[53]

Tocolytics have not been sufficiently studied in multiple gestations (no specific trials) with PTL or PPROM to assess their efficacy in PTB prevention. They should be used judiciously due to higher incidence of side effects (e.g. pulmonary edema) compared with singleton gestations.

Preterm premature rupture of membranes

Deliver if any of the following: ≥ 34 weeks' gestation, fetal lung maturity, PTL, chorioamnionitis, or non-reassuring testing.

If < 34 weeks and none of the above criteria are present, then expectant management with antibiotics, usually ampicillin and erythromycin, together with corticosteroids, as above, is indicated.

Fetal growth restriction/ discordant twins

If neither fetus is SGA (EFW <10% for gestational age), no significant change in management needs to be done. If one fetus is SGA, then: review of all prenatal exposures; specialized ultrasound examination for anomalies; consider amniocentesis for karyotype;[43] consider twice-weekly non-stress tests (NSTs) and weekly umbilical artery Doppler velocimetry (see also Chapter 39). Consider deliver for reversed end-diastolic flow of the umbilical artery (REDF of UA) at > 30–32 weeks.

Single fetal death

Management depends on chorionicity and gestational age.

Dichorionic gestation

- At < 12 weeks, usually no consequences, and so no intervention is needed.
- At > 12 weeks, immediate delivery has no benefit for the remaining fetus and the often-quoted maternal risk has not been demonstrated.

Monochorionic gestation

- At < 12 weeks, associated with high risk of loss of other twin, with no intervention studied.
- At > 12 weeks, associated with about 10% risk of intrauterine death and additional 25% risk of neurological complications in the other twin. These risks seem to occur from hypotension due to transfusion of blood from the other twin to the already demised twin. At the time the demise is discovered, the greatest harm has most likely already occurred in the remaining fetus, and there seems to be no benefit in immediate delivery, especially if the surviving fetus(es) are very preterm and otherwise healthy. In such cases, allowing the pregnancy to continue may provide the most benefit.[43] The coagulopathy risk for the mother is minimal, probably <2%.

Twin–twin transfusion syndrome

Work-up

Upon diagnosis of TTTS, other possible etiologies should be ruled out, by obtaining a detailed anatomy survey with ultrasound of both twins, including umbilical artery Doppler and echocardiography, fetal chromosomes by amniocentesis, infectious studies (e.g. cytomegalovirus [CMV], parvovirus, toxoplasmosis) on amniotic fluid and maternal serum, and maternal glucose tolerance testing.

Therapy

As prognosis with expectant management is poor, termination of pregnancy should be discussed, especially with advanced stages (Table 38.3) diagnosed before 24 weeks. Several therapies have been proposed for TTTS, with insufficient data for secure recommendation. The only therapies studied in trials are amnioreduction, laser, and septostomy.

Amnioreduction

This therapy involves removing, with a 20–22 gauge needle, excess fluid from the polyhydramniotic sac, so as to restore MVP < 8 cm. While in 20% of cases one amnioreduction is sufficient to resolve TTTS, in the other cases it might need to be performed serially, as fluid often reaccumulates quickly. The theory behind its efficacy is that it prevents preterm delivery due to polyhydramnios and also helps to stabilize the flow in AV connections and thereby slows the rate of blood transfer and fluid reaccumulation.[54]

Laser therapy

Direct coagulation of the placental vessels identified in the recipient twin and crossing the membrane to the other twin (semiselective), or of only those vessels thought to be responsible for the imbalance, such as AV anastomoses, is achieved by laser therapy. The techniques can be more or less selective or non-selective of certain AV, AA, or VV anastomoses.

In the first randomized controlled trial (RCT) comparing these two techniques, **endoscopic laser coagulation of anastomoses and amnioreduction was associated with higher perinatal survival (57 vs 41%), higher survival (76 vs 56%) of at least one twin to 28 days of age, and lower incidence (7 vs 17%) of neurological complications among survivors than serial amnioreduction for TTTS diagnosed before 26 weeks of gestation.**[55] It should be noted that there were 11 elective terminations (16%) in the amnioreduction group and none in the laser group; excluding these pregnancies, no differences in outcomes are present. The 41% perinatal survival rate of the amnioreduction group is much lower than the usual 60–65% reported in most series and another RCT.[56] A second recent small trial showed no significant differences in perinatal survival between laser therapy and amnioreduction.[57] Improved neurological outcome with laser has been confirmed by most other non-RCT reports comparing these two interventions. There is insufficient information to assess if the semiselective technique used for laser is beneficial or not compared with other techniques. It is important to counsel parents that, with laser therapy, they have a 12% procedure-related chance of loss, and 66% chance of delivering a dead or a brain-injured baby.[58] Also, 5% of TTTS spontaneously resolve, and about 20% also resolve after the first amnioreduction.

Septostomy

This technique involves purposefully perforating the inter-twin membrane under ultrasound guidance with a 22-gauge needle. Compared with amnioreduction with an 18-gauge needle, septostomy (at times with amnioreduction) is associated with similar **perinatal survival (70 vs 64%) and similar survival (80 vs 78%) of at least one twin to 28 days of age for TTTS diagnosed before 24 weeks of gestation, with neurological and long-term complications among survivors not reported.** Women undergoing septostomy are more likely to require just a single procedure compared with amnioreduction (64 vs 46%). This trial was also stopped before planned recruitment.[56] Other studies are not randomized and include too few patients for meaningful assessment.[59]

Selective fetocide

Selective fetocide via bipolar diathermy can allow the survival of one twin without neurological complications.[60] The most common indication for selective fetocide in TTTS is one of the twins has an anomaly or hydrops with impending fetal death. There are no trials available. The rate of loss or PPROM within 2–3 weeks of the procedure of the remaining twin is about 20%.

Other interventions

There is insufficient evidence to evaluate the efficacy of other interventions reported for TTTS, such as transfusion therapy, indomethacin, and digoxin.

Multiple treatment options for **acardiac twin** have been described. In a recent systematic review, intrafetal ablation was determined to be the treatment of choice.[61]

Monoamniotic twins

Due to rarity of the condition, there are no trials available. Several controlled series have suggested: first trimester

screening with NT measurement; fetal echocardiography at 22–24 weeks; ultrasound every 3–4 weeks until 24 weeks to assess cord entanglement; corticosteroids in the standard dose at 24–26 weeks; daily NSTs initiated at viability; admission at 24–26 weeks with continuous monitoring (allow bathroom and shower privileges). After 24 weeks, serial ultrasound should be performed every 2 weeks for fetal biometry, size discordance, and amniotic fluid volume, and umbilical cord Doppler should be performed weekly. In the presence of a persistent non-reactive fetal heart tracing (once documented as reactive) or abnormal biophysical profile (BPP), poor or discordant growth, and/or abnormal umbilical artery Doppler velocimetry, in-hospital continuous monitoring should be initiated.

Timing of delivery

Consider delivery for obstetric indications including abnormal fetal testing or impaired fetal growth < 32 weeks, or electively around 32 weeks.

Single intrauterine death

If gestational age is < 28–30 weeks, can continue to monitor. If gestational age is > 30 weeks, urgent delivery is warranted.

Mode of delivery

Cesarean section at 32 weeks is the preferred mode of delivery due to the risks of: fetal interlocking and cord entanglement, inadvertently clamping and dividing the cord of the second twin during the delivery of the first twin, premature placental separation, and cord prolapse.

Acardiac twin

Due to the rarity of the condition, there are no trials available. As cardiac failure is more common when the EFW of the acardiac twin is > 70% of the EFW of the pump twin, interventions to 'terminate' the acardiac twin in utero have been proposed for EFW of acardiac twin > 70% and also 'pump' twin compromise. Of all the proposed techniques, ultrasound-guided laser coagulation or radiofrequency ablation of intrafetal vessels seem to be the first line treatment in centers experienced with these techniques. Cord ligation and occlusion have also been reported with some success.[62]

Conjoined twins

Due to rarity of the condition, there are no trials available. Elective termination would be considered if cardiac (thoracopagus) or cerebral (craniopagus) fusion due to poor outcome,[32] or if the pregnancy outcome due to the level of deformity is unacceptable. If pregnancy is continued, elective cesarean at term is recommended.

Antepartum testing
Ultrasound

An ultrasound should be performed in the first trimester to assess viability, gestational age, and chorionicity.

An ultrasound should be performed between 18 and 20 weeks to assess gestational age, chorionicity (if not done previously), placental cord insertion sites, fetal anatomic surveys, fetal gender, and (possibly) cervical length.

Fetal growth

Twins grow at the same rate as singletons up to 28–32 weeks, and then the growth of twins slows, so that fetal twin charts are best used for management. Sonographic assessment can be performed every 4 weeks from 18–20 weeks until delivery; if discordance or IUGR is diagnosed, the frequency is increased to every 3 weeks.

Amniotic fluid

Multiple methods to access amniotic fluid by ultrasound in multiples have been described, including subjective assessment, total amniotic fluid index (AFI), individual AFI, single deepest pocket (SDP, aka maximum vertical pocket) and two-diameter pocket. Whereas the SDP technique, using < 2 cm for oligohydramnios and > 8 cm for hydramnios, is accurate in assessing amniotic fluid volume in normal pregnancies, it is not very accurate in detection of oligohydramnios in multiple pregnancies.

Fetal surveillance

Routine antepartum testing has not proven to be valuable in the management of multiple gestations. Antepartum fetal surveillance in multiple gestations is recommended in all situations in which surveillance would ordinarily be performed in a singleton pregnancy (e.g. FGR, maternal disease, decreased fetal movement, etc.).[43] Some clinicians start NSTs in all twin gestations at around 34 weeks, but there is no firm evidence for or against this intervention. Doppler flow studies are not routinely beneficial,[63] but probably have the same benefit in fetal morbidity and mortality in cases of twin FGR as in cases of singleton FGR (See Chapter 39).

Delivery
Assessment of fetal lung maturity

As disparity in lung maturity usually occurs in only 5% of twins, just one gestational sac may be sampled for assessment of lung maturity. In certain circumstances, such as diabetes or growth discordance, a bigger difference in maturity discordance may necessitate sampling both sacs.

Timing of delivery

Fetal and neonatal morbidity and mortality begin to increase in twins at 37 completed weeks and triplets at 35 completed weeks. There are **insufficient data available** to assess any effect of elective delivery at around 37 weeks' gestation for women with an otherwise uncomplicated twin pregnancy, since only a small ($n = 36$) trial has assessed this question.[64] There are no statistically significant differences between elective induction of labor at 37 weeks and expectant management with regards to CD (trend for decrease of 44%), CD for fetal distress (trend for decrease of 53%), perinatal death (zero in both groups), or any other outcome.[64] If the fetuses are AGA with evidence of sustained growth, with normal AFI and reassuring testing without maternal disease, the pregnancy can be delivered at **37 or 38 weeks**, with the woman allowed to influence this decision. However, if the woman is experiencing morbidities that would not usually mandate delivery (e.g. dyspnea, inability to sleep, severe edema, painful varicosities), delivery may be considered at 37 weeks.[43]

Route of delivery

Twins
There is insufficient evidence to assess the best mode of delivery for twins. Trial of labor (TOL) after CD is associated with similar risks with twin as with singleton gestations. (See also Chapter 13 in *Obstetric Evidence Based Guidelines*.)

There are **no trials for twins presenting vertex/vertex** (40% of twin pregnancies). TOL is usually suggested, as this has been shown to be safe.

Compared with TOL, elective CD for the **non-cephalic second twin** (about 34% of twin pregnancies) had no benefit in neonatal outcome with increased maternal febrile morbidity in one small trial.[65] However, when all twins at 36 weeks or beyond, not just those with a non-cephalic second twin, were examined, it has been reported that the term second twin has a higher rate of perinatal mortality when delivered vaginally as opposed to scheduled cesarean delivery.[66] The rate of low 5-minute Apgar score is less frequent in twins delivered by CD.[67] Attempts at vaginal twin delivery have been supported, especially for twins with EFW of > 1500 g, and can only be performed by an adequately experienced obstetrician, with continuous availability of expert anesthesia, and usually in or very close to an operating room. The interval between the first and second twin deliveries is not critical, as long as the second twin is monitored continuously and accurately. Oxytocin may need to be (re)started, as contractions often diminish, and amniotomy should be performed only when the presenting part is engaged. The total breech extraction is associated with shorter maternal stay and lower neonatal pulmonary disease, infection, and neonatal intensive care unit (NICU) stay than the podalic version in retrospective studies.[67,68]

There are no trials for twins presenting with **first twin non-vertex** (about 26%), with recommendation for CD made based mostly on data from singleton gestations.

Triplets and higher-order multiples

Because vaginal delivery of triplets is usually associated with an increased risk for stillbirth and neonatal and infant deaths compared with cesarean delivery,[69] **cesarean section is the route of choice.** Some centers have recently reported similar outcomes for TOL or CD for triplets, but these series are small and not RCTs.

Delayed interval delivery

Preterm labor or PPROM can result in the delivery of only one twin or other multiple gestation fetus. Delaying the delivery of the remaining fetus(es) may result in decreased morbidity and mortality of these remaining fetuses, with no trials to fully assess the effect of this intervention. Delayed delivery should not be attempted if MC gestation, abruption, preeclampsia, chorioamnionitis, need of CD, or other indications for delivery are present. Therefore only about 25% of multiple deliveries in the second trimester are candidates for this attempt. Delayed delivery is not very successful and does not result in significant improvements at > 28 weeks (delay < 2 weeks even with success). Whereas tocolytics, antibiotics, and cerclage are often used, there is no firm evidence of their benefit. Delayed delivery is associated with decreases in perinatal and infant mortality, with average gains of about 2–5 weeks if successful. The interval between delivery is inversely correlated with gestational age of first delivery.[70]

NEONATAL

There is probably no significant difference between multiples and singletons in odds of death and long-term outcomes (intraventricular hemorrhage, retinopathy of prematurity, necrotizing enterocolitis) at a given gestational age in those unaffected by FGR.[71]

REFERENCES

1. Benirschke K, Kim CK. Multiple pregnancy. 1. N Engl J Med 1973; 288(24): 1276–84. [II-3]
2. Martin JA, Hamilton BE, Sutton PD, et al. Births: final data for 2002. Natl Vital Stat Rep 2003; 52(10): 1–102. [II-3]
3. www.MarchofDimes.com/peristats [epidemiological data]
4. Wenstrom KD, Syrop CH, Hammitt DG, van Voorhis BJ. Increased risk of monochorionic twinning associated with assisted reproduction. Fertil Steril 1993; 60: 510–14. [III]
5. LeFevre ML, Bain RP, Ewigman BG et al. A randomized trial of prenatal ultrasonographic screening: impact on maternal management and outcome. RADIUS (Routine Antenatal Diagnostic Imaging with Ultrasound) Study Group. Am J Obstet Gynecol 1993; 169(3): 483–9. [I]
6. Finberg HJ. The "twin peak" sign: reliable evidence of dichorionic twinning. J Ultrasound Med 1992 ; 11(11): 571–7. [II-3]
7. Dickey RP, Taylor SN, Lu PY, et al. Spontaneous reduction of multiple pregnancy: incidence and effect on outcome. Am J Obstet Gynecol 2002; 186(1): 77–83. [II-2]
8. Meyers C, Adam R, Dungan J, Prenger V. Aneuploidy in twin gestations: when is maternal age advanced? Obstet Gynecol 1997; 89: 248–51. [II-2]
9. Rodis JF, Egan JFX, Craffey A, et al. Calculated risks of chromosomal abnormalities in twin gestations. Obstet Gynecol 1990; 76(6): 1037–41. [II-2]
10. Malone FD, D'Alton ME. Multiple gestation clinical characteristics and management. In: Creasy RK, Resnik R, Iams JD (eds.) Maternal-Fetal Medicine Principles and Practice, 5th edn. Philadelphia: WB Saunders; 2004. [III]
11. Jones KL. Smith's Recognizable Patterns of Human Malformation, 5th edn. Philadelphia: WB Saunders; 1997; 654. [III]
12. Yinon Y, Mazkereth R, Rosentzweig N, et al. Growth restriction as a determinant of outcome in preterm discordant twins. Obstet Gynecol 2005; 105: 80–4. [II-3]
13. D'Alton ME, Simpson LL. Syndromes in twins. Semin Perinatol 1995; 19(5): 375–86. [II-3]
14. Nassar AH, Usta IM, Rechdan JB, et al. Pregnancy outcome in spontaneous twins versus twins who were conceived through in vitro fertilization. Am J Obstet Gynecol 2003; 189: 513–18. [II-2]
15. Magee BD. Role of multiple births in very low birth weight and infant mortality. J Reprod Med 2004; 49(10): 812–16. [II-2]
16. Petterson B, Nelson KB, Watson L, Stanly F. Twins, triplets and cerebral palsy in births in Western Australia in the 1980s. BMJ 1993; 307: 1239–43. [II-2]
17. Chasen ST, Madden A, Chervenak FA. Cesarean delivery of twins and neonatal respiratory disorders. Am J Obstet Gynecol 1999; 181 (5 Pt 1): 1052–6. [II-2]
18. Wen SW, Demissie K, Yang Q, Walker MC. Maternal morbidity and obstetric complications in triplet pregnancies and quadruplet and higher-order multiple pregnancies. Am J Obstet Gynecol 2004; 191: 254–8. [II-2]
19. Sibai BM, Hauth J, Caritis S, et al. Hypertensive disorders in twin versus singleton gestations. National Institute of Child Health and Human Development Network of Maternal-Fetal Medicine Units. Am J Obstet Gynecol 2000; 182: 938–42. [I]
20. Al-Kouatly HB, Chasen ST, Kalish RB, Chervenak FA. Causes of thrombocytopenia in triplet gestations. Am J Obstet Gynecol 2003; 189(1): 177–80. [II-2]
21. Malone FD, Kaufman GE, Chelmow D, et al. Maternal morbidity associated with triplet pregnancy. Am J Perinatol 1998; 15: 73–7. [II-3]
22. Schwartz DB, Daoud Y, Zazula P, et al. Gestational diabetes mellitus: metabolic and blood glucose parameters in singleton versus twin pregnancies. Am J Obstet Gynecol 1999; 181(4): 912–14. [II-2]
23. Silvan E, Maman E, Homko CJ, et al. Impact of fetal reduction on the incidence of gestational diabetes. Obstet Gynecol 2002; 99: 91–4. [II-3]
24. Francois K, Ortiz J, Harris C, et al. Is peripartum hysterectomy more common in multiple gestations? Obstet Gynecol 2005; 105(6); 1369–72. [II-3]
25. Quintero RA, Morales WJ, Allen MH, et al. Staging of twin–twin transfusion syndrome. J Perinatol 1999; 19: 550–5. [II-2]
26. Berghella V, Kaufmann M. Natural history of twin–twin transfusion syndrome. J Reprod Med 2001; 46(5): 480–4. [II-3]
27. Slotnick RN, Ortega JE. Monoamniotic twining and zona manipulation: a survey of U.S. IVF centers correlating zona manipulation procedures and high-risk twinning frequency. J Assist Reprod Genet 1996; 13: 381–5. [II-3]
28. Bromley B, Benacerraf B. Using the number of yolk sacs to determine amniocity in early first trimester monochorionic twins. J Ultrasound Med 1995; 14: 415–19. [II-2]

29. Demaria F, Goffinet F, Kayem G, et al. Monoamniotic twin pregnancies: antenatal management and perinatal results of 19 consecutive cases. BJOG 2004; 111(1): 22–6. [II-3]

30. Roque H, Young BK, Lockwood CJ. Perinatal outcomes in monoamniotic gestations. J Matern Fetal Neonatal Med 2003; 13(6): 414–21. [II-3]

31. Van Gemert MJ, Umur A, van den Wijngaard JP, et al. Increasing cardiac output and decreasing oxygenation sequence in pump twins of acardiac twin pregnancies. Phys Med Biol 2005; 50(3): N33–42. [II-3]

32. Spitz L, Kiely EM. Conjoined twins. JAMA 2003; 289(10): 1307–10. [II-3]

33. Mackenzie TC, Crombleholme TM, Johnson MP, et al. The natural history of prenatally diagnosed conjoined twins. J Pediatr Surg 2002; 37(3): 303–9. [II-3]

34. Sebire N, Snijders R, Hughes K, et al. Screening for trisomy 21 in twin pregnancies by maternal age and fetal nuchal translucency thickness at 10–14 weeks of gestation. Br J Obstet Gynaecol 1996; 103(10): 999–1003. [II-2]

35. Wapner RJ, Johnson A, Davis G. Prenatal diagnosis in twin gestations: a comparison between second trimester amniocentesis and first trimester chorionic villus sampling. Obstet Gynecol 1993; 82(1): 49–56. [II-2]

36. Wapner RJ. Genetic diagnosis in multiple pregnancies. Semin Perinatol 1995; 19: 351–62. [III]

37. O'Brien J, Dvorin E, Yaron Y. Differential increases in AFP, hCG, and uE3 in twin pregnancies: impact on attempts to quantify Down syndrome screening calculations. Am J Med Genet 1997; 73(2): 109–12. [II-1]

38. Ghidini A, Lynch L, Hicks C, et al. The risk of second-trimester amniocentesis in twin gestations: a case-control study. Am J Obstet Gynecol 1993; 169(4): 1013–16. [II-2]

39. McMahon KS, Neerhof MG, Haney EI, et al. Prematurity in multiple gestations: identification of patients who are at low risk. Am J Obstet Gynecol 2002; 186: 1137–41. [II-3]

40. Goldberg R, Iams J, Miodovnik M. The preterm prediction study: risk factors in twin gestations. National Institute of Child Health and Human Development; Maternal-Fetal Medicine Units Network. Am J Obstet Gynecol 1996; 175(4 Pt 1): 1047–53. [II-2]

41. Eddleman KA, Stone JL, Lynch L, Berkowitz RL. Selective termination of anomalous fetuses in multifetal pregnancies: two hundred cases at a single center. Am J Obstet Gynecol 2002; 187: 1168–72. [II-3]

42. Miller V, Ransom S, Shalhoub A, et al. Multifetal pregnancy reduction: perinatal and fiscal outcomes. Am J Obstet Gynecol 182; 6: 1575–80. [II-3]

43. Multiple gestation: complicated twin, triplet, and higher-order multifetal pregnancy. ACOG Practice Bull No. 56, October 2004. [III]

44. Crowther CA. Hospitalization and bed rest for multiple pregnancy. Cochrane Database Syst Rev 2005; 4. [meta-analysis: 4 RCTs, >1000 women. Mostly in Harare, Zimbabwe]

45. Crowther CA, Neilson JP, Verkuyl DAA, Bannerman C, Ashurst HM. Preterm labour in twin pregnancies: can it be prevented by hospital admission? Br J Obstet Gynaecol 1989; 96: 850–3. [RCT, n = 139]

46. Dor J, Shalev J, Mashiach S, et al. Elective cervical suture of twins pregnancies diagnosed ultrasonically in the first trimester following induced ovulation. Gynecol Obstet Invest 1982; 13(1): 55–60. [RCT, n = 50]

47. Berghella V, Odibo AO, To MS, Rust OA, Althuisius SM. Cerclage for short cervix on ultrasonography: meta-analysis of trials using individual patient-level data. Obstet Gynecol 2005; 106(1): 181–9. [meta-analysis: 4 RCTs, n = 49 twin gestations]

48. Rebarber A, Roman AS, Istwan N, Rhea D, Stanziano G. Prophylactic cerclage in the management of triplet gestations. Am J Obstet Gynecol 2005; 193: 1193–6. [II-2]

49. Colton T, Kayne H, Zhang Y. A meta-analysis of home uterine activity monitoring. Am J Obstet Gynecol 1995; 173(5); 1499–505. [I]

50. Hartikainen-Sorri AL, Kauppila A, Tuimala R. Inefficacy of 17 alpha-hydroxyprogesterone caproate in the prevention of prematurity in twin pregnancy. Obstet Gynecol 1980; 56(6): 692–5 [II-2]

51. Yamasmit W, Chaithongwongwatthana S, Tolosa JE, et al. Prophylactic oral betamimetics for reducing preterm birth in women with a twin pregnancy. Cochrane Database Syst Rev 2005 4 [meta-analysis; 5 RCTs, n = 344]

52 Fuchs I, Tsoi E, Henrich W, et al. Sonographic measurement of cervical length in twin pregnancies in threatened preterm labor. Ultrasound Obstet Gynecol 2004 ; 23: 42–5. [II-3]

53. Effect of corticosteroids for fetal maturation on perinatal outcomes. NIH Consensus Statement 1994; 12: 1–24. [III]

54. Bower SJ, Flack NJ, Sepulveda W, et al. Uterine artery blood flow response to correction of amniotic fluid volume. Am J Obstet Gynecol 1995; 173: 502–7. [II-3]

55. Senat M, Deprest J, Boulvain M, et al. Endoscopic laser surgery versus serial amnioreduction for severe twin-to-twin transfusion syndrome. N Engl J Med 2004; 351(2): 136–44. [RCT, n = 142]

56. Moise KJ Jr, Dorman K, Lamvu G, et al. A randomized trial of amnioreduction versus septostomy in the treatment of twin-twin transfusion syndrome. Am J Obstet Gynecol 2005; 193(3 Pt 1): 701–7. [RCT, n = 73]

57. Crombleholme T, Shera D, Porter F, et al. NIH-sponsored prospective randomized trial of amnioreduction versus selective fetoscopic laser photocoagulation for twin–twin transfusion syndrome. Am J Obstet Gynecol 2006; 195: s21. [RCT, n = 42]

58. Fisk N, Galea P. Twin-twin transfusion – as good as it gets? N Engl J Med 2004; 351(2): 182–4. [III]

59. Johnson JR, Rossi KQ, O'Shaughnessy RW. Amnioreduction versus septostomy in twin-twin transfusion syndrome. Am J Obstet Gynecol 2001; 185: 1044–7. [II-2]

60. Taylor MJ, Shalev E, Tanawattanacharoen S, et al. Ultrasound guided umbilical chord occlusion using bipolar diathery for stage III/IV twin-twin transfusion syndrome. Prenat Diagn 2002; 22: 70–6. [II-3]

61. Tan TY, Sepulveda W. Acardiac twin: a systemic review of minimally invasive treatment modalities. Ultrasound Obstet Gynecol 2003; 22(4): 409–19. [review of II-2 and II-3 studies]

62. Wong AE, Sepulveda W. Acardiac anomaly: current issues in prenatal assessment and treatment. Prenat Diagn 2005; 25: 796–806. [II-3]

63. Giles W, Bisits A, O'Callaghan S, Gill-A. The Doppler assessment in multiple pregnancy randomised controlled trial of ultrasound biometry versus umbilical artery Doppler ultrasound and biometry in twin pregnancy. BJOG 2003; 110(6): 593–7. [I]

64. Suzuki S, Otsubo Y, Sawa R, Yoneyama Y. Clinical trial of induction of labor versus expectant management in twin pregnancy. Gynecol Obstet Invest 2000; 49: 24–7. [RCT, n = 36]

65. Rabinovici J, Barkai G, Reichman B, Serr D, Mashiach S. Randomized management of the second twin: vaginal delivery or cesarean section. Am J Obstet Gynecol 1987; 156: 52–6. [RCT, n = 60]

66. Smith GC, Pell JP, Dobbie R. Birth order, gestational age, and risk of delivery related perinatal death in twins: a retrospective cohort study. BMJ 2002; 325(7371): 1004. [II-2]

67. Hogle KL, Hutton EK, McBrien KA, Barrett JFR, Hannah ME. Cesarean delivery for twins: a systematic review and meta-analysis. Am J Obstet Gynecol 2003; 188: 220–7. [meta-analysis: 4 studies – only 1 RCT, Ref. 65.]

68. Maudin JG, Newman RB, Mauldin PD. Cost-effective delivery management of the vertex and non-vertex twin gestation. Am J Obstet Gynecol 1998; 179: 864–9. [II-2]

69. Vintzileos AM, Ananth CV, Kontopoulos E, Smulian JC. Mode of delivery and risk of stillbirth and infant mortality in triplet gestations: United States, 1995 through 1998. Am J Obstet Gynecol 2005; 192: 464–9. [II-3]

70. Oyelese Y, Ananth CV, Smulian JC, Vintzileos AM. Delayed interval delivery in twin pregnancies in the United States: impact on perinatal mortality and morbidity. Am J Obstet Gynecol 2005; 192: 439–44. [II-3]

71. Garite TJ, Clark RH, Elliot JP, Thorp JA. Twins and triplets: the effect of plurality and growth on neonatal outcome compared with singleton infants. Am J Obstet Gynecol 2004; 191: 700–7. [II-2]

39

Fetal growth restriction

Juan Carlos Sabogal and Stuart Weiner

KEY POINTS

- Small for gestational age (SGA) is defined as an estimation of fetal weight < 10th percentile for gestational age. **Fetal growth restriction (FGR) is SGA with failure to reach growth potential.**
- **Risk factors associated with FGR** are (**maternal**) pregnancy-related hypertension; pregestational diabetes; autoimmune, cardiac or other maternal diseases; toxic exposure (smoking, alcohol, cocaine, drugs); malnutrition; living at high altitudes or in a developing country; low socioeconomic status; race; family, or prior history; and (**fetal**) genetic diseases (e.g. aneuploidy); fetal malformations (1–2%); multiple gestation; placental abnormalities (abruption, mosaicism, chorioangiomas, etc.); and fetal infection (cytomegalovirus [CMV], rubella, toxoplasmosis).
- **Complications** of FGR manifest as fetal (**oligohydramnios**, non-reassuring fetal heart rate (**NRFHR**), and **death**), neonatal (**preterm birth** and its consequences – respiratory distress syndrome [**RDS**], intraventricular hemorrhage [**IVH**], necrotizing enterocolitis [**NEC**], **sepsis**, etc. – **hypoglycemia, electrolyte disturbances, hyperviscosity syndrome, neurodevelopmental delay, and death**), infant and child (**impaired gross motor development, cerebral palsy, lower intelligence quotient, mental retardation, speech/reading disabilities, learning deficits, poor academic achievement, and suicide**), as well as long-term adult consequences (**hypertension, coronary artery disease, diabetes, obesity, and problems with social and financial issues**).
- **The incidence of FGR can be reduced** with appropriate dating by **early (< 20 weeks) ultrasound**, as well as **identification and treatment of risk factors** (e.g. smoking and other toxic exposures, medical disorders, etc.). A **low-dose aspirin** reduces the incidence of FGR by 10%, especially if > 75 mg aspirin is started before 20 weeks.
- The **best screening test**, as well as **diagnostic test**, for FGR is **ultrasound**.
- **Work-up** for FGR includes **maternal history** for any risk factor, as well as **ultrasound** with assessment of **biometry,** detailed anatomy, amniotic fluid assessment, placental grade and appearance, and (at least) **umbilical artery Doppler** analysis. **Amniocentesis** should be offered to rule out aneuploidy (karyotype) and infection (polymerase chain reaction [PCR] for CMV and toxoplasmosis). **Infectious work-up** can also include maternal serum immunoglobulins IgG and IgM for CMV and toxoplasmosis. Rubella immunity should be ascertained. **Antiphos- pholipid antibodies** may be checked. **Maternal work-up** for pre-eclampsia, or evaluation for any disease possibly associated with FGR, should be done.
- Fetal therapy is limited, since interventions studied have not been shown to be beneficial or have been insufficiently studied. **Control or elimination of risk factors** (e.g. stop drug abuse or smoking, control maternal disease) should be performed.
- **Doppler ultrasound of the umbilical artery is the cornerstone of FGR follow-up and management**, since it is associated with a **decreased risk of perinatal mortality**.
- **Steroids** should be given if fetal testing in the FGR fetus suggests the need for delivery at 24–34 weeks in the next 2–7 days.
- The timing of delivery should be individualized, and **based on gestational age** and **all antepartum tests**. Delivering early at < 32 weeks for hypothetical avoidance of fetal hypoxia might not improve outcome.

DEFINITIONS

Small for gestational age (SGA) is defined as an estimation of fetal size (usually weight) < 10th **percentile** for gestational age for the relevant population. Cut-offs of < 3rd or < 5th percentiles have also been described. This condition has also been called 'small fetus'. It can be divided into three subgroups:

- normal SGA (e.g. normal anatomy and Doppler ultrasound);
- abnormal SGA (structural or genetic fetal anomaly);
- **fetal growth restriction (FGR)** is defined as SGA with failure to reach growth potential (e.g. abnormal Doppler ultrasound)

Table 39.1   *Risk factors associated with FGR*

Maternal

Pregnancy-related hypertension (20–30%)
Pregestational diabetes
Autoimmune disease (APS, SLE)
Maternal cardiac disease (complex cyanotic congenital heart diseases)
Other maternal diseases (especially if poorly controlled)
Toxic exposure (smoking, alcohol, cocaine, drugs)
Malnutrition
Living at high altitudes
Living in developing country
Low socioeconomic status
Race (Afro-American)
Family or prior history of FGR
Extremes of maternal age

Fetal

Genetic diseases[a] (5–20%)
Fetal malformations (1–2%)
Multiple gestation (3%)
Placental abnormalities (abruption, mosaicism, chorioangiomas, etc.)
Fetal infection (CMV, rubella, toxoplasmosis) (5–10%)
Malaria

[a]May include aneuploidy, uniparental disomy, growth factor mutations, etc.
FGR, fetal growth restriction; APS, antiphospholipid syndrome; SLE, systemic lupus erythromatosus; CMV, cytomegalovirus.

Severe FGR can be defined as that associated with fetal weight < 3rd percentile with abnormal Doppler ultrasound. FGR is also called IUGR (intrauterine growth restriction).

Low birth weight (LBW) is defined as < 2500 g. For SGA or FGR in a multiple gestation, please refer to Chapter 38.

EPIDEMIOLOGY/INCIDENCE

By definition, there is a 10% incidence of SGA fetuses in the general population. Normal SGA fetuses represent about 70% of SGA fetuses, FGR about 20–25%, and abnormal SGA < 10%. FGR is related to the cut-off chosen, and to specific risk factors of the population (Table 39.1).

GENETICS/INHERITANCE/RECURRENCE

The majority of FGR fetuses do not have a genetic change that can help predict inheritance and recurrence. If the comprehensive work-up reveals a genetic change, proper counseling is indicated. The identification of the etiology can help with assessing recurrence risks. For example, identification of intrauterine infection as an etiology signifies future immunity and therefore usually no recurrence risk of the particular infection-related FGR.

TERATOLOGY/ETIOLOGY/BASIC PATHOPHYSIOLOGY

There are two scenarios which can lead to an SGA baby, and it is very important to distinguish between them. The so-called **constitutional SGA** fetus is the one with an estimated fetal weight (EFW) below the 10th percentile for GA, but otherwise healthy. This baby characteristically grows at a constant speed that usually parallels a specific percentile throughout the pregnancy. More importantly, this baby is not prone to develop any fetal or perinatal complications, has a normal postnatal outcome, and does not need therapy. Ultrasound shows normal amniotic fluid and Doppler patterns. Some ethnic groups are more likely to show SGA babies if race-adjusted charts are not used.

The conditions in which an SGA fetus is **not healthy** because of one or more disorders (see Table 39.1) contributing to the SGA weight is termed FGR, or abnormal SGA if related to genetic or structural anatomic abnormalities. While the causes of FGR are diverse, most of them lead to a common pathway: **compromise of the uteroplacental perfusion**. This feature constitutes the hallmark of FGR. Over time, the supply of nutrients and oxygen mismatch the fetal requirements that the normal process of growth entails. Then, the normal accretion of tissue decreases, and components of fetal structure and physiology are removed from tissue to undertake abnormal biochemical paths (proteolysis, gluconeogenesis, and beta-oxidation), which are the results of an adaptive attempt to maintain a supply of energy substrates to support vital functions in an adverse environment, giving up on fetal growth. Placental apoptosis is increased. Such biochemical phenomena translate into sonographically recognizable traits, such as decreased growth. Often altered fetal proportion is evident, since places of normal fat accretion such as abdominal wall will show lack of it, with the resultant small abdominal circumference (AC) at ultrasound. At the same time, in an attempt to maintain blood supply to critical tissues (brain, heart, adrenals), the fetal circulation decreases in some not-so-critical organs like the splanchnic circulation and fetal kidneys, often generating oligohydramnios. This pattern of redistribution of the fetal blood flow is detected by Doppler analysis, showing less diastolic flow (increased impedance) in the umbilical artery (UA). At times, increased diastolic flow in the middle cerebral artery (MCA) develops as 'brain-sparing' changes try to maintain adequate oxygenation and nutrition to the fetal brain circulation. Compared with an adequate for gestational age (AGA) fetus, metabolic changes associated with the FGR fetus are **lower pH, pO_2, glucose,** lactate dehydrogenase (LDH), **cholesterol, fatty acids, triglycerides, growth factors (e.g. insulin-like growth factor), insulin, most amino acids, and increased pCO_2, lactic acid, and bilirubin.** Finally, the process may be so severe that **heart failure** ensues and the fetus can die in utero.

CLASSIFICATION

FGR has been classified as asymmetric or symmetric. This classification has been proposed to aid in identification of etiology, but is not associated with changes in outcome, and has **limited clinical value** today, also because many FGR fetuses do not fit these definitions and are therefore difficult to classify.

Asymmetric FGR is characterized by a significant reduction in AC compared with other biometric parameters. The usual etiology is placental insufficiency, often related to maternal hypertensive disease, and manifesting late in pregnancy.

Symmetric FGR is characterized by a similar reduction in all biometric measurements. Usually, the etiology is present right from the beginning of the pregnancy, and can include aneuploidy, other genetic diseases, drug/toxic exposure, and others. This symmetric 'sick' FGR is sometimes difficult to differentiate from the constitutional 'healthy' SGA baby.

RISKS FACTORS/ASSOCIATIONS

See Table 39.1. This is a very heterogeneous disorder, which represents the final common pathway of several mechanisms.

COMPLICATIONS

FGR fetuses are at increased risk for **oligohydramnios, non-reassuring fetal heart rate (NRFHR),** and **fetal death,** and as neonates for iatrogenic or spontaneous **preterm birth** and its consequences (respiratory distress syndrome [RDS], intraventricular hemorrhage [IVH], necrotizing enterocolitis [NEC], **sepsis,** etc.), **hypoglycemia, electrolyte disturbances, hyperviscosity syndrome, neurodevelopmental delay,** and **death.**[1,2] When considered as a group, FGR babies have a risk as high as 100 times of perinatal mortality compared with AGA babies. Compared with AGA controls, FGR fetuses followed for at least 5–11 years grow to have more chronic conditions and functional limitations.[3] These include higher rates of **impaired gross motor development, cerebral palsy, lower intelligence quotient, mental retardation, speech/reading disabilities, learning deficits, poor academic achievement, and suicide.**[4] The Barker hypothesis on the fetal origin of adult disease has been confirmed by data from cohorts of adults that were born at low birth weights. Comparing outcomes with paired normal subjects of similar socioeconomic background, lifelong handicaps from FGR/LBW include higher incidence of **hypertension, coronary artery disease, diabetes, obesity, and problems with social and financial issues.**[5]

MANAGEMENT

Prevention

Early (< 20 weeks) ultrasound can accurately date the pregnancy, and better identify FGR later in pregnancy. Early-dating ultrasound probably decreases both false-positive and false-negative cases of SGA fetus. Several of the risk factors (see Table 39.1) can be identified preconceptionally or at the first prenatal visit and modified/avoided so as to prevent FGR: i.e. **smoking and other toxic exposures. Medical disorders** should be well-controlled, as this can prevent FGR (e.g. diabetes, hypertension, etc.).

Overall, low-dose aspirin given as prevention during pregnancy is associated with a **significant but small (10%) reduction of FGR.**[6] In low- and moderate-risk women this is significant, while in high-risk women there is a lower (3%) non-significant decrease. **If started < 20 weeks, low-dose aspirin decreases SGA** by 18% (6% vs 8%), while it has no effect if started after 20 weeks. **A dose of > 75 mg** is associated with the largest benefit (incidence of SGA 14% vs 21%, a 32% decrease).[6]

Balanced energy (about 500–1000 calories with <25% protein) supplementation prevents FGR in women with nutritional deficiencies. Antimalarian prophylaxis effectively prevents FGR in women living in areas endemic for malaria.

Screening for fetal growth restriction

Increased levels of maternal serum **alpha fetoprotein (MSAFP)** in early second trimester are associated with the subsequent development of FGR.[7] While several other serum factors are associated with FGR, biochemical screening for FGR is not indicated. **Fundal height measurements** at each prenatal visit have **poor sensitivity and a very high false-positive rate for FGR.**[8,9]

First trimester **ultrasound dating** is associated with the most reliable dating of a pregnancy: proper diagnosis of FGR implies evidence of a growth pattern that is below expectations based on GA, which should best be based on exact (i.e. based on first trimester ultrasound) dates. The **best screening test**, as well as **diagnostic test**, for FGR is **ultrasound**. Early (< 20 weeks) ultrasound first establishes GA (see Chapter 3 of *Obstetric Evidence Based Guidelines*). It is important to understand that a first trimester crown–rump length (CRL) of 2–6 days less than expected is associated with an increased risk for LBW.[10] Biometric measurements such as biparietal diameter, head circumference, AC, and femur length are used for estimation of fetal weight. AC is the single sonographic measurement most predictive of fetal growth. 'Customized or personal growth charts' mean that software is able to generate a gestation-related optimal weight that uses a regression analysis based on variables such as maternal height, weight in early pregnancy, parity, ethnic group, and the baby's sex, avoiding misdiagnosis with standard charts.[11] The effect of the use of these personal growth charts, with the diagnosis of FGR based on a change in an already-established pre-existing growth pattern, has not been assessed in any trial. Race/gender-specific nomograms of weight for GA make the diagnosis of FGR more accurate, but there are no trials to show change in outcome. There is insufficient evidence to support routine screening for FGR with **Doppler ultrasound**, because of lack of proven interventions once the Doppler is found to be abnormal. Patients with a UA high resistance index between 10 and 14 weeks' gestation have a 5.5-fold greater risk of developing FGR later in pregnancy.[12] **Uterine artery** bilateral notching at 12–14 weeks' gestation is associated with 75% sensitivity in the prediction of FGR in high-risk women.[13]

Diagnosis

An estimation of fetal weight < 10% for gestational age by ultrasound biometry is the diagnosis for an SGA fetus. **FGR** is the subgroup of **SGA fetuses** suspected of having a pathological condition associated with placental dysfunction responsible for the SGA, such as those **with abnormal UA Doppler**. As the majority of fetuses with EFW between 5 and 10% are constitutionally SGA and do not have FGR, some clinicians define FGR or SGA as EFW < 5th, or even < 3rd percentile for GA. Other clinicians diagnose FGR based on AC < 5% for gestational age. Cerebellar diameter is preserved in size even in FGR fetuses, and may help diagnosis in the second or early third trimester (see Chapter 3 of *Obstetric Evidence Based Guidelines*).

Work-up

Maternal history should be reviewed for any risk factor (see Table 39.1), including detailed medical, infection, and drug history. Every fetus identified as having biometry consistent with EFW < 10th percentile, or AC < 5th percentile, should have ultrasound by properly trained staff, with assessment of **biometry, detailed anatomy**, amniotic fluid (AF) **assessment, placental grade and appearance**, and at least UA **Doppler** analysis. For biometry, particular attention should be paid to **AC**, and to the **HC/AC** (head circumference/ abdominal circumference) ratio. A **fetal echocardiogram** should be considered if inadequate heart views are obtained. Some advanced fetal centers perform Doppler ultrasound of the umbilical vein, MCA, ductus venosus, and other vessels, but there is not enough information to justify routine use of these Doppler studies. Placental analysis might reveal an echogenic, 'aged', or thick placenta, or the presence of abnormality (e.g. abruption, etc.).

Amniocentesis should be offered to rule out aneuploidy (karyotype) and infection (polymerase chain reaction [PCR] for cytomegalovirus [CMV], toxoplasmosis), especially if no other causes are identifiable and the FGR is severe (e.g. EFW < 5%), diagnosed at early GA such as < 24 weeks, and/or is associated with congenital anomalies and/or polyhydramnios. If placental image on ultrasound is abnormal, **placental biopsy** (late chorionic villus sampling [CVS]) may be considered to evaluate for placental mosaicism. **Infectious work-up** should include either PCR from amniotic fluid, or maternal serum immunoglobulins IgG and IgM of CMV and toxoplasmosis. Rubella immunity should be ascertained. There is insufficient evidence to recommend a thrombophilia work-up (see Chapter 27). **Antiphospholipid antibodies** (anticardiolipin IgG and IgM, lupus anticoagulant, and anti-β_2 glycoprotein I) may be checked, especially for counseling regarding etiology and a future pregnancy. **Maternal work-up** for pre-eclampsia, including at least blood pressure and urine protein, and evaluation for any disease possibly associated with FGR (see Table 39.1), should be done.

Counseling (prognosis, complications, and pregnancy considerations)

Prognosis is very much dependent on associated risk factors and underlying etiology, if one can be identified. Worse prognosis is for fetuses with most severe growth restriction, absent or reversed UA Doppler, other abnormal Doppler study (e.g. ductus venosus), oligohydramnios, or early GA at diagnosis.[1,2]

Fetal intervention

Avoidance of toxins

Once diagnosis is made, whenever possible an effort to **control or eliminate the triggering factor** should be made (e.g. stop drug abuse or smoking).

Therapy for medical conditions

Proper treatment of chronic hypertension, pre-eclampsia, diabetes, or other medical conditions is important, but there are no trials to prove a beneficial effect on FGR.

Bed rest

There is insufficient evidence to evaluate the use of a bed rest in-hospital policy for women with suspected impaired fetal growth. Compared with ambulation, bed rest in the hospital was **not associated with differences** in fetal growth parameters (relative risk [RR]=0.43, 95% CI 0.15–1.27) and neonatal outcomes in a small study.[14] Hospitalization for bed rest is **possibly dangerous** (associated with venous thromboembolism, etc.), expensive, and is inconvenient for the pregnant woman.

Nutrient therapy

There is **not enough evidence** to evaluate the use of nutrient therapy such as carnitine, solcoseryl, glucose, or galactose for suspected impaired fetal growth, as trials are too small and/or had methodological limitations.[15] Carnitine was associated with a 2-week shorter pregnancy duration, with no other differences found. Iron, vitamins, and high protein supplements seem to have no major impact on fetal growth.

Beta-mimetics

The theoretical basis for using beta-mimetic therapy for impaired fetal growth is promoting fetal growth by increasing the availability of nutrients and by decreasing vascular resistance. Compared with a control group, beta-mimetic therapy was **not associated with changes** in LBW, other anthropometric measures, or neonatal morbidity and mortality in two small trials.[16] Beta-mimetics are associated with several complications, and therefore should not be used for this indication.

Calcium channel blockers

There is **not enough evidence** to evaluate the use of calcium channel blockers for impaired fetal growth. Compared with smoking controls, smoking women receiving flunarizine had a higher birth weight in a small trial.[17] No other significant differences were found.

Aspirin

In women with abnormal uterine Doppler (either notch or abnormal pulsatility index [PI]), aspirin does not reduce SGA or LBW compared with placebo.[18–20]

Oxygen

There is **insufficient evidence** to evaluate the benefits and risks of maternal oxygen therapy for suspected impaired fetal growth. Compared with no oxygenation, oxygenation is associated with a lower perinatal mortality rate (33 vs 65%; a 50% reduction) in women with suspected impaired growth and abnormal UA Doppler studies.[21] In all studies, birthweights were higher in the oxygen group, despite similar (average range=10–20 days) intervals to delivery. No significant side effects or adverse outcomes have been reported. Higher GA in the oxygenation groups may have accounted for the difference in mortality rates. Also, two of the studies didn't use placebos, no blinding was made, and finally, the number of patients overall does not allow us to assess the effect.[21]

Volume expansion

There is **insufficient evidence** to assess the effect of increase in maternal fluid intake (either intravenous [IV] or orally) on FGR. In a very small trial, compared with no volume expansion, volume expansion in women with FGR fetuses with absent end-diastolic flow of umbilical artery (AEDF of UA) was associated with a decrease (2/7 vs 6/7) in perinatal mortality.[22]

Abdominal decompression

Abdominal decompression consists of a rigid dome placed about the abdomen and covered with an airtight suit, with the space around the abdomen decompressed to −50 to −100 mmHg for 15–30 seconds out of each minute for 30 minutes once to thrice daily, or with uterine contractions during labor. This is thought to 'pump' blood through the intervillous space. There is **insufficient evidence** to assess the effect of this intervention, as all trials are old, and have the possibility of containing serious bias. Therapeutic abdominal decompression is associated with the following reductions: persistent pre-eclampsia; 'fetal distress' in labor; LBW; Apgar scores < 6 at 1 minute; and perinatal mortality (7 vs 40%).[23]

Antepartum testing and follow-up

See Chapter 51.

Ultrasound

Biometry.   Repeated **biometry** is part of the assessment of the fetal condition, and should be performed **every 2–3 weeks**. Ultrasound biometry at 2-week intervals is associated with higher false-positive rates than at ≥ 3-week intervals.[24]

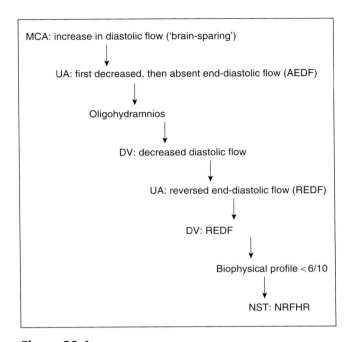

MCA: increase in diastolic flow ('brain-sparing')

↓

UA: first decreased, then absent end-diastolic flow (AEDF)

↓

Oligohydramnios

↓

DV: decreased diastolic flow

↓

UA: reversed end-diastolic flow (REDF)

↓

DV: REDF

↓

Biophysical profile <6/10

↓

NST: NRFHR

Figure 39.1
Progressive pattern of changes in testing parameters associated with FGR. MCA, middle cerebral artery Doppler; UA, umbilical artery Doppler; AEDF, absent end diastolic flow; DV, ductus venosus Doppler; REDF, reverse end diastolic flow; NST, non-stress test; NRFHR, non-reassuring fetal heart rate testing.

Doppler ultrasound

Doppler ultrasound **is the cornerstone of FGR follow-up and management**, since using Doppler ultrasound in management of FGR is associated with a decreased risk of perinatal mortality.[25] Compared with no Doppler ultrasound, **Doppler ultrasound** of the UA in high-risk pregnancy (especially those complicated by hypertension or presumed impaired fetal growth) is associated with a trend to a reduction in perinatal deaths (1.5 vs 2.1%, a 38% decrease).[26] The use of Doppler ultrasound is also associated with **fewer inductions of labor**, and **fewer admissions to hospital**, without reports of adverse effects. No difference is found for NRFHT in labor or cesarean delivery.[26]

Fetal kick counts

There is insufficient evidence (no trials) to assess the effect of fetal kick counts for FGR fetuses.

Non-stress tests (NSTs; cardiotocography)

Compared with no cardiotocography or concealment of information, knowledge of antenatal cardiotocography results appears to have **no significant effect** on perinatal mortality or morbidity in high- or intermediate-risk pregnancies

managed inpatient or outpatient. There is a trend to an increase in perinatal deaths in the cardiotocography group (1.8 vs 0.6%).[27] There is no increase in the incidence of interventions such as induction of labor or cesarean delivery.

Biophysical profile

Compared with other fetal testing (usually NST), biophysical profile (BPP) increases the incidence of induction, but does not affect incidences of cesarean delivery, admission to a neonatal intensive care unit (NICU), or perinatal mortality.[28]

Estriol levels

Compared with concealed levels, knowledge of plasma estriol levels does not affect perinatal mortality (3% in each group) in women with FGR, hypertension, or adverse obstetric history.[29]

Changes in testing parameters

The changes in testing parameters can follow a progressive pattern (Figure 39.1).[30,31] Unfortunately, **very few fetuses follow this progression exactly**. Non-reassuring fetal heart rate (NRFHR) testing and BPP< 6 are usually late changes in the deterioration of the FGR fetus. Late changes such as UA or ductus venosus (DV) reversed end-diastolic flow (REDF) are associated with higher risk of perinatal morbidity and mortality, as is fetal monitoring showing decreased variability. The changes in fetal Doppler ultrasound are usually present earlier than changes in fetal monitoring or BPP,[30] and might be classified as either early, with affection of UA or MCA (affected about 15–16 days prior to delivery), or late, with affection of UA in the form of reversed flow, and abnormal tracings in DV, aortic, and pulmonary outflow tracts (affected about 4–5 days prior to delivery). Whereas perinatal mortality is about 10% with early findings only, this figure may increase to more than 50% if late findings are also present.[30,31]

Interval in fetal testing

In terms of interval of fetal testing, no evidence is available on the optimal interval, although recommendations may change according to fetal condition. Testing should start either on the diagnosis of FGR or at ≥ 28–30 weeks, depending on the clinical scenario. In the presence of normal Doppler findings, testing can be performed once a week with Doppler, as long as the tests remains reassuring. If Doppler findings are abnormal, more frequent testing with twice per week NST and/or BPP might be suggested, depending on the clinical scenario, if the fetus is not delivered.

Delivery

Preparation: steroids for fetal lung maturity

When fetal testing in the FGR fetus suggests need for delivery at 24–34 weeks in the next 2–7 days, steroids for fetal lung maturity (FLM) should be administered. Betamethasone 12 mg intramuscular (IM) q24h × 2 doses is associated with decrease in IVH, NEC, and perinatal mortality (see Chapters 15 and 16 of *Obstetric Evidence Based Guidelines*). Steroids can temporarily affect NST, BPP, and Doppler testing.

Timing

The timing of delivery should be individualized, and **based on GA and all antepartum testing factors**, and in general not just one test. There is only one trial[32,33] so far on timing of delivery of the FGR fetus. For fetuses with growth restriction and compromise at 24–36 weeks, **immediate delivery is associated with similar incidence of perinatal death** (10%) **compared with delayed delivery** (9%): delayed delivery was an average of only 4 days later. Incidence of fetal (0.7 vs 3.1%) and neonatal (7.7 vs 4.1%) deaths,[32] as well as death and disability at 2 years of age (19 vs 16%) are similar in the two groups.[33] Trends for ventilation > 24 hours, IVH, and NEC tended to favor delayed delivery. **Disability in babies younger than < 31 weeks was higher in those delivered immediately** (13%) compared with those in the delayed group (5%).[33] As no specific protocol/Doppler change was followed in either group, specific recommendations cannot be made from this important trial, except that delivering early for hypothetical avoidance of fetal hypoxia might not improve outcome, with the authors recommending that the 'obstetrician should delay'. The following recommendations are based mostly on non-trial evidence.

At any GA
NRFHR consisting of recurrent late decelerations or brady-cardia on monitoring should prompt decision for delivery. Absent/minimal (< 5 beats) variability from 32 weeks on in the presence of FGR should also be an indication for considering delivery. If biophysical profile testing is employed, a BPP < 6 is an indication for delivery.

At about ≥ 35 weeks (term or near term)
FGR with abnormal fetal testing (such as AEDF or REDF in UA, BPP < 6, oligohydramnios with AFI < 5, etc.) may warrant **delivery before** estimated date of confinement (EDC). Some clinicians recommend delivery at 39 weeks of the SGA fetus with otherwise normal testing if dating is accurate (i.e. based on first trimester ultrasound).

At 32–34 weeks
Forty-eight hours after steroids have been given, usually AEDF or REDF in the UA, BPP < 6, and (if known) AEDF or REDF in the DV are indications for delivery. Usually tocolysis should not be used for preterm labor (PTL) or preterm premature rupture of membranes (PPROM) in the presence of FGR, unless fetal heart rate (FHR) tracing is reassuring and 48 hours are needed for steroids for fetal lung maturity at < 34 weeks.

At 24–31 weeks
FHR may not show accelerations or more than minimal variability even in normal fetuses, but delivery is always indicated for recurrent late decelerations or bradycardia on monitoring. It is unclear when in the progression of pathological changes (see Figure 39.1) delivery is best indicated at this GA, since a very preterm delivery could prevent in-utero deterioration but be associated with the morbidity and mortality of extreme prematurity. Whenever possible (in the absence of recurrent late decelerations or bradycardia), delivery should be postponed after 48 hours of steroids for FLM.

At < 24 weeks
FGR is associated with poor outcome, and counseling regarding termination can be offered. Transfer to a tertiary care center is recommended if pregnancy is continued.

Mode

There is insufficient evidence to assess the mode of delivery associated with the best outcomes for the FGR fetus, since there are no trials. The decision for either induction of labor or elective cesarean section should account for numerous variables such as fetal hemodynamic status, monitoring, cervical ripening, and parent desires. A TOL for the vertex FGR fetus can only be attempted if fetal monitoring is reassuring.

Neonatology management

FGR neonates frequently require assistance with ventilation and feeding, especially if born preterm. FGR neonates < 32 weeks or < 1500 g require special care, usually in a tertiary care center. Work-up should be completed if not already done prenatally. Hypoglycemia, polycythemia, and coagulopathies are common, and may need treatment. Etiology of FGR dictates management. Long-term, there is yet not sufficient evidence to assess the effect of growth hormone therapy on postnatal growth of SGA babies, probably also because of the heterogeneous nature of the causes of SGA.[34]

FUTURE PREGNANCY PRECONCEPTION COUNSELING

A prior SGA infant is associated with higher risk (20%) of recurrent SGA infant, as well as (especially if preterm FGR) with higher risk of fetal death.[35]

REFERENCES

1. Craigo SD, Beach ML, Harvey-Wilkes KB, D'Alton ME. Ultrasound predictors of neonatal outcome in intrauterine growth restriction. Am J Perinatol 1996; 13: 465–71. [II-3]

2. Dashe JS, McIntire DD, Lucas MJ, Leveno KJ. Effects of symmetric and asymmetric fetal growth on pregnancy outcomes. Obstet Gynecol 2000; 96(3): 321–7. [II-2]

3. Hack M, Taylor HG, Drotar D, et al. Chronic conditions, functional limitations, and special needs of school-aged children born with extremely low birth weight in the 1990s. JAMA 2005; 294(3): 318–25. [II-2]

4. Gembruch U, Gortner L. Perinatal aspects of preterm intrauterine growth restriction. Ultrasound Obstet Gynecol 1998; 11: 233–9. [II-3]

5. Mittendorfer-Rutz E, Rasmusen F, Wassertman D. Restricted fetal growth and adverse maternal and psychosocial and socioeconomic conditions as risk factor for suicidal behavior of offspring: a cohort study. Lancet 2004: 364: 1135–40. [II-2]

6. Aickin DR, Duff GB, Evans JJ, et al. Antenatal biochemical screening to predict low birth weight infants. Br J Obstet Gynaecol 1983; 90: 129–33. [II-3]

7. Knight M, Duley L, Henderson-Smart DJ, King JF. Antiplatelet agents for preventing and treating pre-eclampsia. Cochrane Database Syst Rev 2005; 4. [meta-analysis: 25 RCTs, $n=>20\,000$]

8. Beazley JM, Underhill RA. Fallacy of the fundal height. BMJ 1970; 4: 404–6. [II-3]

9. Lindhard A, Nielsen PV, Mouritsen LA, et al. The implications of introducing the symphyseal-fundal height-measurement. A prospective randomized controlled trial. Br J Obstet Gynaecol 1990; 97: 675–80. [RCT, $n=1639$]

10. Smith GC, Smith MF, McNay MB, Fleming JE. First-trimester growth and the risk of low birth weight. N Engl J Med 1998; 339: 1817–22. [II-2]

11. Gardosi J, Chang A, Kalyan B, Sahota D, Symonds EM. Customised antenatal growth charts. Lancet 1992; 339(8788): 283–7. [II-2] www.gestation.net/main.htm.

12. Dugoff L, Lynch AM, Cioffi-Ragan D, et al. First trimester uterine artery Doppler abnormalities predict subsequent intrauterine growth restriction. Am J Obstet Gynecol 2005; 193(3 Pt 2): 1208–12. [II-2]

13. Vainio M, Jujansuu E, Koivisto AM, Maenpaa J. Bilateral notching of uterine arteries at 12–14 weeks of gestation for prediction of hypertensive disorders of pregnancy. Acta Obstet Gynecol Scand 2005; 84(11): 1062–7. [II-2]

14. Laurin J, Persson PH. The effect of bedrest in hospital on fetal outcome in pregnancies complicated by intra-uterine growth retardation. Acta Obstet Gynecol Scand 1987; 66: 407–11. [RCT, $n=107$. Allocation of treatment was by odd or even birth date]

15. Say L, Gulmezoglu AM, Hofmeyr GJ. Maternal nutrient supplementation for suspected impaired fetal growth. Cochrane Database Syst Rev 2005; 4. [meta-analysis: 3 RCTs, $n=121$]

16. Say L, Gulmezoglu AM, Hofmeyr GJ. Betamimetics for suspected impaired fetal growth. Cochrane Database Syst Rev 2005; 4. [meta-analysis: 2 RCTs, $n=118$]

17. Janssens D. Prevention of low birth weight by flunarizine given to smoking mothers. Arch Gynecol 1985; 237(Suppl 1): 397. [RCT, $n=100$]

18. Yu CK, Papageorghiou AT, Parra M, Palma Dias R, Nicolaides KH. Randomized controlled trial using low-dose aspirin in the prevention of pre-eclampsia in women with abnormal uterine artery Doppler at 23 weeks' gestation. Ultrasound Obstet Gynecol 2003; 22(3): 233–9. [RCT, $n=560$; plus meta-analysis of 5 prior studies]

19. Subtil D, Goeusse P, Houfflin-Debarge V, et al. Randomised comparison of uterine artery Doppler and aspirin (100 mg) with placebo in nulliparous women: the Essai Regional Aspirine Mere-Enfant study (Part 2). BJOG 2003; 110(5): 485–91. [RCT, $n=239$ vs 617]

20. Vainio M, Kujansuu E, Iso-Mustajarvi M, Maenpaa J. Low dose acetyl-salicylic acid in prevention of pregnancy-induced hypertension and intrauterine growth retardation in women with bilateral uterine artery notches. BJOG 2002; 109(2): 161–7. [RCT, $n=90$]

21. Say L, Gulmezoglu AM, Hofmeyr GJ. Maternal oxygen administration for suspected impaired fetal growth. Cochrane Database Syst Rev 2005; 4. [meta-analysis: 3 RCTs, $n=94$]

22. Karsdorp VH, van Vugt JM, Dekker GA, van Geijn HP. Reappearance of end-diastolic velocities in the umbilical artery following maternal volume expansion: a preliminary study. Obstet Gynecol 1992; 80: 679–83. [RCT, $n=14$]

23. Hofmeyr GJ. Abdominal decompression for suspected fetal compromise/preeclampsia. Cochrane Database Syst Rev 2005; 4. [meta-analysis: 3 RCTs, $n=367$]

24. Mongelli M, Sverker E, Tambyrajia R. Screening for fetal growth restriction: a mathematical model of the effect of time interval and ultrasound error. Obstet Gynecol 1998; 92: 908–12. [III]

25. Alfirevic Z, Neilson JP. Doppler ultrasonography in high risk pregnancies: systematic review with meta-analysis. Am J Obstet Gynecol 1995; 172: 1379–87. [meta-analysis]

26. Neilson JP, Alfirevic Z. Doppler ultrasound for fetal assessment in high risk pregnancies. Cochrane Database Syst Rev 2005; 4. [meta-analysis: 11 RCTs, $n=$ about 7000]

27. Pattison N, McCowan L. Cardiotocography for antepartum fetal assessment. Cochrane Database Syst Rev 2005; 4. [meta-analysis: 4 RCTs, $n=1588$]

28. Alfirevic Z, Neilson JP. Biophysical profile for fetal assessment in high risk pregnancies. Cochrane Database Syst Rev 2005; 4. [meta-analysis: 4 RCTs, $n=2828$]

29. Duenhoelter JH, Whalley PJ, MacDonald PC. An analysis of the utility of plasma immunoreactive estrogen measurements in determining delivery time of gravidas with a fetus considered at high risk. Am J Obstet Gynecol 1976; 125: 889–98. [RCT, $n=622$ women with high-risk pregnancies, including fetal growth restriction, hypertension, adverse obstetric history. RCT by hospital no. to plasma estriol level either revealed or concealed]

30. Baschat AA, Gembruch U, Harman CR. The sequence of changes in Doppler and biophysical parameters as severe fetal growth restriction worsens. Ultrasound Obstet Gynecol 2001; 18: 571–7. [II-2]

31. Ferrazzi E, Bozzo M, Rigano S, et al. Temporal sequence of abnormal Doppler changes in the peripheral and central circulatory systems of the severely growth-restricted fetus. Ultrasound Obstet Gynecol 2002; 19: 140–6. [II-2, $n=26$]

32. GRIT Study Group. A randomized trial of timed delivery for the compromised preterm fetus: short term outcomes and Bayesian interpretation. BJOG 2003; 110: 27–32. [RCT, $n=588$]

33. GRIT Study Group. Infant well being at 2 years of age in the Growth Restriction Intervention Trial (GRIT): multicentered randomized controlled trial. Lancet 2004; 364: 513–20. [RCT follow-up, $n=588$]

34. Donaldson M. What is the role of growth-hormone therapy in short children who were small for gestational age? Lancet 2001; 358: 347–8. [review]

35. Surkan PJ, Stephansson O, Dickman PW, Cnattingius S. Previous preterm and small-for-gestational-age births and the subsequent risk of stillbirths. N Engl J Med 2004; 350: 777–85. [II-2]

40

Fetal macrosomia

Suneet P Chauhan and Everett F Magann

KEY POINTS

- Although **clinical and sonographic estimated fetal weight** can identify newborns with weights > 4000 g, both methods **are poor at detecting neonates that will weigh ≥ 4500 g.**
- **Prevention of macrosomia** is obtained with **diet and glucose monitoring with insulin** if needed compared with no treatment or diet only in gestational diabetes, **postprandial** vs preprandial **blood sugar (glucose) monitoring in gestational diabetics requiring insulin therapy**, and strict conventional **management of gestational diabetics (fasting blood sugar < 90 mg/dl and 2-hour postprandial blood sugar < 120 mg/dl).**
- Among uncomplicated pregnancies, **induction for suspected macrosomia is not indicated.**
- There is insufficient evidence to recommend best management of suspected macrosomia among pregnancies complicated by diabetes mellitus, prior cesarean delivery, or shoulder dystocia, because of the lack of randomized trials and the inaccuracy of predicting birth weight.

DEFINITION

A fetus with **estimated fetal weight** (EFW) ≥ **4000 g** can be presumed to be macrosomic. Macrosomic newborns can be classified as grades I (birth weight 4000–4499 g), II (4500–4999 g), and III (≥ 5000 g).[1] This classification is clinically relevant, for the grades are associated with different types of complications.

EPIDEMIOLOGY/INCIDENCE

The prevalence of macrosomia has decreased significantly in the USA,[2] although it is increasing in other countries such as Denmark.[3] The rate of neonates weighing ≥ 4000 g was 10.2% in 1996 and 9.2% in 2002, a decrease of 10% in 7 years. For newborns weighing ≥ 5000 g, the decrease in the prevalence has been 19% (from 0.16% in 1996 to 0.13% in 2002).[2] In Denmark,[3] the rate of grade I macrosomia has increased from 17% in 1990 to 20% in 1999. The rate of macrosomia in other countries has ranged from 1% in Thailand[4] to 5% in Antigua and Barbuda[5] and 20% in the Republic of Croatia.[6]

RISK FACTORS

Hispanic women, maternal obesity, maternal birth weight > 8 lbs (3629 g), grand multiparity (≥ 5 deliveries), prior macrosomic fetus, abnormal 50 g glucose screen but normal 3-hour glucose test, diabetes (pregestational or gestational), gestational age ≥ 40 weeks, and excessive weight gain during pregnancy are well-known risk factors.[7] Intrapartum hydramnios[8] and second stage of labor > 120 minutes[9] are other risk factors for macrosomia. The majority of newborns with birth weights ≥ 4500 g do not have any known risk factors.[7]

COMPLICATIONS

The *maternal* complications with macrosomic fetuses include prolonged labor, operative vaginal delivery, cesarean delivery, postpartum hemorrhage, and vaginal lacerations.[7]

Compared with newborns with birth weights of 3000–3999 g, *neonatal* complications for grade I macrosomia include breech presentation, induction, meconium staining, dysfunctional/prolonged labor, cephalopelvic disproportion, and cesarean delivery. For grade II macrosomia, the complications are also Apgar scores ≤ 3 at 5 minutes, assisted ventilation > 30 minutes, birth injuries, meconium aspiration, and hyaline membrane disease. For grade III macrosomia, there is also a significantly higher likelihood of neonatal and infant mortality.[1]

MANAGEMENT
Prevention

A significant decrease in the rate of macrosomia is obtained with:

- **Diet and glucose monitoring with insulin** if needed compared with no treatment or diet only in gestational diabetes.[10]
- **Postprandial** vs preprandial **blood glucose monitoring in gestational diabetics requiring insulin therapy.**[11]
- **Conventional management of gestational diabetics (fasting blood sugar < 90 mg/dl and 2-hour postprandial blood sugar < 120 mg/dl)** vs modified blood sugar goal based on whether the abdominal circumference is < vs > 75% for gestational age (if abdominal circumference ≥ 75%, the fasting blood sugar should be < 80 mg/dl and 2-hour postprandial < 100 mg/dl).[12]

The rate of macrosomia was **not** significantly decreased with:

- Among pregestational and gestational diabetes, administering insulin twice daily vs four times daily.[13]
- Use of glyburide compared to insulin in the management of gestational diabetics not controlled adequately on diet.[14]
- Induction of labor vs expectant management for pregnancy at > 41 weeks.[15]

Screening

During labor, the detection of neonates weighing at least 4000 g is similar with clinical or sonographic EFWs, although the likelihood ratio with clinicians' estimate was 15, while with measurements of biometric parameters it was 42.[16]

Neither clinical nor sonographic EFW can accurately identify neonates that weigh ≥ 4500 g.[2,17,18]

Management of suspected macrosomia

Whenever macrosomia is suspected, the pregnancy should be classified into one of the following groups: (1) uncomplicated; (2) pregestational or gestational diabetes; (3) prior cesarean delivery; or (4) history of shoulder dystocia.

Uncomplicated

Induction of labor for suspected fetal macrosomia in non-diabetic women has not been shown to alter the risk of maternal or neonatal morbidity, but the power of the included studies to show a difference in rare neonatal morbidity is limited. Compared with expectant management, **induction of labor** at around 40 weeks for suspected macrosomia (EFW > 4000 g) **has not been shown to reduce the risk of cesarean or instrumental delivery.**[19] Perinatal morbidity, including shoulder dystocia, is similar between the groups. Labor induction for suspected macrosomia results in an increased rate of cesarean delivery without

an improved outcome.[20] Thus, there is no indication for induction for suspected macrosomia among uncomplicated pregnancies.

While the ACOG practice bulletin on fetal macrosomia[7] suggests that elective cesarean delivery should be considered if the EFW is at least 5000 g, there is insufficient evidence to assess this intervention, and there are no reports on the peripartum outcomes when the fetus is suspected of having grade III macrosomia.[2]

Diabetes

In insulin-requiring diabetic pregnancies, **induction at 38 weeks,** compared with expectant management until 42 weeks, is associated with a significant decrease in the rate of macrosomic fetuses, but the limited sample size does not permit drawing 'firm conclusions.'[21]

A retrospective study concluded that a protocol involving induction for EFW ≥ 90% but < 4250 g and cesarean delivery for sonographic weight ≥ 4250 g decreases the rate of shoulder dystocia by 50% but increases the rate of cesarean delivery by 16%.[22] While the American College of Obstetricians and Gynecologists (ACOG) practice bulletin on fetal macrosomia[7] suggests that cesarean delivery among diabetics is indicated if the EFW is ≥ 4500 g, other clinicians have set the threshold at ≥ 4000 g[17,18] or at ≥ 4250 g (see Chapter 4).[22]

Prior cesarean delivery

The majority of patients attempting vaginal birth after cesarean delivery (VBAC) can successfully deliver a macrosomic fetus.[23–25] The rate of uterine rupture may be higher (3.6%) for a macrosomic trial of labor with prior cesarean delivery, if the patient has not delivered vaginally before.[26] Thus, obstetric factors (prior deliveries, need for induction, etc.) should be considered when attempting VBAC with suspected macrosomia. (see Chapter 13 in *Obstetric Evidence Based Guidelines*.)

Prior shoulder dystocia

Women with prior shoulder dystocia are at much higher risks of recurrence (about 15%) and of injury to the newborn.[27,28] (see Chapter 21 of *Obstetric Evidence Based Guidelines*). There are no randomized trials[2] on how to manage these pregnancies, but it is reasonable to offer cesarean delivery at term when managing a patient with a prior shoulder dystocia and now suspected fetal macrosomia, considering the vagaries of EFW.

REFERENCES

1. Boulet SL, Alexander GR, Salihu H, Pass MA. Macrosomic birth in the United States: determinants, outcomes, and proposed grades of risk. Am J Obstet Gynecol 2003; 188: 1372–8. [II-1]

2. Chauhan SP, Grobman WA, Gherman RA, et al. Suspicion and treatment of the macrosomic fetus: a review. Am J Obstet Gynecol 2005; 193: 332–46. [III]

3. Orskou J, Henriksen TB, Kesmodel U, Secher NJ. Maternal characteristics and lifestyle factors and the risk of delivering high birth weight infants. Obstet Gynecol 2003; 102: 115–20. [II-3]

4. Serirat S, Deerochanawong C, Sunthornthepvarakul T, Jinayon P. Gestational diabetes mellitus. J Med Assoc Thai 1992; 75: 315–19. [II-3]

5. Martin TC, Clarke A. A case control study of the prevalence of perinatal complications associated with fetal macrosomia in Antigua and Barbuda. West Indian Med J 2003; 52: 231–4. [II-3]

6. Mikulandra F, Stojnic E, Perisa M, et al. Fetal macrosomia – pregnancy and delivery. Zentralbl Gynakol 1993; 115: 553–61. [II-3]

7. American College of Obstetricians and Gynecologists. Fetal macrosomia. ACOG Practice Bulletin No. 22. Washington, DC: ACOG; 2000. [III]

8. Chauhan SP, Martin RW, Morrison JC. Intrapartum hydramnios at term and perinatal outcome. J Perinatol 1993; 13: 186–9. [II-2]

9. Myles TD, Santolaya J. Maternal and neonatal outcomes in patients with a prolonged second stage of labor. Obstet Gynecol 2003; 102: 52–8. [II-2]

10. Crowther CA, Hiller JE, Moss JR, et al. Effect of treatment of gestational diabetes mellitus on pregnancy outcomes. N Engl J Med 2005; 352: 2477–86. [RCT, $n=1000$. Impaired glucose tolerance (defined following 75 g OGTT as fasting < 7.0 mmol/L, 2 hours between 7.8 mmol/L and 11.0 mmol/L). Diet, glucose monitoring, and insulin as needed vs routine care]

11. de Veciana M, Major CA, Morgan MA, et al. Postprandial versus preprandial blood glucose monitoring in women with gestational diabetes mellitus requiring insulin therapy. N Engl J Med 1995; 333: 1237–41. [RCT, $n=66$]

12. Bonomo M, Cetin I, Pisoni MP, et al. Flexible treatment of gestational diabetes modulated on ultrasound evaluation of intrauterine growth: a controlled randomized clinical trial. Diabetes Metab 2004; 30: 237–44. [RCT, $n=229$]

13. Nachum Z, Ben-Shlomo I, Weiner E, Shalev E. Twice daily versus four times daily insulin dose regimens for diabetes in pregnancy: randomised controlled trial. BMJ 1999; 319: 1223–7. [RCT, $n=392$]

14. Langer O, Conway DL, Berkus MD, Xenakis EM, Gonzales O. A comparison of glyburide and insulin in women with gestational diabetes mellitus. N Engl J Med 2000; 343: 1134–8. [RCT, $n=404$]

15. A clinical trial of induction of labor versus expectant management in postterm pregnancy. The National Institute of Child Health and Human Development Network of Maternal-Fetal Medicine Units. Am J Obstet Gynecol 1994; 170: 716–23. [RCT, $n=440$]

16. Hendrix NW, Grady CS, Chauhan SP. Clinical vs sonographic estimate of birth weight in term parturients: a randomized clinical trial. J Reprod Med 2000; 45: 317–22. [RCT, $n=758$]

17. Gonen R, Spiegel D, Abend M. Is macrosomia predictable, and are shoulder dystocia and birth trauma preventable? Obstet Gynecol 1996; 88: 526–9. [II-1]

18. Gonen R, Bader D, Ajami M. Effects of a policy of elective cesarean delivery in cases of suspected fetal macrosomia on the incidence of brachial plexus injury and the rate of cesarean delivery. Am J Obstet Gynecol 2000; 183: 1296–300. [II-1]

19. Irion O, Boulvain M. Induction of labour for suspected fetal macrosomia. Cochrane Database Syst Rev 2007; 1. [meta-analysis: 2 RCTs, $n=313$]

20. Sanchez-Ramos L, Bernstein S, Kaunitz AM. Expectant management versus labor induction for suspected fetal macrosomia: a systematic review. Obstet Gynecol 2002; 100: 997–1002. [meta-analysis: 11 studies, of which 2 RCTs; $n=3751$]

21. Boulvain M, Stan C, Irion O. Elective delivery in diabetic pregnant women. Cochrane Database Syst Rev 2007; 1. [meta-analysis: 1 RCT, $n=200$]

22. Conway DL, Langer O. Elective delivery of infants with macrosomia in diabetic women: reduced shoulder dystocia versus increased cesarean deliveries. Am J Obstet Gynecol 1998; 178: 922–5. [II-1]

23. Phelan JP, Eglinton GS, Horenstein JM, Clark SL, Yeh S. Previous cesarean birth. Trial of labor in women with macrosomic infants. J Reprod Med 1984; 29: 36–40. [II-1]

24. Flamm BL, Goings JR. Vaginal birth after cesarean section: is suspected fetal macrosomia a contraindication? Obstet Gynecol 1989; 74: 694–7. [II-1]

25. Zelop CM, Shipp TD, Repke JT, Cohen A, Lieberman E. Outcomes of trial of labor following previous cesarean delivery among women with fetuses weighing > 4000 g. Am J Obstet Gynecol 2001; 185: 903–5. [II-1]

26. Elkousy MA, Sammel M, Stevens E, Peipert JF, Macones G. The effect of birth weight on vaginal birth after cesarean delivery success rates. Am J Obstet Gynecol 2003; 188: 824–30. [II-1]

27. Lewis DF, Raymond RC, Perkins MB, Brooks GG, Heymann AR. Recurrence rate of shoulder dystocia. Am J Obstet Gynecol 1995; 172: 1369–71. [II-2]

28. Ginsberg NA, Moisidis C. How to predict recurrent shoulder dystocia. Am J Obstet Gynecol 2001; 184: 1427–30. [II-2]

41
CMV

Marianne Vendola

KEY POINTS

- Cytomegalovirus (CMV) is the most common cause of viral intrauterine infection, affecting **0.5–2.5% of all neonates.**
- In most cases, pregnant women acquire CMV by **exposure to children** in their home or from occupational exposure to children.
- Approximately **2% of immunoglobulin G (IgG)-negative women acquire CMV infection during pregnancy.** Approximately **40%** (range 30–60%) **of pregnant women with a primary infection transmit CMV infection to their fetus.** The rate of transmission increases with increase in gestational age (highest in third trimester), but the severity of disease is instead inversely proportional to gestational age (the infant is most affected when maternal infection is in the first trimester). Overall, about **15–20% of infected infants develop sequelae** (so about 5–8% of infants of infected mothers have sequelae).
- Complications of affected infants with congenital CMV infection include jaundice, petechiae ('blueberry muffin baby'), thrombocytopenia, hepatosplenomegaly, growth restriction, microcephaly, intracranial calcifications, non-immune hydrops, and preterm birth, as well as late complications such as hearing loss, mental retardation, delay in psychomotor development, chorioretinitis, optic atrophy, seizures, expressive language delays, and learning disabilities. Long-term mortality is about 10–30%.
- Prevention **(including avoiding intimate contact with children, frequent handwashing, and glove use) is associated with an 84% decrease in CMV seroconversion during pregnancy.**
- CMV screening in pregnancy is not routinely recommended in most countries, until an appropriate fetal intervention is proven to decrease neonatal disease in cases of maternal CMV infection.
- Maternal diagnosis of CMV infection is by serum **IgM+.**

- Fetal diagnosis of CMV infection is by detection of virus in amniotic fluid by polymerase chain reaction (PCR) testing.
- There are no trials to assess the effectiveness of any intervention aimed at preventing congenital CMV. Ganciclovir and CMV-specific hyperimmune globulin are not supported by sufficient evidence for recommendation, but are the most promising interventions reported so far.

PATHOGEN

Cytomegalovirus (CMV) is a double-stranded DNA virus of the herpes family.[1]

INCIDENCE/EPIDEMIOLOGY

CMV is the most common cause of viral intrauterine infection, affecting **0.5–2.5% of all neonates** in different parts of the world.[2] The prevalence of CMV infection varies according to socioeconomic background. In the USA, the seropositivity rate is 50–60% for women of middle and 70–80% for women of lower socioeconomic background.

RISK FACTORS/ASSOCIATIONS

Risk factors are low socioeconomic status; exposure to infective individuals; multiple partners; extremes of age; multiparity; and blood transfusion. Only cellular blood products which contain leukocytes are capable of transmitting CMV, and the risk factor is 0.1–0.4%/unit in immunocompetent recipients.[3] The incidence of cases with congenital disease following maternal recurrent infection has been shown to be increased with immunodeficiency, hormonal exposure, nutritional deficiency, and genital tract infections.[4] Although sexual transmission of CMV can occur, **in most cases pregnant women acquire CMV by exposure to**

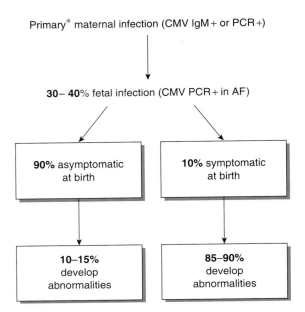

Figure 41.1
Natural history of CMV perinatal infection. *The prognosis is better for mothers with recurrent disease, with the fetus having a low risk of infection and a low risk of developing sequelae. In fact, vertical transmission after recurrent infection is 0.5–2%. CMV, cytomegalovirus; IgM, immunoglobulin M; PCR, polymerase chain reaction; AF, amniotic fluid.

children in their home or from occupational exposure to children.

SYMPTOMS

CMV is usually asymptomatic or with symptoms mild enough that it goes undiagnosed. The symptoms might include a mononucleosis-like or flu-like syndrome, malaise, fatigue, lymphadenopathy, or persistent fever, and abnormal laboratory values (lymphocytosis, or increased aminotransferase levels). There is no jaundice or hepatosplenomegaly. The presence of symptoms or laboratory abnormalities is highly suggestive of primary infection.[5]

PATHOPHYSIOLOGY/ CLASSIFICATION

General

The CMV virus leads to infected large cells with intranuclear inclusions. It has a 4–8-week period of incubation, and 3–12-month-long viremia (infants can shed virus for up to 6 years). Serious disease occurs only in immunocompromised adults, or fetuses. The transmission of the virus to the

fetus can follow either a primary or recurrent infection. Approximately 2% of immunoglobulin G (IgG)-negative women acquire CMV infection during pregnancy. Approximately 40% (range 30–60%) of pregnant women with a primary infection transmit CMV infection to their fetus (Figure 41.1.) Even periconceptional infection a week before or up to 5 weeks after last menstrual period (LMP) is associated with this rate of transmission. **The rate of transmission increases with increase in gestational age (highest in third trimester), but the severity of disease is instead inversely proportional to gestational age (infant most affected when maternal infection in first trimester).** The risk of congenital CMV disease at birth is mainly associated with maternal primary infection, but the presence of maternal antibodies before conception does not prevent transmission in all cases, even if it is protective in most cases.

Primary infection (see Figure 41.1)

Fetal infection generally (99.5%) occurs following maternal primary infection, and rarely following recurrent CMV infection. Of the women who are not immune (IgG–, IgM–) for CMV at the beginning of pregnancy, about 2% acquire maternal infection. Transplacental transmission may occur weeks or months after primary maternal CMV infection, and can be isolated from the amniotic fluid (AF) by a polymerase chain reaction (PCR) DNA technique to positively identify intrauterine transmission of CMV. **Overall, about 15–20% of infected infants develop sequelae (so about 5–8% of infants of infected mothers have sequelae).**

Recurrent infection

Recurrent infections can occur with immunosuppression and during pregnancy. Recurrent infections during pregnancy are most often asymptomatic and primarily caused by the reactivation of the endogenous virus, but can also be caused by a low-grade chronic infection or reinfection by a different strain of CMV.[6] The risk of vertical transmission with recurrent infection is about 0.5–2%. Recurrent infection is responsible for only 0.5% of CMV congenital infections. Neonates infected from recurrent maternal infection have no symptoms at birth, do not have CMV in urine, and have a < 8% risk of sequelae (hearing loss and chorioretinitis).

CLINICAL NEONATAL FINDINGS/COMPLICATIONS

Clinical findings of symptomatic congenital CMV infection include jaundice, petechiae ('blueberry muffin baby'), thrombocytopenia, hepatosplenomegaly, growth restriction, microcephaly, intracranial calcifications, non-immune hydrops, and preterm birth.[1] CMV diseases have late

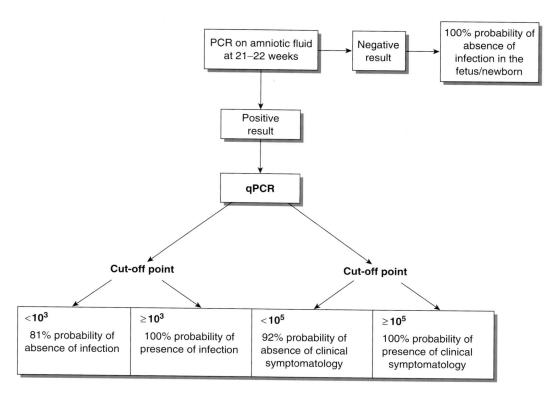

Figure 41.2
Assessment of chance of fetal infection and long-term complications by quantitative polymerase chain reaction (qPCR) in amniotic fluid (AF).[8]

complications such as hearing loss, mental retardation, delay in psychomotor development, chorioretinitis, optic atrophy, seizures, expressive language delays, and learning disabilities.[2] CMV is the most common cause of congenital sensorineural hearing loss.[7] Long-term mortality is about 10–30%.

PREGNANCY MANAGEMENT

Counseling/prognosis

Counseling should include at least the natural history of the disease, the chances of vertical transmission, prognosis, and complications (see Figure 41.1). A quantitative polymerase chain reaction (PCR) count of $\geq 10^3$ genome equivalents per ml of amniotic fluid (AF) is a certain sign of congenital infection, and $\geq 10^5$ genome equivalents per ml can predict symptomatic infection[8] (Figure 41.2). In cases of severely injured fetus on ultrasound, there is a high likelihood of sequelae, and pregnancy termination can be offered as a management option.[9] When no ultrasonographic abnormalities are detected, the incidence of postnatal neurological abnormalities is about 15–20%.[8,10]

Prevention

Hygiene

Compared with no prevention, **prevention (including avoiding intimate contact with children, frequent handwashing, and glove use) is associated with an 84% decrease in CMV seroconversion during pregnancy,** especially in women in contact with children in day care facilities.[11]

Vaccines

A live-attenuated CMV vaccine is available, but may be reactivated, and safety issues have not been resolved. A glycoprotein B construct vaccine is in the late phases of testing.

Screening

Serum

CMV screening in pregnancy is not routinely recommended in most countries, even in women who are seronegative.[4] *If an appropriate fetal intervention is proven to decrease neonatal disease in case of CMV,* screening with IgM and IgG levels should be performed to all pregnant women between 8 and 12 weeks. IgM is 75% sensitive, and persists for 4–8 months. Seronegative women should be provided with basic information on how to avoid infection. A second and possibly a third antibody control at 18–20 weeks and at 30–32 weeks should be recommended. IgG-positive and IgM-negative women with high IgG avidity index could be assured of no risk of primary infection, which causes the majority of sequelae in the fetus. No further controls would be necessary.[2]

Ultrasound fetal findings

These findings are growth restriction, ventriculomegaly, oligohydramnios, echogenic bowel, choroid plexus cyst (unilateral), pleural effusion, brain and liver calcification, and hydrops fetalis.[8] Microcephaly, hydrocephaly, and intracranial calcifications are signs of high risk for neonatal sequelae.[2] The limitations of ultrasound are well known. Fetal abnormalities may become evident late, change, or disappear during pregnancy, and not all symptoms of congenital inclusion disease are detectable by ultrasound, which has just a 5% sensitivity for detecting congenital CMV.

Investigations/diagnosis/work-up

Maternal primary CMV infection is diagnosed by IgM + serum, which persists for 4–8 months. Although seroconversion is a reliable method for diagnosing primary CMV infection, the diagnosis can be problematic. The rise in CMV-specific antibodies may be delayed for up to 4 weeks, and the presence of CMV-specific IgM can be found in up to 10% of women with recurrent disease. Although CMV can be transmitted to the fetus both by primary and secondary (recurrent) infection, invasive prenatal diagnosis should be offered to women with primary infection, as they are at higher risk for fetus infection. In recurrent infection, the presence of maternal CMV IgG offers good protection, and fetal infection occurs only in 0.5–1% of cases.[12]

At present, **detection of virus in AF by PCR testing is the most accurate means of diagnosis for CMV infection in the fetus,** with sensitivities ranging from 80% to 100%.[10] Amniocentesis provides a direct method of diagnosing intrauterine CMV infection because the infected fetus excretes the virus via urine into AF. The sensitivity of detecting a true infection by sampling the AF increases after 21 weeks' gestation and after a minimum 6 weeks interval following maternal primary infection, so that if an amniocentesis is performed before this interval, it should be repeated later.[4,10]

CMV DNA detected in AF reveals a history of viremia but it does not directly demonstrate the current fetal condition.[7] Quantitative PCR in amniotic fluid can help predict infection and later sequelae (see Figure 41.2). Infected fetuses may also have abnormal ultrasound findings. Normal fetal ultrasound does not rule out severe neurological damage. Percutaneous umbilical blood sampling (PUBS) should be avoided, and has been used in the past to diagnose the fetus with a high suspicion for CMV and negative PCR. The use of viral culture has decreased, also because it takes 2–6 weeks to obtain final results.

Neonatal diagnosis is based on detection of PCR in body fluids, in particular in the urine.

Therapy

There has been no randomized trial on intervention to prevent maternal and/or fetal CMV infection in pregnancy.

CMV-specific hyperimmune globulin

There is insufficient evidence to recommend CMV-specific hyperimmune globulin for prevention or treatment of CMV congenital infection. In a non-randomized study, CMV hyperimmune globulin IV 100 U/kg every month until delivery to the mother for prevention of vertical transmission in primary maternal CMV infection was associated with a decrease in the incidence of infected neonates from 40% in controls to 16%.[13] Maternal CMV hyperimmune globulin 200 U/kg IV to the mother (with additional AF or umbilical cord infusions for persistent ultrasound findings) for therapy of known CMV DNA + fetuses was associated with a decrease in the incidence of symptomatic CMV disease at birth from 50% in controls to 3%.[13] It is unclear how this in-utero therapy would 'cure' abnormal ultrasound findings already present in these fetuses. Almost all these women were infected in the first or second trimester, so efficacy in the third trimester is unknown. Hyperimmune globulin appeared less effective for the prevention of fetal infection than for the treatment of fetuses already infected. An explanation to this outcome is that the mechanism of action of hyperimmune globulin differs in the prevention and in the therapy group. For the prevention of fetal infection, it presumably reduces maternal systemic or placental viral loads. Once the fetus is infected, hyperimmune globulin reduces placental or fetal inflammation, or both, resulting in increased fetal blood flow with enhanced fetal nutrition and oxygenation. Treatment with hyperimmune globulin acts by decreasing the number and percentage of both NK (natural killer) cells and HLA (human leukocyte antigen)-DR + cells.[13] Interestingly, this therapy is not effective in prevention of vertical transmission of HIV.

Ganciclovir

Ganciclovir inhibits viral DNA polymerase, and has been used successfully in adults, especially immunocompromised (AIDS, transplant, etc.) patients. A trial demonstrated reduction of hearing loss in neonates with proven congenital CMV infection with CNS involvement when treatment was begun within 1 month of birth.[14] There are no trials evaluating fetal therapy with ganciclovir. Ganciclovir administration into the umbilical vein and anti-CMV IgG injections into the fetal abdominal cavity have been reported in case reports,[7] but the evaluation of the prognosis is not well established.

REFERENCES

1. American College of Obstetricians and Gynecologists. Perinatal viral and parasitic infections. Clinical Management Guidelines for Obstetrician-Gynecologists. ACOG Practice Bulletin. No 20, September 2000. [review]
2. Azam AZ, Vial Y, Fawer CL, Zufferey J, Hohlfeld P. Prenatal diagnosis of congenital CMV infection. Obstet Gynecol 2001; 97: 443–8. [II-2]
3. Triulzi DJ. Transfusion transmitted cytomegalovirus. www.itxm.org/archive/tmu8-94.htm. [II-3; web document]
4. Henrich W, Meckies J, Dudenhausen JW, Vogel M, Enders G. Recurrent CMV infection during pregnancy: ultrasonographic diagnosis and fetal outcome. Ultrasound Obstet Gynecol 2002; 19: 608–11. [II-3]
5. Nigro G, Anceschi MM, Cosmi EV. Clinical manifestations and abnormal laboratory findings in pregnant women with primary cytomegalovirus infection. BJOG 2003; 110: 572–7. [II-3]
6. Boppana SB, Rivera LB, Fowler KB, Mach M, Britt WJ. Intrauterine transmission of cytomegalovirus to infants of women with preconceptional immunity. N Engl J Med 2001; 344: 1366–71. [II-3]
7. Matsuda H, Kawakami Y, Furaya K, Kikuchi Y. Intrauterine therapy for a cytomegalovirus-infected symptomatic fetus. BJOG 2004; 111: 756–7. [II-3]
8. Lipitz S, Achiron R, Zalel Y, et al. Outcome of pregnancies with vertical transmission of primary cytomegalovirus infection. Obstet Gynecol 2002; 100: 428–33. [II-3]
9. Liesnard C, Donner C, Brancart F, et al. Prenatal diagnosis of congenital cytomegalovirus infection: prospective study of 237 pregnancies at risk. Obstet Gynecol 2000; 95: 881–8. [II-2]
10. Oshiro BT. CMV infection in pregnancy. Contemp Obstet Gynecol 1999; 11: 16–24. [review]
11. Adler SP, Finney JW, Manganello AM, Best AM. Prevention of child-to-mother transmission of cytomegalovirus among pregnant women. J Pediatr 2004; 145: 485–91. [RCT, $n=166$]
12. Guerra B, Lazzarotto T, Quarta S, et al. Prenatal diagnosis of symptomatic congenital cytomegalovirus infection. Am J Obstet Gynecol 2000; 183: 476–82. [II-2]
13. Nigro G, Adler SP, La Torre R, Best AM. Passive immunization during pregnancy for congenital cytomegalovirus infection. N Engl J Med 2005; 353: 1350–62. [II-1]
14. Kimberlin DW, Lin CY, Sanchez PJ, et al. Effect of ganciclovir therapy on hearing in symptomatic congenital cytomegalovirus disease involving the central nervous system: a randomized, controlled trial. J Pediatr 2003; 143: 16–25. [RCT, $n=42$]

42

Toxoplasmosis

Marianne Vendola

KEY POINTS

- Maternal infection starts with **ingestion** (from food, water, hands, or insects) **of cysts from uncooked/undercooked meat of infected animals** *or* **contact with oocysts from infected cats or contaminated soil.**
- Fetal/neonatal disease is **more severe if maternal infection occurs in the first trimester,** and the **incidence of maternal–fetal transmission is directly proportional to gestational age** (low in first trimester, high in third trimester).
- **Prevention** has been shown to **decrease the incidence of the disease,** and remains the **most important of interventions.**
- **Prenatal and/or neonatal screening** is controversial and is not adopted in most countries, because of low incidence, concerns with poor/difficult diagnosis, availability of diagnostic and therapeutic services, population compliance, and high risk of terminating false-positive fetuses.
- The principal method used to diagnose and evaluate timing of congenital infection is based on detection of specific antibodies and monitoring the immune response. *Maternal infection* is diagnosed by sending maternal serology to a reference laboratory. *Fetal congenital infection* is diagnosed by amniotic fluid (AF) polymerase chain reaction (PCR).
- **Correct interpretation** of serological testing carried out in a reference laboratory **decreases unnecessary anxiety and even terminations.**
- If maternal infection is confirmed by a reference laboratory, **start spiramycin 3–4 g/day.**
- If AF PCR is positive, start **sulfadiazine, pyrimethamine,** and **folinic acid.**

PATHOGEN

Toxoplasma gondii (TG) is an obligate intracellular protozoan (parasite).

INCIDENCE/EPIDEMIOLOGY

The incidence of *primary acute maternal infection* is 0.01–0.1% in the USA and UK. The prevalence of past infection is approximately 20–30% in the USA and UK, 50–80% in continental Europe (87% in France), 50–70% in Latin American countries, 5–35% in Asia, as in Scandinavian countries. Once immune, immunity lasts for life.

The incidence of *congenital infection* is 2–3 cases per 1000 live births in France and Belgium and 1 in 1000 to 1 in 10 000 live births in the USA.[1]

SYMPTOMS

Most of the times (almost always) there are no maternal symptoms; occasionally flu/mononucleosis-like fever, fatigue, rash, and lymphadenopathy (around head and neck) can be associated with maternal infection.

PATHOPHYSIOLOGY

TG can infect any mammals, who serve as intermediate host. The definitive host is the cat (only one that can support both sexual and asexual reproduction). The parasite can exist as:

1. Trophozoite (invasive form).
2. Cyst (latent form).
3. Oocyst (only in cats: result of sexual reproduction, which occurs in the small intestine of a cat who has eaten outside tissue cysts containing *T. gondii*).

Only during this first exposure is the cat infectious, as these oocysts are produced for 2 weeks and contain infectious sporozoites; the oocysts require 1–5 days to become infected; after 2 weeks the cat becomes immune and not infectious. In soil, oocysts can remain infectious for years. Human infection starts with **ingestion** (from food, water, hands, or insects) **of cysts from uncooked/undercooked**

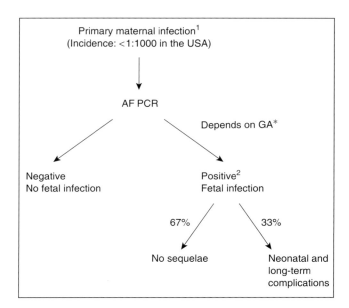

Figure 42.1
Natural history of toxoplasmosis in pregnancy. AF, amniotic fluid; PCR, polymerase chain reaction; GA, gestational age.

*See text for diagnosis, and Table 42.1 for transmission.
[1] Start spiramycin.
[2] Stop spiramycin; start sulfadiazine, pyrimethamine, folinic acid (except in first trimester).

meat of infected animals (e.g. lamb, mutton, etc.) *or* contact with oocysts from infected cats (who get it from infected mice, etc.) **or contaminated soil.** The infected oocysts become infective inside the pregnant woman in 4–10 (average 7) days, leading to parasitemia. Eventually, TG can infect and live forever in striated muscle or brain. Only very few cases of congenital toxoplasmosis transmitted by mothers who were infected prior to conception have been reported; they can be attributed to either reinfection with a different strain or to reactivation of chronic disease. This reactivation is very rare, but can occur especially in an immunocompromised woman. Immunocompetent women with prior toxoplasmosis can be reassured that the risks to the subsequent fetus/neonate are miniscule, especially >9 months after infection.[1]

MATERNAL–FETAL TRANSMISSION (FIGURE 42.1)

Primary maternal TG infection in pregnancy can lead to fetal infection, with this rate highly dependent on gestational age of maternal infection[1] (Table 42.1).

Of the congenitally infected fetuses – PCR (polymerase chain reaction) positive by amniocentesis – about 67%

Table 42.1 *Maternal–fetal transmission*[1]	
Maternal infection	**Probability of congenital infection (%)**
Preconception[a]	<1
First trimester	10–25
Second trimester	30–55
Third trimester	60–80

[a]Usually within 9 months of conception.

manifest only subclinical infection (only serologically positive), whereas 33% have fetal/neonatal illness. Overall, about 7% of fetuses of primary infected mothers are affected. **Fetal/neonatal disease is more severe if maternal infection occurs in the first trimester** (but fetus has a <1/1000 risk of getting affected if ≤4 weeks gestational age at time of maternal infection), but more common if maternal infection occurs in the third trimester.

COMPLICATIONS

Fetal/neonatal complications (check by prenatal ultrasound) include: ventriculomegaly (75%), increased placental thickness (32%), hepatomegaly (12%), ascites (15%), intracranial calcifications (18%), hydrocephalus (4%), microcephaly (5%), and hepatosplenomegaly (4%). Additionally, in the neonate, TG congenital infection is associated with neonatal chorioretinitis (22%), deafness, decreased IQ, and subsequent blindness, seizure disorders, and delay in neuropsychomotor development.[1] Congenital infection is also associated with an increased risk of preterm birth (PTB), but not intrauterine growth restriction (IUGR), when seroconversion occurs before 20 weeks.

PREGNANCY MANAGEMENT
Principles

Counseling regarding basic pathophysiology, maternal–fetal transmission, complications, and preventive/therapeutic management should be done. Termination can be offered, especially if the fetus is definitively positive (PCR-positive amniotic fluid [AF]) and the infection occurred in the first trimester (worse prognosis).

Prevention

Prevention has been shown to decrease the incidence of the disease, and remains the most important of interventions (Table 42.2).

Table 42.2 *Prevention of congenital toxoplasmosis*
• Avoid raw or undercooked meat (or eggs) of any origin
• Avoid contact with raw meat or soil
• Wash fruits and vegetables before eating
• Cats: avoid changing cat litter. Handwash after handling cats. Do not let cats outside the house (could eat infected mice). No stray cats in the house. No feeding raw meat to cats. Avoid raw milk

Screening

Serum

Routine toxoplasmosis screening programs for pregnant women have been established in some European countries such as France and Austria. In the UK and the USA no prenatal or neonatal screening for TG is formally recommended by appropriate medical societies, not without controversy.[2] Prenatal maternal screening has not been recommended in the USA because of low incidence, concerns with poor/difficult diagnosis, availability of diagnostic and therapeutic services, population compliance, and high risk of terminating false-positive fetuses. If prenatal screening is implemented, it should start preconceptionally or at least in the first trimester, and be repeated every month (or at least every trimester) in all IgG-negative mothers (Figure 42.2). Neonatal screening in the USA would detect about one positive neonate for 12 000 screened mothers, with the possibility that treatment may prevent severe sequelae, but would probably not be cost-effective.

Ultrasound

Ultrasound findings associated with TG congenital infection can include intracranial calcifications, microcephaly, ventricular dilatation and hydrocephalus, ascites, hepatosplenomegaly, IUGR, and increased placental thickness.[3]

Work-up/diagnosis (see Figure 42.2)

The principal method used to diagnose and evaluate timing of congenital infection is based on detection of specific antibodies and monitoring the immune response.

IgG antibodies usually appear within 2 weeks of infection and persist in the body indefinitely.

IgM antibodies are considered to be a sign of recent infection and can be detected by enzyme immunoassays (EIAs) or an immunosorbent agglutination assay test (IAAT) within 2 weeks of infection. They often remain positive for up to 1–2 years. *IgA antibodies* may also persist for more than 1 year and their detection is informative mainly for the

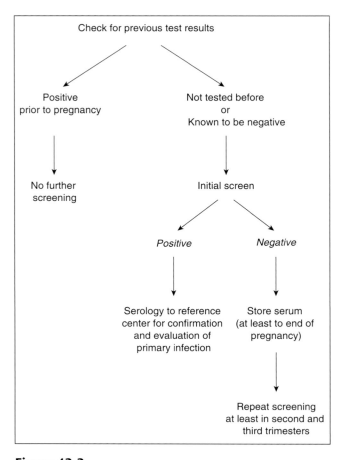

Figure 42.2
Laboratory diagnosis of congenital toxoplasmosis. (Adapted from Rorman et al.[1])

diagnosis of congenital toxoplasmosis. *IgE antibodies* increase rapidly and remain detectable for less than 4 months after infection, which is a very short time to use them for diagnostic test.

The **Sabin–Feldman dye test (SFDT) is still considered the 'gold standard'.**[1] It detects the presence of anti TG-specific antibodies (total Ig). The absolute antibody titer is also important: values over 250 IU/ml are considered highly suggestive of a recent infection. IgG avidity testing is based on the increase in functional affinity (avidity) between TG-specific IgG and antigen over time, as the host immune response evolves. Pregnant women with high avidity antibodies are those who have been infected at least 3–5 months earlier.[4] Current testing cannot define which specific strain of TG caused the antibody response, so that reinfection with the same or different strains cannot be determined.

Maternal infection is diagnosed by sending maternal serology to a reference laboratory (in the USA: Jack Remington, Palo Alto: Tel. 650-853-4828; Fax 650-614-3292; www.pamf.org/serology/clinicianguide.html). It is best to make the diagnosis based on two different serum specimens collected at least 4 weeks apart. Usually, the reference laboratory reports many serology results, with a high possibility of infection if:

- seroconversion during pregnancy
- increase in both specific IgG titer (> three fold) and dye test titer (> three fold)
- presence of specific IgM and dye test ≥ 300 IU/ml.

Correct interpretation of serological testing performed in a reference laboratory decreases unnecessary anxiety and even terminations.[5]

Fetal congenital infection is diagnosed by AF PCR. The specificity and positive predictive value on AF samples are close to 100%; the sensitivity is around 70–80%, but is best when maternal infection occurs between 17 and 21 weeks of pregnancy. Therefore, a negative AF PCR does not completely rule out congenital infection. AF PCR should obviously be performed after 15 weeks. Ultrasound can also aid in diagnosis of fetal infection (see under Complications), but it has very poor sensitivity and specificity.

Therapy

If maternal infection, counsel regards risks, possibility of termination (especially in first trimester), management.

If maternal infection is confirmed by a reference laboratory, start spiramycin 3–4 g/day. This is available in the USA only by the Food and Drug Administration (FDA) when Palo Alto serology is positive. Spiramycin concentrates in the placenta.

If AF PCR is positive, start **sulfadiazine** 1–1.5 g po qid, **pyrimethamine** 25–100 mg po qd, and **folinic acid** (leucovorin) 10–25 mg with each dose of pyrimethamine (decreases bone marrow toxicity) 6 mg po 3×/week: all for 28 days;

then, half-dose for 28 days. Treatment with pyrimethamine and sulfadiazine to prevent fetal infection is contraindicated during the first trimester (pyrimethamine is teratogenic), but at this time sulfadiazine can be used alone.[6,7] This treatment should be stopped in the last few weeks of pregnancy. This is the basic treatment protocol recommended by the World Health Organization (WHO) and Center for Disease Control (CDC).[1] Other drugs such as spiramycin (3–4 g/day × 3–4 weeks) are recommended in certain circumstances. Spiramycin is used to prevent placental infection; it is used in European countries, but in the USA it is not approved by the FDA. Treatment decreases complications of TG, but possibly not fetal infection.

REFERENCES

1. Rorman E, Zamir CS, Rilkis I, Ben-David H. Congenital toxoplasmosis – prenatal aspects of *Toxoplasma gondii* infection. Reprod Toxicol 2006; 21: 458–72. [review]
2. Neto EC. Newborn screening for congenital infectious diseases. Emerg Infect Dis 2004; 10: 1068–73. [II-3]
3. El Ayoubi M, de Bethmann O, Monset-Couchard M. Lenticulostriate echogenic vessels: clinical and sonographic study of 70 neonatal cases. Pediatr Radiol 2003; 33: 697–703. [II-3]
4. Montoya JG, Liesenfeld O, Kinney S, Press C, Remington JS. VIDAS test avidity of Toxoplasma-specific immunoglobulin G for confirmatory testing of pregnant women. J Clin Microbiol 2002; 40: 2505–8. [II-3]
5. Liesenfeld O, Montoya JC, Tathinemi NJ, et al. Confirmatory serologic testing for acute toxoplasmosis and rate of induced abortions among women reported to have positive Toxoplasma immunoglobulin M antibody titers. Am J Obstet Gynecol 2001; 184: 140–5. [II-2]
6. Drugs Used in Parasitic Diseases, 2nd edn. Geneva: World Health Organization; 1995. [review]
7. Chin J. Toxoplasmosis. In: Control of Communicable Disease Manual, 17th edn. Washington, DC: American Public Health Association; 2000: 500–3. [review]

43

Parvovirus

Marianne Vendola

KEY POINTS

- The **incidence of acute primary maternal parvovirus B19** infection during pregnancy in susceptible women is about **3–4%**.
- The major means of infection is by **contact with young infected children**. The infection is usually **asymptomatic** in the adult (and pregnant woman).
- About 25–33% of fetuses of mothers with primary parvovirus B19 infection become infected themselves by vertical transmission.
- Perinatal complications of fetal infection occur in about 10% of fetuses, and include **fetal anemia, and myocarditis**, leading to **hydrops** (2–6%), **and** occasionally **fetal death** if infection occurs < 20 weeks.
- Screening is not recommended, since 1/5000 screened women would be at risk for fetal hydrops from parvovirus B19.
- **Maternal infection is usually diagnosed by IgM +, or by IgG seroconversion.**
- **Fetal ultrasound** can screen for development of anemia and/or hydropic changes in infected mother by increased **peak systolic velocity (PSV) of the middle cerebral artery (MCA)** using a **threshold of ≥ 1.50 multiples of the median (MoM)**. If MCA PSV values are < 1.50 MoM, it is suggested to **continue weekly ultrasound scans for 10–12 weeks after the exposure.**
- If MCA PSV is >1.50 or fetal hydrops is seen on ultrasound, **fetal transfusion is indicated**, even if the incidence of spontaneous resolution of hydrops is about 30%, since survival with transfusion is >90%.
- Even in cases of fetuses transfused in utero for parvovirus B19-induced hydrops, **long-term outcome seems to be similar to normal controls.**

PATHOGEN

Human parvovirus B19 is a single-stranded DNA virus. Parvovirus B19 is the only known parvovirus which is a human pathogen.

INCIDENCE/EPIDEMIOLOGY

The **incidence of acute primary maternal parvovirus B19** infection during pregnancy in susceptible women is about 3–4%.[1,2] The parvovirus B19-specific immunoglobulin (IgG) seroconversion incidence in susceptible pregnant women (primary infection) goes from 1.5–6% during endemic to 13–16% during epidemic periods.[1] Approximately 50–75% of women of reproductive age are IgG + (immune) for parvovirus B19.

RISK FACTORS/ASSOCIATIONS

The infection is more common in the winter and spring. The risk of infection is associated with the level of **contact with young infected children**. The highest infection rates occur in schoolteachers, day care workers, and women with nursery or school-age children in the home. Around 50–80% of susceptible household members and 20–30% of individuals exposed in a classroom acquire acute infection from an infected child. Adverse prognostic factors are older maternal age, maternal immunity and seroconversion, raised maternal serum alpha fetoprotein (MSAFP), and ultrasound findings.

SYMPTOMS

In adults at least half of the infections are **asymptomatic**. About 30% may have flu-like symptoms, arthralgias, and adenopathy. Parvovirus B19 causes a common exanthematous disease in children 5–14 years old, called fifth disease or erythema infectiosum. Children have symptoms such as low-grade fever and 'slapped-cheeks' rash, and are usually diagnosed just based on these symptoms.

PATHOPHYSIOLOGY (FIGURE 43.1)

Parvovirus B19 is mainly transmitted by respiratory droplets. The incubation period for erythema infectiosum

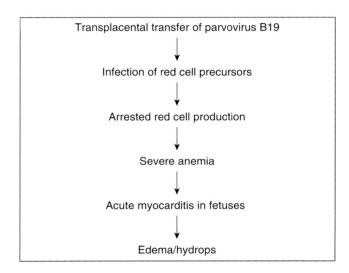

Figure 43.1
Pathophysiology of parvovirus B19 fetal infection.

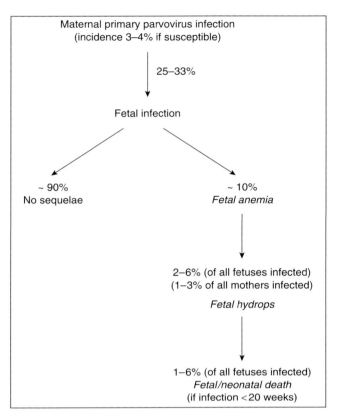

Figure 43.2
Natural history of parvovirus infection in pregnancy.

is 13–18 days, and infectivity is greatest 7–10 days before onset of symptoms. The major target cells for parvovirus B19 are erythroid progenitors bearing the main cellular parvovirus B19 receptor P blood group antigen globoside on their surface. The virus is believed to cause arrest of maturation of red blood cell (RBC) precursors at the late normoblast stage and causes a decrease in the number of platelets. The virus causes infection and lysis of erythroid progenitor cells by apoptosis, leading to hemolysis and transient aplastic crisis. Subsequent fetal anemia is thought to be responsible for the development of skin edema and effusions. Myocarditis leading to heart failure may contribute to the development of fetal hydrops.[1,3] Parvovirus B19 has been demonstrated to carry an apoptosis-inducing factor and to induce cell cycle arrest. Cells in the S-phase of DNA mitosis are particulary vulnerable to parvovirus B19 and the fetus is at particular risk because of the vast number of cells in active mitosis, shorter half-life of RBCs, and immature immune system.

MATERNAL–FETAL TRANSMISSION (FIGURE 43.2)

About **25–33% of fetuses of mothers with primary parvovirus B19 infection become infected themselves by vertical transmission.** About 90% have no sequelae from this intrauterine infection. Although it is not easy to determine the exact timing of transmission of parvovirus B19 infection to the fetus, it is likely that parvovirus B19 infects the fetus during or immediately after maternal viremia, even in the early stages of gestation. Parvovirus B19 can persist until term or after birth, even when infection occurs early in gestation.

COMPLICATIONS (SEE FIGURE 43.2)

Of the infected fetuses, about 5–20% can develop **anemia,** of which 30–50% develop **hydrops fetalis** (about 2–6% of all infected fetuses). Some have reported a rate of 1–3% for fetal hydrops in infected mothers.[1] The risk of **fetal death** is 1–6% of all infected fetuses.[4] Fetal death occurs almost exclusively in hydropic cases diagnosed at < 20 weeks, especially if cases > 20 weeks are treated with timely transfusion (90% survival).[4] Early embryonic/fetal death may manifest as miscarriage (about 10% of infected mothers < 20 weeks). Although acute parvovirus infection may occur relatively commonly during pregnancy, an adverse fetal outcome is an uncommon complication.[3] Rarely, parvovirus has been detected in fetuses with hydrocephalus (possibly from vasculitis), but it is unclear if malformations seen with parvovirus are just coincidental, and not related to the viral infection. Parvovirus B19 may be an important cause of fetal death, not always associated with fetal hydrops. **All cases of fetal death should be tested for parvovirus B19 by polymerase chain reaction (PCR).** Maternal serology might be a less-sensitive determinant for parvovirus B19-associated fetal death, since immunoglobulin M (IgM) response generally lasts 2–4

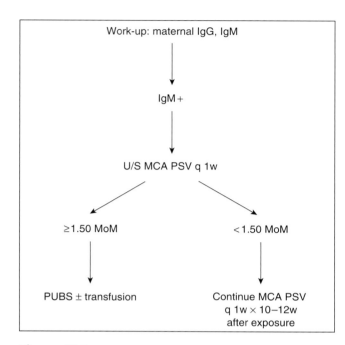

Figure 43.3
Management of parvovirus infection in pregnancy. IgG, immunoglobulin G; IgM, immunoglobulin M; U/S, ultrasound; MCA, middle cerebral artery; PSV, peak systolic velocity; MoM, multiples of the median; PUBS, percutaneous umbilical blood sampling; w, week.

months, and parvovirus B19 infection can already be persistent in fetuses during the early stages of pregnancy, eventually leading to fetal death months later. The more mature immune response in older fetuses could delay any pathogenic consequences of parvovirus B19 infection, resulting in a lower rate of hydrops than in younger fetuses.[5,6]

ULTRASOUND FETAL FINDINGS

Sonographically detectable markers of fetal compromise include pericardial or pleural effusion, ascites, abdominal wall/skin edema, bilateral hydroceles, oligohydramnios or hydramnios, increased (> 95th centile) cardiac biventricular outer diameter, and, rarely, hydrocephalus, microcephaly, and intracranial and hepatic calcifications.[1,3]

PREGNANCY MANAGEMENT

Counseling/prognosis

Counseling should include the natural history of the disease, including vertical transmission, chances of fetal disease (anemia and hydrops), prognosis, and possible interventions. The long-term outcome of fetuses affected after 20 weeks is very good.

Prevention

Avoidance of contact with infected children – or (better) children in general – is best prevention. This is not always feasible. Active immunization with vaccine is not available. **Intravenous immunoglobulin (IVIG) prophylaxis** is reasonable to consider for documented exposures in immunocompromised patients. It is not currently recommended for prophylaxis in pregnancy.

Screening

Universal screening is not recommended, as the risk of fetal hydrops from parvovirus infection is about 1/5000 screened pregnancies, making screening not warranted.[1] Screening may be warranted in pregnant women who take care of young children, especially during epidemics.[1]

Work-up/diagnosis

Work-up includes determination of serum IgG and IgM. **Maternal infection is usually diagnosed by IgM +, or by IgG seroconversion.** IgM appears by 3 days of an acute infection, peaks at 25–30 days, and disappears by 4 months. Serum IgG appears a few days after IgM, and coincides with resolution of maternal symptoms. The detection of viral DNA by PCR is another means of diagnosis. Electron microscopy (EM) is also possible, whereas virus culture usually fails. Increased MSAFP has also been used as a prognostic factor for poor outcome.[7]

Once maternal infection has been diagnosed, **fetal ultrasound** can screen for development of anemia and/or hydropic changes. Anemia can be detected by increased **peak systolic velocity (PSV) of the middle cerebral artery (MCA)** prior to the appearance of sonographically detectable markers of hydrops.[8] This is based on the observation (first in rhesus immunization, where the mechanism leading to anemia is different) that with fetal anemia there is an increase of fetal cardiac output to maintain adequate oxygen delivery to tissues, leading to increased blood flow velocities also in anemic fetuses with hydrops from parvovirus B19. MCA PSV using a **threshold of ≥ 1.50 MoM** (multiples of the median) has a high sensitivity (100%) and specificity (100%) for detecting fetal anemia.[8] If MCA PSV values are < 1.50 MoM, it is suggested to **continue weekly ultrasound scans for 10–12 weeks after the exposure** to follow those fetuses that potentially are at high risk for anemia and hydrops (Figure 43.3). The peak incidence of hydrops is at about 4–6 weeks after maternal infection. In cases of elevated MCA PSV but no hydrops, surveillance should be increased with ultrasound scans 2–3 per week to detect any sign of hydrops, or umbilical cord sampling performed.

Fetal diagnosis is by amniotic fluid (AF) PCR +. There is at present no need for percutaneous umbilical blood sampling (PUBS) for diagnosis.

Therapy

There are **no trials** evaluating therapeutic interventions. **No antiviral therapy is available.**

Treatment should be directed at fetuses with abnormal MCA PSV and/or hydropic changes. In these fetuses, anemia and even hydrops can resolve spontaneously over 4–6 weeks (about **30% spontaneous resolution for hydrops**).[9] Resolution is more common in older (> 20 weeks) fetuses, because of a more mature immune system.

Intervention for anemic and/or hydropic fetuses is gestational-age dependent:

- Between 24 and 33 6/7 weeks, steroids for fetal lung maturity should be given. Fetal cordocentesis to document anemia, and transfusion as necessary improves outcome in anemic and/or hydropic fetuses.
- Before 24 weeks, with severe hydrops, termination may be offered, but transfusion can be beneficial, with apparently no significant sequelae if successful.
- After 33 6/7 weeks, delivery should be considered.

If cordocentesis is performed, anemia could be detected before a critical decrease of hemoglobin of <6 g/dl and before the development of severe hydrops. Blood sampling can allow testing for fetal hemoglobin/hematocrit and leukocyte and platelet counts. **Once sonographic signs of hydrops are present, transfusion is indicated** using erythrocytes and possibly platelets. Several non-randomized but controlled studies suggest a significant benefit of transfusion of fetuses with anemia and/or hydrops from parvovirus infection compared with conservative treatment.[3,4,10] Intracardiac transfusion is a last resort alternative to intra-umbilical cord transfusion, particularly when intra-umbilical cord transfusion is not possible, because of risks of bradycardia and cardiac arrest of this procedure.[11]

NEONATE

Infants born to IgM + mothers are born IgG + (mostly maternal), and 25% stay IgG + at 1 year, as they were infected and have become immune. Long-term outcome includes incidence of **developmental delay similar** to the general population, **even in cases of fetuses transfused in** utero for parvovirus B19-induced hydrops.[12,13] Two phases of the infantile infection are described: a first phase of viremia of 2–3 days, accompanied by fever and myalgia; a second phase that can last several weeks, with dermatological signs such as erythema infectiosum, vasculitis, arthralgias, or arthritis. Long-term persistence of the virus in the neonate organism may be responsible for chronic manifestations.

REFERENCES

1. Van Gessel PH, Gaytant MA, Vossen AC, et al. Incidence of parvovirus B19 infection among an unselected population of pregnant women in the Netherlands: a prospective study. Eur J Obstet Gynecol Reprod Biol 2006; 128: 46–9. [II-3]
2. Wong A, Tan KH, Tee CS, Yeo GS. Seroprevalence of CMV, toxoplasma and parvovirus in pregnancy. Singapore Med J 2000; 41(4): 151–5. [II-3]
3. Von Kaisenberg CS, Jonat W. Fetal parvovirus B19. Ultrasound Obstet Gynecol 2001; 18: 280–8. [II-3]
4. Enders M, Weidner A, Zoellner I, Searle K, Enders G. Fetal morbidity and mortality after acute human parvovirus B19 infection in pregnancy: prospective evaluation of 108 cases. Prenatal Diagn 2004; 24: 513–18. [II-2]
5. Tolfvenstam T, Papadogiannakis N, Norbeck O, Petersson K, Broliden K. Frequency of human parvovirus B19 infection in intrauterine fetal death. Lancet 2001; 357: 1494–7. [II-2]
6. Skjoldebrand-Sparre L, Tolfvenstam T, Papadogiannakis N, et al. Parvovirus B19 infection: association with third-trimester intrauterine fetal death. BJOG 2000; 107: 476–80. [II-2]
7. Bernstein IM, Capeless EL. Elevated maternal serum alpha-fetoprotein and hydrops fetalis in association with fetal parvovirus B-19 infection. Obstet Gynecol 1989; 74: 456–7. [II-2]
8. Cosmi E, Mari G, Delle Chiaie L, et al. Noninvasive diagnosis by Doppler ultrasonography of fetal anemia resulting from parvovirus infection. Am J Obstet Gynecol 2002; 187: 1290–3. [II-2]
9. Rodis JF, Borgida AF, Wilson M, et al. Management of parvovirus infection in pregnancy and outcomes of hydrops: a survey of members of the Society of Perinatal Obstetricians. Am J Obstet Gynecol 1998; 179: 985–8. [II-3]
10. Schild RL, Bald R, Plath H, et al. Intrauterine management of fetal parvovirus B19 infection. Ultrasound Obstet Gynecol 1999; 13: 161–6. [II-2]
11. Galligan BR, Cairns R, Schifano JV, Selbing A, Bernvil SS. Preparation of packed red cells suitable for intravascular transfusion in utero. Transfusion 1989; 29(2): 179–81. [II-3]
12. Dembinski J, Haverkamp F, Maara H, et al. Neurodevelopmental outcome after intrauterine red cell transfusion for parvovirus B19-induced fetal hydrops. BJOG 2002; 109: 1232–4. [II-2]
13. Rodis JF, Rodner C, Hansen AA, et al. Long-term outcome of children following maternal human parvovirus B19 infection. Obstet Gynecol 1998; 91: 125–8. [II-2]

44

Herpes

Marianne Vendola

KEY POINTS

- Around 20–30% of pregnant women have IgG for herpes simplex virus (HSV)-2 (prior infection) and are therefore infected with it, with intermittent shedding from the vaginal mucosa. About 2–4% of IgG-negative women seroconvert (acquire HSV and convert to IgM+) during pregnancy, and 90% of these women are undiagnosed.
- Neonatal HSV infection occurs in > 90% of cases from contact with infected maternal genital secretions. **Primary first episode infection,** defined as herpes simplex virus confirmed in a person without prior HSV-1 or HSV-2 antibodies, **can lead to a 40–50% vertical transmission rate if delivery occurs vaginally** during this episode, and therefore represents the most important clinical scenario to avoid.
- Vaginal delivery during **recurrent infection is associated with a 0–3% incidence of neonatal HSV infection.** Transplacental HSV vertical transmission is rare.
- Neonatal HSV causes **disseminated or central nervous system (CNS) disease** (seizures, lethargy, irritability, tremors, poor feeding, temperature instability, and bulging fontanelle) **in approximately 50% of cases. Up to 30% of infants will die and up to 40% will have neurological damage despite antiviral therapy.**
- **Prevention of maternal infection** is the most important management strategy. Universal maternal screening with HSV-1 and HSV-2 specific serology has not been tested in a trial and is controversial. If the woman is seronegative, the partner should be tested. If he is seropositive, avoidance of direct orogenital contact, use of condoms, the possibility of abstinence, and medical suppression of partner should be discussed. If the woman is seropositive, suppression with acyclovir or valacyclovir from 36 weeks until delivery, examination for lesions in labor with cesarean delivery (CD) if they are present, and avoidance (if possible) of artificial rupture of membranes (AROM), scalp electrodes, vacuum extractors, and forceps should be recommended. **If any genital lesion suspicious for HSV is seen at time of labor, a CD should be performed.**

- Diagnosis of genital herpes is most sensitive with polymerase chain reaction (**PCR**) **assay** of genital lesions (typed to determine whether HSV-1 or HSV-2 is the cause of the infection). Type-specific (**HSV-1 and HSV-2**) glycoprotein G-based **serological testing** should also be sent.
- **Women with primary or first episode genital HSV in pregnancy** should receive **acyclovir 400 mg po tid×7–14 days, or valacyclovir (Valtrex) 1 g po bid×7–14 days,** and receive suppression with **acyclovir 400 mg po bid or valacyclovir 500 mg po qd at 36 weeks until delivery.**
- **Women with reactivation (recurrent) symptomatic HSV should receive either acyclovir 400 mg po tid×5 days, or valacyclovir (Valtrex) 500 mg po bid×5 days,** and receive suppression with acyclovir or valacyclovir at 36 weeks until delivery.

PATHOGENS

Herpes simplex virus type 1 (HSV-1) and type 2 (HSV-2) are both DNA viruses.

INCIDENCE/EPIDEMIOLOGY

Genital herpes is an infection of HSV-1 or HSV-2 that causes ulceration in the genital area. **Around 20–30% of pregnant women have immunoglobulin G (IgG) for HSV-2 (prior infection) and are therefore infected with it, with intermittent shedding from the vaginal mucosa.** Approximately 15–25% of couples in early pregnancy are discordant for HSV status, with the woman at risk of getting primary infection from her partner.[1-3] **About 2–4% of IgG-negative women seroconvert (acquire HSV) during pregnancy, and 90% of these women are undiagnosed because of minimal or no symptoms.**[1] Approximately 0.1–1% of pregnant women carry HSV in their genitalia. The incidence of neonatal herpes is 2 in 100 000 live births annually in the UK and 1–3 in 10 000 live births annually in the USA.[1]

RISK FACTORS/ASSOCIATIONS

Risk factors for maternal HSV infection are immunocompromise, other sexually transmitted diseases (STDs) and risk factors for STDs. Risk factors for neonatal HSV infection are HSV in the genital tract at the time of delivery, primary HSV infection, and invasive obstetric procedures.[1]

SYMPTOMS

About 70% of newly acquired HSV infections among pregnant women are asymptomatic, and 30% of women have clinical presentations that range from minimal lesions to widespread genital lesions associated with severe local pain, dysuria, sacral paresthesia, tender regional lymph node enlargement, fever, malaise, and headache (rarely meningitis).

CLASSIFICATION/ PATHOPHYSIOLOGY

HSV infection causes intranuclear inclusion bodies and multinucleated giant cells. HSV-1 causes about 90% of oral and 10% of genital infections. HSV-2 causes 10% of oral and 90% of genital infections. Types of infection include the following:

Primary first episode

Primary first episode infection is **defined as herpes simplex virus confirmed in a person without prior HSV-1 or HSV-2 antibodies.** About 2–4% of these seronegative women seroconvert to HSV-1 or HSV-2 during pregnancy (only 30% have symptoms – if symptoms are present, they are severe – and 50% have recurrence within 6 months), with no fetal consequences unless they convert shortly before labor and deliver vaginally; viral shedding is very high with primary infection.

Non-primary first episode

Non-primary first episode infection is HSV-2 confirmed in a person with prior findings of HSV-1 antibodies, or vice versa. About 1.5–2% of HSV-1 IgG+ women seroconvert to HSV-2+, whereas the risk of conversion from HSV-2 IgG to HSV-1+ is < 1%. If symptoms are present, they are usually milder than first episode primary infection.

Reactivation (recurrent) genital herpes

Reactivation (recurrent) genital herpes is caused by **reactivation of latent herpes simplex virus, usually HSV-2.** If symptoms are present, they last 7–10 days, are mild, with low viral load shedding for 3–5 days. Some clinicians distinguish

another category within this one, called first recognized recurrence, which is HSV-1 (or HSV-2) confirmed in a person with prior findings of HSV-1 (or HSV-2) antibodies, but this is not clinically different from reactivation disease.

Over 90% of HSV episodes in pregnancy are either recurrent or non-primary first-episode HSV. Intimate contact between a susceptible person (without antibodies against the virus) and an individual who is actively shedding the virus or with body fluids containing the virus is required for HSV infection to occur. Contact must involve mucous membranes or open or abraded skin. HSV invades and replicates in neurons as well as in epidermal and dermal cells. Virions travel from the initial site of infection on the skin or mucosa to the sensory dorsal root ganglion, where latency is established. Viral replication in the sensory ganglia leads to recurrent clinical outbreaks. These outbreaks can be induced by various stimuli, such as trauma, ultraviolet radiation, extremes in temperature, stress, immunosuppression, or hormonal fluctuations. Viral shedding, leading to possible transmission, occurs during primary infection, during subsequent recurrences, and during periods of asymptomatic viral shedding.

MATERNAL–FETAL TRANSMISSION

Maternal–fetal transmission of HSV usually occurs at delivery from contact with infected genital secretions. Approximately 1% of women with a history of HSV have asymptomatic viral shedding at delivery. **Vaginal delivery during first episode primary infection is associated with a 40–50% incidence of neonatal HSV infection.** Vaginal delivery during **recurrent infection is associated with a 0–3% incidence of neonatal HSV infection.**[1] The infant of the mother with primary HSV in the third trimester lacks the protection of transplacental type-specific antibodies (which take 6–12 weeks to fully protect the infant), and is at risk of exposure during delivery when viral shedding could be of greatest load. The major sites of intrapartum viral entry are the neonatal eyes, nasopharynx, or a break in skin.

Transplacental infection is rare. First episode primary infection during pregnancy can lead to microcephaly, ventriculomegaly, spasticity, echogenic bowel, hepatosplenomegaly, and flexed extremities.[4]

COMPLICATIONS

In the mother, primary infection can lead to severe symptoms, and occasionally to disseminated disease, hepatitis, and encephalitis.

Factors that influence the risk of fetal infection include primary maternal infection, gestational age, delivery mode, status of membranes, and maternal antibodies. Primary, rather than recurrent genital HSV, is the main risk factor for

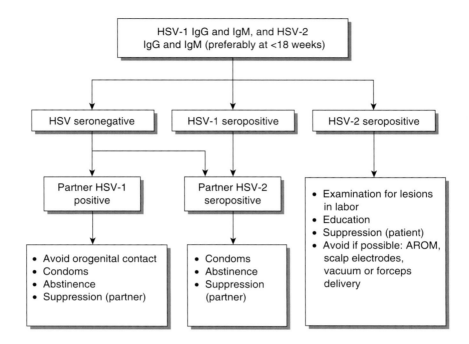

Figure 44.1
Proposed testing and counseling of pregnant women regarding HSV. (Adapted from Brown et al.[1]) HSV, herpes simplex virus; AROM, artificial rupture of membranes.

neonatal herpes. In the first episode, if genital herpes lesions are present at the time of delivery and the baby is delivered vaginally, the risk of **neonatal herpes** is 40–50%, calculated in different studies.[5] The risk of neonatal infection in women with established infection and recurrence at term is 0–3%. The risk of neonatal infection from postnatal transmission without prevention is 15%.[6] Neonatal HSV causes **disseminated or central nervous system (CNS) disease (seizures, lethargy, irritability, tremors, poor feeding, temperature instability, and bulging fontanelle) in approximately 50% of cases. Up to 30% of infants will die and up to 40% will have neurological damage despite antiviral therapy.**[1] Prenatal ultrasonography can detect **microcephaly, hydrocephaly, intracranial calcification, and placental calcifications** that result from a chronic fetal infection.[4]

PREGNANCY MANAGEMENT

Pregnancy considerations

The course of HSV infection in pregnancy is similar to that in non-pregnant women.

Counseling/prognosis

Prevention, natural history, incidence of vertical transmission and sequelae, prognosis, and therapeutic options

should all be reviewed for the pregnant woman with maternal HSV infection, especially if primary.

Prevention

Prevention of maternal infection includes avoidance of sexual contact with infected individuals. A **preventive strategy for maternal infection** involving universal screening has been proposed (Figure 44.1). Condoms seem to prevent infection from infected male partners. For prevention of fetal/neonatal infection, **avoidance of vaginal delivery at times of primary infection is most important. If any genital lesion suspicious for HSV is seen at the time of labor, a cesarean delivery (CD) should be performed.** About 46% of these lesions test positive by polymerase chain reaction (PCR). Clinical diagnosis by visual examination fails to identify all women with HSV in their genital secretions.[7] No scalp electrode, forceps, or vacuum should be used if viral shedding is possible. **Prevention of neonatal infection is critical, as neonatal treatment is poorly effective at avoiding long-term CNS complications.** See also Therapy section below.

Screening

Universal screening is not generally offered to pregnant women, but has been recently proposed (see Figure 44.1).[1] There has been no evidence that screening women to identify pregnancies at risk of new infections will effectively decrease the incidence of infection at term, as such a study would require thousands of women. Screening to identify pregnant women with asymptomatic herpes infections may have no value at present without any known safe and effective interventions to prevent an already unlikely neonatal transmission. **All pregnant women should be asked about their own and their partners' histories of genital (and oral) herpes and examined for evidence of active herpes at delivery.** Asymptomatic pregnant women with positive partners, as well as HIV-positive pregnant women, should be offered type-specific serological testing.

Work up/diagnosis

Diagnosis of genital herpes relies on laboratory confirmation with **HSV culture** or **PCR assay** of genital lesions (typed to determine whether HSV-1 or HSV-2 is the cause of the infection). Type-specific (**HSV-1 and HSV-2**) glycoprotein G-based **serological testing** should also be sent. **PCR assays are more sensitive,** but lack of HSV detection by PCR does not indicate lack of HSV infection, because viral shedding is intermittent. HSV culture should be done within 48–72 hours of appearance of the lesion. If a new infection is suspected and the virus is not isolated from the lesion, serological testing should be repeated in 6 weeks. HSV antibodies appear during the first weeks after infection, and persist for life.[1] Tzanck smear (Wright's stain with material from the vesicle) is diagnostic with multinucleated giant cells and viral inclusions.

Therapy[1]

Antiviral drugs

Acyclovir and the other HSV antivirals have, as mechanism of action, the specific inhibition of viral thymidine kinase. They cross the placenta but do not accumulate in the fetus. All these antivirals are safe for the fetus (category B).

Valacyclovir (Valtrex) is the prodrug of acyclovir and requires hepatic metabolism to become active. As for famciclovir, valacyclovir has better absorption, longer half-life, decreased duration of pain, and shedding compared with acyclovir.

Famciclovir is the prodrug of penciclovir and also requires hepatic metabolism to become active. As there are no specific studies in pregnancy, acyclovir and valacyclovir should be preferred.

Trials in non-pregnant adults show no differences in outcomes with any of these drugs for primary HSV.

Primary or first episode HSV

Women with primary or first episode genital HSV in pregnancy should be treated with:

- Analgesia (topical and systemic).
- Hygienic support to avoid secondary yeast and bacterial infection.
- Antiviral therapy (hastens lesion healing and decreases viral shedding) with either:
  - **acyclovir 400 mg po tid × 7–14 days** or
  - **valacyclovir (Valtrex) 1 g po bid × 7–14 days.**

They should receive suppression with acyclovir **400 mg po bid or valacyclovir 500 mg po qd at 36 weeks until delivery.** Suppression decreases the incidence of recurrent genital lesions at term, viral shedding, and therefore the need for CD. There is insufficient evidence to justify suppression based on neonatal HSV, since this outcome is so rare.

First episode within 6–12 weeks of delivery

Women who develop **first episode** (possible primary) genital herpes lesions **at or within 6–12 weeks of delivery** should receive:

- **Intravenous acyclovir** given intrapartum to the mother and subsequently to the neonate, as this may reduce the risk of neonatal herpes.
- Daily suppressive acyclovir or valacyclovir from 36 weeks until delivery.

Complicated CMV infection

Women with **disseminated genital HSV, pneumonitis, hepatitis, or CNS complications** should receive:

- **Intravenous (IV) acyclovir 5–10 mg/kg body weight q8h until clinical improvement, followed by oral antiviral therapy for 10 days of total therapy.**

History of HSV

Women with a history of HSV and **reactivation (recurrent) symptomatic HSV** should be treated with:
- Analgesia (topical and systemic).
- Hygienic support to avoid secondary yeast and bacterial infection.
- Antiviral therapy (hastens lesion healing and decreases viral shedding) with either:
  - **acyclovir 400 mg po tid × 5 days** or
  - **valacyclovir (Valtrex) 500 mg po bid × 5 days.**

They should receive suppression with acyclovir or valacyclovir at 36 weeks until delivery, or starting even earlier if frequent recurrent episodes.

There is insufficient evidence to assess suppression in women with **history of genital HSV and no recurrence during pregnancy,** but suppression might be a reasonable option after counseling.[1]

Mode of delivery

- For active genital lesions, or prodromal symptoms of HSV (either primary or reactivation), especially in women presenting with first episode genital herpes lesions at the time of delivery, cesarean section is recommended.[1,5] Some clinicians advocate CD even for women with primary HSV in third trimester, despite maternal therapy.[1]
- A reactivation/**recurrent episode** of genital herpes occurring **during pregnancy** is not an indication for delivery by cesarean section. In women with **established genital HSV** but without active genital lesions or prodromal symptoms at the time of labor, CD is not indicated. In women with **symptomatic** genital herpes, antiviral suppressive medication initiated from 36 weeks until delivery reduces the need for CD for lesions and viral detection.[8]

Postpartum/neonate

Seventy percent of mothers of HSV-infected neonates are asymptomatic. Neonates with infection manifest symptoms at the end of the first week of life, with skin lesions, cough, tachypnea, cyanosis, jaundice, seizures, and disseminated intravascular coagulation (DIC). The classic triad is skin lesions, chorioretinitis, and CNS abnormalities. Severe HSV neonatal infection leads to a 30% incidence of death and up to 40% incidence of mental problems/neurological damage in survivors.

Mother with HSV at the time of delivery should wash their hands but can handle their neonate. Acyclovir is compatible with breastfeeding.

REFERENCES

1. Brown ZA, Gardella C, Wald A, Morrow RA, Corey L. Genital herpes complicating pregnancy. Obstet Gynecol 2005; 106: 845–56. [review]
2. Gardella C, Brown ZA, Wald A, et al. Risk factors for herpes simplex virus transmission to pregnant women: a couples study. Am J Obstet Gynecol 2005; 193: 1891–9. [II-1]
3. Leone P, Fleming DT, Gilsenan AW, Li L, Justus S. Seroprevalence of herpes simplex virus-2 in suburban primary care offices in United States. Sex Transm Dis 2004; 31: 311–16. [II-2]
4. Lanouette JM, Duquette DA, Jacques SM, et al. Prenatal diagnosis of fetal herpes simplex infection. Fetal Diagn Ther 1996; 11: 414–16. [II-3]
5. RCOG 2002. Management of genital herpes in pregnancy. Clinical Guideline No. 30. [review]
6. Jungmann E. Genital herpes. Clin Evid 2004; 11: 2073–88. [II-2]
7. Gardella C, Brown ZA, Wald A, et al. Poor correlation between genital lesions and detection of herpes simplex virus in women in labor. Obstet Gynecol 2005; 106: 268–74. [II-2]
8. Sheffield JS, Hollier LM, Hill JB, Stuart GS, Wendel GD. Acyclovir prophylaxis to prevent herpes simplex virus recurrence at delivery: a systematic review. Obstet Gynecol 2003; 102: 1396–403. [meta-analysis; 5 RCTs, *n*=799]

45

Varicella

Marianne Vendola

KEY POINTS

- As about 90% of pregnant women are immune (VZV IgG +) to varicella, **primary maternal varicella zoster virus (VZV) infection (chickenpox)** occurs in **about 0.5–3/1000 pregnancies.**
- **Pneumonia** can occur in up to **10% of pregnant women with chickenpox.**
- **Congenital varicella syndrome (CVS)** occurs in 0.4–2% **of all maternal infections, usually if maternal VZV infection occurs at < 20 weeks of gestation.**
- CVS includes congenital limb hypoplasia, dermatomal skin scarring, rudimentary digits, intrauterine growth restriction (IUGR), and occasionally damage to the eyes (chorioretinitis, cataracts) and central nervous system (microcephaly, cortical atrophy, leading to mental retardation).
- All pregnant (and preconception reproductive-age) women should be asked at their first prenatal visit if they have had a chickenpox infection. All women who have not had chickenpox in the past or are unsure should have VZV IgG and IgM serology. VZV IgG-negative women should receive the vaccine postpartum.
- Diagnosis of **maternal chickenpox** is usually made based on clinical findings alone, and confirmed by **VZV IgM.**
- **Ultrasound** can help in the diagnosis and estimation of the probability of CVS. **At least 5 weeks should be allowed between the onset of maternal symptoms and fetal ultrasound.** Fetal infection can be diagnosed by VZV DNA in amniotic fluid, but this does not predict risk of CVS.
- **VZV-seronegative pregnant women exposed to VZV** should receive **VZV IgG (aka VZIG).**
- Pregnant women who develop **chickenpox** should receive oral (or intravenous [IV] if severe) **acyclovir** within 24 hours of rash, and should avoid contact with susceptible individuals such as other pregnant women or children. Varicella zoster immune globulin (VZIG) has no therapeutic effect once chickenpox has developed.
- **Delivery should be delayed until 5 days after the onset of maternal illness,** to allow for passive transfer of maternal IgG. **Infants delivered within 5 days of maternal**

symptoms or 2 days after delivery should receive VZIG. If neonatal infection occurs, the neonate should receive acyclovir.
- Pregnant women who develop **pulmonary chickenpox** should be immediately hospitalized in isolation, and should receive intravenous **(IV) acyclovir.**
- **Maternal shingles is not a risk for the infant** who is protected from passively acquired maternal antibodies.
- **Non-immune women should be offered postpartum varicella vaccination.** The vaccine is considered safe in breastfeeding women. Conception should be delayed until 1 month after the VZV vaccine was given (live attenuated vaccine).

PATHOGEN

Varicella zoster virus (VZV) is a DNA virus of the herpes family.

INCIDENCE/EPIDEMIOLOGY

As about 90% of pregnant women are immune (VZV IgG +) to varicella, **primary maternal VZV infection (commonly called chickenpox, or VZD)** is uncommon, and estimated to **complicate about 0.5–3/1000 pregnancies.** Women from tropical areas are more susceptible (50% immunity only) to the development of chickenpox. The availability of VZV vaccine is expected to decrease the incidence of varicella.

RISK FACTORS/ASSOCIATIONS

Maternal varicella infection is associated with contact with infected individuals, which usually are children, if not immunized. Risk factors for varicella pneumonia are cigarette smoking, > 100 skin lesions, advanced gestational age, history of chronic obstructive pulmonary disease (COPD), immunosuppression, and household contact.

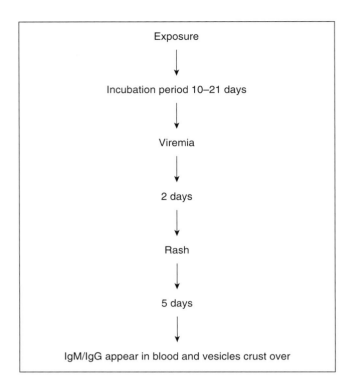

Figure 45.1
VZV infectious sequence.

SYMPTOMS

Pruritic rash with maculopapular skin lesions in crops, which become vesicles and pustules, and later crust over, along with fever and malaise.

PATHOPHYSIOLOGY

VZV is highly contagious and transmitted by respiratory droplets and direct personal contact with vesicle fluid or indirectly via fomites. The incubation period is about 15 (10–21) days. The disease is infectious 48 hours before the rash appears, and continues to be infectious until the vesicles crust over (Figure 45.1). The rash lasts 7–10 days. Chickenpox (or primary VZV infection) is a common childhood disease which usually causes a mild infection, leading to the 90% seropositivity of pregnant women. After the primary infection the virus remains dormant in sensory nerve root ganglia and can be reactivated to cause a vesicular erythematous skin rash known as herpes zoster (commonly called shingles).

MATERNAL–FETAL TRANSMISSION

Primary maternal infection leads to an about **8% vertical transmission,** causing primary fetal infection. Of these,

about 10% develop congenital varicella syndrome (CVS) **(0.4–2% of all maternal infections), usually if maternal VZV infection occurs < 20 weeks of gestation.**[1]

COMPLICATIONS
Maternal

Although varicella infection is much less common in adults than in children, in adults it is more often associated with pneumonia, hepatitis, and encephalitis. **Pneumonia can occur in up to 10% of pregnant women with chickenpox** and the severity seems increased in later gestation. Pulmonary symptoms start 2–6 days after the rash, with a mild cough leading to hemoptysis, chest pain, dyspnea, and cyanosis. The mortality rate with treatment for varicella pneumonia is now only < 1%.

Fetal

Sequelae are dependent on fetal age at the time of infection. In up to 98% of cases of maternal infection, the fetus remains healthy without clinical signs of illness, but when infection occurs, it can result in CVS, neonatal varicella, or asymptomatic seroconversion.

The overall rate for CVS **when maternal infection occurs in the first 20 weeks of gestation** has been demonstrated to be about **0.4–2%.**[1–3] CVS is characterized by **congenital limb hypoplasia, dermatomal skin scarring, rudimentary digits, intrauterine growth restriction (IUGR), and occasionally damage to the eyes (chorioretinitis, cataracts) and central nervous system (CNS: microcephaly, cortical atrophy, leading to mental retardation).** These defects are secondary to recurrent in-utero herpes zoster. **Prenatal ultrasound findings** can include limb deformity, microcephaly, hydrocephalus, soft tissue calcification, and IUGR.[4]

CVS with **maternal infection > 20 weeks** is very rare, as it has only been reported in < 10 case reports (< 1/1000 risk).[2] Maternal infection after 20 weeks and up to 36 weeks may present as shingles in the first few years of infant life, as a reactivation of the virus after a primary infection in utero.

If maternal infection occurs **1–4 weeks before delivery,** up to 50% of babies are infected and up to 23% of these develop clinical varicella. **Severe chickenpox occurs more often if the infant is born within 7 days of onset of the mother's rash** when cord blood VZV IgG is low. Both intrauterine and peripartum VZV infection predispose to development of childhood zoster. Neonates born to mothers who contract chickenpox between 5 days before delivery and 2 days after delivery have a 17–30% chance of developing **neonatal varicella.**[5]

There are no fetal consequences for herpes zoster, since the viral load is very low, and the mother already has VZV IgGs that cross the placenta and protect the fetus.

Table 45.1 *Counseling advice for pregnant women at risk[2]*

Maternal rash appears	Risk for varicella embryopathy	Suggested management
First 20 weeks	0.5–2% above the baseline risk	VZIG within 96 hours after contact if the woman is seronegative Ultrasound 5 weeks after maternal rash appears to detect defects
21–28 weeks	Rare	VZIG within 96 hours after contact if the woman is seronegative Ultrasound 5 weeks after maternal rash appears to detect defects
After 28 weeks	None	VZIG within 96 hours after contact if the woman is seronegative to prevent varicella complication Explain baseline risk
5 days before or 2 days after delivery	None	If possible, delay the delivery until 5–7 days after onset of maternal rash Administer VZIG to neonate if exposed IV acyclovir is warranted for severe cases
Maternal varicella pneumonia		IV acyclovir 10–15 mg/kg every 8 hours for 5–10 days and antibacterial Blood gas, mechanical ventilation, and supportive therapy as needed

VZIG, varicella zoster immune globulin; IV, intravenous.

PREGNANCY MANAGEMENT

Pregnancy considerations

Chickenpox is a more severe disease in the adult than in the child. In pregnant women, frequency of VZV, frequency of pneumonia, and mortality are not increased compared with non-pregnant adults. Pneumonia may be more severe in pregnant women.

Counseling (Table 45.1)

Natural history, incidence of vertical transmission, and sequelae (mostly occurring if maternal infection occurs < 20 weeks), prognosis, and therapeutic options should all be reviewed with the pregnant woman with primary maternal VZV infection.

Prevention

VZV-seronegative pregnant women should avoid exposure to individuals with chickenpox. A live attenuated varicella vaccine (Varivax, Merck) has been demonstrated as safe in preventing chickenpox in adults. In the USA and in some European countries, seronegative women presenting for preconception counseling or women undergoing infertility treatment may be offered vaccination. The vaccine is not available in the UK for these indications. Varicella vaccine is contraindicated in pregnant women. If a woman accidentally receives VZV vaccine within 1 month of conception or in pregnancy, the incidence of fetal infection and complications

is extremely low, and termination should not be recommended (see also Chapter 37).[6] Non-immune health workers exposed to VZV should minimize patient contact from days 8–21 post-contact.

Screening

Routine serological screening of all pregnant women is currently not recommended. **All pregnant (and preconception reproductive-age) women should be asked at their first prenatal visit if they have had a chickenpox infection.** Over 95% of women who report a prior varicella infection have VZV IgG and are therefore immune. **All women who have not had chickenpox in the past or are unsure should have VZV IgG and IgM serology.** Of women who were uncertain, > 90% have VZV IgG; of women who give negative histories, about 50% have IgG. If testing is done in the preconception period, women can be offered two doses of varicella vaccine at least 1 month apart. Pregnancy should be delayed 1 month after vaccination. Based on a decision model, the above prenatal screening (selective serotesting) with postpartum vaccination of susceptibles would seem cost-effective.[7]

Work-up/diagnosis

Diagnosis of **maternal chickenpox** is usually made based on clinical findings alone. Diagnosis can be confirmed by **VZV IgM** newly positive by ELISA (enzyme-linked immunosorbent assay), or by VZV antigen (Ag) in skin/vesicular lesions by immunofluorescence antibody (Ab) to membrane Ag. **Fetal infection can be diagnosed by VZV DNA** detected by polymerase chain reaction (PCR) in amniotic fluid, but its presence is not synonymous with the development of CVS. The presence of fetal varicella-specific IgM, which remains in the blood for 4–5 weeks, is diagnostic.[8] **Ultrasound** can help in diagnosis and estimation of probability of CVS. **At least 5 weeks should be allowed between the onset of maternal symptoms and fetal ultrasound,** to avoid false-negative results. Initial PCR testing of amniotic fluid at 17–21 weeks may be negative with normal ultrasound, suggesting low risk of CVS. Positive PCR at 17–21 weeks with normal ultrasound should lead to repeat ultrasound at 22–26 weeks. A normal ultrasound at that stage makes CVS very unlikely. In contrast, abnormal ultrasound suggests a high likelihood of CVS.[9,10]

Therapy

Exposure

VZV-seronegative pregnant women exposed to VZV:

- should receive **VZV IgG** 625 U IM within 72–96 hours of exposure. VZV IgG may not prevent but may attenuate symptoms up to 10 days after exposure. It probably does not affect fetal infection, and it is expensive.

Chickenpox

Pregnant women who develop chickenpox:

- should receive oral **acyclovir** within 24 hours of rash. Oral acyclovir reduces the duration of fever and symptoms of varicella infection in immunocompetent adults if commenced within 24 hours of the onset of rash.[11] Administration of acyclovir does not appear to be teratogenic. Acyclovir is prescribed to treat extensive varicella at the high dose of 12.4 mg/kg of body weight or 500 mg/m² IV every 8 hours. Major side effects often include local tissue irritation, transient elevation of hepatic transaminases, CNS toxicity, and renal dysfunction. Transplacental passage of acyclovir is prompt, and therapeutic levels reach the placenta and fetal blood.[8]
- should **avoid contact with susceptible individuals** such as other pregnant women or children.
- should undergo symptomatic treatment and maintain hygiene to avoid bacterial superinfection.
- VZIG has no therapeutic effect once chickenpox has developed.
- If maternal infection occurs at term, there is a significant risk of varicella in the newborn. **Delivery should be delayed until 5 days after the onset of maternal illness,**

to allow for passive transfer of maternal IgG. Infants delivered within 5 days of maternal symptoms or 2 days after delivery are at 15–20% risk of getting neonatal varicella, and of these, about 30% can die. **Neonates born to women who develop chickenpox between 5 days before and 2 days after delivery should receive VZIG.** If neonatal infection occurs, the neonate should receive acyclovir.

- If there is neonatal exposure in the first 7 days of life (e.g. from an infected sibling), no intervention is required if the mother is immune; however, the neonate should be given VZIG if the mother is not immune to varicella. Neonates who develop chickenpox in the first 14 days of life should receive intravenous (IV) acyclovir.

Pregnant women who develop pulmonary chickenpox

- They should be immediately hospitalized in isolation.
- They should receive **IV acyclovir** 10–15 mg/kg × 7 days within 72 hours of symptoms (decreases severity and mortality).

Maternal shingles

Maternal shingles is **not a risk for the infant,** who is protected from passively acquired maternal antibodies.[3]

Non-immune women

Non-immune women should be offered **postpartum varicella vaccination.** The vaccine is considered safe in breast-feeding women. Conception should be delayed until 1 month after the VZV vaccine was given (live attenuated vaccine).

CLINICAL NEONATAL FINDINGS OF CVS[10]

- Skin scarring in a dermatomal distribution, 73%
- Neurological abnormalities (microcephaly, cortical atrophy, mental retardation), 62%
- Eye defects (microphthalmia, chorioretinitis), 52%
- Hypoplasia of the limbs, 46%
- Muscle hypoplasia, 20%
- Gastrointestinal abnormalities, 19%
- Genitourinary abnormalities, 12%
- Internal organs effects, 13%
- Developmental delay, 12%

REFERENCES

1. Harger JH, Ernest JM, Thurnau GR, et al. Frequency of congenital varicella syndrome in a prospective cohort of 347 pregnant women. Obstet Gynecol 2002; 100: 260–5. [II-3]
2. Tan MP, Koren G. Chickenpox in pregnancy: revisited. Reprod Toxicol 2006; 21: 410–20. [review]
3. Royal College of Obstet and Gynecol. Clinical Green Top Guideline: Chickenpox in pregnancy. January 17, 2005. [guideline]
4. Pretorius DH, Hayward I, Jones KL, Stamm E. Sonographic evaluation of pregnancies with maternal varicella infection. J Ultrasound Med 1992; 11: 459–63. [II-3]
5. National Advisory Committee on Immunization update on varicella. Can Common Dis Rep 2004; 30: 1–26. [review]
6. Gershon AA, Steinberg SP. Live attenuated varicella vaccine: protection in healthy adults compared with leukaemic children. National Institute of Allergy and Infectious Diseases Varicella Vaccine Collaborative Study Group. J Infect Dis 1990; 161: 661–6. [III]
7. Smith WJ, Jackson LA, Watts DH, Koepsell TD. Prevention of chickenpox in reproductive-age women: cost-effectiveness of routine prenatal screening with postpartum vaccination of susceptibles. Obstet Gynecol 1998; 92: 535–45. [III]
8. McGregor JA. Varicella zoster infection in pregnancy. Contemp Obstet Gynecol 2002; 4: 47–55. [review]
9. Enders G, Miller E. Varicella and Herpes Zoster in Pregnancy and in Newborn. Cambridge: Cambridge University Press; 2000: 317–47. [review]
10. Koren G. Congenital varicella syndrome in the third trimester. Lancet 2005; 366: 1591–2. [review]
11. Wallace MR, Bawler WA, Murray NB, Brodine SK, Oldfield EC III. Treatment of adults varicella with oral acyclovir. A randomized placebo-controlled trial. Ann Intern Med 1992; 117: 358–63. [RCT, non-pregnant adults]

46

Fetal death

Irina D Burd

KEY POINTS

- **Ultrasound examination** should be performed **for confirmation of fetal death.**
- The most informative examinations **to find the etiology** of fetal death are **autopsy** and **chromosomal analysis.**
- **Induction of labor** in patients with fetal death is recommended unless the patient is already in labor.
- **Misoprostol (e.g.** 400 µg vaginally every 4 hours) is the **most cost-effective method of delivery for fetal death <28 weeks, with acceptable side effects.**
- High-dose Prostin E2 (prostaglandin E_2; dinoprostone) suppositories are contraindicated >28 weeks' gestation.

DEFINITIONS

A fetal death is defined by the World Health Organization (WHO) as:

> death prior to the complete expulsion or extraction from the mother of a product of human conception, irrespective of the duration of pregnancy and which is not an induced termination of pregnancy.[1]

The WHO definition of fetal death does not exclude spontaneous abortion at <12 weeks, which has different etiologies and management than fetal death occurring in the second or third trimester. Substantial differences exist not only internationally but even in the USA on the definition of fetal death (Table 46.1).[2] The US National Center for Health Statistics (NCHS), a division of the Centers for Disease Control and Prevention (CDC), recommends defining **fetal death** as that of **intrauterine death occurring in fetuses weighing ≥350 g or at ≥20 weeks of** gestation,[1] and this is the definition used in this guideline.

Embryonic death is defined as death occurring at ≤12 weeks. *Early fetal death* is defined as death occurring at 13–19 6/7 weeks of gestation. *Intermediate fetal death* is defined as death occurring at 20–27 weeks of gestation. *Late fetal death* is defined as death occurring at >28 weeks of gestation. *Unexplained fetal death* is death before delivery with no identifiable cause after work-up. *Fetal demise* (often abbreviated IUFD, or intrauterine fetal demise) is defined as loss of fetus (≥12 weeks) at any stage. *Stillbirth* is defined as the birth of a neonate with absence of breathing, heartbeat, pulsation of the umbilical cord, or definite movements of voluntary muscles,[1] and has been used interchangeably at times with fetal death.

DIAGNOSIS

The diagnosis of fetal death should be **confirmed by ultrasound**, with absence of heart movements.

EPIDEMIOLOGY/INCIDENCE

In 2002 the fetal death rate was 6.4 per 1000 live births plus fetal deaths in the USA.[3] Close to one-half of these deaths occurred in the third trimester. When compared with 1990 data, the rate of early or intermediate fetal death remained stable at 3.2 per 1000, while the rate of late fetal death decreased from 4.3 to 3.2 per 1000.[4]

ASSOCIATIONS/RISK FACTORS/ POSSIBLE ETIOLOGIES (TABLE 46.2)

Many maternal and fetal factors have been associated with fetal death. Up to 50% of fetal deaths are not associated with any of these risks, and are called 'unexplained'. Fetal death rate is an important marker of quality of health care. Other factors associated with fetal demise are maternal age (both high and low), unmarried status, low socioeconomic status, black race,[5] low education, maternal obesity, male fetal sex, multiple gestation, multiparity (>5), and non-vertex presentation.[6–9]

Table 46.1 *Definitions of fetal deaths varying by state and location in the United States and territories (1997 reporting requirements)*

	All products of conception	Gestation of 16 weeks or longer	Gestation of 20 weeks or longer	Gestations of 5 months or longer	Birth weight of 350 g or more	Birth weight of 400 g or more	Birth weight of 500 g or more
Alabama, Alaska, California, Connecticut, Florida, Illinois, Indiana, Iowa, Maine, Maryland, Minnesota, Nebraska, Nevada, New Jersey, North Carolina, North Dakota, Ohio, Oklahoma, Oregon, Texas, Utah, Vermont, Washington, West Virginia, Wyoming			X				
American Samoa, Arkansas, Colorado, Georgia, Hawaii, New York, Northern Mariana Islands, Rhode Island, Virginia, Virgin Islands	X						
Arizona, Delaware, Guam, Idaho, Kentucky, Louisiana, Massachusetts, Mississippi, Missouri, Montana, New Hampshire, South Carolina, Wisconsin			X		X		
Michigan			X			X	
District of Columbia			X				X
Kansas					X		
Pennsylvania		X					
New Mexico, South Dakota, Tennessee							X
Puerto Rico				X			

Adapted from Lindsey.[2]

Smoking and alcohol abuse are two of the most common identifiable preventable causes of fetal death. Pesticides, radiation, and fertility drugs have also been associated with fetal death.

PREGNANCY MANAGEMENT
Counseling

Counseling should include review of possible etiologies, work-up, delivery options, as well as possible complications. Grieving counseling should be included, in addition to option for referral to grieving help groups, etc. Review of risk of recurrence, prevention of recurrence, and best management for a future pregnancy should be done mainly and accurately postpartum.

Work-up (Table 46.3)[10–18]

Evaluation of the etiology of fetal death is essential to counsel regarding recurrence risks, facilitate the grieving process, and improve understanding to facilitate therapeutic measures. The evaluation can be emotionally difficult, and should be multidisciplinary (obstetrician, maternal–fetal specialist, pathologist, geneticist, radiologist, etc.). Communication between all these members is most important. Work-up should include:

1. Review all **risk factors** to help identify specific possibilities (see Table 46.2). See the specific guideline (chapter) if a specific factor is identified as the probable cause. In family history, particular attention should be paid to pregnancy losses, consanguinity, mental retardation, diabetes, and congenital anomalies.

Table 46.2   *Associations/risk factors/possible etiologies of fetal death*

Maternal risk factors	Fetal risk factors	Other
Chronic hypertension[a]	**Congenital malformations** (up to 35%)	**Unexplained fetal death** (up to 50%)
Pre-eclampsia	**Chromosomal/genetic abnormalities** (up to 12%)	
Metabolic diseases (**diabetes mellitus,** thyroid disease, etc.)	IUGR Placental abruption, placenta and vasa previa	
Chronic renal disease	Placental pathology:	
Antiphospholipid syndrome	Chronic villitis Massive chorionic intervillositis	
Substance abuse (especially cocaine, alcohol, coffee: >3 cups/day, etc.)	Twin–twin transfusion syndrome Umbilical cord complications (nuchal cord or	
Smoking	knotted cord) Oligohydramnios	

Viral infections:
  Parvovirus B19
  Cytomegalovirus
  HSV-1, HSV-2
  Coxsackievirus
  HIV
	Fetomaternal hemorrhage
	Intrauterine asphyxia
	Uteroplacental insufficiency
	PPROM
	Male sex
	Postdates
	Autosomal metabolic disorders	

Bacterial infections:
  Listeria monocytogenes
  Escherichia coli
  Group B streptococci
  Ureaplasma urealyticum
  Treponema pallidum		

Parasitic infections: *Toxoplasma gondii*		
Severe anemia Cholestasis Cyanotic heart disease Inherited thrombophilias Isoimmunization		

[a] In bold, most common associations. IUGR, intrauterine growth restriction; PPROM, preterm premature rupture of membranes. Adapted from Lindsey.[2]

Table 46.3   *Maternal and fetal investigation for fetal death**

Maternal and fetal investigation	References
Pre-delivery	
Amniotic fluid for cytogenetics	10
Anticardiolipin antibody (ACA) and lupus anticoagulant (LA)	11
Kleihauer–Betke (fetal cell count)	12,13
Screen for coagulopathy (especially if fetal death >4 weeks from delivery)	14
Post-delivery	
Cord blood for culture and cytogenetics	15
Autopsy and placental examination	16–18
Fascia cytogenetics	15

* See text for additional information

All records should be reviewed for any possible association.

2. Before delivery, **detailed ultrasound**, fetal echocardiogram, 3D ultrasound, and whole-body X-rays, and/or magnetic resonance imaging (MRI) can be considered. These examinations should be recommended especially if a detailed autopsy will not be available. An **amniocentesis** (and/or chorionic villus sampling [CVS]) should be offered for karyotype and fetal infection work-up. About 5–10% of cells from amniotic fluid (AF) of fetal deaths fail to grow, but this yield is much higher than that obtained from postnatal study of karyotype.[19]

3. Before delivery, **obtain consent for fetal autopsy**. If consent is not given for a full autopsy, ask the parent to consider a limited autopsy such as external examination by a pathologist/clinical geneticist or an internal examination limited to brain and/or spinal cord, chest organs or abdominal organs as appropriate, or an MRI.[20]

4. At delivery, **examine the baby and placenta carefully.** Pictures, radiological evaluation (e.g. MRI, etc.), and a clinical geneticist evaluation may also be helpful.

5. Prior to autopsy, obtain tissue (e.g. skin with dermis, muscle/fascia from the fetal thigh; at least 1×1 cm specimen) for **cytogenetic and molecular genetic studies.** Skin surface should be cleansed with Betadine (povidone-iodine) or Hibiclens (chlorhexidine) prior to obtaining a specimen. Tissue should be placed in Hanks' solution (pink), or normal saline, if Hanks' solution is not available, not in formalin. A cytogenetic form should be completed with pertinent details.

6. **Autopsy** is the **most useful** step in identifying the cause of fetal death. It reduces the number of unexplained fetal deaths by at least 10%.[16] Autopsy should include X-rays of the fetus and photographs, and should follow College of American Pathologists guidelines (www.cap.org). Clinical information, all records including ultrasound reports regarding the case, and any specific requests should be made available to the pathologist. It is suggested to call the pathologist assigned to autopsy for discussion of the case. A perinatal pathologist with experience in fetal death cases should perform the autopsy.

7. Obtain tissue for **placental karyotype** (rule out confined placental mosaicism). Obtain a specimen from the fetal side of the placenta in a similar manner of No. 5 in a separate labeled container.

8. Consider obtaining **placental cultures** to rule out infectious cause (aerobic/anaerobic cultures).[21]

9. Send **placenta for pathological examination.** Consider asking the pathologist for estimation of placental infarcts.

10. Consider obtaining cord blood for culture, if possible.

11. Labs:
   a   complete blood count (CBC), antibody screen, urine drug screen (UDS)
   b   maternal toxoplasmosis, cytomegalovirus, herpesviridae, and parvovirus titers (IgM and IgG); check rapid plasma reagin (RPR) and rubella status
   c   Kleihauer–Betke (K-B)
   d   glucose (if glucose screening not done in pregnancy)
   e   anticardiolipin antibody (ACA), lupus anticoagulant (LA), and anti-β_2 glycoprotein-I.
   f   suggested thrombophilia work-up, in particular if placental thrombosis and/or infacts present, and no other etiology identified. (mother – antithrombin III, factor V Leiden, protein C, protein S, prothrombin gene mutation; fetus – factor V Leiden, methylenetetrahydrofolate reductase deficiency, prothrombin gene mutation).

12. Consider any other work-up, depending on risk factor identified in Table 46.2.

Up to 50% of fetal deaths will remain unexplained despite an adequate evaluation.[2,6] This is a diagnosis of exclusion.

For fetal demise before 20 weeks, consider individualized work-up and refer to recurrent pregnancy loss guidelines (Chapter 14 of *Obstetric Evidence Based Guidelines*).

Delivery/anesthesia

Once diagnosis is confirmed and counseling and work-up initiated, options for delivery should be discussed. Options include expectant management, induction, or dilation and evacuation (D&E).

Expectant management

Between 80 and 90% of women with fetal death will spontaneously enter labor within 3 weeks of fetal demise.[8] Duration of labor is shorter in patients with spontaneous labor.[22] However, the endomyometritis rate is reported higher in the spontaneous labor group (6% vs 1%). There is no difference in the frequency of postpartum hemorrhage, retained placenta, or need for blood transfusion. Retention of a dead fetus can cause chronic consumptive coagulopathy due to gradual release of thromboplastin from the placenta into the maternal circulation.[14] This usually occurs after 4 weeks, but may occur earlier. Coagulation abnormalities occur in about 3–4% of patients with uncomplicated fetal deaths over the next 4–8 weeks, and this number rises in the presence of abruption or uterine perforation.[14] Another disadvantage of expectant management is a long interval between fetal death and spontaneous labor, limiting the amount of information that can be obtained about the cause of death from a postmortem examination or autopsy of the baby. Moreover, women with fetal death find it difficult psychologically to continue a pregnancy with a known fetal death. In patients opting for spontaneous labor (especially **with a >4-week interval between fetal death and time of delivery**), **screen for coagulopathy** with fibrinogen level and platelet count measurement should be obtained prior to administration of neuraxial anesthesia, as well as other invasive procedures; a prothrombin time and activated partial thromboplastin time are optional as long as the patient has no obvious signs of bleeding.[14]

Induction

Induction of labor in women with fetal death is usually recommended, unless the patient is already in labor, given the problems mentioned with expectant management. Induction of labor is typically initiated soon after diagnosis of fetal death. **Drugs such as oxytocin and/or prostaglandins administered for induction of labor at or near term can be given according to standard obstetric protocols.** However, these regimens are often unsuccessful remote from term, and have been associated with long and painful labors since the uterus is less sensitive to oxytocin before term. Options for induction of labor at about 16 to 32–34 weeks include:

- misoprostol (prostaglandin 1, PGE_1)
- prostaglandins E_2 (PGE_2)
- high-dose oxytocin
- hypertonic saline.

These substances have been used as alternatives to oxytocin in the second and early third trimester inductions, especially in cases where the cervix is unfavorable and not ready to commence labor.[15]

For gestations < 28 weeks, misoprostol (200 µg vaginally every 4 hours, 400 µg vaginally or orally every 4 hours, or 600 µg vaginally every 12 hours) is the most effective agent for induction of labor and results in successful expulsion (mostly within 24 hours) in 80–100% of cases.[23–28] Misoprostol 400 µg given orally every 4 hours is more effective than misoprostol 200 µg given vaginally every 12 hours for the induction of second and third trimester pregnancy with intrauterine fetal death, but has more gastrointestinal side effects.[23] Misoprostol 600 µg administered vaginally at 12-hour intervals is associated with fewer adverse effects and is as effective as dosing at 6-hour intervals.[28] Misoprostol 200 mg intravaginal is associated with a shorter **mean induction–abortion interval than dinoprostone (prostaglandin E_2) 0.5 mg intracervical,**[29] **with a complete abortion rate of 87.5% in the misoprostol group and 60.6% in the dinoprostone group.** While the American College of Obstetricians and Gynecologists (ACOG) recommends that misoprostol should not be used for cervical ripening or labor induction in women with prior uterine incisions,[30] the risk of uterine rupture is 0% with one prior low-transverse (LT) cesarean delivery (CD), about 5–10% with ≥ two prior LT CD, and about 50% with prior vertical CD.[31]

PGE_2 suppositories (20 µg inserted vaginally every 4 hours) can also be administered until labor is induced. Pretreatment with acetaminophen, Compazine (prochlorperazine), and diphenoxylate is useful to minimize fever, nausea, vomiting, and diarrhea, which invariably occur. The PGE_2 dose should be reduced to 5–10 mg if used at a more advanced gestation (off-label use) as uterine sensitivity and the risk of uterine rupture increase with gestational age.[32] **High-dose prostaglandin E_2 suppositories are contraindicated > 28 weeks' gestation.**[33]

High-dose oxytocin (200 units in 500 ml saline at 50 ml/hour) may also be used for induction of labor remote from term.[34] **The mother should be observed for signs of water intoxication, and maternal electrolyte concentrations should be monitored at least every 24 hours.** Nausea and malaise are the earliest findings of hyponatremia, and may be seen when the plasma sodium concentration falls below 125–130 mEq/L. This may be followed by headache, lethargy, obtundation, and eventually seizures, coma, and respiratory arrest. Misoprostol 50 µg, with the dose doubled every 6 hours

until effective contractions, is associated with a success rate within 48 hours of induction of 100% compared with 96.7% to oxytocin infusion titrated based on patient response, with **mean induction to delivery time significantly longer (almost double) in the oxytocin group compared with the misoprostol group (23.3 vs 12.4 hours). Misoprostol is also cheaper (one-tenth the price of oxytocin).**[35]

The efficacy and tolerance of **mifepristone** (RU 486), a progesterone antagonist, was investigated in a double-blind controlled multicenter study involving 94 patients with an intrauterine fetal death.[36] Success of treatment was defined as the occurrence of fetal expulsion within 72 hours after the first drug intake. Mifepristone treatment (600 mg/day for 2 days) was considered to be effective in 29 of 46 patients (63%). There were only eight successes in 48 patients (17.4%) in the placebo group ($p = 0.001$). Tolerance was good in the mifepristone group. In the placebo group, disseminated intravascular coagulation (DIC) occurred in one woman for whom the investigator waited several weeks for spontaneous expulsion. Mifepristone is of interest in the management of intrauterine fetal death, **with more studies needed to compare the above methods, in particular misoprostol, with mifepristone.**

To date, there are no studies evaluating **Laminaria** for ripening of cervix in conjunction with other methods of induction.

Dilation and evacuation

There are no trials comparing surgical D&E with medical forms of induction in the second trimester. Comparing complication rates of patients who undergo D&E or medical induction **between 14 and 24 weeks of gestation,** D&E is a safe method in this time frame, especially if **done by experienced operators, under continuous ultrasound guidance.**[37]

POSTPARTUM

Before the patient's discharge, she needs to be counseled that results of all investigations may take 2 or 3 months for completion and that, despite extensive evaluation, a cause of death may not be found. **Grief counseling** should be initiated prior to discharge from hospital. No information is available from randomized trials to indicate whether there is or is not a benefit from providing specific psychological support or counseling after perinatal death.[38]

Prevention of recurrence and management in a future pregnancy

A **special outpatient visit** should be set up to review the results of the complete work-up, and discuss possible etiology and future management. If a particular medical problem is identified in the mother, it should be addressed prior to next conception (see specific guidelines). For example, tight control of blood glucose prior to conception can substantially reduce the risk of congenital anomalies in the fetus of a diabetic mother. Preconception counseling is helpful if congenital anomalies or genetic abnormalities are found. In the future, comparative genomic hybridization, FISH (fluorescent in-situ hybridization), and other novel genetic techniques will provide better ways to work-up the myriad genetic causes of fetal death. A woman with a prior fetal loss and either factor V or prothrombin heterozygocity, or protein S deficiency, might benefit from enoxaparin 40 mg subcutaneously daily, starting at 8 weeks.[39] In some cases, such as cord occlusion, the patient can be assured that recurrence is very unlikely.[40,41] Fetal death of unknown cause has a low risk of recurrence. Overall, there is a slightly increased incidence of other common pregnancy complications, such as preterm birth and intrauterine growth restriction (IUGR), in subsequent pregnancies (odds ratio [OR] = ~ 2–3). Most patients find increased fetal surveillance with the next pregnancy reassuring. Frequent ultrasound is reassuring, but has not been evaluated in trials, with false-positive results possibly detrimental. Weekly biophysical profile or fetal heart rate testing can be combined with maternal kick counts starting at 32 weeks. Elective induction can be discussed with the patient in terms of risks and benefits, at 39 weeks, or earlier if fetal lung maturity has been proven.

REFERENCES

1. Procedures for coding fetal cause of death (2003 revision). Available at: http://www.cdc.gov/nchs/about/major/fetaldth/abfetal.htm#Data%20Highlights. [review]
2. Lindsey JL. Evaluation of fetal death. E-medicine. Last updated 9/17/04. [review]
3. Martin JA, Kochanek KD, Strobino DM, Guyer B, MacDorman MF. Annual summary of vital statistics – 2003. Pediatrics 2005; 115: 619–34. [Health statistics]
4. Centers for Disease Control and Prevention (CDC). Racial/ethnic trends in fetal mortality – United States, 1990–2000. MMWR Morb Mortal Wkly Rep 2004; 53: 529–32. [data review]
5. Vintzileos AM, Ananth CV, Smulian JC, Scorza WE, Knuppel RA. Prenatal care black-white fetal death disparity in the United States: heterogeneity by high-risk conditions. Obstet Gynecol 2002; 99(3): 483–9. [II-3]
6. Centers for Disease Control and Prevention, National Center for Health Statistics, National Vital Statistics System: Arias E, Anderson RN, Kung HC, Murphy SL, Kochanek KD. Deaths: final data for 2001. National Vital Statistics Reports; 52(3). Hyattsville, Maryland: National Center for Health Statistics; 2003. [data review]
7. Froen JF, Arnestad M, Frey K, et al. Risk factors for sudden intrauterine unexplained death: epidemiologic characteristics of singleton cases in Oslo, Norway, 1986–1995. Am J Obstet Gynecol 2001; 184: 694–702. [II-2]
8. ACOG. Diagnosis and management of fetal death. ACOG Technical Bulletin No. 176, January 1993. [review]
9. Oron T, Sheiner E, Shoham-Vardi I, et al. Risk factors for antepartum fetal death. J Reprod Med 2001; 46(9): 825–30. [II-2]
10. Brady K, Duff P, Harlass FE, Reid S. The role of amniotic fluid cytogenetic analysis in the evaluation of recent fetal death. Am J Perinatol 1991; 8: 68–70. [II-2]
11. Lockwood CJ, Rand JH. The immunobiology and obstetrical consequences of antiphospholipid antibodies. Obstet Gynecol Surv 1994; 49: 432–41. [II-3]
12. Laube DW, Schauberger CW. Fetomaternal bleeding as a cause for "unexplained" fetal death. Obstet Gynecol 1982; 60: 649–51. [II-3]
13. Owen J, Stedman CM, Tucker TL. Comparison of predelivery versus postdelivery Kleihauer–Betke stains in cases of fetal death. Am J Obstet Gynecol 1989; 161: 663–6. [II-2]
14. Maslow AD, Breen TW, Sarna MC, et al. Prevalence of coagulation abnormalities associated with intrauterine fetal death. Can J Anaesth 1996; 43(12): 1237–43. [II-3]
15. ACOG. Genetic evaluation of stillbirths and neonatal deaths. ACOG Committee Opinion. No. 178, November 1996. Committee on Genetics. American College of Obstetricians and Gynecologists. [review]
16. Incerpi MH, Miller DA, Samandi R, Settlage RH, Goodwin TM. Stillbirth evaluation: what tests are needed. Am J Obstet Gynecol 1998; 178: 1121–5. [II-3]
17. Ahlenius I, Floberg J, Thomassen P. Sixty-six cases of intrauterine fetal death. A prospective study with an extensive test protocol. Acta Obstet Gynecol Scand 1995; 74(2): 109–17. [II-2]
18. Langston C, Kaplan C, Macpherson T, et al. Practice guideline for examination of the placenta: developed by the Placental Pathology Practice Guideline Development Task Force of the College of American Pathologists. Arch Pathol Lab Med 1997; 121: 449–76. [review]
19. Khare M, Howarth E, Sandler J, Healey K, Konje JC. A comparison of prenatal versus postnatal karyotyping for the investigation of intrauterine fetal death after the first trimester of pregnancy. Prenat Diagn 2005; 25: 1192–5. [II-2]
20. Woodward PJ, Sohaey R, Harris DP, et al. Postmortem fetal MR imaging: comparison with findings at autopsy. AJR Am J Roentgenol 1997; 168(1): 41–6. [II-2]
21. Goldenberg RL, Thompson C. The infectious origins of stillbirth. Am J Obstet Gynecol 2003; 189: 861–73. [II-2]
22. Salamat SM, Landy HJ, O'Sullivan MJ. Labor induction after fetal death. A retrospective analysis. J Reprod Med 2002; 47(1): 23–6. [II-2]
23. Bugalho A, Bique C, Machungo F, Bergstrom S. Vaginal misoprostol as an alternative to oxytocin for induction of labor in women with late fetal death. Acta Obstet Gynecol Scand 1995; 74: 194–8. [II-2]
24. Bugalho A, Bique C, Machungo F, Faaundes A. Induction of labor with intravaginal misoprostol in intrauterine fetal death. Am J Obstet Gynecol 1994; 171(2): 538–41. [II-2]
25. Merrell DA, Koch MA. Induction of labour with intravaginal misoprostol in the second and third trimesters of pregnancy. S Afr Med J 1995; 85(10 Suppl): 1088–90. [II-2]
26. Eng NS, Guan AC. Comparative study of intravaginal misoprostol with gemeprost as an abortifacient in second trimester missed abortion. Aust N Z J Obstet Gynaecol 1997; 37(3): 331–4. [II-1]
27. Chittacharoen A, Herabutya Y, Punyavachira P. A randomized trial of oral and vaginal misoprostol to manage delivery in cases of fetal death. Obstet Gynecol 2003; 101(1): 70–3. [RCT, *n* = 80]
28. Herabutya Y, Chanrachakul B, Punyavachira P. A randomised controlled trial of 6 and 12 hourly administration of vaginal misoprostol for second trimester pregnancy termination. BJOG 2005; 112(9): 1297–301. [RCT, *n* = 279]
29. Kara M, Ozden S, Eroglu M, Cetin A, Arioglu P. Comparison of misoprostol and dinoproston administration for the induction of labour in second trimester pregnancies in cases of intrauterine fetal loss. Ital J Gynaec Obstet 1999; 11(1): 13–16. [RCT, *n* = 65]
30. American College of Obstetricians and Gynecologists. Induction of labor with misoprostol. ACOG Committee Opinion No. 228. Washington, DC: American College of Obstetricians and Gynecologists; 2000. [review]

31. Airoldi J, O'Neill AM, Einhorn K, Hoffman M, Berghella V. Misoprostol for second trimester labor induction in women with prior cesarean deliveries: does the type and number of incisions matter? Obstet Gynecol 2006; 107: 59–60s [II-2 and review of the literature]

32. Kent DR, Goldstein AI, Linzey EM. Safety and efficacy of vaginal prostaglandin E$_2$ suppositories in the management of third-trimester fetal demise. J Reprod Med 1984; 29: 101–2. [II-2]

33. PROSTIN E2 ® Vaginal Suppository package insert. [III]

34. Toaff R, Ayalon D, Gogol G. Clinical use of high concentration drip. Obstet Gynecol 1971; 37: 112–20. [II-3]

35. Nakintu N. A comparative study of vaginal misoprostol and intravenous oxytocin for induction of labour in women with intra uterine fetal death in Mulago Hospital, Uganda. Afr Health Sci 2001; 1(2): 55–9. [RCT, $n = 120$]

36. Cabrol D, Dubois C, Cronje H, et al. Induction of labor with mifepristone (RU 486) in intrauterine fetal death. Am J Obstet Gynecol 1990; 163(2): 540–2. [II-2]

37. Autry AM, Hayes EC, Jacobson GF, Kirby RS. A comparison of medical induction and dilation and evacuation for second-trimester abortion. Am J Obstet Gynecol 2002; 187(2): 393–7. [RCT; $n = 297$]

38. Chambers HM, Chan FY. Support for women/families after perinatal death. Cochrane Database Syst Rev 2007; 1. [meta-analysis]

39. Gris JC, Mercier E, Quere I, et al. Low-molecular-weight heparin versus low-dose aspirin in women with one fetal loss and a constitutional thrombophilic disorder. Blood 2004; 103(10): 3695–9. [RCT, $n = 160$]

40. Verdel MJ, Exalto N. Tight nuchal coiling of the umbilical cord causing fetal death. J Clin Ultrasound 1994; 22(1): 64–6. [II-2]

41. Carey JC, Rayburn WF. Nuchal cord encirclements and risk of stillbirth. Int J Gynaecol Obstet 2000; 69(2): 173–4. [II-2]

47

Hemolytic disease of the fetus/neonate

Giancarlo Mari, Farhan Hanif and Kathryin Drennan

KEY POINTS

- The formation of maternal antibodies to fetal red blood cell (RBC) antigents is called **RBC alloimmunization,** and can lead to hemolytic disease and anemia of the fetus/neonate.
- Maternal **Rh(D) alloimmunization** is the most common RBC alloimmunization, and occurs when a pregnant woman develops an immunological response to a paternally derived Rh(D) antigen foreign to the mother and inherited by the fetus. The IgG antibodies cross the placenta, bind to the antigens on the fetal RBCs, and can cause hemolysis.
- **Anti-D immunoglobulin** prophylaxis properly given prevents >99% of cases of alloimmunization if given **both antepartum and postpartum.** It should be given to all Rh(D)-negative women with a negative antibody screen **at 28 weeks,** and, if the neonate is Rh(D) positive, within 72 hours **after birth.** Anti-D immunoglobulin can be given **as late as 28 days postpartum** if previously not given but indicated. **Anti-D immunoglobulin prophylaxis is 300 μg** (1 μg = 5 IU) at 28 weeks, **as well as after delivery if the neonate is Rh(D) positive.** A 100 μg dose administered at 28 and 34 weeks is also used. However, there are no trials to directly compare the different regimes. Mothers who are **weak D** positive (formerly called Du) **do not need anti-D prophylaxis.** A Kleihauer–Betke (KB) test should be ordered **to determine** the amount of fetal cells that has entered the maternal circulation, and hence **the appropriate dose of anti-D immunoglobulin** in certain high-risk situations (abdominal trauma, abruption, manual extraction of the placenta, etc.) or, if the 100 μg dose is used, after every delivery of an Rh(D) negative, non-alloimmunized woman.
- If **Rh(D) antibodies are detected in the maternal circulation on the antibody screen, the patient is considered alloimmunized.** Management of the **alloimmunized** pregnancy is shown in Figure 47.1. This is based initially on genotyping of the fetus' father, and, if necessary, fetal Rh(D) status determination, usually by polymerase chain reaction (PCR) from amniocytes. Maternal blood for fetal DNA testing is also available. **The critical titer for Rh(D) antibody should be determined in each laboratory.**
- **Ultrasound** using the **middle cerebral artery peak systolic velocity (MCA PSV)** has 100% sensitivity for detecting significant fetal anemia (95% CI: 0.86–1.00), **and is the screening method of choice in RBC alloimmunized pregnancies,** if available and quality assurance can be confirmed. **Compared with amniocentesis for** ΔOD_{450}, **MCA PSV assessment is associated with about a 70–80% reduction in the number of invasive tests. Screening with MCA PSV can be started as early as 15 weeks. If MCA PSV is ≥1.5 MoM, fetal blood sampling (FBS) is indicated.** When a cordocentesis is performed at >24 weeks' gestation, Corticosteroids for fetal maturation should be considered before the procedure, and blood tranfusion initiated for fetal hemoglobin < 5th percentile.
- If adequately trained sonologists are not available, screening for anemia should be done with amniocentesis using ΔOD_{450} values.
- In **Kell** alloimmunized pregnancies, **maternal titers do not correlate** well with fetal alloimmune disease. ΔOD_{450} levels also **do not correlate** with fetal anemia. **MCA PSV screening, instead, is predictive and accurate for the diagnosis of fetal anemia from Kell alloimmunization.**

DEFINITION

The formation of maternal antibodies to fetal red blood cell (RBC) antigens is called **RBC alloimmunization** or isoimmunization. Both terms are at times used interchangeably to describe this disease. Erythroblastosis fetalis is an older term for the same condition.[1] Maternal RBC alloimmunization can cause hemolytic disease of the fetus/neonate.

EPIDEMIOLOGY/INCIDENCE

The most common RBC antigen for alloimmunization is Rh(D).[2] The Rh(D)-negative blood group is found in about

15% of whites, 3–5% of black Africans, and is rare in Asians. The risk of Rh(D) alloimmunization during or immediately after a first pregnancy is about 0.7–1%. The risk of fetal anemia from RBC alloimmunization is about 0.35%, of which about 10% require transfusion. Rh(D) alloimmunization affects 6.7 out of every 1000 live births.[3]

GENETICS

Most Rh(D)-negative pregnant women have a deletion of the sequence on both copies of chromosome 1.

ETIOLOGY/BASIC PATHOPHYSIOLOGY

Maternal Rh(D) alloimmunization occurs when a pregnant woman develops an immunological response to a paternally derived RBC antigen – e.g. Rh(D) – foreign to the mother and inherited by the fetus. The immunoglobulin G (IgG) antibodies cross the placenta, bind to the antigens on the fetal RBCs, and can cause hemolysis. Hemolysis then causes anemia, which, if severe, leads to fetal cardiac failure, edema, hydrops, and eventually fetal death. Other antigens ('irregular antigens') than Rh(D) can cause RBC alloimmunization (see below).

NATURAL HISTORY

About 17% of Rh(D)-negative women who do not receive prophylaxis become immunized. Over 90% of this immunization occurs from fetomaternal hemorrhage at delivery, and the majority of the remaining 10% occurs in the third trimester. Most of this immunization is caused by just < 0.1 ml of fetomaternal hemorrhage. Before anti(D) immunoglobulin prevention, hemolytic disease of the fetus/ neonate affected 9–10% of pregnancies, and was a major cause of perinatal mortality. Risk of RBC alloimmunization from different clinical situations is shown in Table 47.1.

PREGNANCY MANAGEMENT
Prevention (Anti-D immunoglobulin)

The ABO, the Rh(D) status, and the antibody screen should be determined in all pregnant women at the initial prenatal visit. If the woman is Rh-negative and the antibody screen is negative, the patient should receive Rh(D) immune globulin. Anti-D immunoglobulin prophylaxis properly given prevents > 99% of cases alloimmunization. It is controversial whether the antibody screen should be repeated at 28 weeks before the administration of immune globulin.

Table 47.1 *Risk of RBC alloimmunization from different clinical situations*

Clinical situation	Risk of RBC alloimmunization (%)
Induced abortions	4–5
First trimester losses	1–2
CVS	14
Amniocentesis	7–15
External cephalic version	2–6
Threatened abortion	↑ (controversial)
Antepartum hemorrhage	↑↑
Placenta previa with bleeding	↑
Suspected abruption	↑
Blunt trauma to abdomen (including motor vehicle accidents)	↑
Fetal death	↑
Fetal blood sampling	↑
Fetal surgery	↑
Ectopic	↑
Partial molar pregnancy	↑

RBC, red blood cells; CVS, chorionic villus sampling.

The advantage of this second screening test is the detection of those rare cases in which immunization occurs early in pregnancy. After delivery if the neonate is Rh(D) positive, the patient should receive immune globulin. If the patient has never received immune globulin and the screening test is positive, the patient is at risk for having an anemic baby in the current pregnancy (if she has not delivered yet) or in a future pregnancy if she has delivered. The anti-D immune globulin affects the antibody screen.[4] Usually the effect of the immune globulin is not present until 12 weeks after its administration.

Anti-D immunoglobulin prophylaxis properly given prevents the majority of cases of alloimmunization. Unfortunately, there is no immunoglobulin available for prevention of RBC antigens other than Rh(D). Anti-D immunoglobulin is extracted by cold alcohol fractionation from plasma of individuals with high-titer D IgG antibodies. The risk of transmissions of viral infections or side effects is minimal to absent, and clinically not a significant factor.

The accepted regimens of **anti-D immunoglobulin prophylaxis are 100 μg at 28 and 34 weeks as well as after delivery if the neonate is Rh(D) positive, or 300 μg at 28 weeks** and after delivery if the neonate is Rh(D) **positive** and delivery occurs at least 3 weeks after the first administration. There are no trials to compare directly these two regimens, but they probably both achieve > 99% prevention of Rh(D) alloimmunization. The half-life of anti-D immunoglobulin is 16–24 days. When the 300 µg dose is used and delivery has not occurred within 12 weeks of injection, a second 300 µg dose of anti-D immunoglobulin should be given. The antibody titer obtained at delivery can occasionally still be positive (1:1, 1:2 titer) after anti-D immunoglobulin at 28 weeks' gestation. When indicated, a second dose of immune globulin is administered after delivery, even in cases of preterm delivery.

Mothers who are **D** positive, with D present in reduced quantities (formerly called Du) **do not need anti-D prophylaxis.** Mothers who are **partial D** positive (lacking some epitopes of D) should receive anti-D immunoglobulin, since they are at risk for hemolytic disease.[5] In those cases where the **father of the fetus/neonate is definitely known to be Rh(D) negative,** neither antepartum nor postpartum anti-D prophylaxis is administered.

Evidence for dosing and timing

After birth (postpartum)

Anti-D immunoglobulin given within 72 hours **after childbirth** is associated with a **96% decreased incidence of Rh(D) alloimmunization 6 months after birth** and a 88% **decreased incidence of Rh(D) alloimmunization in a subsequent pregnancy** in Rh(D)-negative women who have given birth to an Rh(D)-positive infant.[6] These benefits are seen, regardless of the ABO status of the mother and baby. **Higher doses (up to 200 µg) are more effective than lower doses (up to 50 µg)** in preventing Rh(D) alloimmunization.[6] Anti-D immunoglobulin can be given **as late as 28 days postpartum** if indicated but previously not given. **Anti-D immunoglobulin is given to all Rh(D)-negative women after confirmation from cord blood of Rh(D)-positive status of the neonate.** Even when immune globulin is correctly administered and with higher doses, alloimmunization can still occur (antepartum) in up to 2% with postpartum anti-D administration only.

Before birth

The addition of anti-D immunoglobulin 100 µg (500 international unit [IU]) prophylaxis at 28 and 34 weeks **lowers this risk to about 0.2%** without any adverse effects.[7–9] When women receive anti-D immunoglobulin at 28 **and** 34 weeks' gestation, there is a trend for less immunization during pregnancy for all women (relative risk [RR] = 0.42, 95% confidence interval (CI) 0.15–1.17); and for women giving birth to an Rh-positive infant (RR = 0.41, 95% CI 0.16–1.04) compared with no prophylaxis.[7–9] In trials that used a 100 µg dose of anti-D immunoglobulin, there was a

non-significant reduction in immunization at 2–12 months following birth of a Rh-positive infant in women who had received anti-D (RR = 0.14, 95% CI 0.02–1.15). However, women receiving anti-D were significantly less likely to have a positive Kleihauer–Betke (KB) test (which detects fetal cells in maternal blood) in pregnancy (RR = 0.60, 95% CI 0.41–0.88) and at the birth of an Rh-positive infant (RR = 0.60, 95% CI 0.46–0.79).[8] No data were available for the risk of Rh(D) alloimmunization in a subsequent pregnancy. No differences were seen for neonatal jaundice.

There are no trials using the 300 µg dose, or trials comparing just 28-week vs both 28- and 34-week prophylaxis.

Even with antepartum and postpartum prophylaxis, the risk of Rh(D) alloimmunization remains because of inadvertent antepartum or postpartum omission, failure to use the drug for other antenatal complications, and insufficient dosing at delivery in cases of large fetomaternal hemorrhage.

Practice guidelines in the United States recommend that anti-D immunoglobulin be administered early in the third trimester, **300 µg at 28 weeks of gestation.** This practice reduces the incidence of antenatal alloimmunization from 2 to 0.1%.[2,3] In the **United Kingdom, 100 µg** of anti-D immunoglobulin is given at 28 and 34 weeks of gestation.[5] **In Canada, 100 to 120 µg** is administered at 28 and 34 weeks.

Special clinical situations

In addition to antepartum and postpartum prophylaxis, other indications for anti-D immunoglobulin include those situations in which there is a significant risk of fetomaternal hemorrhage. These indications are listed in Table 47.1. Anti-D immunoglobulin should be given for threatened abortion probably only in cases with significant bleeding. A repeat dose is unnecessary after prophylaxis if delivery occurs < 3 weeks from the last dose.

Anti-D immunoglobulin 300 µg protects against 30 ml of fetal whole blood or 15 ml of fetal RBCs in the maternal circulation. In certain high-risk situations in which excessive fetomaternal bleeding may have occurred (e.g. abruption, manual removal of placenta, abdominal trauma), this dose may be inadequate, and a **KB test** should be done **to determine** the amount of fetal cells that have entered the maternal circulation and hence **the appropriate dose of anti-D immunoglobulin** to be given. Some clinicians have advocated the KB test for all Rh(D)-negative women at delivery, since 50% of cases requiring more than the standard posPartum dose of anti-D immunoglobulin can be missed by high-risk situation screening only.[10] **The risk of fetal–maternal hemorrhage > 30 ml is about 0.1–0.2%.**

The anti-D immunoglobulin available in the USA (e.g. RhoGam, Rhophylac, WinRho; and BabyRho-D) and other countries are all very effective, with none shown to be significantly more effective in prevention of hemolytic disease than the others; thus, cost and route of administration – e.g. intramuscular (IM) and intravenous (IV) – may be the only factors determining choice.

Management of RBC allommunized pregnancies

Counseling

If Rh(D) antibodies are detected in the maternal circulation on the antibody screen (e.g. positive indirect Coombs' test), **the patient is considered alloimmunized.** Among Rh(D)-alloimmunized pregnancies, mild-to-moderate hemolytic anemia and hyperbilirubinemia occur in 25–30% of fetuses/neonates, and 25% of these can develop hydrops.[11] With correct management, the **perinatal survival rate in cases of anemia is >90%;** when fetal hydrops is present, survival is often >80%. There is no trial that has assessed the best management for RBC alloimmunized pregnancies, but fetal transfusion is probably the most beneficial of all fetal therapies available. Although it is reported that the risk of fetal demise is between 1% and 2% for each fetal blood sampling, there are situations in which the risk is much higher (for example, when cordocenteses and transfusions are performed at gestational ages as early as 15–18 weeks).

Work-up/investigations required

Management of the **alloimmunized** pregnancy is shown in Figure 47.1. In patients at risk for fetal anemia because of RBC alloimmunization, it is important to perform a first trimester ultrasound to establish the gestational age. Assessment for risk of fetal anemia depends on history of Rh complications in previous pregnancies, titer of RBC antibodies, and MCA PSV values.[12–13]

The genotype of the fetus' father should be determined by zygosity testing. The most likely zygosity can also be predicted by evaluating the pattern of C, D, and E loci, since they are inherited together and some combinations are more common than others, but this is not 100% exact and not very useful now clinically. If the father is Rh(D) negative, no further testing or intervention is necessary. If the father is heterozygous for the Rh(D) antigen, fetal Rh(D) testing is indicated. If the father is Rh(D) homozygous, the fetus is assumed to be Rh(D) positive, and no fetal Rh(D) status testing is necessary. Of course the paternity should be certain, otherwise fetal testing is indicated.

Fetal Rh(D) status can be determined by polymerase chain reaction **(PCR) from amniocytes** with >95% accuracy (sensitivity and specificity). This is available in the USA in several centers: one of them is the Blood Center of Southeastern Wisconsin (www.bloodcenter.com). This is also available for many other antigens, such as c, E, Kell, M, N, etc. Chorionic villus sampling (CVS) is not advised, as it results in a high risk of worsening alloimmunization from fetomaternal hemorrhage. Determination of fetal Rh(D) status can **also** now be obtained **non-invasively,** with fetal DNA analysis from maternal blood.[14,15] This can be done through the International Blood Group Reference Laboratory in Bristol, UK, or, under research basis, the Blood Center of Southeastern Wisconsin.

Rh(D) antibody titers correlate somewhat with risk of anemia/hydrops, with 1:16 = 10%, 1:32 = 25%, 1:64 = 50%, and 1:128 = 75% risk of anemia. **The critical titer should be determined in each laboratory.** Unfortunately, large differences in titer can be seen in the same woman between laboratories. In most laboratories, the critical titer is ≥ 1:16 in albumin or ≥ 1:32 in indirect antiglobulin (indirect Coombs' test). If the titer is less than 1:16, the fetus is not in jeopardy at that time. However, serial titers should be obtained every 4 weeks. If the patient has had a prior affected pregnancy, and the fetus is known to be Rh(D) positive, titers are not necessary. The MCA PSV is used to detect those fetuses that are going to develop anemia.[16] The presence of additional antibody(ies) with anti-D increases the need for intrauterine fetal transfusions.

Ultrasound is the screening method of choice for fetal anemia. With fetal anemia, decreased blood viscosity leads to increased venous return, consequent increase in cardiac output, with increased blood flow velocity in all vessels. Degrees of anemia correlate with blood velocity. The vessel to study is the **middle cerebral artery (MCA).** The main advantage of the MCA is that it is easy to measure at a 0° angle. In the biparietal diameter view, the MCA can be visualized with color Doppler. The MCA **peak systolic velocity (MCA PSV)** should be measured at its proximal point, after the origin from the internal carotid artery, at a 0° angle (avoiding angle correction). Measurement at this point allows the lowest intra- and inter-observer variability as well as standardization of the measurement.[18] Multiples of the median (MoM) for the **hemoglobin concentration** (Table 47.2) and **MCA PSV** (Table 47.3 and Figure 47.2) correct for the effect of gestational age (GA) on the measurements.[13] The MCA PSV has a sensitivity of 100% (95% CI 0.86–1.0) for detection of significant fetal anemia with a false positive rate of 12% at 1.50 MoM.[13] The number of false positive increases following 35 weeks' gestation.[19] The number of false positive cases after 35 weeks may be decreased by looking at the trend of the MCA PSV.[16]

Compared with amniocentesis for ΔOD_{450}, the MCA PSV assessment is associated with a 70–80% reduction in the

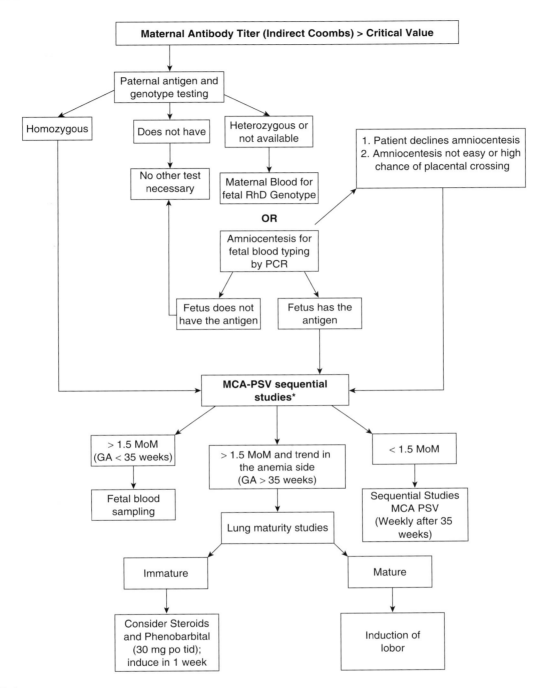

Figure 47.1
Managing a first sensitized pregnancy. MCA PSV, middle cerebral artery peak systolic velocity; PCR, polymerase chain reaction; MoM, multiples of the median; GA, gestational age; PO, orally; tid, three times per day; *The MCA PSV is more accurate tha the delta OD450 for the diagnosis of fetal anemia. When the MCA PSV is not available, delta OD450 is used.

number of invasive tests.[13] The MCA PSV is more accurate than amniocentesis in detecting fetal anemia.[20–23]

The correction of fetal anemia with intrauterine transfusion decreases significantly and normalizes the value of fetal MCA PSV,[24–25] because of an increased blood viscosity and an increased oxygen concentration in fetal blood. The MCA PSV may be used in fetuses previously transfused.[26–27]

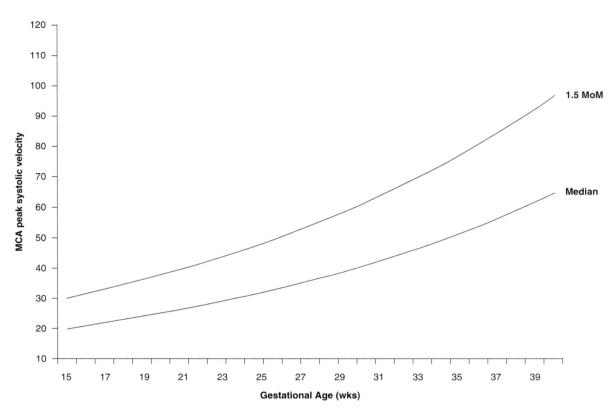

Figure 47.2
Graph of MCA PSV correlated to gestational age. MCA, middle cerebral artery; MoM, multiples of the median.
See also Table 47.3 for exact values of MoMs.

The accuracy with MCA PSV can only be achieved with appropriate training and quality assurance. If adequately trained sonographers are not available, screening for anemia should be done with amniocentesis (see below). Screening with MCA PSV can be started as early as 15 weeks.[28] MCA PSV can also be used for other causes of anemia, including parvovirus infection, non-immune hydrops, fetal maternal hemorrhage, and twin-twin transfusion syndrome.

The steps for the correct measurement of the MCA PSV are the following: (A) an axial section of the head is obtained at level of the sphenoid bones; (B) color Doppler evidences the Circle of Willis; (C) the circle of Willis is enlarged; (D) the color box is placed around the MCA; (E) the MCA is zoomed; (F) the MCA flow velocity waveforms are displayed and the highest point of the waveform (PSV) is measured. The waveforms should be all similar. The above sequence is repeated at least three times in each fetus.

Severe intra-uterine growth restriction (IUGR) has also an increased MCA PSV.[29] Therefore, this should be taken into account when the MCA PSV is used. However, it is very unlikely that an anemic fetus is also a severe IUGR fetus. Moderate to severe fetal anemia may also be suggested by hydropic signs (at least two out of pericardial or pleural effusion, ascites, skin edema), or increase in size of fetal liver or placental thickness, or tricuspid regurgitation.

Amniocentesis for ΔOD_{450} measurement is used if accurate MCA screening is not available. The ΔOD_{450} measurement can be evaluated using either the Liley[30] or Queenan[31] charts. There is controversy over which one is best before 27 weeks, the 'extended' Liley curve or the Queenan curve.[32] The guidelines for the amniocentesis are arbitrary and serial MCA PSV measurements are superior in terms of sensitivity, specificity, and positive and negative predictive values to both the Liley and the Queenan curves.[23] If the MCA PSV test cannot be done and the patient opts for an amniocentesis, the

Table 47.2 *Reference ranges for fetal hemoglobin concentrations as a function of gestational age[a]*

Week of gestation	Fetal hemoglobin concentration (g/dl) Multiples of the median				
	1.16	1.00 (median)	0.84	0.65	0.55
18	12.3	10.6	8.9	6.9	5.8
20	12.9	11.1	9.3	7.2	6.1
22	13.4	11.6	9.7	7.5	6.4
24	13.9	12.0	10.1	7.8	6.6
26	14.3	12.3	10.3	8.0	6.8
28	14.6	12.6	10.6	8.2	6.9
30	14.8	12.8	10.8	8.3	7.1
32	15.2	13.1	10.9	8.5	7.2
34	15.4	13.3	11.2	8.6	7.3
36	15.6	13.5	11.3	8.7	7.4
38	15.8	13.6	11.4	8.9	7.5
40	16.0	13.8	11.6	9.0	7.6

[a]The values at 1.16 and 0.84 multiples of the median (MoM) correspond to the 95th and 5th percentiles, respectively (the normal range):
- mild anemia – hemoglobin concentration between 0.84 and 0.65 MoM
- moderate anemia – hemoglobin concentration between 0.65 and 0.55 MoM
- severe anemia – hemoglobin concentration < 0.55 MoM.

From Mari et al,[13] with permission. Copyright © 2000 Massachusetts Medical Society. All rights reserved.

Table 47.3 *Expected peak velocity of systolic blood flow in the middle cerebral artery as a function of gestational age[a]*

Week of Gestation	MCA PSV (cm/s) Multiples of the median			
	1.00 (median)	1.29	1.50	1.55
18	23.2	29.9	34.8	36.0
20	25.5	32.8	38.2	39.5
22	27.9	36.0	41.9	43.3
24	30.7	39.5	46.0	47.5
26	33.6	43.3	50.4	52.1
28	36.9	47.9	55.4	57.2
30	40.5	52.2	60.7	62.8
32	44.4	57.3	66.6	68.9
34	48.7	62.9	73.1	75.6
36	53.5	69.0	80.2	82.9
38	58.7	75.7	88.0	91.0
40	64.4	83.0	96.6	99.8

MCA PSV, middle cerebral artery peak systolic velocity; MoM, multiples of the median.
[a]Mild anemia – MCA PSV between 1.29 and 1.49 MoM
Moderate anemia – MCA PSV between 1.50 and 1.54 MoM
Severe anemia – MCA PSV ≥ 1.55 MoM.
From Mari et al,[13] with permission. Copyright © 2000 Massachusetts Medical Society. All rights reserved.

followings are general guidelines for managing the Liley curve readings:

- **Zone 1:** repeat amniocentesis in 2–4 weeks. If zone 1, follow with ultrasound every 1 or 2 weeks until delivery.
- **Zone 2 (low/middle third):** repeat amniocentesis in about 2 weeks. If low zone 2, follow with ultrasound every week until delivery. If upper third zone 2, consider FBS.
- **Zone 2 (upper third):** consider FBS, or repeat amniocentesis in 7 days. If again upper third zone 2 or higher, FBS.
- **Zone 3:** FBS.

The advantage of using Queenan's curve is that it can be used following 14 weeks' gestation. Amniocentesis is also associated with a **2–3% (up to 15%) incidence of fetomaternal hemorrhage.** Following fetal transfusions the maternal antibody titer rises significantly.

Fetal intervention

IV transfusion is indicated when an **MCA PSV is ≥ 1.5 MoM.** Other ultrasonographic signs of hydrops may also suggest fetal anemia, or, if ΔOD_{450} is being used for screening instead of MCA PSV, a value in the upper third of zone 2 or zone 3 is an indication for FBS. Transfusion is performed at the umbilical vein either at the placental insection or inside the abdomen. Intraperitoneal transfusion is rarely performed and is contraindicated in the hydropic fetus, because of poor absorption of blood. **Corticosteroids for fetal maturation should be given before the procedure** when FBS is performed after 24 weeks. Type O, Rh(D)-negative, cytomegalovirus-negative, washed, leukoreduced, irradiated packed RBCs cross-matched against maternal blood should be used. The blood usually contains 75–85% RBCs, to allow minimal blood volume for the transfusion.[33]

The procedure is performed under continuous ultrasound guidance. Prophylactic antibiotics can be given (no trial has evaluated their efficacy). Following 24 weeks the procedure should be performed in a location close to the operating room and the anesthesiologist consulted should an emergency occur. Tubing and syringes should be heparinized. Maternal skin can be anesthetized with 1% lidocaine at point of needle entry. A 20- (or 22-) gauge needle is usually used. After entering the umbilical vein, a sample of fetal blood is withdrawn and the hemoglobulin immediately (within 1 or 2 minutes) determined. Fetal blood is confirmed by a mean corpuscular volume (MCV) $> 110\,\mu m^3$. Then, the fetus is given a paralytic agent (e.g. pavulon 0.1 ml/kg) to stop fetal movement. **If the hematocrit is** below the fifth percentile (0.84 MoM) for gestational age, **blood is transfused** in a sterile fashion. A computer program is used to estimate the amount of blood to transfuse based on the initial fetal hematocrit, the estimated fetal weight and the concentration of the blood transfused.[34–35] A final fetal blood sample is taken a few seconds after the transfusion has been completed. If the fetus is hydropic, it is better to perform more than one transfusion at a distance of 3–5 days to increase the hematocrit to the median hematocrit value for gestational age. Following 24 weeks' gestation, the fetal heart rate should be monitored for the next 2–3 hours until fetal movements resume. The risk of fetal death is 1–2% per procedure, even with ultrasound guidance, expert operators, and accurate management.

Hematocrit decreases about 1% per day post-transfusion in the anemic alloimmunized fetus, and this knowledge helps to assess when to repeat the transfusion. If the fetus is non-hydropic, the second transfusion is often necessary 14 days after the first, but after the second/third transfusion, longer intervals of 3 weeks may be possible, as the fetal RBCs are replaced by donated RBCs. Following three transfusions, 99% of the fetal blood is represented by the adult transfused blood. Maternal phenobarbital 30 mg three times per day for 7–10 days to enhance fetal liver maturity and ability to conjugate bilirubin is still unconfirmed by large studies.[36]

Fetal monitoring/testing

Fetal testing with non-stress tests (NSTs), or biophysical profiles (BPP), can start at around 32 weeks or earlier if indicated. The benefit of these tests has not been confirmed in a specific trial. Fetuses with very severe anemia (hemoglobin $\leq$2g/dl) due to RBC alloimmunization may have brain injury (e.g. intracerebellar hemorrhage); therefore, fetal neuroimaging by ultrasound and/or magnetic resonance imaging (MRI) may be indicated.[37]

The surfactant: albumin ratio for fetal lung maturity (FLM) cannot be used since high amniotic fluid bilirubin can affect this result. The other tests for FLM are reliable (see also Chapter 52).

Delivery/anesthesia

See Figures 47.1 and 47.2 for timing of delivery. Mode of delivery depends on obstetric indications. If fetal anemia is suspected during trial of labor, procedures such as scalp FHR monitoring, scalp pH, and operative delivery should be avoided if possible. There are no specific anesthesia precautions.

Neonatology management

Anemic neonates are usually treated with transfusions or exchange transfusions as necessary. They often need light therapy for hyperbilirubinemia. Breastfeeding is not contraindicated. A hearing screen may be indicated as a neonate and at 2 years of age, given that hyperbilirubinemia can cause sensorineural hearing loss. Children who survive even severe hemolytic disease (with hydrops and/or necessitating transfusions) have a normal neurological outcome.[38]

OTHER 'ATYPICAL' ANTIBODIES

There are many atypical blood group antibodies that are capable of producing hemolytic disease. Given their rarity, and the absence of large studies or any trial, the management of antibodies known to cause hemolytic disease other than Rh(D) is based on poor evidence. Many aspects of management are unknown or similar to Rh(D) alloimmunization, except for the details below. It should be acknowledged that the critical titer for antibodies other than Rh(D) has not been well established.

Kell alloimmunization

The incidence of Kell alloimmunization is about 0.1–0.2% in pregnant women. Kell alloimmunization is usually caused by prior transfusion. Over 90% of partners of Kell-immunized women are Kell negative. In the white population, only 9% of fathers are Kell positive, and only 0.2% are homozygous. **Maternal titers do not correlate well with fetal alloimmune disease.** Severe anemia can be diagnosed in fetuses whose mothers had a titer as low as 1:2. ΔOD_{450} **levels also do not correlate with fetal anemia.** This is because fetal anemia is not caused mainly by hemolysis, but by suppression of erythropoiesis at the progenitor cell level. Anti-Kell antibodies specifically inhibit the growth of Kell-positive erythroid burst-forming units and colony-forming units.[39] In fact anti-Kell anemic fetuses have lower reticulocyte counts and bilirubin levels than anti-D anemic fetuses. Kell blood group is complex, consisting of over two dozen antigens. Kell 1 (Kell, or K1) and its allelic partner Kell 2 (Cellano, or K2) are strong immunogens. Poor fetal outcome occurs in about 1.5–3% of Kell-alloimmunize pregnancies, an incidence that is possibly higher than that of other RBC antigens. The management of Kell sensitization is somewhat controversial. Genotypyping of the father of the baby (FOB) is extremely important: most will be Kell negative, and, if paternity is certain, no further testing is necessary. The vast majority of Kell-positive FOBs are heterozygote, so that then the fetal Kell status needs to be determined, usually by amniocentesis PCR. **MCA PSV screening is predictive and accurate for the diagnosis of fetal anemia from Kell alloimmunization.**[13,40] MCA PSV monitoring should start at 15 weeks, and be done as reported in Figures 47.1 and 47.2. ΔOD_{450} measurements from amniocentesis are inaccurate, and should not be used.

Other CDE system antigens

- c (small): 65% risk of hemolytic disease; 80% of FOBs are positive, of which half are homozygous and half are heterozygous.
- C (big): 32% risk of hemolytic disease.
- E (big): 31% risk of hemolytic disease. Maternal titers do not correlate well with fetal hemolytic disease.

MNS system

Only 1% of titers ever rise to $\geq 1:64$. There are only about five cases of severe anemia from anti-M alloimmunization ever reported, so that, even if sensitized, the incidence of severe anemia is probably $< 1\%$.

Others

Other rare but potentially lethal antigens are **Duffy (Fya, Fyb, Fy3, etc)**, **Kidd**, as well as others.

REFERENCES

1. Levine P, Katzin EM, Burnham L. Isoimmunization in pregnancy: its possible bearing on the etiology of erythroblastosis fetalis. JAMA 1941; 116: 825–7. [II-3]
2. Landsteiner K, Weiner AS. An agglutinable factor in human blood recognized by immune sera for Rhesus blood. Proc Soc Exp Biol Med 1940; 43: 223. [II-3]
3. Martin JA, Hamilton BE, Ventura SJ, et al. Births: final data for 2001. Natl. Vital Stat. Rep. 2002; 51: 1–102. [II-3]
4. Moise KJ. Rh disease: it's still a threat. Contemp Obstet Gynecol 2004; 49: 34–48. [review]
5. Lurie S, Rotmensch S, Glezerman M. Prenatal management of women who have partial Rh(D) antigen. BJOG 2001; 108: 895–7. [review]
6. Crowther C, Middleton P. Anti-D administration after childbirth for preventing Rhesus alloimmunisation. Cochrane Database Sys Rev 2007; 1. [meta-analysis: 6 RCTs, n = >10 000. Both low- and high-quality trials]
7. Crowther CA, Middleton P. Anti-D administration in pregnancy for preventing Rhesus alloimmunisation. Cochrane Database Syst Rev 2007; 1. [meta-analysis: 2 RCTs, n = >4,500]
8. Huchet J, Dallemagne S, Huchet C, et al. [Ante-partum administration of preventive treatment of Rh-D immunization in rhesus-negative women. Parallel evaluation of transplacental passage of fetal blood cells. Results of a multicentre study carried out in the Paris region]. Gynecol Obstet Biol Reprod (Paris) 1987; 16: 101–11. [RCT, n = 1882 primiparous Rh(D)-negative women. Administration of 100 μg (500 IU) anti-D immune globulin at 28 weeks and 34 weeks of pregnancy (n = 927). No placebo was given to the control group (n = 955)]. [in French]
9. Lee D. Rawlinson VI. Multicentre trial of antepartum low-dose anti-D immunoglobulin. Transfus Med 1995; 5: 15–19. [RCT, n = 2541 Rh(D)-negative primigravidae. 50 μg (250 IU) anti-D IM at 28 and 34 weeks' gestation (n = 952). Control group had no placebo (n = 1068)].
10. Ness PM, Baldwin ML, Niebyl JR. Clinical high-risk designations does not predict excess fetal–maternal hemorrhage. Am J Obstet Gynecol 1987; 156: 154–8. [II-2]
11. American College of Obstetricians and Gynecologists. Prevention of Rh D alloimmunization. ACOG Practice Bulletin No. 4, May 1999. [review]
12. Mari G, Adrignolo A, Abuhamad AZ, et al. Diagnosis of fetal anemia with Doppler ultrasound in the pregnancy complicated by maternal blood group immunization. Ultrasound Obstet Gynecol 1995; 5: 400–5. [II-2]
13. Mari G, Deter RL, Carpenter RL, et al. Noninvasive diagnosis by Doppler ultrasonography of fetal anemia due to maternal red-cell allimmunization. N Engl J Med 2000; 342: 9–14. [II-2]
14. Bianchi DW, Avent ND, Costa JM, van der Schoot CE. Noninvasive prenatal diagnosis of fetal Rhesus D. Ready for prime(r) time. Obstet Gynecol 2005; 106: 841–4. [review]
15. Harper TC, Finning KM, Martin P, Moise KJ. Use of maternal plasma for noninvasive determination of fetal RhD status. Am J Obstet Gynecol 2004; 191: 1730–2. [II-3]
16. Detti L, Mari G, Akiyama M, et al. Longitudinal assessment of the middle cerebral artery peak systolic velocity in healthy fetuses and in fetuses at risk for anemia. AmJ Obstet Gynecol 2002; 187: 937–39. [II-2]
17. Spong CY, Porter AE, Queenan JT. Management of isoimmunization in the presence of multiple maternal antibodies. Am J Obstet Gynecol 2001; 185; 481–4. [II-2]
18. Mari G, Abuhamad A, Cosmi E, Segata M, Akiyama M. Middle cerebral artery peak systolic velocity – Technique and variability. J Ultrasound Med 2005; 24: 425–30. [II-2]
19. Zimmermann R, Durig P, Carpenter RJ Jr, Marig. Longitudinal measurement of peak systolic velocity in the fetal middle cerebral artery for monitoring pregnancies complicated by red cell alloimmunisation: a prospective multicentre trial with intention-to-treat. Br J Obstet Gynaecol 2002; 109: 746–52. [II-2]
20. Mari G, Penso C, Sbracia M, D'Ancona RL, Copel J. Delta OD 450 and Doppler velocimetry of the middle cerebral artery peak velocity in the evaluation for fetal alloimmune hemolytic disease. Which is the best? Proceedings, Society for Perinatal Obstetricians, Anaheim, CA. Am J Obstet Gynecol 1997; 176: S18. [II-3]
21. Nishie EN, Brizot ML, Liao AW, et al. A comparison between middle cerebral artery peak systolic velocity and amniotic fluid optical density at 450 nm in the prediction of fetal anemia. Am J Obstet Gynecol 2003; 188(1): 214–9. [II-2]
22. Pereira L, Jenkins TM, Berghella V. Conventional management of maternal red cell alloimmunization compared with management by Doppler assessment of middle cerebral artery peak systolic velocity. Am J Obstet Gynecol 2003; 189: 1002–6. [II-2]
23. Oepkes D, Seaward PG, Vandenbussche FP, et al. Doppler ultrasonography versus amniocentesis to predict fetal anemia. N Engl J Med 2006; 355: 156–64. [II-1]
24. Mari G, Rahman F, Oloffson P, Oczan T, Copel JA. Increase of fetal hematocrit decreses the middle cerebral artery peak systolic velocity in

pregnancies complicated by rhesus alloimmunization. J Maternal Fetal Med 1997; 6: 206–8. [II-3]

25. Stefos T, Cosmi E, Detti L and Mari G. Correction of fetal anemia and the middle cerebral artery peak systolic velocity. Obstet Gyneol 2002; 99: 211–5. [II-2]

26. Detti L, Oz U, Guney I, et al. Doppler ultrasound velocimetry for timing the second intrauterine transfusion in fetuses with anemia from red blood cell alloimmunization. Am J Obstet Gynecol 2001; 185: 1048–51. [II-2]

27. Mari G, Zimmermann R, Moise KJ Jr., Deter RL. Correlation between middle cerebral artery peak systolic velocity and fetal hemoglobin after 2 previous intrauterine transfusions. Am J Obstet Gynecol 2005; 193: 1117–20. [II-3]

28. ACOG Practice Bulletin No. 75: Management of alloimmunization. Obstet Gynecol 2006; 108: 457–64. [review]

29. Mari G, Hanif F, Kruger M, et al. Middle cerebral artery peak systolic velocity: a new Doppler parameter in the assessment of growth restricted fetuses. Ultrasound Obstet Gynecol 2007; 29: 310–6. [II-3]

30. Liley AW. Liquor amnii analysis in the management of the pregnancy complicated by rhesus sensitization. Am J Obstet Gynecol 1961; 82: 1359–70. [II-3]

31. Queenan JT, Tomai TP, Ural SH, King JC. Deviation in amniotic fluid optical density at a wavelength of 450 nm in Rh-immunized pregnancies from 14 to 40 weeks' gestation: a proposal for clinical management. Am J Obstet Gynecol 1993; 168: 1370–6. [II-3]

32. Sikkel E, Vandenbussche PH, Oepkes D, et al. Amniotic fluid delta OD 450 values accurately predict severe fetal anemia in D-alloimmunization. Obstet Gynecol 2002; 100: 51–7. [II-3]

33. el-Azeem SA, Samuels P, Rose RL, Kennedy M, O'Shaughnessy RW. The effect of the source of transfused blood on the rate of consumption of transfused red blood cells in pregnancies affected by red blood cell alloimmunization. Am J Obstet Gynecol 1997; 177: 753–7. [II-2]

34. Nicolaides KH, Soothill PW, Clewell WH, et al. Fetal haemoglobin measurement in the assessment of red cell isoimmunisation. Lancet 1988; 1(8594): 1073–5. [II-3]

35. Mandelbrot L, Daffos, F, Forestier F, et al. Assessment of fetal blood volume for computer-assisted management of in utero transfusion. Fetal Ther 1988; 3: 60–6. [II-3]

36. Trevett T, Dorman K, Lamvu G, et al. Does antenatal maternal administration of phenobarbital prevent exchange transfusion in neonates with alloimmune hemolytic disease? Am J Obstet Gynecol 2003; 189: s214. [II-3]

37. Ghi T, Brodelli L, Simonazzi G, et al. Sonographic demonstration of brain injury in fetuses with severe red blood cell alloimmunization undergoing intrauterine transfusions. Ultrasound Obstet Gynecol 2004; 23: 428–31. [II-3]

38. Hudon L, Moise K, Hegemier SE, et al. Long-term neurodevelopmental outcome after intrauterine transfusion for the treatment of fetal hemolytic disease. Am J Obstet Gynecol 1998; 179: 858–63. [II-3]

39. Vaughan JI, Manning M, Warwick RM, et al. Inhibition of erythroid progenitor cells by anti-Kell antibodies in fetal alloimmune anemia. N Engl J Med 1998; 338: 798–803. [II-3]

40. van Dongen H, Klumper FJC, Sikkel E, Vandenbussche FP, Oepkes D. Non-invasive tests to predict fetal anemia in Kell-alloimmunized pregnancies. Ultrasound Obstet Gynecol 2005; 25: 341–5. [II-2]

48

Neonatal alloimmune thrombocytopenia

Jason K Baxter

KEY POINTS

- Neonatal alloimmune thrombocytopenia (NAIT) is a fetal/neonatal thrombocytopenia ($< 150\,000/mm^3$) due to **maternal sensitization to incompatible fetal platelet antigens.**
- The most significant complication of NAIT is the 10–30% fetal/neonatal risk of **intracranial hemorrhage (ICH)**, of which 45% occurs antenatally, most often in the third trimester at around 30–35 weeks, but as early as 20 weeks. There is also a 5–13% risk of **neonatal mortality.**
- Only **HPA-1a antigen** and a **past history of ICH** predict a more severe thrombocytopenia.
- The **goal** of management is to **prevent ICH** in the fetus and neonate. Keeping fetal/neonatal platelets $> 20\,000/\mu Lmm^3$ achieves this goal.
- Routine universal maternal screening is in general not recommended.
- Intravenous immunoglobulin (IVIG) is associated with a **75% response rate, and a very rare risk of ICH,** with half of non-responders improved with the addition of high-dose prednisone.
- **Fetal blood sampling (FBS)** is associated with a 1–2% risk of fetal loss per procedure, and 5–10% cumulative.
- **Management is usually based on IVIG therapy, with FBS as needed,** as determined by prior history of ICH (or not), and its timing (**Figure 48.1**).
- An **alternative approach,** using **FBS at 20 weeks** for all pregnancies, is described in **Figure 48.2.** There is insufficient evidence to compare these two approaches, but this second approach may be associated with a higher risk of fetal loss and preterm birth from early FBS.

DEFINITION

Neonatal alloimmune thrombocytopenia (NAIT) is fetal/neonatal thrombocytopenia due to **maternal sensitization to incompatible fetal platelet antigens.** It is also called alloimmune thrombocytopenia (AIT), or fetal maternal alloimmune thrombocytopenia (FMAIT).

EPIDEMIOLOGY/INCIDENCE

The incidence of NAIT is 1:1000–1500 births.[1] NAIT is the most common reason for severe thrombocytopenia and/or intracranial hemorrhage (ICH) in term newborns.

ETIOLOGY/BASIC PATHOPHYSIOLOGY

Maternal alloimmunization occurs against fetal platelet antigen (Ag) lacked by the mother's own platelets.

Platelet disease similar to RBC Rh disease

- Like red blood cells (RBCs), platelets have specific surface proteins called antigens
- Mother lacks platelet antigen possessed by father
- Mother is exposed to antigen by fetal platelets
- **Maternal sensitization to incompatible fetal (platelet) antigens**
- Transplacental transfer of maternal antiplatelet antibody to the fetus
- Subsequent antibody-coating and sequestration of platelets in the fetal reticuloendothelial system.

Different from Rh disease

- **Firstborn children are often affected** (primiparas account for 20–60% of cases)
- Maternal antibody titers are not predictive of outcome
- Antiplatelet immunoglobulin G (IgG) production can occur in first pregnancy.

Table 48.1 *New nomenclature for NAIT*

Old nomenclature	New nomenclature (in order of discovery)	Incidence
Pl^{A1}, PLA-1, ZW^A	HPA-1a	Most common (> 75%) (2% whites, 0.4% blacks, < 0.1% Asians are negative)
Pl^{A2}, PLA-2	HPA-1b	Worse severity
Ko^b	HPA-2a	
Ko^a	HPA-2b	
Bak^a, Lek^a	HPA-3a	Second most common (15% whites are negative)
Bak^b, Lek^b, PLA-3	HPA-3b	
Pen^a, Yuk^b	HPA-4a	
Pen^b, Yuk^a	HPA-4b	More common in Asians
Br^b	HPA-5a	
Br^a, PLA-5	HPA-5b	Third most common (< 1% whites are negative) Most common in Japan

a = high-frequency antigen; b = low-frequency antigen.

Maternal platelet count and function is normal (although 10% of women with NAIT may have gestational thrombocytopenia). **Most incompatibilities will not become sensitized.**[1]

GENETICS

HPA-1b is due to a single base pair change of cytosine to thymine at position 196 (proline to leucine) in platelet glycoprotein IIIA.[2]

CLASSIFICATION

There are five major biallelic systems of platelet-specific antigens (which differ by single amino acids). The **new nomenclature** is described in Table 48.1.

- Whites: 97% HPA-1a +: 68% homozygotes (HPA-1a/HPA-1a), 29% heterozygotes (HPA-1a/HPA-1b); 2–3% HPA-1b/HPA-1b.
- HLA class II determinant DRW52a (HLA-DR3) or HLA-B8 are more likely to develop antibodies vs HPA-1a; 1/42 pregnancies have platelet Ag incompatibility, but only 1/30 of these get NAIT.
- Other rare causes of NAIT are **HLA class I** (but not class II) antigens, which are also expressed by platelets. Gov (HPA-15) is unstable, making serological testing difficult.

NATURAL HISTORY/COMPLICATIONS

The fetus/neonate develops decreased platelets. This can lead to:

- 90% affected neonates have diffuse petechiae
- 10–30% ICH, of which 45% occur antenatally, most often in third trimester at around 30–35 weeks, but as early as 20 weeks:
  - mostly intraparenchymal, leading to encephalomalacia
  - may result in porencephalic cysts (which may be seen by ultrasound)
  - sometimes intraventricular hemorrhage (IVH), leading to arachnoiditis ± hydrocephalus.
- 5–13% **neonatal mortality**
- first case in family usually detected shortly after birth (due to petechiae, bleeding, or incidentally).

RECURRENCE RISK

- Clinical history of affected sibling is best indicator of risk in current/future pregnancy.
- **Recurrence** in subsequent pregnancy **is generally of greater severity.** It is about 100% for **HPA-1a** (usually **worst Ag**).[2]
- There is no correlation between platelet count at cordocentesis and degree of thrombocytopenia in previously

affected infant. How severe NAIT was in the last pregnancy is not as predictive.

- Only **HPA-1a antigen** and **past history of ICH** predict a more severe thrombocytopenia.
- **Prior ICH**: greatest risk, only true predictor of severity.
- Fetal platelets in first monitored pregnancy: **70% < 50 000/mm³** at first percutaneous umbilical blood sampling (PUBS); 50% < 20 000/mm³, 50% < 24 weeks. If > 50 000/mm³ on first PUBS, still possible decrease later (in HPA-1a, fetal platelets decrease as much as about 23 000/mm³ per week).[2]

MANAGEMENT
Principles

- **Goal: prevent hemorrhage, specifically ICH, in fetus and neonate.**
- ICH is rare with platelets >20 000/mm³; therefore, **goal is to keep platelets >20 000/mm³**. The normal platelet count of a fetus ≥ 18 weeks is ≥ 150 000/mm³, as in an adult.
- Fetal cord blood sampling (FBS) with direct measurement of fetal platelet count is the only method to assess disease severity.
- Optimal management of NAIT has not been determined by any randomized trial, and no one therapy is proven 100% effective.

Prevention

Some clinicians have advocated routine universal maternal serological screening for platelet antigens for identifying pregnancies at risk for NAIT, before it occurs in the first pregnancy without warning.

Rationale against routine maternal serological screening

- About 25% of NAIT is not caused by the most common antigen.
- Maternal immune response is influenced by other factors (e.g. HLA type).
- Only a minority of infants of mothers negative for platelet antigen will develop significant thrombocytopenia.
- Many false negatives and false positives.
- No adequate risk/benefit ratio or cost-effectiveness analyses have been performed. The incidence of ICH is low.

Screening by maternal ultrasound is futile, as fetal thrombocytopenia cannot be detected by ultrasound, and when it is so severe as to cause fetal ICH, it is too late for effective intervention.

Since there is no consensus regarding utility of screening unaffected women for alloimmune antiplatelet antibodies, active **management of the disease is usually confined to women who have had a previously affected fetus.**

Work-up for suspected NAIT
Indications for testing

- Neonate with petechiae and ecchymosis, unexplained thrombocytopenia
- Fetus with unexplained ICH, hydrocephalus, or porencephalic cyst
- Woman incidentally found to be HPA-1a negative
- Family history of NAIT.

NAIT serological testing

- Test parents in a reference laboratory (e.g. Blood Center of Southeastern Wisconsin)
- Initial testing: maternal platelet antibody; paternal antigen typing (usually HPA-1, 3, 5) if maternal antibody positive.

Diagnosis

- The mother is **antibody positive** (specific to father and fetal platelet antigen) and **antigen negative.**
- The **father's antigen zygosity** and **neonatal antigen** determines the risk of recurrence in subsequent pregnancies: 100% if father is homozygous, 50% if heterozygous.
- This documentation of maternal, paternal, and neonatal serological diagnosis should always be reviewed to guide management in the next pregnancy.

Counseling

Prognosis, natural history and complications, and management criteria should all be reviewed with the family. **All patients should be advised that the optimal management of alloimmune thrombocytopenia has *not* been determined and that no one therapy has proven 100% effective.**

Investigations and consultations

With a heterozygous father, consider **amniocentesis to determine fetal antigen** status by polymerase chain reaction

(PCR). Chorionic villus sampling (CVS) should be considered only if mother would terminate affected fetus. Multidisciplinary management should involve a hematologist and the blood bank.

Fetal therapy

There are insufficient data to assess different types of interventions for the pregnancy with NAIT.

There are two main antenatal treatments (IVIG and intrauterine transfusion).

Intravenous immunoglobulin

Intravenous immunoglobulin (IVIG) (> $1000/dose) is most common in North America:

- Pooled blood product, increasing hepatitis and HIV risks (donor screening and viral inactivation procedures decrease risk).
- Usually given as a **weekly infusion** over 6–12 hours.
- IVIG has an unclear mechanism of action, but is theorized to work via:
  - Fc-receptor **saturation in the placenta** with a reduction of antibody transfer across the placenta (most probable main mechanism).
  - Fc-receptor blockade on macrophages, leading to inhibition of uptake of the antibody-coated platelets by fetal macrophages. Endothelial stabilization prevents damage by maternal platelet antibodies (low platelets are not a cause of ICH).
  - Suppression of maternal IgG antibody production.
- IVIG not only can prevent/improve thrombocytopenia in the majority of cases but also prevents ICH. There are only very rare (possibly only two in the literature) reports of IVIG failures to prevent ICH.[3]
- Side effects – headaches and febrile reactions: pretreat with Benadryl (diphenhydramine) and acetaminophen.
- Only way to monitor efficacy of IVIG treatment is via FBS.
- **Seventy-five percent respond to weekly IVIG, half of non-responders being improved with addition of high-dose prednisone** (1 mg/kg = 60 mg/day).[4] Dexamethasone has been associated with oligohydramnios and fetal growth restriction (FGR).[4]
- When the IVIG dose is 2 g/kg/week, it can be infused at doses of 1 g/kg twice a week.
- If this fails, consider weekly in-utero platelet transfusions via FBS until birth.

Intrauterine transfusion

Repeated intrauterine transfusion of antigen-compatible platelets via FBS is more popular in Europe:

- Weekly in-utero transfusion of platelets via FBS may be required from 20 weeks until delivery.
- Risk of increasing sensitization due to fetomaternal hemorrhage.
- **Risk of fetal hemorrhage** is at least 1–2% per procedure, and 5–10% cumulative loss for each pregnancy.[5–7] To minimize fetal hemorrhage at FBS, always begin transfusing platelets immediately after obtaining platelet sample.[5–7]
- Transfuse maternal platelets (antigen negative), obtained by plasmapheresis a day or two earlier (packed, washed, and irradiated).

$$\text{Volume infused} = \frac{\begin{array}{c}(\text{Estimated fetoplacental volume}) \times \\ (\text{desired increase in platelet count})\end{array}}{\text{Platelet infusion concentration}}$$

- **Goal: keep platelets > 50 000/mm³** if being treated concurrently (usually 3–10 ml required).
- Due to risk of emergent delivery, corticosteroids for fetal lung maturity before FBS are suggested at > 24–34 weeks.
- In fetuses with platelets > 80 000/mm³ at first FBS and not treated, follow-up FBS showed decreases of at least 10 000/mm³ per week.

Many centers use IVIG as initial treatment, with FBS to monitor response, with the addition of oral steroids for refractory cases, as suggested in Figure 48.1. Management depends on history of prior ICH or not. This is an empirical approach, which tries to avoid a 20-week FBS, associated with significant complications as just discussed.

Previous sibling without in-utero ICH

In cases where **previous siblings did *not* have in-utero ICH** (Figure 48.1):

A. Begin IVIG at 1 g/kg/week at 20 weeks. Some advocate also adding prednisone 0.5–1.0 mg/kg/day, or a higher dose of IVIG (2 g/kg/week), but there is insufficient evidence to assess the effectiveness of these approaches.[7]

B. Assess adequacy of therapy by FBS at 30–32 weeks: (a) have platelets ready at any FBS, with slow transfusion started after sampling even before platelet count (PC) available; (b) compatible (mother's preferred) platelets; (c) transfusion volume – aim for 200 000–400 000 platelets, by using following equation:

Transfusion volume = Estimated fetal blood volume × [(Final PC − initial PC)/Donor PC]:

1. If adequate (platelet count ≥ 30 000/mm³), continue IVIG weekly to term. If the first fetal platelet count is > 20 000/mm³ while on IVIG, the chance

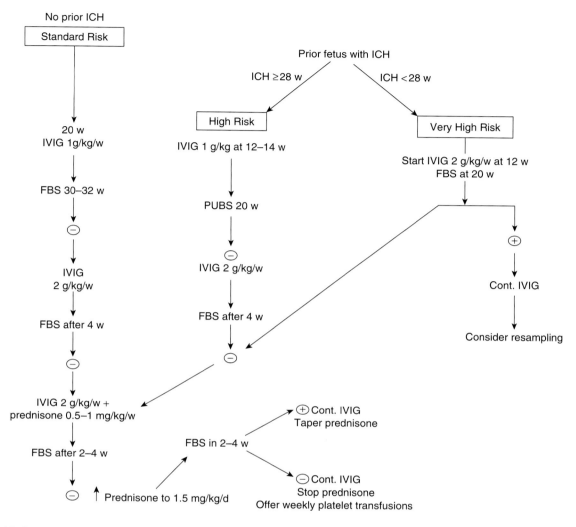

Figure 48.1

Suggested antenatal management for prior NAIT.
⊖ = fetal platelet count < 30 000/mm³; ⊕ = fetal platelet count ≥ 30 000/mm³.
ICH, intracranial hemorrhage; IVIG, intravenous immunoglobulin therapy; FBS, fetal blood sampling; PUBS, percutaneous umbilical blood sampling; Cont., continue; w, week; d, day; k = thousand.

of platelet count > 20 000/mm³ at a later sampling is 89%, while if the first count is ≤ 20 000/mm³, this chance is only 51%.[8] Therefore, if the response is adequate (> 20 000/mm³), a second FBS may not be required, provided IVIG is continued, given the risks of FBS.[8]

2. If inadequate fetal platelet count (< 20 000), start IVIG 2 g/kg/week (some suggest adding prednisone at this point, too). The chance that this initial platelet count is < 20 000/mm³ is < 20%.

3. Resample after 4 weeks of therapy. If inadequate, add prednisone 0.5–1 mg/kg/day to term.

4. Resample after 4 weeks of therapy. If inadequate, intensify therapy to IVIG 2 g/kg/week and prednisone 1.5 mg/kg/day and resample in 2 weeks. If response occurs, prednisone can be tapered.

5. If above salvage therapy fails, continue IVIG, stop prednisone, begin weekly in-utero platelet transfusions and deliver early with mature amniocentesis.

C. Follow with serial (every 2–4 weeks) ultrasound assessments.

D. Delivery mode management options:
   1. Cesarean section (no evidence it decreases incidence of ICH).
   2. FBS. If platelet count > 50 000/mm³, vaginal delivery is considered safe.

Previous sibling with in-utero ICH

In cases where **previous sibling had in-utero ICH** (see Figure 48.1):

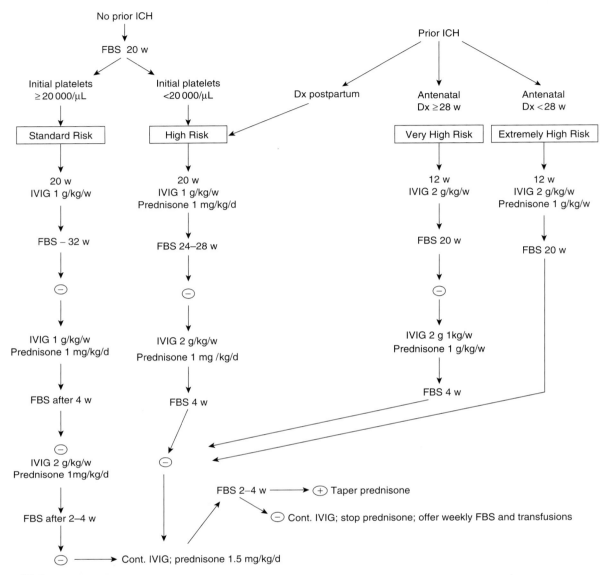

Figure 48.2
Alternative antenatal management for prior NAIT with initial FBS.
⊖ = fetal platelet count ≤ 25 000/mm³ or fetal platelet count ≤ 40 000/mm³ (*and* not increased > 10 000/mm³ compared with prior FBS). ⊕ = fetal platelet count > 25 000/mm³ *and* increased > 10 000/mm³ compared to prior FBS, or fetal platelet count ≥ 40 000/mm³.
ICH, intracranial hemorrhage; IVIG, intravenous immunoglobulin therapy; FBS, fetal blood sampling; Dx, diagnosis; w, week; d, day.

A. Begin IVIG at 1–2 g/kg/week at 12–14 weeks (see Figure 48.1: if prior ICH < 28 weeks: suggest IVIG 2 g/kg/week).
B. Assess adequacy of therapy by FBS at 20 weeks.
   1. If adequate (≥ 30 000/mm³), continue IVIG (platelet count falls if IVIG stopped).
   2. If inadequate (< 30 000/mm³): IVIG 2 g/kg/week and resample in 4 weeks. If still inadequate, add prednisone 0.5–1.5 mg/kg/day (see Figures 48.1 and 48.2).

If medical management fails, offer weekly in-utero platelet transfusions (half-life is 5–7 days).

C. Follow with serial (every 2–4 weeks) ultrasound assessments.
D. Delivery early with mature amniocentesis.
E. Delivery mode management options:
   1. Cesarean section (no evidence it decreases incidence of ICH).
   2. FBS. If platelet count > 50 000/mm³, vaginal delivery is considered safe.

Early FBS

An **alternative approach**, using **FBS at 20 weeks** for all pregnancies, is described in Figure 48.2. This approach has the benefit of knowing the fetal platelet count early in pregnancy, and therefore offers more directed therapy; however, it is associated with the complications of an early FBS.[7]

General issues regarding therapy

* Patients should be instructed to avoid activities (i.e. sports) that could result in potential trauma.
* External cephalic versions and non-steroidal anti-inflammatory drugs (NSAIDs) are contraindicated.
* Patients should receive IVIG and antenatal steroids several days prior to each FBS to maximize beneficial effects.
* Fetal IVIG therapy is not efficacious, since it increases antibody levels, but it does not always increase the fetal platelet count.
* There are **reported cases of ICH while receiving IVIG treatment,**[3,7] so that IVIG should be considered a highly effective but not perfect therapy to prevent ICH (and therefore FBS and possible transfusions are still necessary).
* Women with prior IVIG administration should have their serum checked for human T cell lymphotropic virus types I and II and hepatitis C antibodies.

Fetal monitoring/testing

FBS is indicated in certain cases, as shown in Figures 48.1 and 48.2. Ultrasound can help detect ICH, but when this is detected it is too late for intervention to prevent severe sequelae.

Anesthesia

No special precautions, since maternal platelets are usually normal.

Delivery

* Avoid fetal trauma: avoid maternal abdominal trauma, external cephalic version, fetal scalp lead, and vacuum or forceps.
* Delivery should occur once fetal lung maturity is confirmed.
* Cesarean delivery is indicated if platelet count is $< 50\,000/mm^3$; consider FBS to confirm adequate platelet count ($\geq 50\,000/mm^3$), which is safe for trial of labor and attempt at vaginal delivery.

Neonatology management

* Maternal platelets (Ag negative, obtained by plasmaphoresis, plasma depleted, washed, irradiated, and packed) should always be available for transfusion after delivery.
* Neonatal treatment is with IVIG, IV steroids, and antigen-compatible platelets until platelet count recovers, usually by 7–10 days of age.
* The volume of platelets transfused = Blood volume $\times$ [(Desired increase in platelet count − Actual platelet count)/Platelet concentration)]. For the term neonate, this usually equates to 1 ml plt = increase platelet count by $5000/mm^3$ (10 ml = 50 000, 20 ml = 100 000). Often the neonatologist chooses to transfuse 10 ml of platelets per neonatal weight (kg).

Future pregnancy preconception counseling

Management, events, and outcome of the pregnancy should be reviewed with the family postpartum (after discharge of the neonate). As stated above, the natural history of NAIT is that, if it recurs (depending on FOB [father of baby] zygocity), it is more severe than in the previous pregnancy.

REFERENCES

1. Davoren A, McParland P, Crowley J, et al. Antenatal screening for human platelet antigen-1a: results of a prospective study at a large maternity hospital in Ireland. BJOG 2003; 110: 492–6. [II-2]
2. Bussel JB, Zabusky MR, Berkowitz RL, McFarland JG. Fetal alloimmune thrombocytopenia. N Engl J Med 1997; 337: 22–6. [II-3]
3. Kroll H, Kiefel V, Giers G, et al. Maternal intravenous immunoglobulin treatment does not prevent intracranial haemorrhage in fetal alloimmune thrombocytopenia. Transfus Med 1994; 4(4): 293–6. [II-2]
4. Bussel JB, Berkowitz RL, Lynch L, et al. Antenatal management of alloimmune thrombocytopenia with intravenous gamma-globulin: a randomized trial of the addition of low-dose steroid to intravenous gamma-globulin. Am J Obstet Gynecol 1996; 174(5): 1414–23. [RCT, *n*=54]
5. Paidas MJ, Berkowitz RL, Lynch L, et al. Alloimmune thrombocytopenia: fetal and neonatal losses related to cordocentesis. Am J Obstet Gynecol 1995; 172: 475–9. [II-3]
6. Overton T, Duncan KR, Jolly M, Letsky, Fisk NM. Serial aggressive platelet transfusion for fetal alloimmune thrombocytopenia: platelet dynamics and perinatal outcome. Am J Obstet Gynecol 2002; 186: 826–31. [II-2]
7. Berkowitz RL, Kolb EA, McFarland JG, et al. Parallel randomized trials of risk-based therapy for fetal alloimmune thrombocytopenia. Obstet Gynecol 2006; 107: 91–6. [RCT, *n*=79]
8. Gaddipati S, Berkowitz RL, Lembet AA, et al. Initial fetal platelet counts predict the response to intravenous gammaglobulin therapy in fetuses that are affected by PLA1 incompatability. Am J Obstet Gynecol 2001; 185: 976–80. [II-2]

49

Non-immune hydrops fetalis

Arianna Bonato and Dennis C Wood Jr

KEY POINTS

- Diagnostic criteria for hydrops are abnormal fluid accumulation in **at least two** fetal spaces, such as: **ascites, pleural effusion, pericardial effusion, and skin edema.**
- Non-immune hydrops (NIH) is the hydrops **not caused by an immune process**, and now represents > 90% of all hydropic cases seen.
- The main associations are with cardiovascular disorders (30–40%), extracardiac anomalies (15–25%), chromosomal abnormalities (15–20%), congenital infections (10–15%), hematological conditions (5–15%), monochorionic twin pregnancies (5–10%), and, rarely, genetic syndromes (1%) or inborn errors of metabolism (0.5–1%).
- In general, perinatal mortality in pregnancies complicated by NIH is 50–100%, depending on the etiology.
- **Basic work-up** includes detailed **history** (personal and especially family), **maternal laboratory tests** (blood group and typing, indirect Coombs' test for antibody screen, CBC, RPR, rubella antibody; IgG and IgM for parvovirus, CMV, toxoplasmosis, coxsackie virus, HSV-1 and HSV-2, *Listeria* [can skip infectious serology if PCR obtained from AF]; Kleihauer–Betke test); fetal **ultrasound**, including accurate anatomic ultrasound, MCA PSV, other Doppler studies, and fetal echocardiogram; and **amniocentesis** for karyotype and PCR for above infections.
- Management, including fetal monitoring, treatment, and delivery, should follow the appropriate guideline for the specific etiology of NIH.

DIAGNOSIS/DEFINITION

Hydrops fetalis is a severe fetal condition, the end stage of many different disorders, leading to accumulation of fluid in body cavities or tissues. Diagnostic criteria for hydrops are abnormal fluid accumulation in **at least two** of the following spaces: **ascites, pleural effusion, pericardial effusion, and skin edema** (> 5 mm measured at the level of skull or chest wall) (Figure 49.1). These diagnostic findings can be associated with polyhydramnios (in 40–75% of cases) and placentomegaly. Immune hydrops is associated in particular with isommunization from a red blood cell (RBC) antigen (e.g. Rh disease) (see Chapter 47 for immune hydrops), whereas non-immune hydrops (NIH) includes all other etiologies except immune ones.

EPIDEMIOLOGY/INCIDENCE

The incidence of NIH is about 1/2000–1/3000 at birth, and as high as 0.5% in tertiary referral centers. The incidence may be as high as 1/150 on ultrasound, since the high rate of intrauterine demise makes the hydrops incidence at birth an underestimation. NIH may account for up to 3% of perinatal mortality. When Potter described NIH for the first time in 1943, its incidence was very low compared with fetal hydrops for isoimmunization. After the introduction of anti-D prophylaxis, NIH represents > 90% of all hydrops cases.

ETIOLOGY/BASIC PATHOPHYSIOLOGY

The pathophysiology of NIH is complex and basically related to three main mechanisms: impaired lymphatic flow, cardiac failure, and extravasation (either increased intravascular hydrostatic pressure, decreased intravascular osmotic pressure, or both) (Figure 49.2). NIH is the final phenotype of hundreds of different disorders. Different etiological factors and complex mechanisms convey to extra-accumulation of fluid in the fetal interstitial space, with 10–20% of hydrops causes still undetermined after extensive work-up.[1] The complex physiopathology of hydrops makes it a challenge for the obstetrician to investigate its etiology and decide upon the management.

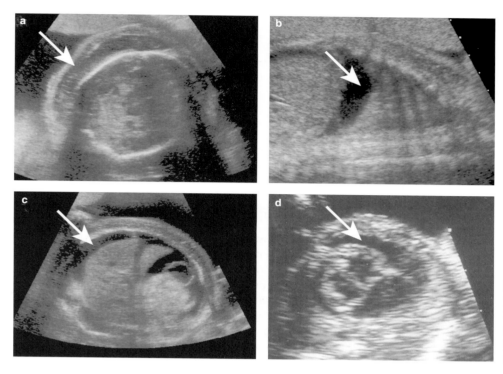

Figure 49.1
Diagnostic criteria for hydrops:
need ≥2 out of these 4: (a) skin
edema; (b) pleural effusion;
(c) ascites; and (d) pericardial
effusion.

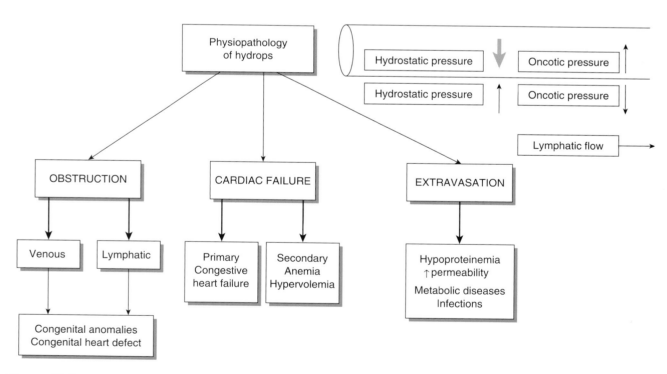

Figure 49.2
The pathophysiology of hydrops.

ASSOCIATIONS/POSSIBLE ETIOLOGIES/DIFFERENTIAL DIAGNOSIS[2]

Cardiovascular disorders (30–40%)

The main causal association of NIH is with fetal cardiovascular disease. Tachyarrhythmias (40%), cardiac structural malformations (20%), high-output cardiac failure (15%), and bradyarrhythmias (6%) resulting from congenital heart malformation or maternal connective disorders are the most common cardiovascular diseases. In the case of abnormal cardiac rhythm, stroke volume can be reduced, producing a systemic venous congestion to the point that the lymphatic system is unable to return interstitial fluid into the vascular compartment. The underlying mechanism in cardiac malformations is attributed to the raising of systemic venous pressure, due either to the obstruction of right heart output or to the transmission of systemic arterial pressure to the right heart through various types of pathological shunts. Primary or secondary closure of foramen ovale is a possible reason for heart failure and hydrops. Cardiac rhabdomyomas, associated in half of the cases with tuberous sclerosis, can also lead to fetal hydrops for ventricular outflow obstruction or for causing a re-entry pathway in the atrioventricular junction. Sacrococcygeal teratoma, large fetal angiomas, and placental chorioangiomas may lead to fetal hydrops by acting as peripheral arteriovenous shunts, increasing fetal cardiac output, producing cardiac hypertrophy, and congestive heart failure. Aneurysm of the great vein of Galen is a large cerebral arteriovenous malformation causing congestive heart failure and hydrops.

Extracardiac anomalies (15–25%)

Thoracic (5–10%)

Thoracic space-occupying lesions can produce a compression of venous return and thereby a heart preload decrease. Cystic adenomatoid malformation (CAM), pulmonary sequestration and congenital diaphragmatic hernia (CDH) are the most common causes of NIH in this category. CDH produces compression of venous return, especially when the liver is herniated in the chest, and a worse prognosis is expected when hydrops is found as an associated factor. Primary hydrothorax is the accumulation of lymphatic fluid in the pleural cavity without any other demonstrated anomaly (mass or chromosomal abnormality). The most common cause of primary hydrothorax in neonates is chylothorax, characterized by a milky pleural fluid from the high concentration of lymphocytes. Prenatal diagnosis (i.e. lymphocytes count > 80% in pleural effusion) is more difficult due to fetal physiological leukocytosis.

Genitourinary (3%)

Urinary tract anomalies may be associated with ascites, but rarely present generalized hydrops. Lower tract obstruction produces bladder overdistention that may leak into the abdominal cavity. More rare causes of ascites are the rupture of a dilated renal pelvis or renal thrombosis. Congenital nephrotic syndrome of Finnish type, a rare fatal autosomal recessive disease, can be associated with fetal hydrops and is characterized by elevated serum and amniotic fluid alpha-fetoprotein.

Gastrointestinal (1%)

Intestinal perforation produces a variable degree of ascites (meconium peritonitis) that is not easy to differentiate from other kinds of intra-abdominal serum effusions. The presence of meconium, seen as bright plaques or echo-poor cystic areas, would lead to the diagnosis even in absence of dilated gut. When meconium peritonitis is not associated with generalized hydrops, the prognosis is good. Prenatal causes of bowel obstructions are atresias ('apple-peel' syndrome), volvulus, and meconium ileus (cystic fibrosis).

Skeletal dysplasias (1%)

Many different skeletal dysplasias can lead to hydrops, with the severe thoracic hypoplasia compressing venous return and polyhydramnios due to poor fetal swallowing.

Chromosomal abnormalities (15–20%)

The incidence of chromosome abnormalities is inversely proportional to gestational age (GA) at diagnosis of NIH, with a 50–75% incidence when NIH is diagnosed < 20 weeks.[3] Turner and Down syndromes account for 90% of all aneuploidies associated with hydrops, although many other chromosomal abnormalities such as trisomy 18 and 13, 45,X/46,XX mosaicism, triploidy, and tetraploidy have been reported. The main features of Turner syndrome are cystic hygroma and tubular coarctation of aorta, suggesting both lymphatic and cardiac etiology in hydrops output. The mere finding of a cystic hygroma in the first trimester strongly suggests aneuploidy (60% of risk).

Congenital infections (10–15%)

Parvovirus B19 is the most common infective agent leading to severe anemia and NIH. It represents about 5% of all cases of NIH, but, when congenital defects are ruled out, parvovirus 19 infection accounts for about 25% of fetal hydrops. Syphilis is a rare cause of fetal hydrops, which develops because of anemia and hepatic dysfunction, resulting in hypoproteinemia and portal hypertension. Other infections such as toxoplasmosis, coxsackie virus, herpes simplex virus (HSV), rubella, and cytomegalovirus (CMV) have been shown to be occasionally associated with NIH in fetuses. The reasons for hydrops in all these conditions are unclear, but infected fetuses tend to present similar biochemical, hematological, and immunological alterations.

Hematological disorders (5–15%)

Anemia, the most frequent cause of NIH from hematological disorders, is produced by excessive erythrocyte loss or underproduction. Hemolysis in alpha-thalassemia is responsible for 86% of fetal hydrops in southeast Asia and is also common in eastern Mediterranean countries.[5] Most rarely, erythrocyte enzyme disorders such as G6PD (glucose-6-phosphate dehydrogenase) deficiency or pyruvate kinase deficiency can lead to fetal NIH. Hemorrhage for fetomaternal transfusion or for twin–twin transfusion syndrome (TTTS) in monochorionic twins can lead to anemia and subsequent NIH. In general, when the fetal hematocrit is < 15%, heart failure ensues, leading to the developing of severe ascites and a lesser degree of edema and pericardial or pleural effusion.

Monochorionic twin pregnancies (5–10%)

TTTS is a severe complication of monochorionic pregnancies that results from unbalanced bilateral blood flow through placental vascular anastomoses. It occurs in 10–15% of monochorionic pregnancies, and both fetuses can become hydropic, the recipient from high-output cardiac failure, and the donor from either anemia or changes in placental blood flow direction that submit the donor's heart to an excessive charge (see Chapter 38).

Metabolic diseases (1%)

Even if metabolic diseases account for only 1% of NIH, up to 15% of the unexplained causes of NIH after negative basic work-up include unknown metabolic disorders. Diagnosis is expensive, and an investigation for metabolic diseases is justified only when other more frequent causes have been ruled out.[6,7]

MATERNAL COMPLICATIONS

Pre-eclampsia ('mirror syndrome'), anemia, preterm labor (from polyhydramnios as well as fetal compromise), gestational diabetes mellitus (GDM), birth trauma, retained placenta, postpartum hemorrhage.

PREGNANCY MANAGEMENT
Counseling/prognosis

NIH is the end stage of many severe diseases whose outcome is related to the etiology and the grade of severity as well as the period of onset. **In general, perinatal mortality in pregnancies complicated by NIH is 50–100%, depending on the etiology.** The worst prognosis is expected with:

- NIH before 24 weeks' gestation (high risk of chromosomal abnormalities)
- NIH and cystic hygroma (associated with 100% mortality)
- NIH and chromosomal anomaly (very high mortality).

NIH associated with metabolic diseases or certain fetal abnormalities is considered to have a poor prognosis, especially when a progressive trend is observed. In such cases, counseling should include the option of termination. After 24 weeks the survival rate, excluding aneuploidies, is nearly 50% when effective treatments are applied. Fetal anemia and fetal arrhythmia are two of the etiologies of NIH associated with > 70–90% survival, if appropriate treatment is instituted.[1]

Work-up/diagnosis (Figure 49.3 and Table 49.1)

After the finding of hydrops by ultrasound, it is important to carry out a systematic assessment of both the fetus and mother to find out the underlying etiology (underlying diagnosis), and define a prognosis. Not all the work-up described below needs to be completed if a sure cause of the NIH is identified during testing.

Elements of basic work-up

1. *History (personal and especially family):* genetic/metabolic disease (e.g. tuberous sclerosis), congenital anomaly, ethnicity, consanguinity, history of recent infection or contact, autoimmune disease, and events of the pregnancy, including previous infection screening and ultrasound findings.
2. *Laboratory:* blood group and typing, indirect Coombs' test for antibody screen, complete blood count (CBC), rapid plasma reagin (RPR), rubella antibody; immunoglobulins IgG and IgM for parvovirus, CMV, toxoplasmosis, coxsackie virus, HSV-1 and HSV-2, *Listeria* (can skip infectious serology if polymerase

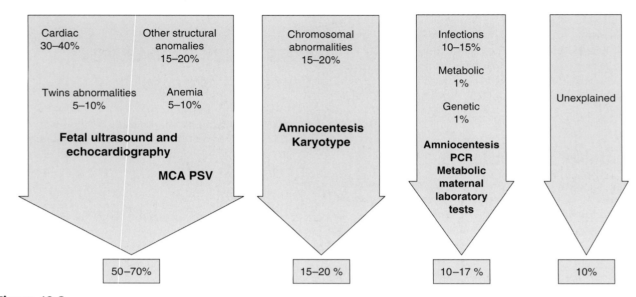

Figure 49.3
Etiology-based work-up of hydrops. MCA PSV, middle cerebral artery peak systolic velocity; PCR, polymerase chain reaction.

chain reaction [PCR] obtained from amniotic fluid [AF]); Kleihauer–Betke test. If mean corpuscular volume (MCV)< 80 μm³, hemoglobin electrophoresis; if patient has lupus, SSA and SSB antibody tests.

3. *Ultrasound:* accurate fetal anatomic ultrasound; middle cerebral artery peak systolic velocity (MCA PSV), and other Doppler studies; fetal echocardiogram.

4. *Amniocentesis:* fluorescent in-situ hybridization (FISH) and culture for karyotype; PCR for CMV, parvovirus, toxoplasmosis, coxsackie virus, HSV-1 and HSV-2, *Listeria.*

5. *Other tests to be considered:* magnetic resonance imaging (MRI; especially if ultrasound suspicious but not diagnostic for anomaly); percutaneous umbilical blood sampling (PUBS) if MCA PSV > 1.50 MoM; freezing amniotic fluid/extra fetal serum for future tests.

If the above work-up is negative, consider: glucose-6-phosphate dehydrogenase (G6PDH) deficiency; metabolic work-up (e.g. lysosomal storage disorders and rare hemoglobinopathies) (should be done especially if positive family history, or recurrent NIH); adenovirus and other infection PCR.

Anatomy ultrasound

Anatomy ultrasound should include assessment of:

- abdomen for ascites, thorax for pleural/pericardial effusion, and skin for edema
- complete anatomy survey
- fetal heart: arrhythmias (M-mode), structural anomalies, function (Doppler)
- Doppler analysis of umbilical artery, MCA PSV, ductus venosus, and possibly other arteries and veins
- liver length, spleen size, amniotic fluid index (AFI)
- placental thickness, malformations.

MCA PSV is > 90% sensitive and specific for fetal anemia, using MoM > 1.50 (see Chapter 48).[8,9] The most likely explanation for the observed increase of MCA PSV is the reduction of blood viscosity, leading to enhanced venous return and preload with consequent increase in cardiac output. Hydrothorax (pleural effusion) is an easily observable collection of fluid in the pleural space. It can be unilateral or bilateral and when severe can lead to pulmonary hypoplasia. In the presence of ascites, liquid is evident all around the abdominal circumference and a thorough observation from different angles is necessary to differentiate real ascites from the hypoechogenic rim produced by dorsal and abdominal musculature just beneath the abdominal wall. In male fetuses, fluid collection in the scrotum (hydrocele) often precedes massive ascites. Pericardial effusion distends the pericardium without any motion during cardiac activity. Occasionally, hypoechogenic ventricular myocardium mimics the presence of fluid collection, but this pitfall is

Table 49.1 *Conditions associated with NIH, and related work-up*

Conditions associated with NIH	Work-up

CARDIOVASCULAR (30–40%)
Structural
HLHS, HRHS, AVC, VSD, ASD, Ebstein anomaly, TGA, TOF, truncus, AV valves or
  AO/pulmonary valve, atresia/stenosis, premature closure of DA or FO, etc.
Arrhythmias
SVT, atrial flutter, heart block, WPW, non-conducted PACs, etc.
Mass
Cardiac rhabdomyoma, pericardial/intrapericardial/intracardial teratoma
High-output cardiac failure
Chorioangioma (>5 cm), sacrococcygeal teratoma, umbilical cord hemangioma,
  neuroblastoma
Vascular disorders
Cardiomyopathy, aneurysm of the vein of Galen, artery calcification, peripheral artery
  thrombosis
	Accurate **fetal echocardiography** for
	  morphological and functional study,
	  including 2D, M-mode, pulse Doppler,
	  color Doppler (3D if available)
	
	Accurate **fetal anatomical ultrasound**
	  (including peripheral vessel Doppler)

EXTRA-CARDIAC ANOMALIES (15–25%)
Thorax
CCAM, pulmonary sequestration, CDH, pulmonary lymphangiectasia, chylothorax,
  brochogenic cyst, any thoracic mass (including tumor)
Urinary
PUV, urethral stenosis/atresia, prune-belly syndrome, congenital nephrosis
Gastrointestinal
Volvulus-atresia, malrotation, duplication, meconium peritonitis, hepatic fibrosis,
  cholestasis, biliary atresia, cloacal dysgenesis, hemochromatosis
Skeletal dysplasias
Thanatophoric dysplasia, short rib-polydactyly, osteogenesis imperfecta,
  achondrogenesis, hypophosphatasia
	Accurate **fetal anatomical ultrasound**
	
	Consider thoracocentesis, or paracentesis, for
	biochemical, cytological, and microbiological
	analysis

Chromosomal abnormalities (15–20%) 45X (or mosaic 45X/46XX), trisomy 21, trisomy 18, trisomy 13, triploidy, etc.	**Amniocentesis**
Infections (10–15%) Parvovirus B19 (5%), CMV, syphilis, coxsackie B, toxoplasmosis, rubella, *Listeria,* adenovirus	RPR, rubella antibody, maternal serologies Amniocentesis: PCR (or culture) of AF

Hematological (5–15%)
Excessive red cell loss
Alpha-thalassemia, G6PD deficiency, fetomaternal transfusion, TTTS, fetal
  hemorrhage, red cell enzyme deficiencies, congenital leukemia, etc.
Underproduction
Fetal liver and bone marrow deficiency, congenital leukemia,
  Parvovirus B19 (or other infection), red cell aplasia
	MCA peak systolic velocity
	
	Maternal testing:
	• Indirect Coombs
	• Mean corpuscular volume
	• Hemoglobin electrophoresis
	• Maternal blood chemistry

Monochorionic twin pregnancy (5–10%) TTTS TRAP sequence	Accurate fetal ultrasound

Genetic syndromes (1%)
Noonan syndrome (congenital lymphedema), myotonic dystrophy, arthrogryposis,
  multiple pterygia, etc.
	Accurate fetal ultrasound, genetic studies
	  from AF

(Continued)

Table 49.1 *(Continued)*	
Conditions associated with NIH	Work-up
Metabolic (0.5–1%) *Lysosomal storage disorders* Gaucher's disease (type 2), Niemann–Pick disease, Tay–Sachs disease, GM1 gangliosidosis, mucopolysaccharidosis, mucolipidosis, sialidosis, galactosialidosis, etc.	Amniocentesis: enzymatic analysis of supernatant and cultivated amniocytes Maternal testing

NIH, non-immune hydrops; HLHS, hypoplastic left heart syndrome; HRHS, hypoplastic right heart syndrome; VSD, ventricular septal defect; TGA, transposition of the great arteries; TOF, tetralogy of Fallot; AV, atrio-ventricular; AO, aortic; DA, ductus arteriosus; FO, foramen ovale; SVT, supraventricular tachycardia; WPW, Wolff-Parkinson-White; PACS, premature atrial contractions; CCAM, congenital cystic adenomatoid malformation; CDH, congenital diaphragmatic hernia; PUV, posterior urethral valves; CMV, cytomegalovirus; RPR, rapid plasma reagin; PCR, polymerase chain reaction; AF, amniotic fluid; G6PD, glucose phosphate dehydrogenase; MCA, middle cerebral artery; TTTS, twin–twin tranfusion syndrome; TRAP, twin reversal arterial perfusion.

ruled out when the hypoechogenic line doesn't overpass the atrioventricular level. Placenta edema is diagnosed when its thickness is > 6 cm, and polyhydramnios is conventionally defined as an AFI above the 95th percentile for GA, or maximal pocket > 8 cm. The finding of isolated ascites with oligohydramnios suggests to a urinary tract anomaly. The presence of more defects can suggest a chromosomal abnormality; fetal face examination and limb movement observation can suggest more complex conditions such as genetic syndromes. Signs of infection are also visible through ultrasound such as ventriculomegaly or hydrocephalus, hyperechogenic bowel, hepatic or brain calcifications, fetal growth restriction. Consider 3D ultrasound if available.

Fetal echocardiography

An accurate fetal echocardiography aims first to examine the position, size, function, and rhythm of the heart. The systematic observation of a four-chamber view, outflow tracts, and great arteries and arches can rule out the majority of congenital heart defects (CHDs) associated with hydrops. The addition of color and pulse Doppler permits a more complete evaluation of heart function and flow across atrioventricular valves and arterial valves, while M-mode allows a more accurate study of heart squeezing, recording of wall thickness and rhythm. Color Doppler investigation can demonstrate atrioventricular valve regurgitation, and insonation of peripheral vessels can show venous pulsatility in ductus arteriosus or hepatic veins as signs of cardiac failure or provide information on right atrium pressure and heart function.

Amniocentesis

Different analyses in amniotic fluid permit investigation of fetal karyotype, congenital infections, and metabolic diseases. FISH (fluorescent in-situ hybridization) and QF-PCR (quantitative fluorescent polymerase chain reaction) can provide a rapid assessment of chromosomes 13, 18, 21, X and Y, assessing about 70% of chromosomal anomalies. A full karyotype from culture of amniocytes rules out all chromosome anomalies.

For a diagnosis of infection, PCR in the amniotic fluid is the most sensitive test, although a negative result does not exclude an infective etiology in 100% of cases. Parvovirus, CMV, and toxoplasmosis are the most common infectious etiologies of NIH, with investigation of other less-frequent infective agents possibly performed in stored amniotic fluid at a later time. Biochemical testing of enzymatic activity in cultured amniotic fluid permits investigation of inborn errors of metabolism. For the high cost of reagents, it seems reasonable to perform these analyses in the absence of other demonstrated etiologies.

Cordocentesis and other invasive procedures

PUBS should not be considered a routine procedure of the work-up of NIH, but a part of it when there is a strong suspicion of fetal anemia (i.e. elevated MCA PSV). The high fetal loss related risk (1–2%) and the limited information it provides suggest a prudent use of this procedure. When it is performed, fetal blood tests should include CBC, blood group and Coombs' test, and serum biochemistry. In special cases, thalassemia screening, total IgM, and G6PD in male fetuses can be performed. Peritoneal fluid, pleural fluid, pulmonary cyst fluid, and urine can be obtained in the attempt at fetal diagnosis and occasionally therapy. Cytological and biochemical analyses of these fluids can orientate to the final diagnosis of NIH. Likewise, karyotype and infective agents can be searched for in these fluids.

Management

Management, including fetal monitoring, treatment, and delivery, should follow the **appropriate guideline for the specific etiology of NIH.**

Fetal monitoring/testing

Doppler studies (especially umbilical artery), non-stress tests (NSTs) and/or biophysical profiles (BPPs) can be performed at weekly intervals (these last two usually ≥ 28 weeks) in the NIH fetus to assess fetal status and best timing for delivery.

Treatment

At 32–34 weeks, delivery and postnatal treatment should be considered, unless NIH has resolved. The **therapeutic approach depends on the differential diagnosis of the etiology of NIH.**

For parvovirus B19 and arrhythmias, treatment is feasible and effective. Intrauterine transfusion of fetuses with severe hydrops due to parvovirus infection reduces the risk of fetal death (Chapter 43). When heart failure and hydrops are associated with supraventricular tachycardia, prompt maternal therapy with an antiarrhythmic agent may be lifesaving. In severe pleural effusion, pulmonary compression may lead to lung hypoplasia and polyhydramnios for the obstruction of fetal swallowing, increasing the risk of preterm labor. Both these conditions, as well as low-output cardiac failure, explain the poor prognosis of severe hydrothorax. In these cases, thoracoamniotic shunting may be indicated. Amniodrainage may be considered in the case of severe polyhydramnios to increase maternal comfort and possibly decrease the risk of preterm labor.

Obstetric management

Steroids for fetal lung maturity (FLM) may be considered between 24 and 33 6/7 weeks if delivery is expected within 7 days. Tocolysis for preterm labor may not be advisable in all cases. Pre-eclampsia may develop in up to 50% of cases.

Delivery/anesthesia

For labor and delivery, cesarean delivery (CD) should be performed for the usual obstetric indications. Sometimes, hydropic spaces need to be drained to allow vaginal delivery, or CD may be necessary given the size of the fetus.

Neonatology management

All NIH fetuses require intubation and mechanical ventilation. It is important to offer all the resources available at a tertiary center to these neonates, since they require expert, intensive, multidisciplinary, complex care. In the case of fetal or neonatal death, an accurate autopsy should be performed. Long-term follow-up shows that the majority of NIH babies who are born and discharged alive have normal long-term follow-up.[10]

Postpartum

A separate postpartum outpatient visit should be set up to discuss the possible etiology of the NIH, including recurrence risks. Recurrent NIH is very rare, and mostly due to inborn errors of metabolism, e.g. lysosomal storage disorders, rare hemoglobinopathies, or other genetic causes.

REFERENCES

1. Sohan K, Carroll SG, De La Fuente S, Soothill P, Kyle P. Analysis of outcome in hydrops fetalis in relation to gestational age at diagnosis, cause and treatment. Acta Obstet Gynecol Scand 2001; 80(8): 726–30. [II-3]
2. Machin GA. Hydrops revisited: literature review of 1,414 cases published in the 1980s. Am J Med Genet 1989; 34(3): 366–90. [review]
3. Iskaros J, Jauniaux E, Rodeck C. Outcome of nonimmune hydrops fetalis diagnosed during the first half of pregnancy. Obstet Gynecol 1997; 90(3): 321–5. [II-3]
4. Ganapathy R, Guven M, Sethna F, Vivekananda U, Thilaganathan B. Natural history and outcome of prenatally diagnosed cystic hygroma. Prenat Diagn 2004; 24(12): 965–8. [II-2]
5. Forouzan I. Hydrops fetalis: recent advances. Obstet Gynecol Surv 1997; 52(2): 130–8. [review]
6. Stone DL, Sidransky E. Hydrops fetalis: lysosomal storage disorders in extremis. Adv Pediatr 1999; 46: 409–40. [II-3]
7. Burin MG, Scholz AP, Gus R, et al. Investigation of lysosomal storage diseases in nonimmune hydrops fetalis. Prenat Diagn 2004; 24: 653–7. [II-3].
8. Hernandez-Andrade E, Scheier M, Dezerega V, Carmo A, Nicolaides KH. Fetal middle cerebral artery peak systolic velocity in the investigation of non-immune hydrops. Ultrasound Obstet Gynecol 2004; 23(5): 442–5. [II-3]
9. Cosmi E, Dessole S, Uras L, et al. Middle cerebral artery peak systolic and ductus venosus velocity waveforms in the hydropic fetus. J Ultrasound Med 2005; 24: 209–13. [II-3]
10. Haverkamp F, Noeker M, Gerresheim G, Fahnenstich H. Good prognosis for psychomotor development in survivors with nonimmune hydrops fetalis. BJOG 2000; 107: 282–4. [II-3]

50

Sonographic assessment of amniotic fluid: oligohydramnios and polyhydramnios

Everett F Magann and Suneet P Chauhan

AMNIOTIC FLUID ASSESSMENT

KEY POINTS

- Ultrasound estimates of amniotic fluid volume (AFV) correlate poorly with dye-determined or directly measured oligohydramnios and polyhydramnios.
- **The single deepest pocket (SDP) is the best ultrasound technique to estimate AFV** in both singleton and twin gestations, since the amniotic fluid index (AFI) over-diagnoses oligohydramnios compared with the SDP, resulting in more interventions and operative deliveries and leading to increased maternal morbidity without any improvement in perinatal outcome.

AMNIOTIC FLUID ASSESSMENT IN SINGLETON PREGNANCIES

Background

- Urine production with urethra patent starts at 8–9 weeks; at 18 weeks, is about 50–100 ml/day; at term, is 800 ml/day, or 5 ml/kg/h. The primary component of amniotic fluid (AF) in the second half of pregnancy is fetal urine.
- The fetus swallows half of AF/day (about 0.5 L/day at term).
- Lungs also produce and absorb AF. Other systems involved in AF dynamics include skin, saliva/nose, and membranes/placenta/cord.
- The fetus with uteroplacental insufficiency will shunt blood flow to the brain, heart, and adrenal glands at the expense of the rest of the organ systems including the kidneys. Inadequate renal perfusion results in decreased urinary output and oligohydramnios.

Indications

AF volume (AFV) can help in the assessment of:
- In the second trimester:
  - evidence of **fetal anomalies** (e.g. urinary obstruction or dysfunction)

- severe **fetal growth restriction** (FGR; associated with fetal aneuploidy)
  - assist in the confirmation of preterm premature rupture of the fetal membranes (**PPROM**).
- In the late second and third trimester of pregnancy, as above, plus:
  - used along with the non-stress test (NST) or with the other components of the biophysical profile (BPP) in the **assessment of fetal well-being** in the pregnancy at risk for an adverse outcome.

Techniques

AFV can be measured precisely antepartum by a dye-dilution technique (the dye marker is placed in the uterine cavity by amniocentesis), and directly at the time of cesarean delivery (CD). These measurement techniques are invasive, time consuming, require laboratory support, and, if measured at cesarean, can only be done at the time of delivery. Because of these limitations, the AFV is estimated antepartum by ultrasound.

Three ultrasound methods of **estimating AFV** are currently being used:

- The subjective assessment evaluates the AFV without measurements, and labels the observed volume as low, normal, or high, usually at the time of the second trimester ultrasound, between 16 and 24 weeks.[1]
- The amniotic fluid index (**AFI**) divides the abdomen into four quadrants and measures the single deepest pocket (**SDP**) in each quadrant without fetal small parts or cord and sums the measurements.[2] AFI ≤ 5 cm can be labeled as oligohydramnios, 5–20 cm as normal, and > 20 cm as hydramnios.[3] The AFI can also be evaluated more accurately by gestational age (GA)-specific charts that label AFV as oligohydramnios (< 5th percentile), normal (5–95th percentile), and hydramnios (> 95th percentile) (Table 50.1).[4]
- The **SDP** technique (aka maximum vertical pocket – MVP) identifies the deepest vertical pocket of fluid that has a horizontal measurement of at least 1 cm and is

without cord or fetal small parts.[5] SDP < 2 cm is labeled as oligohydramnios, 2–8 cm as normal, and > 8 cm as hydramnios.

Originally,[3] the pocket of fluid was measured if it did not have an aggregate of cord or small parts. There is a significantly greater number of low dye-determined AFVs identified using the '**to the cord**' measurement technique rather than 'through the cord' and without any difference for normal and high dye-determined volumes.[6] Therefore, the 'to the cord' measurement is recommended.

AMNIOTIC FLUID ASSESSMENT IN MULTIPLE GESTATIONS

Background

In twin pregnancies the AFV of each sac is about the same as that for normal singleton pregnancies of similar third trimester gestational age.[7]

Technique

The most consistent method of estimating AFV in twin pregnancies is the **SDP** technique. The dividing membrane is identified and the SDP of amniotic fluid in each amniotic sac is measured. Since the AFVs of twin pregnancies are similar to singleton pregnancies, the same categories of oligohydramnios (SDP < 2 cm), normal (2–8 cm), and hydramnios (> 8 cm) can be used. The summated AFI technique,[8,9] which sums the 4 SDPs identified without regard to membrane placement or fetal position, is inaccurate. When correlated to known AFVs in twin pregnancies, this technique has low sensitivity for intertwin differences in AFV and cannot identify twin pairs with either oligohydramnios or hydramnios.[10] The subjective evaluation of the amount of fluid surrounding each fetus, when correlated with dye-determined AFVs in diamniotic twins, has been found to be as accurate as the AFI and SDP in the identification of oligohydramnios (all of the sonographic techniques poorly identify abnormal AFVs).[11]

ACCURACY OF THE ULTRASOUND ESTIMATES OF AMNIOTIC FLUID VOLUME TO IDENTIFY OLIGOHYDRAMNIOS IN SINGLETON PREGNANCIES

By direct measurements at the time of cesarean delivery or dye-determined fluid volumes, all three of the ultrasound

Table 50.1 *Evaluation of amniotic fluid index (AFI) by gestational age*

Week	AFI percentile values		
	5th	50th	95th
16	7.9	12.1	18.5
17	8.3	12.7	19.4
18	8.7	13.3	20.2
19	9.0	13.7	20.7
20	9.3	14.1	21.2
21	9.5	14.3	21.4
22	9.7	14.5	21.6
23	9.8	14.6	21.8
24	9.8	14.7	21.9
25	9.7	14.7	22.1
26	9.7	14.7	22.3
27	9.5	14.6	22.6
28	9.4	14.6	22.8
29	9.2	14.5	23.1
30	9.0	14.5	23.4
31	8.8	14.4	23.8
32	8.6	14.4	24.2
33	8.3	14.3	24.5
34	8.1	14.2	24.8
35	7.9	14.0	24.9
36	7.7	13.8	24.9
37	7.5	13.5	24.4
38	7.3	13.2	23.9
39	7.2	12.7	22.6
40	7.1	12.3	21.4
41	7.0	11.6	19.4
42	6.9	11.0	17.5

Adapted from: Moore TR, Cayle JE. The amniotic fluid index in normal human pregnancy. Am J Obstet Gynecol 1990; 162: 1168–73; with permission from Elsevier.

techniques used to estimate AFV (subjective evaluation, AFI, and SDP) can identify normal volumes but poorly identify oligohydramnios and hydramnios.[12] The cumulative world's literature shows that the association between ultrasound measurements and normal actual volume is good (sensitivity of 70–98%), but in the clinically concerning area of oligohydramnios the association between an ultrasound-estimated AFV and the actual volume is poor (sensitivity of 6–18%).[1,12] A comparison of the 3rd and 5th percentiles of the AFI and SDP adjusted for GA and the fixed cut-offs of an AFI of < 5 cm, and the SDP of < 2 cm, all compared with actual AFVs,[21] showed that the percentiles were no better predictors of actual oligohydramnios. Additionally, the normal values and percentiles for one specific patient population do not correlate with different patient populations, and, if percentiles are used, then normative values should be established for each patient population.[4]

ACCURACY OF THE ULTRASOUND ESTIMATES OF AMNIOTIC FLUID TO PREDICT PREGNANCY OUTCOMES

Although the subjective estimation of AFV is as accurate as the AFI and SDP in the identification of dye-determined low, normal, and high AFVs[1], nearly all ultrasound evaluations and studies use either the AFI or the SDP technique.

The role of the AFI in classifying a pregnancy as high risk on antenatal testing remains uncertain. An AFI of < 5 cm is associated with an increased risk of non-reassuring fetal heart tracing (NRFHT) in labor, meconium-stained amniotic fluid, cesarean delivery for NRFHT, and low Apgar scores.[3,22] Some clinicians have found no association with an AFI < 5 cm and adverse pregnancy outcomes.[23,24] In postdates pregnancies, comparing the SDP with the AFI, the AFI labels more pregnancies as having oligohydramnios, resulting in more labor inductions and subsequent cesarean deliveries, without any improvement in perinatal outcome.[25]

Cesarean deliveries for NRFHT and Apgar scores of < 7 cm at 5 minutes occur in a significantly greater number of women if the AFI is < 5 cm compared with controls.[26] Both the Apgar score < 7 at 5 minutes and cesarean delivery for NRFHT are subjective evaluations and can be influenced by a number of factors. The most objective assessment, umbilical cord pH, has not been linked with an AFI ≤ 5 cm.[22]

SHOULD WE ESTIMATE AMNIOTIC FLUID VOLUME WITH THE SDP OR THE AFI?

Both the AFI as a component of the modified BPP (NST + AFV estimation) and the SDP as part of the BPP (fetal movement, fetal breathing, fetal tone, NST, AFV estimation) are used extensively to monitor at-risk preterm pregnancies. Whereas both fluid estimations have been linked with fetal intolerance of labor, cesarean deliveries for NRFHT, and low Apgar scores, **only the SDP as a component of the BPP has been correlated with the umbilical cord pH.**[27] In addition, as a stand-alone test, the SDP has been linked with perinatal morbidity and mortality,[28] whereas the AFI has never been evaluated as a stand-alone test for this outcome. No investigations have evaluated the AFI with the NST in the prediction of cerebral palsy. A low BPP is associated with antenatal asphyxial events, and may be of use in selected pregnancies to prevent poor pregnancy outcomes.[29,30]

The AFI has been compared with the SDP as a component of the modified BPP (NST + AFI or SDP), or the BPP (fetal movement, fetal tone, fetal breathing movement, NST, and AFI or SDP) in the antepartum evaluation of at-risk pregnancies and as a fetal admission test. In high-risk pregnancies monitored using the BPP,[31] the AFI and SDP are similar in their predictability of adverse antepartum or intrapartum outcomes; however, the AFI labels twice as many women with low fluid compared with the SDP, resulting in more interventions, without any improvement in outcome. In high-risk pregnancies undergoing *modified* BPP, more women are labeled as having low fluid by the AFI with more interventions without any improvement in outcome compared with the SDP.[32] As intrapartum screening tests, neither the AFI nor the SDP are found to be predictive of adverse intrapartum outcomes.[33]

In summary, **both the AFI and the SDP poorly predict oligohydramnios.** The AFI + NST have been linked to perinatal morbidity and mortality, but not to umbilical cord pH at delivery. The AFI as a stand-alone test has not been linked to perinatal morbidity or mortality. The SDP as a component of the BPP has been correlated to perinatal morbidity and mortality, umbilical cord pH at delivery, and cerebral palsy, and as a stand-alone test the SDP has been independently linked with perinatal mortality.[34] Directly compared, the AFI and SDP are similar in their prediction of outcomes, but the AFI overcalls the diagnosis of oligohydramnios, leading to increased interventions and more operative deliveries without any improvement in perinatal outcomes. For these reasons, **the SDP appears to be the better ultrasound estimator of AFV to use with the NST or the BPP.**

MANAGEMENT

In pregnancies at risk for an adverse pregnancy outcome, antenatal surveillance can be undertaken with either the **NST and SDP or** the **BPP and SDP** to assess the AFV. If an estimation of the AFV is undertaken on admission to Labor and Delivery to identify those pregnancies that will have a greater risk of intrapartum complications, then the SDP techniques should also be used.

OLIGOHYDRAMNIOS

KEY POINTS

- Mild oligohydramnios is defined as an **AFI < 5th percentile.** Severe oligohydramnios is an **SDP of < 2 cm. SDP < 2 cm has the best correlation with abnormal neonatal outcome, with the least false-positive rate.**
- **Question** the woman **concerning** (P)PROM.
- **Document,** by ultrasound, **normal fetal kidneys, bladder, and fetal weight.**
- **Suggest hydration** with 2 L of water orally.

At 16–24 weeks:

- Consider **amniocentesis.**
- Consider amnioinfusion for better diagnostic visualization. The role of amnioinfusion as therapy for pregnancy prolongation and prevention of pulmonary hypoplasia has not been tested in a trial.

At 24–40 weeks:

- Consider interventions as for 16–24 weeks if severe oligohydramnios and fetal karyotype and anatomy have not been checked before.
- At ≥ 28 weeks, perform NST and/or BPP to assure fetal well-being. If reassuring, continue SDP/NST weekly/twice weekly, depending on fetal status.
- At ≥ 36 weeks, consider induction/delivery if SDP is < 2 cm and Bishop score is ≥ 9.

At ≥ 40 weeks:

- Consider induction/delivery if AFI < 5 cm.
- Transcervical amnioinfusion should be offered to women at or near term with oligohydramnios.

DIAGNOSIS/DEFINITION

Oligohydramnios should be defined as that low AFV that is linked with an adverse pregnancy outcome, but is commonly defined just as low AFV. **Mild** oligohydramnios can be defined as an AFI < 5th percentile for GA. **Severe** oligohydramnios can be defined as an SDP of < 2 cm measured vertically.

EPIDEMIOLOGY/INCIDENCE

The true incidence of oligohydramnios appears to be approximately 0.2% in the second trimester and 3–5% in the third trimester.

ETIOLOGY

Rupture of membranes (ROM), renal hypofunction, urinary obstruction, and placental insufficiency with/without FGR.

COMPLICATIONS

Fetal anomalies (up to 30% in the second trimester, up to 50% if severe). Oligohydramnios, in particular SDP < 2 cm, has been associated with FGR, NRFHT, CD for NRFHT, endometritis, etc., but the true natural history is not well known since many intervene for oligohydramnios.

MANAGEMENT (FIGURE 50.1)

Question the woman concerning (P)PROM, and perform a clinical examination if (P)PROM is suspected.

The ultrasound should document normal **fetal kidneys, bladder, and fetal weight.**

At 16–24 weeks

At 16–24 weeks consider amniocentesis. Also consider amnioinfusion for better diagnostic visualization. The role of amnioinfusion as therapy for pregnancy prolongation and prevention of pulmonary hypoplasia has not been tested in a trial.

At 24–40 weeks

At 24–40 weeks, consider interventions as for 16–24 weeks in presence of severe oligohydramnios if fetal karyotype and anatomy have not been checked before.

At ≥ 28 – < 36 weeks

At ≥ 28 weeks to < 36 weeks, perform NST and/or BPP to assure fetal well-being. If reassuring, continue SDP/ NST weekly/twice weekly, depending on fetal status:

- If SDP is ≥ 2 cm, follow with weekly NST/SDP.
- If SDP < 2 cm, manage individually (suggest at least twice-weekly NST/SDPs). Consider delivery only if there are substantial signs of fetal compromise such as abnormal BPP, umbilical artery (UA) Doppler flow, NST, etc.
- If SDP normalizes in the subsequent ultrasounds, these patients can be followed with routine care.
- For any oligohydramnios, strongly encourage maternal hydration with 2 L of water.

At 36 weeks

At ≥ 36 weeks, consider induction/delivery if the Bishop score ≥ 9. IF the SDP is < 2 cm and the Bishop score is < 9, continue close monitoring if no other abnormal testing or significant fetal/maternal disease; consider delivery otherwise. If the SDP is ≥ 2 cm and the Bishop score is < 9, follow with NST/SDP.

At 40 weeks

At ≥ 40 weeks, consider induction/delivery if the AFI is < 5 cm.

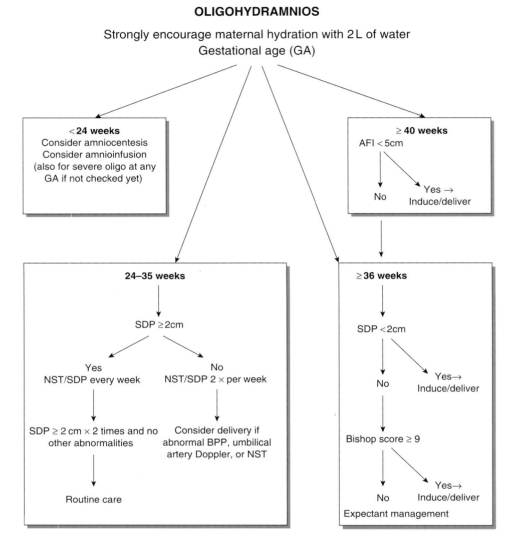

OLIGOHYDRAMNIOS

Strongly encourage maternal hydration with 2 L of water
Gestational age (GA)

<24 weeks
Consider amniocentesis
Consider amnioinfusion
(also for severe oligo at any
GA if not checked yet)

≥40 weeks
AFI <5cm

No   Yes →
            Induce/deliver

24–35 weeks

SDP ≥2cm

Yes   No
NST/SDP every week   NST/SDP 2 × per week

SDP ≥ 2 cm × 2 times and no   Consider delivery if
other abnormalities   abnormal BPP, umbilical
                               artery Doppler, or NST

Routine care

≥36 weeks

SDP <2cm

No   Yes→
                Induce/deliver

Bishop score ≥ 9

No   Yes→
                Induce/deliver

Expectant management

Figure 50.1
Management of oligohydramnios. Oligo, oligohydramnios; AFI, amniotic fluid index; SDP, single deepest pocket; NST, non-stress test; U/S, ultrasound; BPP, biophysical profile; UA, umbilical artery.

Maternal hydration

The effects of oral hydration on the AFV, as estimated by an increase in the AFI or an increase in fetal urine production, are well documented.[34–37] **Drinking 2 L of water** over 2–4 hours before repeat ultrasound examination later that day or the next day **increases the AFI** compared with the control group in women with either oligohydramnios (2 studies, 78 women)[36,38] or normal AFV (1 study, 40 women).[35] Hypotonic but not isotonic intravenous (IV) infusion increases the AFV at a level similar to that of oral hydration (1 trial, 42 women).[38] Following an IV infusion of a 1 L solution, using a dye-dilution technique at CD, the median increase in the AFI is 1.7 cm and in the AFV is 188 ml. The length of time

that this AFV remains increased is uncertain.[39] No adverse effects on the mother or infant have been reported in the four studies, but maternal satisfaction was not studied. Unfortunately, maternal and, especially, fetal/neonatal outcomes were not assessed. Given these limitations, plus the small sample size of the studies, the clinical utility of this intervention is still not fully determined, but there is potential to avoid unnecessary interventions.

Amnioinfusion

If oligohydramnios (without PROM) is detected just before labor, or in **labor near or at term:**

- **Transabdominal amnioinfusion:** reduces NRFHT (from 42% to 5%) and CD for NRFHT (from 25% to 5%).[40]
- **Transcervical amnioinfusion:** in term women with oligohydramnios (usually AFI < 5 cm), amnioinfusion of usually about 500 ml of normal saline and more as needed decreases CD for NRFHT by 77%, overall CD by 48%, umbilical artery pH < 7.20 by 60%, NRFHT by 76%, and low Apgar scores < 7 at 5 minutes by 48%. The rate of endometritis tended to be lower with amnioinfusion.[41–43]

Given better results and a lot more data with this latter technique, prophylactic **transcervical amnioinfusion should be offered to women at or near term with oligohydramnios.**

POLYHYDRAMNIOS (AKA HYDRAMNIOS)

KEY POINTS

- Polyhydramnios is defined as an **SDP of ≥ 8 cm**, or an **AFI of ≥ 95th percentile for gestational age** (AFI >24 cm is polyhydramnios at any GA). Severe polyhydramnios is an SDP of ≥ 15 cm, or an AFI of ≥ 30 cm.
- **Major associations are diabetes and fetal malformation, but up to 50% of mild polyhydramnios is of unknown cause.**
- **Risk of major anomaly at birth after normal ultrasound is 1% with AFI < 30 cm, 2% with AFI 30–34.9 cm, and 11% with AFI ≥ 35 cm.**
- Polyhydramnios is associated with higher rates of **macrosomia, malpresentation, cord prolapse, abruption, primary cesarean delivery, and uterine atony.**
- **Work-up should include** (at least) a **glucose screening test,** antibody screen if not done in the last 4 weeks, RPR, **and accurate fetal anatomy ultrasound.** Parvovirus, toxoplasma, and CMV IgM and IgG can be included. Amniocentesis should be strongly considered if there is severe polyhydramnios, polyhydramnios with fetal anomaly on ultrasound, polyhydramnios associated with FGR, or detected < 24 weeks.

DIAGNOSIS/DEFINITION

SDP ≥ 8 cm, or an AFI of ≥ 95th percentile for GA (AFI >24 mm is polyhydramnios at any GA). Severe polyhydramnios: SDP ≥ 15 cm, or AFI ≥ 30 cm.

EPIDEMIOLOGY/INCIDENCE

The incidence is 1–5% of pregnancies, depending on definition, but <1% for severe polyhydramnios.

ETIOLOGY

Increased production (most commonly maternal diabetes) or decreased clearance (obstruction or poor swallowing). Most common causes are: maternal diabetes (20–30%); fetal malformations (10–15%); multiple gestations (5%); Rh or other isoimmunization; 'mirror syndrome'; others; unknown cause (about 50%, especially for mild polyhydramnios). Severe polyhydramnios is usually pathologic.

COMPLICATIONS

Fetal anomalies may be present (risk of major anomaly on prenatal ultrasound): 8% with AFI < 30 cm, 12% with AFI 30–34.9 cm, and 31% with AFI ≥ 35 cm. **Risk of major anomaly at birth after normal ultrasound is: 1% with AFI < 30 cm, 2% with AFI 30–34.9 cm, and 11% with AFI ≥ 35 cm.** The fetus may have a chromosomal abnormality (risk of aneuploidy: ≤ 1% if normal ultrasound, about 10% if major anomaly present). Detailed ultrasound should detect about 60–80% of major anomalies associated with polyhydramnios. Perinatal mortality for normal anatomy fetuses is < 5%. For anomalous fetuses, perinatal mortality is 10–80% depending on anomaly.[44] Preterm birth (PTB) by preterm labor (PTL) or PPROM is increased especially with severe polyhydramnios. Polyhydramnios is associated with higher rates of **macrosomia, malpresentation, cord prolapse, abruption, primary CD, and uterine atony.**

WORK-UP (DIFFERENTIAL DIAGNOSIS)

History

- **Diabetes mellitus**
- Rh isoimmunization, and diabetes insipidus
- Family history of myotonic dystrophy or inborn errors of metabolism
- Ask regarding maternal discomfort.

Ultrasound

Multiple gestation, in particular twin–twin transfusion syndrome.

CNS/neuro. Anencephaly, holoprosencephaly, Dandy–Walker malformation, lissencephaly, agenesis of corpus callosum, neural tube defects (NTD), etc.

Neuromuscular. Arthrogryposis.

Cardiac. Septal defects,* truncus arteriosus, aortic coarctation, arch interruption, arrhythmias, etc.

Thoracic.   Congenital diaphragmatic hernia (CDH), congenital cystic adenomatoid malformation (CCAM), sequestration, chylothorax, tracheal atresia.

Gastrointestinal.   Cleft lip/palate,* transesophageal (TE) fistula,* esophageal or intestinal atresia, imperforate anus,* abdominal wall defects, annular pancreas.

Skeletal.   Achondroplasia, thanatophoric dysplasia, campomelic dysplasia, osteogenesis imperfecta (OI), hypophosphatasia, etc.

Other.   Cystic hygroma, neck masses, goiter, sacrococcygeal teratoma (SCT).
  Rule out hydrops. Perform umbilical and middle cerebral artery pulsatile index and peak systolic velocity Doppler.

Laboratory

One-hour glucola and antibody screen if not done in last 4 weeks. Parvovirus IgM and IgG; toxoplasmosis IgM and IgG; CMV IgM and IgG; rapid plasma reagin (RPR) (rule out syphilis).

Amniocentesis

Strongly consider if **severe polyhydramnios, polyhydramnios with fetal anomaly on ultrasound, polyhydramnios associated with intrauterine growth restriction (IUGR) or detected < 24 weeks.** Some clinicians advocate offering amniocentesis to all women with polyhydramnios given the 0.5–1% incidence of aneuploidy. If *amniocentesis* is performed:

1. Karyotype (T21, T18, 45X: most common abnormalities).
2. PCR for parvovirus, CMV, toxoplasmosis, syphilis.
3. Myotonic dystrophy study if positive family history or ultrasound evidence of hypotonia, e.g. clubbed feet or positional abnormalities of the extremities.[45]
4. Inborn errors of metabolism: Gaucher disease, gangliosidoses, mucopolysaccharidoses, etc. (consider especially if positive family history or above work-up negative and severe polyhydramnios).

LABOR PRECAUTIONS

For appropriate management to decrease complications from polyhydramnios – associated macrosomia, malpresentation, cord prolapse, abruption, primary CD and uterine atony, see appropriate chapters. Consider delaying or avoiding artificial ROM to avoid cord prolapse, or at least 'needling' the membranes.

(* = Most common anomalies with polyhydramnios).[44]

MANAGEMENT

- Appropriate **counseling** regarding complications as above.
- **Work-up** as above.
- Manage anomaly/aneuploidy/maternal or fetal disease detected during work-up.
- GA < 24 weeks: consider amniocentesis.
- GA 24–40 weeks:
  - AFIs < 30 cm: AFIs every 2–3 weeks. At ≥ 32 weeks, NSTs every week.
  - AFIs ≥ 30 cm: AFIs and evaluations to rule out fetal hydrops weekly. At ≥ 28 weeks, weekly NSTs. Consider amniocentesis.
- AFI ≥ 40 cm, SDP ≥ 12 cm, and/or maternal symptoms: as per severe polyhydramnios, plus consider the following options: (1) Amnioreduction – goal is to normalize AFV. There is a 1.5% complication rate, such as PPROM, chorioamnionitis, abruptio placentae, membrane detachment. Associated with PTL/PPROM, and also abruptio if >2 L taken out at one time. (2) Non-steroidal anti-inflammatory drug (NSAID) therapy – indomethacin and sulindac. (a) Indomethacin: 75–200 mg/day (25–50 mg po every 6–8 hours); mechanism of action: decreases fetal urine production by increasing proximal tubular resorption of water and sodium; side effects: oligohydramnios and ductal closure (see Chapters 15 and 16 of *Obstetric Evidence Based Guidelines*). Only treat for 48 hours and at < 32 weeks to avoid/minimize side effects. (b) Sulindac: 200 mg every 12 hours; same mechanism of action and side effects as indomethacin.
- GA ≥ 39 weeks: induction/delivery for maternal discomfort in severe polyhydramnios. Cesarean delivery for obstetric indications only.

REFERENCES

1. Magann EF, Perry KG, Chauhan SP, et al. The accuracy of ultrasound evaluation of amniotic fluid volume in singleton pregnancies. The effect of operator experience and ultrasound interpretive technique. J Clin Ultrasound 1997; 25: 249–53. [II-2]
2. Phelan JP, Ahn MO, Smith CV. Amniotic fluid index measurements during pregnancy. J Reprod Med 1987; 32: 601–4. [II-3]
3. Rutherford SE, Smith CV, Phelan JP, Jacobs N. The four quadrant assessment of amniotic fluid volume; an adjunct to antepartum fetal heart rate testing. Obstet Gynecol 1987; 87: 353–6. [II-3]
4. Magann EF, Sanderson M, Martin JN Jr, Chauhan SP. The amniotic fluid index, single deepest pocket, and two-diameter pocket in normal human pregnancy. Am J Obstet Gynecol 2000; 182: 1581–8. [II-2]
5. Manning FA, Platt LD, Sipos L. Antepartum fetal evaluation: development of a fetal biophysical profile. Am J Obstet Gynecol 1980; 136: 787–95. [II-3]
6. Magann EF, Chauhan SP, Washington W, Martin JN Jr, Morrison JC. Ultrasound estimation of amniotic fluid volume using the largest vertical pocket containing umbilical cord: measure to or through the cord? Ultrasound Obstet Gynecol 2002; 20: 464–7. [II-2]

7. Magann EF, Whitworth NS, Bass JD, et al. Amniotic fluid volume of third-trimester diamniotic twins. Obstet Gynecol 1995; 85: 857–60. [II-2]

8. Porter TF, Dildy GA, Blanchard JR, Kochenour NK, Clark SL. Normal values for amniotic fluid index during uncomplicated twin pregnancy. Obstet Gynecol 1996; 87: 699–702. [II-2]

9. Chau AC, Kjos SC, Kovacs BW. Ultrasonographic measurement of amniotic fluid volume in normal diamniotic twin pregnancies. Am J Obstet Gynecol 1996; 174: 1003–7. [II-2]

10. Magann EF, Chauhan SP, Whitworth NS, et al. Accuracy of the summated AFI in evaluating amniotic fluid volume in diamniotic twin pregnancies. Am J Obstet Gynecol 1997; 177: 1041–5. [II-2]

11. Magann EF, Chauhan SP, Whitworth NS, et al. Determination of amniotic fluid volume in twin pregnancies: ultrasonographic evaluation versus operator estimation. Am J Obstet Gynecol 2000; 182: 1606–9. [II-2]

12. Magann EF, Nolan TE, Hess LW, et al. Measurement of amniotic fluid volume: accuracy of ultrasonography techniques. Am J Obstet Gynecol 1992; 167: 1533–7. [II-2]

13. Croom CS, Banias BB, Ramos-Santos E, et al. Do semiquantitative amniotic fluid indexes reflect actual volume? Am J Obstet Gynecol 1992; 167: 995–9. [II-2]

14. Dildy GA 3rd, Lira N, Moise KJ Jr, Riddle GD, Deter RL. Amniotic fluid volume assessment: comparison of ultrasonographic estimates versus direct measurements with a dye-dilution technique in human pregnancy. Am J Obstet Gynecol 1992; 167: 986–94. [II-2]

15. Horsager R, Nathan L, Leveno KJ. Correlation of measured amniotic fluid volume and sonographic predictions of oligohydramnios. Am J Obstet Gynecol 1994; 83: 955–8. [II-3]

16. Sepulveda W, Flack NJ, Fisk NM. Direct volume measurement at midtrimester amnioinfusion in relation to ultrasonographic indexes of amniotic fluid volume. Am J Obstet Gynecol 1994; 170: 1160–3. [II-3]

17. Magann EF, Morton ML, Nolan TE, et al. Comparative efficacy of two sonographic measurements for the detection of aberrations in the amniotic fluid volume and the effect of amniotic fluid volume on pregnancy outcome. Obstet Gynecol 1994; 83: 959–62. [II-2]

18. Magann EF, Nevils BD, Chauhan SP, et al. Low amniotic fluid volume is poorly identified in singleton and twin pregnancies using the 2×2 pocket technique of the biophysical profile. South Med J 1999; 92: 802–5. [II-2]

19. Chauhan SP, Magann EF, Morrison JC, et al. Ultrasonographic assessment of amniotic fluid volume does not reflect actual volume. Am J Obstet Gynecol 1997; 177: 291–7. [II-2]

20. Magann EF, Chauhan SP, Martin JN Jr. Oligohydramnios at term and pregnancy outcome. Fetal Maternal Med Rev 2001; 12: 209–27. [II-3]

21. Magann EF, Doherty DA, Chauhan SP, et al. How well do the amniotic fluid index and single deepest pocket indices (below the 3rd and the 5th and above the 95th and 97th percentiles) predict oligohydramnios and hydramnios? Am J Obstet Gynecol 2004; 190: 164–9. [II-2]

22. Miller DA, Rabello YA, Paul RH. The modified biophysical profile: antepartum testing in the 1990s. Am J Obstet Gynecol 1996; 174: 812–17. [II-3]

23. Magann EF, Chauhan SP, Kinsella MJ, et al. Antenatal testing among 1001 high risk women: the role of the ultrasonographic estimate of amniotic fluid volume. Am J Obstet Gynecol 1999; 180: 1330–6. [II-3]

24. Garmel SH, Chelmow D, Sha SJ, Roan JR, D'Alton ME. Oligohydramnios and the appropriately grown fetus. Am J Perinatol 1997; 14: 359–63. [II-3]

25. Alfirevic Z, Luckas M, Walkinshaw SA, McFarland M, Curran R. A randomized comparison between amniotic fluid index and maximum pool depth in the monitoring of post term pregnancies. Br J Obstet Gynaecol 1997; 104: 207–11. [II-2]

26. Chauhan SP, Sanderson M, Hendrix NW, Magann EF, Devoe LD. Perinatal outcome and amniotic fluid index in the antepartum and intrapartum periods: a meta-analysis. Am J Obstet Gynecol 1999; 181: 1473–8. [meta-analysis; 18 studies, $n = 10\,551$]

27. Manning FA, Harman CR, Morrison I, et al. Fetal assessment based on fetal biophysical profile scoring IV. An analysis of perinatal morbidity and mortality. Am J Obstet Gynecol 1990; 162: 703–9. [II-2]

28. Chamberlain PR, Manning FA, Morrison I, Menticoglou SM, Lange IR. Ultrasound evaluation of amniotic fluid. I The relationship of marginal and decreased amniotic fluid volumes to perinatal outcomes. Am J Obstet Gynecol 1984; 150: 245–9. [II-3]

29. Manning FA, Bondaji N, Harman CR, et al. Fetal assessment based on the fetal biophysical profile score: relationship of the last BPS result to subsequent cerebral palsy. J Gynecol Obstet Biol Reprod 1997; 26: 720–9. [II-3]

30. Manning FA, Bondaji N, Harman CR, et al. Fetal assessment based on fetal biophysical scoring VIII. The incidence of cerebral palsy in tested and untested perinates. Am J Obstet Gynecol 1998; 178: 696–706. [II-2]

31. Magann EF, Doherty DA, Field K, et al. Biophysical profile with amniotic fluid volume assessments. Obstet Gynecol 2004; 104: 5–10. [II-3]

32. Chauhan SP, Doherty DA, Magann EF, et al. Amniotic fluid index vs. single deepest pocket technique during modified biophysical profile: a randomized clinical trial. Am J Obstet Gynecol 2004; 191: 661–7. [RCT, $n = 1080$]

33. Moses J, Doherty DA, Magann EF, Chauhan SP, Morrison JC. A randomized clinical trial of the intrapartum assessment of amniotic fluid volume: amniotic fluid index versus the single deepest pocket. Am J Obstet Gynecol 2004; 190: 1564–9. [RCT, $n = 1000$]

34. Magann EF, Chauhan SP, Bofill JA, Martin JN Jr. Comparability of the amniotic fluid index and single deepest pocket measurements in clinical practice. Aust N Z J Obstet Gynaecol 2003; 43: 75–7. [II-2]

35. Kilpatrick SJ, Safford SL. Maternal hydration increases the amniotic fluid index in women with normal amniotic fluid volume. Obstet Gynecol 1993; 81: 49–52. [RCT, $n = 40$]

36. Kilpatrick SJ, Safford SL, Pomeroy T, et al. Maternal hydration increases the amniotic fluid index. Obstet Gynecol 1991; 78: 1098–102. [RCT, $n = 36$]

37. Oosterhof H, Haak MC, Aarnoudse JG. Acute maternal rehydration increases the urine production rate in the near-term fetus. Am J Obstet Gynecol 2000; 183: 226–9. [II-3]

38. Doi S, Osada H, Seki K, Sikiya S. Effect of maternal hydration on oligohydramnios. A comparison of three volume expansion methods. Obstet Gyncol 1998; 92: 525–9. [RCT, $n = 84$]

39. Magann EF, Doherty DA, Chauhan SP, et al. Effect of maternal hydration on amniotic fluid volume. Obstet Gynecol 2003; 101: 1261–5. [II-3]

40. Vergani P, Ceruti P, Strobelt N, et al. Transabdominal amnioinfusion in oligohydramnios at term before induction of labor with intact membranes: a randomized clinical trial. Am J Obstet Gynecol 1996; 175: 465–70. [RCT; $n = 79$]

41. Pitt C, Sanchez-Ramos L, Kaunitz AM, Gaudier F. Prophylactic amnioinfusion for intrapartum oligohydramnios: a meta-analysis of randomized controlled trials. Obstet Gynecol 2000; 96: 861–6. [meta-analysis: 14 RCTs; $n = 793/740$]

42. Amin AF, Mohammed MS, Sayed GH, Abdel-Razik S. Prophylactic transcervical amnioinfusion in laboring women with oligohydramnios. Int J Gynecol Obstet 2003; 81: 183–9. [RCT; $n = 160$; not included in Ref. 41]

43. Hofmeyr GJ. Amnioinfusion for umbilical cord compression in labour. Cochrane Database Syst Rev 2007; 1. [meta-analysis: 14 RCTs, most with < 200 women each – see also Chapter 9 of *Obstetric Evidence Based Guidelines*].

44. Dashe JS, McIntire DD, Ramus RM, Santos-Ramos R, Twickler DM. Hydramnios: anomaly prevalence and sonographic detection. Obstet Gynecol 2002; 100: 134–9. [II-3, $n = 672$, largest series of hydramnios]

45. Esplin MS, Hallam S, Farrington PF, et al. Myotonic dystrophy is a significant cause of idiopathic polyhydramnios. Am J Obstet Gynecol 1998; 179: 974–7. [II-3]

51

Antepartum testing

Christopher R Harman, Michelle L Kush, and Ahmet A Baschat

ANTEPARTUM TESTING

KEY POINTS

- There are no randomized trial data proving that antepartum testing reduces long-term neurologic deficits.
- Although entrenched in high-risk pregnancy management, most antenatal testing schemes are not supported by sufficient evidence. There are insufficient trials to compare adequately different fetal tests of well-being. Therefore recommendations regarding which pregnancies to test and at what gestational age testing should start cannot be made given lack of sufficient evidence.
- **Multiple parameter testing schemes** have **better correlation with fetal condition** than do single-parameter tests.
- The **non-stress test** used alone is not adequate to exclude several important sources of perinatal injury. The non-stress test is associated with a trend for an increase in perinatal deaths in the cardiotocography group (1.8 vs 0.6%). There is no increase in the incidence of interventions.
- **Biophysical profile score (BPS)** surveillance may be beneficial in reducing cerebral palsy, with insufficient trial evidence. Compared to other fetal testing (usually NST), **biophysical profile increases the incidence of induction, but does not affect incidences of cesarean delivery, admission to ICN, or perinatal mortality.** Individual components have been compared in some trials, but the value of that evidence is limited.
- **Umbilical artery Doppler decreases perinatal mortality in antenatal management of FGR fetuses, and should be routinely used in these pregnancies.** Compared to no Doppler ultrasound, **Doppler ultrasound in high-risk pregnancy** (especially those complicated by hypertension or presumed FGR) is associated with a **trend to a reduction in perinatal deaths**, with 17% **fewer inductions of labor** and 44% **fewer admissions to hospital.**
- Identification of FGR fetuses at highest risk of stillbirth may be accomplished by combined arterial and venous Doppler, while **timing of their delivery at critical gestational ages** may be best directed by multiple tests.

- **Testing frequency and complexity** should be adjusted to reflect the stability of the clinical situation.
- Ancillary tests such as contraction stress test, oxytocin challenge test, and vibroacoustic stimulation, may have specific uses, but limited applicability.
- Formal maternal counting of fetal movement appears effective in one study but not in another for prevention of fetal death.

BACKGROUND

Evaluation of fetal health is pivotal in pregnancy management: reliable reassurance of fetal health means the pregnancy can safely be extended; proven fetal compromise dictates delivery, down to the margins of viability. We rely on accurate fetal testing to initiate action, including accelerating fetal lung maturity, transfer to high-risk centers, increased frequency of testing, and addition of testing modalities. Concern with long-term consequences of fetal compromise has dictated a shift in outcome measures, from perinatal mortality to neurologic and other developmental morbidities. Optimizing the testing program means choosing methods, frequency, disease-specific components, and accounting for gestational-age limitations, drug interactions, test variability, and even the interaction of test components. Such individualized fetal testing must be applied in a resource-conscious way, while addressing the ever-increasing public expectation of ideal results. This guideline focuses on the important factors in selecting the best fetal assessment strategy for each pregnancy.

ENDPOINTS IN FETAL MONITORING

Evaluating modalities of fetal monitoring is complex, depending on the interaction of maternal, fetal, placental, uterine, and gestational age factors. The choice of endpoints for comparison will often dictate the results of the comparison. Although many studies exist evaluating fetal testing, including comparing results using different methods, endpoints are seldom uniform. If, for example, fetal testing is designed to prevent cerebral palsy, then the test best at predicting fetal acidosis (umbilical venous pH <7.20) may be the test of choice, because of the high correlation between neonatal acidosis and long-term neurologic handicap.[1] However, the large majority of children with cerebral palsy had normal cord gases, and normal Apgars,[2,3] so the impact of that test's correlation would be hard to prove in a population-based study. This weakness is found in almost all newborn criteria – the resilience of individual babies, the continuing improvements in the excellence of neonatal care, the profound influence of remote antenatal factors on fetal brain development, all mean that neonatal outcome factors are lightweight, at best.[4] Perinatal death, in particular fetal death, is an important outcome when evaluating fetal testing. Given the rarity of this outcome, there are very few trials large enough to be able to meaningfully assess any effect of fetal testing on the incidence of death. For example, even if the quoted false-negative rate (for perinatal death) for BPS is often reported as 0.6/1000, in some populations this may be the baseline incidence of this outcome. There are few randomized controlled trials which evaluate a program of surveillance, carried out over the course of many complicated pregnancies, and determine the impact in meaningful long-term parameters. Even considering non-random clinical trails, the evidence is sparse. Two notable examples illustrate these difficulties.

Growth Restriction Intervention Trial (GRIT)[5–7]

Obstetric caregivers enrolled patients in this randomized management trial when they were uncertain whether to deliver the patient or not, based on a perception of fetal compromise. Umbilical artery Doppler was required before enrollment, but the degree of compromise was not specifically quantified for study entry. The trial was designed to answer the question – can early intervention (immediate delivery) prevent fetal deterioration and avoid hypoxemic brain injury? Cases were allocated to immediate delivery or to delivery delayed until worsening testing results made caregivers certain of the need to proceed. Neonatal and two-year results are summarized in Table 51.1.

This study demonstrated that a policy of 'automatic' delivery based on the risk (or fear) of fetal hypoxemia, without clear testing evidence of a requirement for delivery, did not prevent subsequent death or permanent neurologic sequelae.

It may be difficult for the obstetric caregiver to put GRIT into practice. Perinatal mortality (PNM) was the same with either approach, because the stillbirth rate favoring immediate delivery (0.67% vs 2.4%), was balanced by the neonatal death rate (9% vs 6%). Delivering immediately avoided stillbirth, but produced more babies who died or had permanent injury later. Gestational age, and not the severity of initial Doppler status, was the dominant factor deciding outcome – one's clinical judgment may not be that important. More perplexing, the decision to delay was terminated by a wide variety of mechanisms, including worsening maternal condition, deterioration in Doppler, heart rate testing, biophysical profile, or when the patient's care was transferred to another center. Considering the infrequency of residual morbidity and the 69 different teams that participated, it may not be surprising that the results seem so individual as to be non-generalizable. In summary, GRIT did not confirm the belief that early delivery based on umbilical artery Doppler and other risk factors produced better results. GRIT did parallel other delayed-intervention trials in suggesting that delaying to achieve more gestational time tended to improve the quality and health of the surviving babies.[8,9]

GRIT focused on a population of 573 high-risk fetuses in a multicenter randomized intervention trial, virtually the only one of its kind. A lower level of evidence is seen in a larger experience with a single surveillance scheme – Biophysical profile scoring.

Biophysical Profile Score (BPS) and cerebral palsy[10]

In this study, at-risk pregnancies were all managed according to the BPS protocol (see below), delivered by a single university-based team. Delivery was according to fixed fetal

Table 51.1	*Results from the Growth Restriction Intervention Trial (GRIT)*		
Endpoint	Immediate delivery	Delayed delivery	Odds ratio
CD rate	91%	79%	2.7 (95% CI 1.6–4.5)
Early PNM	10%	9%	1.1 (95% CI 0.61–1.8)
Late PNM	2%	2%	1.0
Cerebral palsy	5%	1%	Not calculated
All disabilities	8%	4%	Not calculated
Death or Disability at 2 years	19% (55/290)	15.5% (44/283)	1.1 (95% CI 0.7–1.8)

CD, cesarean delivery; PNM, perinatal mortality; CI, confidence interval.

criteria, which do account for gestational age in some of the variables.[11] The 26 290 monitored cases were compared to 58 657 non-monitored controls delivered during the same 5-year period in the same healthcare jurisdiction. Cerebral palsy and other neurologic injuries were determined by computerized review of healthcare records and secondary analysis of all index cases, at age 4. The diagnoses were proven in the acquired cases, but an unknown number of cases left the jurisdiction altogether or were unreported for other reasons. Neonatal data were available only on the BPS-monitored cases, and were not reported in this study (Table 51.2).

The large number of subjects meant there was no significant difference in birthweight (2.09 vs 2.28 kg) or mean gestational age at delivery (33.4 vs 34.4 weeks) between groups. Small differences in extremes included babies under 1.0 kg (14% vs 6.7%) and births before 28 weeks (13.5% vs 10.9%) reflecting a somewhat higher acuity, and a significantly higher rate of intervention, comparing monitored vs non-monitored pregnancies.

Before accepting this management scheme as directly transferable to current high-risk practices, however, recall that this was a clinical study using a cohort of undocumented pregnancies. Referral indications included history of stillbirth, suspected FGR and abnormal Doppler (all GRIT criteria) but also included post-dates pregnancy, and diabetic macrosomia. At the time of this study, many non-monitored women had very limited ultrasound evaluation – the current high rate of detection of FGR, anomalies, malpresentation and so on, may diminish the apparent advantage of ultrasound-based BPS. The frequency of abnormal scores prompting intervention (567/26 290, 2.2%) is likely not a solely sufficient explanation for the different rates of neurologic deficit – 51% of those with cerebral palsy had normal BPS and had no intervention. It seems likely that the role of normal BPS in delaying intervention, because practitioners were reassured about the safety of waiting, is also active. In summary, consistent application of the biophysical profile scoring management algorithm appears associated with a significant reduction in long-term neurologic handicap, but the quality of the evidence merits reservation.

MECHANISMS OF PERINATAL INJURY

Permanent fetal injury or death may occur as the result of multiple initial events. The primary focus of antenatal testing has been on the timely detection of fetal hypoxemia and acidosis, but lack of oxygen is seldom the sole cause of injury. Current concepts place increasing emphasis on hemodynamic issues – ischemia and oxidative stress following reperfusion are at least as important as reduced oxygen in the generation of fetal neurologic injury.[12] Many of these events lead to loss of functional placental surface, with increasing placental resistance leading to detectable changes in umbilical artery Doppler velocimetry.[13] Further, as maladaptation to worsening conditions occurs, many fetal efforts to compensate fail.[14] In that scenario, initial fetal responses detectable by monitoring may disappear, meaning the monitoring techniques become irrelevant as the condition worsens. This is shifting ground, and the following stepwise fetal responses to worsening oxygenation become only a rough approximation.

Improve oxygen availability

This is limited, as the fetus cannot directly influence placental transport. Increased hemoglobin concentration, increased oxygen extraction, and (nearer term) improved capacity to tolerate short-term oxidative stress, coupled with circulatory responses such as mild cardiac dilation and baseline tachycardia, may make 14–16% more oxygen available.[15] Such compensation likely can account for the decline in pO_2 over the course of gestation and delivery. Subtle changes in these parameters are unlikely to be important fetal monitoring markers as most of the variance is within the normal variability of fetal behavior, including the normal fluctuations observed in placental and fetal systemic Doppler indices.

Table 51.2 *Comparison of cerebral palsy rates in pregnancies managed and not managed by biophysical profile scoring (BPS) protocol*

Endpoint	BPS monitored	Non-monitored	Odds ratio*
Cerebral palsy	1.33	4.74	3.6, $p<.001$
Cortical blindness	0.66	1.04	1.6, $p<.01$
Cortical deafness	0.90	2.2	2.4, $p<.005$
Mental retardation	0.80	3.1	3.9, $p<.001$
ADHD	4.7	28.1	6.0, $p</001$
EDoC	1.2	1.0	1.2, NS

Rates are per 1000 live births. ADHD, attention-deficit hyperactivity disorder; EDoC, emotional disorders of childhood (control variable).
*Non-monitored vs BPS-monitored.

Differentiate oxygen use

As the normal fetus develops, the ductus venosus restricts centralized nutrient-rich umbilical venous blood flow, deflecting it to the right lobe of the liver. In the compromised fetus, diversion of flow to essential organs and away from non-essential vascular beds is accomplished by two primary mechanisms – mechanical diversion of flow toward the coronary arteries, brain, liver, and placenta (via ductus venosus and foramen ovale), and segmental vasoconstriction in splanchnic, pulmonary, and distal aortic outflows. Secondary hemodynamic changes including dilatation of cerebral blood vessels ('brain sparing' – see below), dilation of coronary arteries ('heart sparing'), and intrahepatic recirculation ('liver sparing') apparently follow progressively. These changes become more dramatic and more exclusive as placental resistance rises, so a significant proportion of the effect may be forced on recipient beds as the placental fraction of cardiac output drops. Differential provision of oxygen-rich blood probably accounts for asymmetric growth and the modest functional limitations of the majority of FGR fetuses (e.g., hematologic indices reflecting relative bone marrow deficiency), who are born with low pO_2 but normal pH and normal long-term development. These changes are illustrated in comprehensive Doppler surveillance, but may be unnoticed if only arterial Doppler is used – precordial venous assessment is required to depict fetal status accurately.[16]

Reduce oxygen consumption

Fetal oxygen consumption falls significantly when the fetus stops moving, but absolute abolition of fetal activity is apparently an end stage of decompensation. In FGR, global reductions in fetal activity may precede abolition of specific behaviors over a long interval, so serial evaluation of behavior gives better detection.[17] As deterioration progresses, intervals of very quiet sleep become longer and longer. Specific fetal behaviors may be lost sequentially – fetal heart rate reactivity is lost before fetal breathing movements, for example.[15] These changes in fetal activity take place on a background of wide variability in time sequence in normal fetuses. These behaviors constitute the basis for behavioral testing including the biophysical profile score (BPS), non-stress fetal heart rate testing (NST), and evocative variants discussed below.

These steps are overlapping, not mutually exclusive, apparently responsive to short-term change such as different maternal positions, maternal exercise, and temporary supplemental maternal oxygen, and reversible if the placental process is not progressive.[18] So, although many early interventions have been based on the emergence of such serious factors (e.g., reversed end-diastolic umbilical artery blood flow mandating immediate cesarean section delivery), it has been amply demonstrated that no single test is reliable enough to dictate management, especially when that means preterm delivery.

PRINCIPLES OF FETAL MONITORING

The ideal antenatal testing regime should:

- Identify impending fetal injury with near-perfect sensitivity, with warning advanced enough to allow effective intervention.
- Distinguish normal variation, benign abnormality, and degrees of significant abnormality, facilitating graded response.
- Identify normal fetal condition with near-perfect predictive value, reliably excluding stillbirth or injury for a clinically relevant interval.
- Exclude grievous fetal abnormality as the source of abnormal testing.
- Be applicable to a variety of common sources of fetal compromise, practicable in common prenatal settings, and reproducible between situations.
- Produce measurable benefits in reduction of perinatal death and long-term neurologic handicap.[19]

FETAL MONITORING METHODS

Fetal heart rate (FHR) testing (also called non-stress test [NST], or cardiotocography [CTG])

This was first formalized as the non-stress test (NST), which is defined as 'reactive' when there are two or more accelerations of at least 15 beats per minute above the baseline, that last for at least 15 seconds, in a 20-minute period of combined FHR and uterine activity monitoring – cardiotocography, or CTG (Figure 51.1). The concordance between fetal movement and accelerations in fetal heart rate is good evidence of fetal wellbeing, with a negative predictive value against fetal demise within 7 days of 99.5–100%.[22] However, in specific circumstances, such as FGR with abnormal placental resistance, the non-stress test may give a false-positive reassurance against acidosis, as high as 15%.[20] Missed anomalies and missed oligohydramnios are major contributors to fetal complications in patients with reactive tracings.

In practical monitoring terms, the false-alarming non-reactive NST is more problematic, occurring in up to 10% of tests at term[21], and up to 50% of the time at 24–28 weeks gestational age. When the subsequent confirmatory test (biophysical profile score, contraction stress test, vibroacoustic stimulation, as examples) is performed, up to 85% will be normal.[22] If performed, the NST should be done in the semi-Fowler ('sitting') position, as it decreases the need for prolonged monitoring compared to the supine position.[23]

Strong evidence, including randomized trial data, supports the position that non-stress fetal heart testing should not be used as a solitary method of monitoring high-risk fetuses.[24–27] Compared to no cardiotocography or

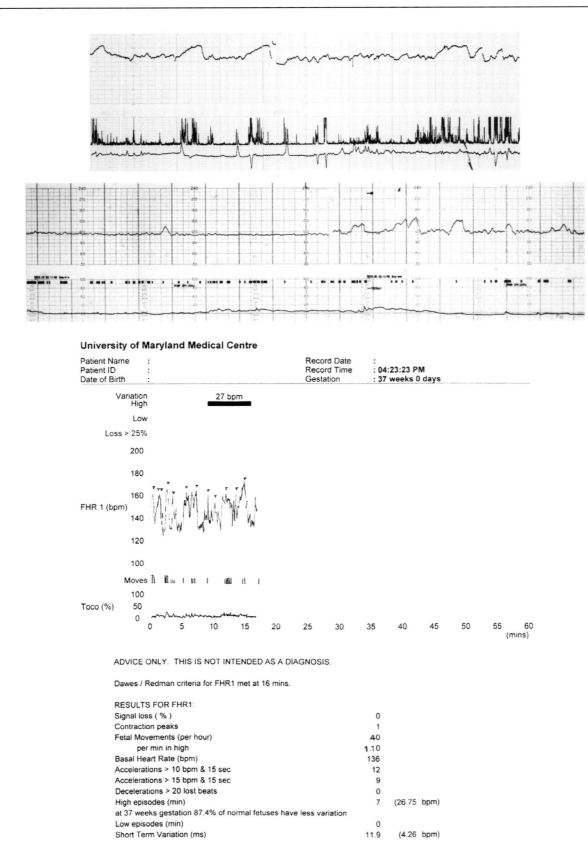

Figure 51.1
Fetal heart rate (FHR) monitoring.

Table 51.3 *Interpretation of BPS variables in 30 minutes*

Fetal variable	Normal behavior (score = 2)	Abnormal behavior (score = 0)
Fetal breathing movements	Intermittent, multiple episodes of more than 30s duration, within 30-min BPS time frame. Hiccups count	Completely absent breathing or no sustained episodes. Continuous breathing without cessation
Body or limb movements	At least four discrete body movements in 30 min. Includes fine motor movements, rolling movements, but not REM or mouthing movements	Three or fewer body/limb movements in a 30-min observation period
Fetal tone/posture	Demonstration of active extension with rapid return to flexion of fetal limbs and brisk repositioning/trunk rotation. Opening and closing of hand, mouth, kicking, and so on	Low-velocity movement only. Incomplete flexion, flaccid extremity positions, abnormal fetal posture. Must score = 0 when FM completely absent
Cardiotocogram	At least two episodes of fetal acceleration of ≥ 15 beats/minute and of ≥ 15 seconds duration. Normal mean variation (computerized FHR interpretation), accelerations associated with maternal palpation of FM (accelerations graded for gestation)	Fetal movement and accelerations not coupled. Insufficient accelerations, absent accelerations, or decelerative trace. Mean variation <20 on numerical analysis of CTG
Amniotic fluid evaluation	At least one pocket ≥ 2 cm with no umbilical cord. Also consider criteria for subjectively reduced fluid	No cord-free pocket ≥ 2 cm, or multiple elements of subjectively reduced amniotic fluid volume definite

BPS, biophysical profile score; CTG, cardiotocogram; FBM, fetal breathing movements; FHR, fetal heart rate; FM, fetal movement; REM, rapid eye movement.

concealment of information, knowledge of antenatal cardiotocography results appears to have no significant effect on perinatal mortality or morbidity in high- or intermediate-risk pregnancies managed in- or out-patient. There is a trend to an increase in perinatal deaths in the cardiotocography group (1.8 vs 0.6%; OR 2.85, 95% CI 0.99–7.12). There is no increase in the incidence of interventions such as elective cesarean delivery or induction of labor.[26]

Computerized interpretation of fetal heart rate monitoring has evolved as a more specific, objective means of maximizing the information obtained from the CTG.[28,29] The computerized CTG (CCTG) analyzes digitized epochs of FHR for numerical criteria, outputting objective data on short-term variability (mean of 4–8 ms) and overall variability, recorded as mean minute variation.[29] Values for short-term variability below 3 ms show strong correlation with fetal acidosis. The CCTG is not as limited by gestational age, and does not require vigorous fetal activity to document a normal result, so it has been adopted as a better version of FHR analysis for a broader range of fetal indications, including incorporation in multiparameter testing regimes.[30] CCTG is superior to simple NST in performance time, positive and negative predictive accuracies, and fewer equivocal test results, but has similar neonatal outcomes.[31] There is reasonably good evidence to support the position that CCTG should also not be used as a solitary method of fetal surveillance.[32]

Response to abnormal test results

In specific circumstances, intervention may be based on FHR testing alone. At term, in a fetus previously documented as having reactive NST with normal variability, delivery should be considered if the tracing shows minimal variability and/or repetitive late decelerations. In other uncommon cases, the first NST may detect a fetal arrhythmia, requiring prompt referral for fetal echocardiography and ultrasound examination. With these exceptions, all non-reassuring CTG results may be followed immediately by full biophysical profile scoring or ultrasound and Doppler assessment as appropriate.[19]

Biophysical profile scoring (BPS)

This ultrasound-based modality uses five parameters of fetal behavior in a protocol-driven format (Table 51. 3) to manage high-risk pregnancies.[33] The parameters have different sensitivities for different fetal outcomes, but the combination of variables consistently gives the best prediction of fetal status, perinatal mortality and neonatal complications (Figure 51.2).[12,34,35]

Fetal breathing movements

These are rhythmic contractions of the fetal diaphragms, unrelated to fetal CO_2 levels, but related to diurnal rhythms,

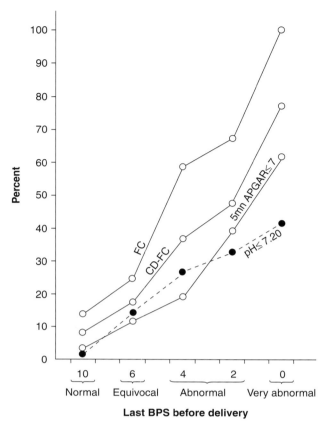

Figure 51.2
Biophysical profile score (BPS) has an exponential relationship to neonatal outcome. Declining scores strongly predict increasing frequency of fetal compromise (FC), cesarean section for fetal compromise (CD-FC), low 5-minute APGAR score and acidotic umbilical vein pH.

Fetal tone

The fetus must move to demonstrate tone – it is not simply a flexed posture. The spasm of fetal activity during startle motions provoked by acoustic stimulation does not constitute normal muscle tone and may give a misleading impression of wellbeing.[39]

Amniotic fluid volume

This is discussed in detail in a separate guideline (Chapter 50). In BPS, the maximum single deepest pocket depth (SDP) is the standard.[40] This has been demonstrated in randomized fashion to give better representation of amniotic fluid volumes than the amniotic fluid index (AFI), with significantly fewer cases being called oligohydramnios, but identical perinatal outcomes in each group.[41] SDP > 2cm meets criteria for BPS score of 2, while a number of criteria, including no SDP >3cm, meet criteria for subjectively reduced amniotic fluid volume (Table 51.4).[11] Reduced amniotic fluid volume is thought to represent reduced fetal

Table 51.4 *Subjectively reduced amniotic fluid*
Uterus tightly follows fetal contour
No single pocket >3 cm
No cord-free pockets of fluid
FHR decelerations with movements
FHR decelerations with transducer pressure
Restricted range of FM

FHR, fetal heart rate; FM, fetal movement

fetal cortisol levels, and demonstrating a maturational pattern. In BPS, fetal hiccups are treated equivalently. Human fetuses can be stimulated to breathe by maternal glucose infusion, a response that contributes directly to the time-efficiency of outpatient BPS, which typically follows mealtimes. FBM are very sensitive to hypoxemia, first illustrating longer periods of fetal apnea between bursts, then being lost altogether.[36] Restoration of fetal pO_2 by intrauterine transfusion or other resuscitation will result in resumption of periodic fetal breathing.[37]

Fetal body movements

Total fetal activity declines when hypoxemia begins, often associated with a gradual drop in amniotic fluid volume.[38] The frequency of fetal movements is a maturational variable – many term fetuses will move during only 10–15 minutes in an hour of observation, while a 28-week fetus who did that would frequently prove abnormal.

urine production in the face of normal fetal swallowing. Hemodynamically mediated redistribution of fetal blood flow, not hypoxemic renal ischemia as once suggested, is the probable mechanism.[18] Randomized data suggest restoring amniotic fluid volume before induction of labor prevents many intrapartum FHR complications – data are insufficient to evaluate the potential of this technique antenatally.[42] The score is not modified for excessive amniotic fluid, while recognizing that the real time ultrasound medium offers an ideal opportunity to investigate the many fetal factors associating polyhydramnios with increased perinatal mortality.

CTG

When fetal compromise occurs, the FHR is a sensitive indicator, with serial loss of NST reactivity, reduced variability, abolition of variability, and appearance of late decelerations. However, almost all fetuses show the first two of these during everyday normal cyclic behavior, so much so that a BPS of 8/8 is just as reliable in indicating normal wellbeing as a score of 10/10, and the NST can be used

Table 51.5   *Systematic application of biophysical profile scoring*

BPS	Interpretation	Predicted PNM/1000[a]	Recommended management
10/10 8/8 8/10 (AFV - normal)	No evidence of fetal asphyxia present	Less than 1/1000	No acute intervention on fetal basis. Serial testing indicated by disorder-specific protocols
8/10 (oligohydramnios)	Chronic fetal compromise possible	89/1000	For absolute oligohydramnios, prove normal urinary tract, disprove asymptomatic rupture of membranes
6/10 (AFV -normal)	Equivocal test, fetal asphyxia is not excluded	Depends on progression (61/1000 on average)	Repeat testing immediately, before assigning final value. If score is 6/10, then 10/10, in two continuous 30-min periods, manage as 10/10. For persistent 6/10, deliver the mature fetus, repeat within 24 hours in the immature fetus, then deliver if less than 6/10
4/10	Acute fetal asphyxia likely. If oligohydramnios, acute or chronic asphyxia very likely	91/1000	Deliver by obstetrically appropriate method, with continuous monitoring
2/10	Acute fetal asphyxia, most likely with chronic decompensation	125/1000	Deliver for fetal indications (usually cesarean section)
0/10	Severe, acute asphyxia virtually certain	600/1000	Deliver immediately by cesarean section

[a]Per 1000 live births, within 1 week of test result shown, without intervention. For scores of 0, 2, or 4, intervention should begin virtually immediately, provided the fetus is viable. AVF, amniotic fluid volume; PNM, perinatal mortality.

Table 51.6.   *Perinatal mortality changes with BPS application*

Program	n	PNM with BPS	PNM without BPS
Ireland[44]	3 200	4.1	10.7
Nova Scotia[45]	5 000	3.1	6.6
Manitoba[22]	56 000	1.9	7.7
California[46]	15 000	1.3	8.8

n, number tested; PNM, perinatal mortality/1000.

selectively – i.e., NST is used sequentially, only in fetuses not demonstrating normal behavior in the ultrasound parameters done first.[11,24]

Management by biophysical profile scoring follows a protocol which relates fetal condition, assumed perinatal risks, gestational age, and recommended action (Table 51.5).[43] Application of BPS has been shown to reduce perinatal mortality (historical controls, Table 51.6),[44–46] and long-term neurologic handicap (concurrent non-randomized controls, as discussed above, Table 51.2). Randomized trials comparing Doppler methods to BPS have been very small, and unable to evaluate such infrequent outcomes.[47–50]

Compared to other fetal testing (usually NST), **biophysical profile increases the incidence of induction, but does not affect incidences of cesarean delivery, admission to ICN, or perinatal mortality.**[51]There are no randomized trials proving BPS alters perinatal outcome, compared to controls.

Responses to abnormal test results

In general, these are indicated in the BPS protocol, and are based on the differential survival rates in and out of the uterus.[52] When BPS is persistently 8/10 on serial testing, that is, one variable is always missing, while the others are always present, specific inquiry should be made about cause. In some cases, that is obvious from the clinical context (e.g., oligohydramnios in preterm premature rupture of membranes with normal fetal status). In other cases, it is not so clear – in a fetus with persistent non-reactive NST despite always having normal ultrasound variables, neurologic anomalies, prior neurologic injury, fetal Down syndrome, or maternal drug ingestion may be underlying. Near term, equivocal or abnormal results almost always call for delivery. As suggested by Table 51.7, equivocal results in the preterm fetus call for repeated testing, transfer to appropriate neonatal resources, antenatal steroid administration and so on, before moving to delivery. In high-risk fetuses, delivery can wait for valuable maturation time – the normal BPS of 8/8 or

Table 51.7 *Risks of stillbirth vs. neonatal death due to prematurity*

BPS	Stillbirth rate[a]	Equivalent neonatal death rate (weeks)
0	560	25.4
2	153	28.3
4	91	29.1
6	61	30.0
8	0.5	Full term
10	0.5	Full term

[a]Death within one week if the fetus remains undelivered. These figures change with time and differ between centers, including differences between inborn and transported babies. Rates are per 1000.

10/10 is proof that the fetus is not acidotic.[53] On the other hand, a BPS of 0–2/10 justifies delivery and neonatal management down to local thresholds of viability.[54]

Modified biophysical profile score

Many modifications have been proposed. The most popular combination suggested has been the AFI–NST combination,[55] including optional use of vibroacoustic stimulation,[56] to shorten observation time. In most of the studies, and virtually all of the actual trials, full BPS (all five variables) was the back-up test required in 15–30% of cases. The primary focus of the simplified test was to reduce the time and complexity of BPS, without altering the negative predictive value (i.e., the safety of non-intervention). The finding that the falsely reassuring stillbirth rate (false-negative rate) was about the same very low rate (3–5 per 10 000 tests), for many of these authors, justifies reducing the number of variables. However, only a few of these trials had enough patients to evaluate the differences in the false-positive rate, that is, the number of fetuses delivered for an incorrect assessment of fetal jeopardy. In the majority of trials, either the data are too few, or the full BPS was superior to the restricted tests, in avoiding unnecessary intervention.

The exceptions are trials of FGR management in which the modified BPS included Doppler information – in those cases, addition of Doppler assessment of umbilical arterial resistance both improved classification of fetal acidosis and reduced interference for false-alarm BPS.[57,58] Modifications to the full BPS protocol are not supported for high-risk fetuses with abnormal Doppler indices, preterm fetuses, postdates pregnancy, fetal anomalies, multiple gestation, or fetuses with arrhythmia, infection, anemia or diabetic macrosomia. Assertions that modified BPS is faster and/or cheaper than full BPS have not been substantiated by controlled studies – in the experience of many BPS teams, the NST is the only component which consumes much time.[11,45] Cost is highly dependent on locale, of course. In many

United States jurisdictions, for example, separate facility fees are charged for the uses of the ultrasound machine generating the AFI, and the FHR monitor generating the NST – total testing costs are very significantly increased with modified BPS compared to selective use of the NST. With the advent of Doppler surveillance and community access to high-resolution ultrasound, argument about the technical expertise needed for evaluation of fetal breathing movements is probably obsolete.

Multivessel Doppler

Placental insufficiency has a large structural component with tertiary stem villous deficiency and progressively smaller perfusion area, leading to progressive rise in resistance in the umbilical artery as depicted in Figure 51.3. Functional aspects of placentation, including placental volume flow, sequential placental flow distribution, and vascular responses to maternal hyperoxygenation, are interesting from the physiologic point of view, but too operator-dependent for clinical monitoring. Umbilical artery Doppler assessment requires careful attention to technical detail, and is usually done in the mid-portion of the free umbilical cord (Figure 51.4).[59] There is a progressive drop in resistance over the length of the cord – too close to the fetal abdomen may misrepresent higher resistance and poorer flow; too close to the placenta may suggest an overly optimistic low resistance. Although each mathematical expression of the Doppler arterial flow velocity waveform has some advantages, the Pulsatility Index (PI) has the advantage of infinite expression (remaining valid even when flow is reversed), and autocorrelation with the volume of the waveform itself. When umbilical artery PI reaches an individualized threshold, higher blood pressure leads to cardiac effects and systemic effects. Initial cardiac effects, including ejection fraction, wall velocity, transvalvular velocity, and so on, are measurable with sophisticated techniques, but the systemic effects are readily demonstrated in a shift toward more cerebral perfusion using the Doppler waveform of the middle cerebral artery (MCA, Figure 51.5). Initially present as a subtle change in the cerebral:placental ratio, this shift is later depicted as a significant decline in the MCA PI as diastolic blood flow rises.[60] The initial change in proportional distribution has been termed centralization, and may simply be due to resistance-mediated diversion of flow away from an ailing placenta. The second change, which has been called brain sparing, may be mediated by hypoxemia-induced cerebral vasorelaxation. The MCA is a straight vessel, usually readily imaged, to allow interpretation of the absolute velocity as well as resistance indices.

As the hemodynamic and respiratory declines continue to interact, oxygen-sensitive interfaces between nutrient-rich and non-rich streams begin to dictate flow.[61] Diversion through an opening ductus venosus is readily depicted as

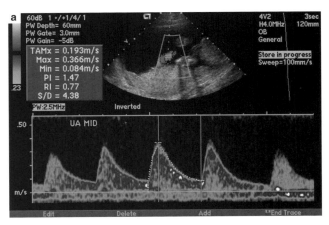

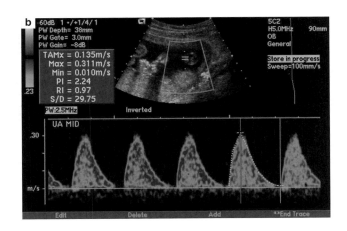

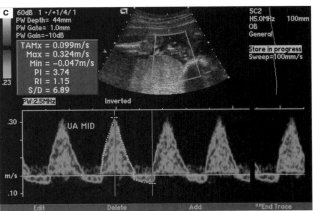

Figure 51.3

Abnormalities in Doppler velocity waveforms of the umbilical artery depict increasing placental resistance. These Doppler examinations are from the same patient as pregnancy progresses. In Figure 51.3a, the umbilical artery resistance is modestly elevated at 18 weeks (PI 1.47). By 24 weeks (Figure 51.3b), end diastolic velocities are absent in most cardiac cycles. By 28 weeks, as shown in Figure 51.3c, reversal of end diastolic flow occupies nearly one quarter of the cardiac cycle. Cesarean section was carried out on the basis of oligohydramnios at 29+ weeks, with umbilical venous pH 7.18.

Table 51.8   *Abnormal umbilical artery Doppler correlates with neonatal compromise**

Cesarean section for fetal compromise
Acidosis
Hypoxemia
Low Apgar-5
Long-term oxygen
Bronchopulmonary dysplasia
Anemia
Increased NRBC
Thrombocytopenia
Prolonged NRBC release
Neutropenia
Transfusions
IVH
NEC
Perinatal mortality

*For all of these outcomes, their frequency rises exponentially from abnormal indices to Absent End-Diastolic Velocities to Reversed End-Diastolic Velocities. BPD, bronchopulmonary dysplasia. NRBC, nucleated red blood cells. IVH, intraventricular hemorrhage. NEC, necrotizing enterocolitis.

progressive changes in waveform pattern (DV, Figure 51.6). Deep reversal of the atrial contraction wave, a-wave, indicates both cardiac impairment (forward volume flow insufficiency forcing the waveform more retrograde) and hypoxemia (dilating the DV itself). DV interrogation is easy to learn, as this vessel contains the highest venous velocities in the fetal abdomen, but when the waveform is abnormal, it must be carefully differentiated from adjacent hepatic venous structures.[62]

Doppler application[63]

Worsening umbilical arterial Doppler correlates well with declining placental function and the emergence of hypoxemia and acidosis.[60] Absent end-diastolic velocities denote an increasing risk of stillbirth, preterm delivery, birthweight below 10th percentile and many neonatal complications (Table 51.8).[60,63–65] Umbilical artery Doppler is useful in directing care – small fetuses with normal Dopplers probably do not need the same level of surveillance, and subsequently of intervention, as do those with abnormal umbilical flow.[66] Perinatal outcome is superior when Doppler is utilized in

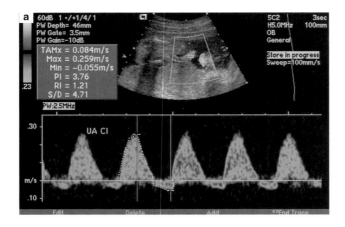

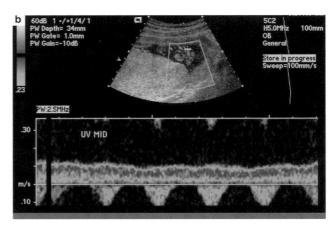

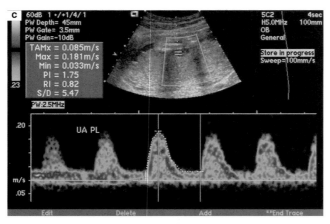

Figure 51.4

It is very important to measure the umbilical artery resistance in mid-cord. (a) At the abdominal cord insertion, resistance is highest, here demonstrating reversal of flow in diastole. (b) Mid-cord is the accepted expression of this high resistance, showing absent end diastolic velocity (note inverted wave forms). (c) The lowest resistance is measurable at the umbilical cord insertion on the surface of the placenta, showing preserved end diastolic flow. It is important to perform these evaluations when the uterus is relaxed.

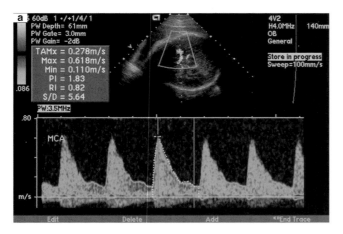

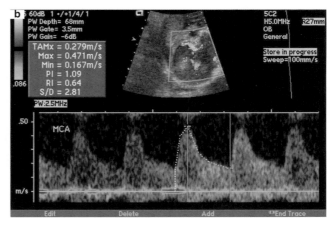

Figure 51.5

Serial MCA Dopplers demonstrate an increase in diastolic blood flow, termed centralization. Normally, the middle cerebral artery shows high resistance with low diastolic velocity (high PI 1.83, a). Diversion of blood flow towards the brain correlates with worsening umbilical artery depiction of increased placental resistance, with falling cerebrovascular resistance, increased end diastolic velocities and PI falling to 1.09 (b).

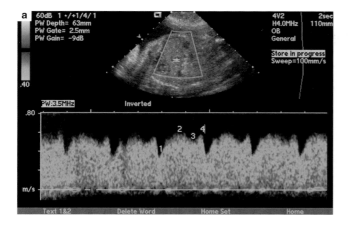

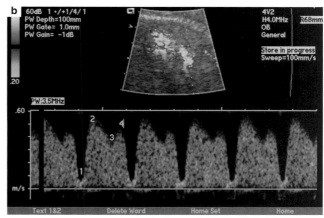

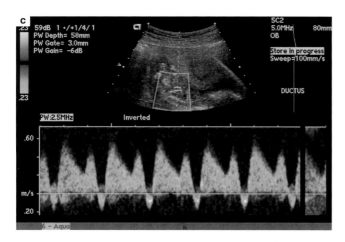

Figure 51.6

Progressive changes in venous return to the heart as depicted in the ductus venosus. (a) There are normally four phases in the wave form, consisting of (1) atrial contraction, (2) ventricular contraction, (3) restitution of the annulus, (4) diastole. Typically, the a-wave (1) shows the only significant downward deflection, a modest reduction in forward flow. (b) Increased afterload, from placental resistance rising, causes abnormal forward cardiac output, with the a-wave nearly retrograde. (c) Further progression in placental insufficiency is associated with cardiac malfunction, with severe retrograde a-waves, as well as distorted cardiac function, producing mid-wave depression as the annulus rises against an over-filled circulation.

decision-making, although interventions based on umbilical Doppler alone have a substantial risk of causing unnecessary prematurity.[67,68] Compared to no Doppler ultrasound, **Doppler ultrasound in high-risk pregnancy** (especially those complicated by hypertension or presumed fetal growth restriction) is associated with a **trend** to a **reduction in perinatal deaths** (1.5 vs 2.1%; OR 0.71, 95% CI 0.50–1.01).[69] The use of Doppler ultrasound is also associated with 17% **fewer inductions of labor** and 44% **fewer admissions to hospital**, without reports of adverse effects. No difference is found for NRFHT in labor or cesarean delivery.[69]

Despite the strong correlations with fetal status, basing delivery decisions on umbilical Doppler alone may lead to unnecessary mortality and morbidity due to prematurity.[2,70–73]

Evaluation of venous Doppler waveforms is pivotal in correct predictions of morbidity and mortality in FGR. The best combination of Doppler techniques in fetuses at risk for placental insufficiency would appear to be the triad of umbilical artery, MCA, and DV.[63]

Response to abnormal test results

The literature includes several series where action solely on the basis of alarming Doppler findings led to iatrogenic prematurity, producing neonatal injury and death, at least partially avoidable if delivery had been postponed a little. With those experiences in mind, GRIT and other trials addressed the potential for adverse effects if delivery were delayed past the point of abnormal Doppler findings. Various steps may be taken during that extended time, including administration of antenatal steroids, transfer to a higher level of neonatal resource, stabilization of maternal conditions, evaluation for vaginal delivery, or retesting with additional Doppler parameters. These studies, constituting Level I-II evidence, have shown no excess liability in the form of perinatal mortality, while adding significantly to intrauterine time.[2,9,71–76] In virtually all Doppler-outcome trials, the single most critical influence on outcome has been gestational age at delivery and its determination of adverse impacts of prematurity. Safe

Table 51.9	Doppler index abnormality suggests BPS surveillance*		
Abnormality†	BPS Frequency‡	Decision to deliver (fetal)§
Elevated indices only	Weekly	BPS ≤ 4 or term or >36 weeks with no change in AC
AEDV	Twice weekly	BPS ≤ 4 or >34 weeks proven maturity or conversion to REDV
REDV	Daily	BPS ≤ 4 or >32 weeks after steroids for FLM
REDV/DV-RAV or REDV/UVP	Three times daily	BPS ≤ 4 or >28–30 weeks after steroids for FLM

*BPS, Biophysical Profile Scoring, determines the timing of intervention; viability thresholds will vary with institution.
†Umbilical artery and precordial venous Doppler. MCA abnormalities confirm the elevated placental resistance, but do not directly alter management according to this scheme.
‡Minimum frequency, increased on basis of severity – maternal condition(s), degree of IUGR, gestational age.
§Neonatology consultation, steroids for fetal lung maturity (FLM), maternal clinical factors, fetal blood sampling parameters, all will impact this collaborative decision.
AC, fetal abdominal circumference; A/REDV, absent or reversed end-diastolic velocity in umbilical artery;
UVP, umbilical venous pulsations; DV-RAV, reversal of atrial contraction wave in ductus venosus.

extension of the pregnancy may be possible by adding other test parameters in sequence.[76–77] An approach to sequential testing, Doppler establishing the appropriate level of intense surveillance, and BPS indicating the timing of delivery, has been proposed by several independent teams. An example is shown in Table 51.9.

Doppler surveillance vs biophysical profile scoring

In addition to comparison between Doppler techniques, there have been several studies comparing the abilities of Doppler and biophysical techniques to predict fetal status (pH, stillbirth) and neonatal outcome. Most of these studies show that both methods have validity, and a small majority show superior correlation between Doppler and outcome values, compared to non-stress testing (with or without computerized analysis) and/or biophysical profile scoring in the management of FGR and diabetic vasculopathy. Of course, statistically superior correlation does not necessarily determine impact – in many of these studies, biophysical changes were the trigger for delivery.[9,27,71,73–77] No management trials directly comparing a Doppler-based method to a biophysical method, used in mutually exclusive fashion, have been completed.

Doppler surveillance and BPS: integrated fetal testing

Fetuses at risk for placental insufficiency are best identified by umbilical artery Doppler indices. However, elevated resistance may exist for months without fetal deterioration. Absent end-diastolic flow may be non-progressive for weeks. Even reversal of end-diastolic flow may persist for many days without fetal decompensation. These issues gave rise to the multivessel Doppler approach – deterioration in precordial venous indices documenting further steps in the pattern of placental insufficiency among FGR fetuses (Figure 51.7).[75] Should reversal of the DV a-wave be the trigger for delivery, then? Experience with the international FGR registry suggests not.[76] In many fetuses, the lag time between the final Doppler status being attained and the BPS deteriorating was clinically significant – days to weeks. Especially in the critical gestational ages before 32 weeks, such an interval may be critical in reducing prematurity impacts.

For BPS, the underlying premise is that reduction in fetal activity reaches clinically detectable levels on a voluntary basis (i.e., responsive to the need for conservation rather than depressive due to a critical central decompensation). If the premise is valid, intervention on the basis of abnormal activity should allow the baby to recover, unharmed, in the neonatal period, if intervention is prompt and effective. If the premise is wrong, then waiting for the challenged fetus to become obtunded (i.e., without activity) would be associated with adverse long-term outcome, despite intervention. A high level of evidence is now available showing that waiting until the need for delivery is certain maximizes intrauterine time, optimizes reduction of prematurity, and at the same time, does not add morbidity or mortality by 'delaying' intervention.[9,73,75–78]

Testing is frequent, complex, and highly individualized. In the evaluation of these fragile FGR fetuses, BPS is a

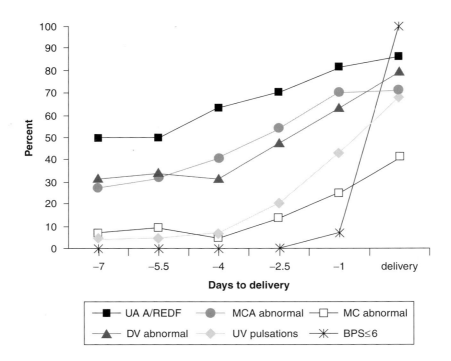

Figure 51.7
Progressive changes in multivessel Doppler occur in sequence before the biophysical profile score (BPS) deteriorates, in many fetuses. Virtually all fetuses were delivered for abnormal BPS (triangles). Most of these IUGR fetuses had reached the end of their Doppler progression before delivery.[75] A/REDV, absent or reversed diastolic velocity in the umbilical artery (UA); MCA, middle cerebral artery; DV, ductus venosus; UV, umbilical vein; BPS, biophysical profile score.

framework, not a rigid scheme, and the decision for delivery reflects not only the BPS parameters, but also the familiarity with fetal status arising from prolonged observation several times every day by the same team. Subtle changes in serial Doppler pattern also play a role in determining intervention. This approach to surveillance in severe FGR (integrated fetal testing) is illustrated in Table 51.10.[79] For management of FGR, see also Chapter 39.

Condition-specific testing

The specific example of IUGR above demonstrates the potential interaction of multiple testing parameters to optimize management. Since other identifiable conditions have increased risks of fetal compromise, but may not have identical patterns of fetal deterioration, it may be necessary/beneficial to modify testing to fit the disorder. The number of trials is growing daily, so the following is a current summary.

Diabetic vasculopathy

The subset of fetuses in diabetic pregnancy at highest risk of adverse outcome has elevated placental resistance as detected by umbilical artery Doppler. This includes women with hypertension, cardiac, renal, and other vascular diabetopathy, and fetuses with FGR. Doppler will correctly stratify the adverse outcomes better than BPS.[80] Prospective randomized evaluation of management has not been reported.

Diabetic fetal macrosomia

Poor glycemic control as judged by maternal blood sugars, or as denoted by fetal macrosomia (estimated fetal weight >90th percentile and polyhydramnios), or both, requires increased surveillance. In the absence of Doppler abnormalities of placentation, management by BPS protocol using twice-weekly testing achieves the same or better perinatal outcome (cord artery pH, mortality, neonatal morbidity) than euglycemic controls.[81] The critical issue is glycemic control – when this is good, antenatal testing is less critical. When diabetic control is poor, identification and monitoring of the macrosomic fetus requires individualized care.[81,82]

Table 51.10   *Protocol for management of intrauterine growth restriction by integrated fetal testing*

IUGR unlikely		
Normal AC, AC growth rate & HC/AC; UA, MCA Doppler, BPS & AVF normal	Asphyxia extremely rare; low risk for intrapartum NRFHT	Delivery for obstetric or maternal factors only, follow growth
IUGR		
AC<5th, low AC growth rate, high HC/AC ratio, abnormal UA, normal MCA, DV, UV Doppler, BPS ≥ 8/10, AFV normal	Asphyxia extremely rare Increased risk for intrapartum NRFHT	Delivery for obstetric or maternal factors only, fortnightly Doppler, weekly BPS
	with blood flow redistribution	
IUGR diagnosed based on above criteria Low MCA, normal DV, UV Doppler BPS ≥ 8/10, AFV normal	Hypoxemia possible, asphyxia rare Increased risk for intrapartum NRFHT	Deliver for obstetric or maternal factors only, weekly Doppler, BPS 2 times/week
	with significant blood flow redistribution	
UA A/REDV Normal DV, UV Doppler BPS ≥ 6/10, oligohydramnios	Hypoxemia common, acidemia or asphyxia possible Onset of fetal compromise	>34 weeks: deliver <32 weeks: antenatal steroids, repeat all testing daily
	with proven fetal compromise	
Significant redistribution present Increased DV pulsatility BPS ≥ 6/10, oligohydramnios	Hypoxemia common, acidemia or asphyxia possible	>32 weeks: deliver <32 weeks: admit, steroids, individualized testing
	with fetal decompensation	
Compromise by above criteria Absent or reversed DV a-wave, pulsatile UV, BPS ≥ 6/10, oligohydramnios	Cardiovascular instability, metabolic compromise, stillbirth imminent, high perinatal mortality irrespective of intervention	Deliver at tertiary care center with the highest level of NICU care

IUGR, intra-uterine growth restriction; AC, abdominal circumference; HC, head circumference; NRFHR, non-reassuring fetal heart rate; MCA, middle cerebral artery; BPS, biophysical profile scoring; AFV, amniotic fluid volume; UA, umbilical artery; A/REDF, absent/reversed end diastolic velocity; DV, ductus venosus; UV, umbilical vein; NICU, neonatal intensive care nursery.

Postdates pregnancy

Data are conflicting. Randomized trials indicate a policy of induction of labor before 42 weeks may reduce incidence of some key outcomes, but those trials have been criticized because they relied on NST alone, and did not take advantage of superior monitoring techniques, including CCTG, Doppler, and BPS.[83] Similar randomized controlled trials have been performed evaluating BPS, CCTG, and Doppler in pregnancy >42 weeks, reaching divergent conclusions.[84] One trial found that intervention was best directed by a combination of single pocket depth and standard visual CTG (versus modified biophysical profile with AFI), while another trial found superior results with computerized CTG (versus either full BPS or umbilical artery Doppler).[85,86] Prior non-randomized cohort studies have demonstrated superior results of full BPS compared to NST alone, and Doppler plus CTG vs. CST/OCT.[87] At present, the best recommendation is made with moderate confidence: pregnancy beyond certain 41+ weeks should be evaluated for delivery. Where delivery is not selected, twice weekly monitoring should include amniotic fluid assessment using the single pocket depth method, CTG analysis and assessment of fetal activity. (See Chapter 23 in *Obstetric Evidence Based Guilidelines*.)

The 'small normal' fetus near term

Late third trimester growth restriction is difficult to identify clinically. When serial sonography does show late growth delay, early placental senescence may be the cause, but such fetuses often have normal placental (umbilical and uterine artery) Doppler. Reduced MCA resistance ('centralization') was associated with increased frequency of intrapartum and neonatal complications.[88] This observation may identify a testing correlate of late hemodynamic compensation, useful in determining which small fetuses should be monitored. However, delivery was determined by the combined results of full BPS, growth, and umbilical artery Doppler – this does not form a basis for reacting to the MCA findings alone. Management by full BPS is recommended, with moderate support.

Preterm premature ruptured membranes (PPROM)

Infection may have an all or none effect on fetal behavior. When the NST is non-reactive and fetal breathing is absent, delivery produces superior neonatal and maternal infectious outcomes – BPS management may be helpful in managing PPROM.[89] A study with similar design, but no intervention for abnormal BPS, could not duplicate the correlations.[90] Further, 48% of fetuses with normal BPS have positive amniotic fluid culture, so abnormal BPS is a poor predictor of amniotic fluid culture results.[91] Differentiation may be on the fetal effects of amniotic fluid infection – while BPS with CCTG did not predict culture results reliably, they did suggest which fetus was likely to show signs of infection.[92] Randomized comparison of BPS and NST alone in this setting did not resolve this issue – neither test had good sensitivity (25.0% and 39.1%, respectively) in predicting infectious morbidity, but both had good predictive accuracy when abnormal (66.7% and 52.9%, respectively).[93] The majority of those with infectious complications were delivered on the basis of onset of labor, clinical evidence of chorioamnionitis, or reaching 32 weeks' gestation – the trial reached negative conclusions based on the 'intent to treat' model, not on failure of the methods to indicate intervention. Recommendation: monitoring in PPROM before 32–34 weeks should not rely on fetal testing alone. Meticulous daily assessment of markers of infection, preterm labor, and BPS may be combined to give best results. Delivery is indicated on reaching gestational age thresholds determined by local experience – passive waiting beyond that is not justified by the weak sensitivity of current antenatal testing. Although not studied in management trials to date, amniocentesis as a means of dictating delivery may be more effective than non-invasive methods.[93] (see also Chapter 16 in *Obstetric Evidence Based Guidelines*)

Fetal anemia

BPS deteriorates as an end-stage effect of visible hydrops, and gray-scale imaging is ineffective in predicting descent to severe anemia in alloimmune cases, so neither should be used alone in monitoring fetuses at risk for anemia.[94] NST or CCTG show correlation with anemia, based on a reduction in variability as anemia worsens, but this relationship is not reliable enough to dictate invasive management. MCA Doppler velocimetry is effective in determining the need for fetal transfusion, the timing between transfusions, and in differentiating degrees of fetal anemia.[95] However, since there is a 1–10% failure rate in detecting severe anemia, and a higher rate of missing mild anemia (which may progress rapidly),[96] MCA should form the core of a comprehensive approach which also includes fetal blood sampling by cordocentesis, and an experienced team familiar with fetal hematology.[97] (see Chapter 47)

Antenatal steroid administration

It is important to recognize effects of antenatal steroids on monitoring parameters, to avoid the conclusion that immediate delivery is required in patients being managed conservatively for preterm labor. Betamethasone given in two injections 24 h apart reduces heart rate variability, body movement and breathing movements in many fetuses, resulting in BPS falling to 6/10 or less, in up to 37%.[50] When monitoring time is extended to 45–60 minutes, most achieved normal scores, indicating this effect is to extend periods of fetal quiescence (Stage 1F, inactive sleep), rather than to delete the behavior. Dexamethasone given in 4 injections 12 h apart does not appear to have the same effects.[98] Neither betamethasone or dexamethasone produce consistent effects on umbilical or MCA Doppler indices. Recommendation: establish fetal wellbeing prior to steroid administration, extend BPS testing time, and do not overreact.

There is insufficient evidence (no trials) to assess the effect of any fetal test of well-being during maternal surgery in any trimester.

ANCILLARY TESTING METHODS

Modified FHR recording methods utilize fetal stimulation to shorten the time to reach reactivity, to convert non-reactive FHR tracings to reactivity, as a confirmatory test for non-reactive NST, and in highest-risk populations, as a more precise test of fetal well being. In the contraction stress test (CST), and the oxytocin challenge test (OCT), spontaneous and induced contractions, respectively, stress the fetoplacental unit, either by placental compression, or by cord compression, producing decelerations in the abnormal test, and no decelerations when the test is normal. These tests have higher negative predictive value than NST alone, similar to biophysical and Doppler methods (3–4 per 10 000 tests), but have high rates of equivocal results, and a high rate of false-alarming results.[34,87,99,100] When BPS is used as the backup test for positive (abnormal) CST, at least 50% of pregnancies can safely continue for at least a week.[99] High cost, requirement of hospital facilities, disagreement on fundamental interpretation of the test, occasional complications resulting from the test methods, and the lack of superior practical performance (same time elapsed, more follow-up tests required) have marginalized these techniques. Despite claims by proponents, CST/OCT are not faster than NST or BPS in clinical application.[44,101] The OCT may have a role in determining the route of delivery when the need for intervention has already been determined (e.g. a positive OCT means proceed to cesarean section), but the data available do not justify any conclusion.

A second type of stimulation is vibroacoustic stimulation (VAS).[102] The fetus is stimulated by external high-amplitude white noise applied to the maternal abdomen. This is capable of causing state change in most fetuses, including provoking conversion to 4F ('frantic fetus'), at term[11]. Occasional side effects include conversion to fixed fetal arrhythmia, and serious concerns about delivery of high-pressure sound (up to 130 decibels) and effects on fetal hearing.[11] Since premature fetuses typically require more sound pressure to elicit responses, and are more susceptible to hearing injury, use of VAS before 32 weeks should be very cautious. VAS has been shown to reduce the time of testing, and reduces the need for backup tests when applied to non-reactive NST.[103] Applied to modified BPS testing, VAS is associated with a 67% false-alarm rate requiring performance of full BPS in any case.[104] More critical, however, is the false-negative rate – 55% of fetuses with subsequent fetal NRFHT had reassuring VAS-NST.[105] Sound responsiveness is reduced in many high-risk groups (less than 32 weeks' gestation, hypertension, depression, severe IUGR, cocaine exposure, treatment with magnesium sulfate or antenatal steroids included).[11] Specific trials have demonstrated superiority of multivariable testing including Doppler, NST, and biophysical variables over either CST or VAS in prolonged pregnancy and IUGR. Both trials concluded CST and VAS could be eliminated from fetal testing regimes.[87,106] The proven effect of VAS to provoke fetal neurologic state change seems outweighed by its ability to generate false reassurance. Routine application in high-risk fetal populations is not recommended.

Compared to mock or no vibroacoustic stimulation, **fetal vibroacoustic stimulation reduces the incidence of non-reactive antenatal cardiotocography test** (from 13 to 8%) and reduces the overall mean cardiotocography testing time by about 10 minutes.[107] Vibroacoustic stimulation compared with mock stimulation evoked significantly more fetal movements when used in conjunction with fetal heart rate testing. While no safety issues have been consistently reported, more data on safety are needed.[107]

Shining a bright halogen light on the mother's abdomen shortens the time to first acceleration on NST.[108]

Compared to no administration, **antenatal maternal glucose administration** (20–50 mg orally, e.g. as orange juice) **does not decrease the incidence** of non-reactive antenatal cardiotocography tests, regardless of prior fasting or non-fasting.[109]

Compared to no manipulation, or to vibroacoustic stimulation, **manual fetal manipulation does not decrease** the incidence of non-reactive antenatal cardiotocography test.[110]

Fetal movement counting in low-risk pregnancy

The **largest randomized trial** of maternal monitoring of fetal movement[111] failed to show any benefit over 'informal inquiry about movement during standard antenatal care.' This trial produced a noticeable effect on control subjects, whose experience in the trial led to improved perinatal performance compared to non-trial participants in the general population. It did not produce a benefit in treated patients, with the **same perinatal mortality in both study and control patients**. Many women do report reduced fetal activity prior to stillbirth, so why did this trial demonstrate no effect? First, decreased movement was not reported promptly by many subjects. Second, the 'rescue' method was simple CTG, where false reassurance of a normal heart rate preceded a large proportion of fetal deaths. So, it may be that maternal awareness of fetal activity can be a useful adjunct in monitoring low-risk situations, if reporting is immediate, and if the rescue method is full biophysical profile scoring or even more complex assessment. The only **other trial**[112] revealed a **decreased incidence of fetal death** from 0.19% (3/1583) in the counting group to 0.76% (12/1569) in the control group. Non-trial data do not support reliance on fetal movement counting between episodes of formal fetal assessment in high-risk pregnancy.[113]

PRACTICAL ANTENATAL TESTING: WHO, WHEN, HOW, AND WHY?

No trial has conclusively proven that antenatal testing lowers long-term adverse neurologic outcomes, so recommendations might be rated as Level B or even C (i.e., consensus, expert opinion, but no clear evidence). Many trials have indicated that specific antenatal monitoring regimes have a possible impact on mortality and short-term outcomes – an inference is apparent. The standard of care, accordingly, is very clear: the definition of any of those factors in Table 51.11 should be attended by antenatal surveillance of appropriate intensity and precision.

Similarly, management trials determining when to start monitoring are not likely – thresholds for viability, knowledge of the disease process, severity of individual cases, past history, all may indicate starting monitoring much earlier (e.g. at 24–26 weeks in severe FGR) than recommended by general guidelines (32–34 weeks for most at-risk fetuses, according to the ACOG). Routine application of testing such as NST or umbilical artery Doppler alone pose substantial risk of iatrogenic prematurity in fetuses with abnormal testing – a blanket proposal of 'testing early and testing often' is potentially more dangerous than helpful. Testing should be timed in recognition of the characteristics of the test and the fetal patient, in context.

The choice of test is determined not only by the specific condition-related advantages above, but also by available personnel and equipment resources, cost, availability of effective treatment for abnormal results, and evidence of

Table 51.11 *Indications for antenatal surveillance*

Primarily maternal conditions	Primarily placental conditions	Primarily fetal conditions	Miscellaneous conditions
Severe hyperthyroidism Symptomatic hemoglobinopathy Cyanotic heart disease Chronic renal disease Type I diabetes Marked uterine anomalies Uterine artery Doppler abnormalities	Antiphospholipid antibody syndrome Systemic lupus erythematosus Hypertensive disorders, including PIH Thrombophilia Marked placental anomalies Umbilical artery Doppler abnormalities	Decreased fetal movement Oligohydramnios Polyhydramnios Intrauterine growth restriction (not placental) Post-dates pregnancy Alloimmunization Macrosomia Fetal anomalies/aneuploidy Multiple gestation (all) Abnormal systemic fetal Doppler	IVF pregnancy Previous stillbirth Previous recurrent abruption Teratogen exposure

outcome impact of the management protocol. For disorders with placental/vascular components (FGR, hypertensive disorders, vascular disease), multivessel Doppler methods are necessary to optimize monitoring. In most situations, including determining delivery timing for IUGR fetuses, multivariable BPS may offer significant benefits over single-variable testing (Table 51.12).

Testing interval will depend on severity (up to three times daily in FGR fetuses with the worst Doppler pattern, according to the integrated fetal testing protocol), but a product of normal Doppler results has been to decrease the frequency of testing and shorten antenatal hospital stays in FGR. There is no apparent high-level evidence supporting the widely practiced uniform protocol of weekly BPS testing, as opposed to some other frequency of assessment – but the important role of maternal compliance with testing schedules should not be overlooked.

PITFALLS IN ASSESSING FETAL MONITORING METHODS

Pregnancy is usually uncomplicated. For instance, if pregnancy termination for lethal anomalies detected at 18–20 weeks were the only management maneuver, normal outcome would occur in >90%. In a population with a low incidence of the target outcome, predictive accuracies arising from large population-based studies, not sensitivity/specificity derived from small groups (even if randomized), are required.[114]

Monitoring is not performed in isolation. For ultrasound-based methods, detection of critical complications such as imminent cord prolapse, abruptio in progress, unsuspected twin complications, and so on, leads to important individual impacts not attributable to the testing scheme itself.[11] Further,

Table 51.12 *Suggested antenatal fetal surveillance**

	Fetal surveillance	
Preeclampsia	At diagnosis	Twice weekly UA Doppler
Chronic HTN	32–34 weeks	Weekly NST/SDP or BPS
IUGR	At diagnosis	Weekly UA Doppler
Gestational diabetes		
A1	At 40 weeks	Weekly NST/SDP
A2	At 36 weeks	Weekly NST/SDP
Pregestational diabetes	At 32 weeks	twice weekly NST/SDP
Postterm	At 41 weeks	Twice weekly NST/SDP
Multiple gestation		
concordant	At 32–34 weeks	Weekly NST/SDP
≥1 fetus IUGR	At diagnosis	Weekly UA Doppler

* Patient care should be individualized. Some patients may require BPS, Doppler flow studies, or other testing in addition to the above. UA, umbilical artery; NST, non-stress test; HTN, hypertension; SDP, single deepest pocket; BPS, biographical profile score; IUGR, intra-uterine growth restriction.

in the context of maternal participation, the interactive nature of monitoring likely benefits from detection of accelerated hypertension, polyhydramnios, or peripheral edema, heightening the acuity of monitoring outside the test parameters.

Experience with new technologies influences results. For instance, as technical expertise with venous Doppler techniques improves, it seems quite likely that more detailed understanding of patterns of fetal disease will further influence monitoring patterns. Such effects undoubtedly occur during the performance of trials – the large numbers of subjects needed to answer research questions take time and often multiple sites – the testing regime may change significantly before results are finalized.

Correlations do not prove impact. A large number of studies, including randomized trials, conclude method superiority based on statistical correlation with fetal or neonatal standards. Such correlations must exist if the testing regime has a significant chance of affecting outcome. Increasingly, attention should be paid to randomized management trials, not randomized studies limited to documentation of associations.

Short-term outcome may be misleading. Focusing on umbilical cord pH at delivery, in relation to either Doppler or BPS testing, may not be informative. Any differences in pH for early intervention were clearly overbalanced by an excess of neurologic handicap at age three years in GRIT (Table 51.1); although the rate of cerebral palsy was lower in the monitored group in the BPS-CP study (Table 51.2), the majority of BPS-monitored CP cases had normal BPS before delivery. In both these examples, the short-term outcome measures incompletely represented the (more important) long-term impacts. Future management trials must define mechanisms and funding for such long-term follow-up.

Prenatal care – the final frontier of antenatal monitoring

Absence of prenatal care is a risk factor for adverse outcome.[115] The provision of adequate prenatal care, evaluation of risks and institution of antenatal monitoring attending those risks will improve the frequency of preterm labor in adolescents[116] and in women in prison,[117] and may facilitate maternal–fetal bonding, with important long-term implications.[118] The means by which this happens are elusive.[119]

Standard prenatal care is unlikely to completely address the important issues of FGR and preterm labor. The identification of specific risk factors and specific mechanisms to address them will likely have measurable impact. Excellent examples of the positive impact of focused care are seen in application of Doppler in FGR and prophylactic regimes in maternal thrombophilia. At the same time, cigarette smoking, teratogen exposure, the anemia of urban malnutrition, and social issues, including workspace hazards, all have proven impacts on perinatal health, opening major opportunities for public intervention.[119,120]

A new focus of risk evaluation and target-specific prenatal care is required. This prenatal care may directly 'treat' many of the causes of adverse outcome. It will also form the basis of new monitoring plans for as yet unsolved issues such as the excess poor outcomes in mild maternal hypothyroidism, IVF pregnancy and first trimester bleeding. As prenatal care and antenatal monitoring have succeeded with many major perinatal problems to date, there are many more still to be addressed.[121]

REFERENCES

1. McCowan LM, Pryor J, Harding JE. Perinatal predictors of neurodevelopmental outcomes in small-for-gestational age children at 18 months of age. Am J Obstet Gynecol 2002; 186(5): 1069–75. [II-3 Upgraded descriptive study due to neurodevelopmental follow-up, 282 subjects].

2. Nelson KB. The epidemiology of cerebral palsy in term infants. Ment Retard Dev Disabil Res Rev 2002; 8(3): 146–50. [review]

3. Schifrin BS. The CTG and the timing and mechanism of fetal neurological injuries. Best Pract Res Clin Obstet Gynecol 2004; 18(3): 437–56. [review]

4. Korst LM, Phelan JP, Wang YM, et al. Acute fetal asphyxia and permanent brain injury: a retrospective analysis of current indicators J Maternal–Fetal Med 1999; 8: 101–6. [II-3; pre-trial survey]

5. GRIT study group. When do obstetricians recommend delivery for high-risk preterm growth-retarded fetus? Growth Restriction Intervention Trial. Eur J Obstet Gynecol Reprod Biol 1996; 67(2): 121–6. [II-3; pre-trial survey]

6. GRIT study group. A randomized trial of timed delivery for the compromised preterm fetus: short term outcomes and Bayesian interpretation. BJOG 2003; 110(1): 27–32. [multicenter RCT]

7. Thornton JG, Hornbuckle J, Vail A, Spiegelhalter DJ, Levene M. Infant wellbeing at 2 years of age in the Growth Restriction Intervention Trial (GRIT): multicentered randomized controlled trial. Lancet 2204; 364(9433): 513–20. [multicenter RCT with neurodevelopmental follow-up]

8. Baschat AA, Gembruch U, Harman CR. The sequence of changes in Doppler and biophysical parameters as severe fetal growth restriction worsens. Ultrasound Obstet Gynecol 2001; 18: 571–7. [II-2]

9. Cosmi E, Ambrosini G, D'Antona D, Saccardi C, Mari G. Doppler, cardiotocography, and biophysical profile changes in growth-restricted fetuses. Obstet Gynecol 2005; 106(6): 1240–5. [II-2]

10. Manning FA, Bondaghi N, Harman CR, Casiro O, Menticoglu S, Morrison I, Berck DJ. Fetal assessment based on fetal biophysical profile scoring VIII. The incidence of cerebral palsy in tested and untested perinates. Am J Obstet Gynecol 1998; 178(4): 696–706. [II-2]

11. Harman, CR. Antenatal Assessment of Fetal Status. In: Creasy R, Iams J, Resnik R. (eds). Maternal-Fetal Medicine. 5th edition. Toronto: WB Saunders. 2004. [review]

12. Berger R, Garnier Y, Jensen A. Perinatal brain damage: underlying mechanisms and neuroprotective strategies. J Soc Gynecol Investig 2002; 220; 9(6): 319–28. [review]

13. Jackson MR, Walsh AJ, Morrow RJ, Mullen JB, Lye SJ, Ritchie JW. Reduced placental villous tree elaboration in small-for-gestational-age pregnancies: relationship with umbilical artery Doppler waveforms. Am J Obstet Gynecol 1995; 172(2 Pt 1): 518–25. [II-2. Placentas from AGA and IUGR, both term and preterm, were assessed by Doppler before delivery and with history and 3-D modeling after delivery, showing the loss of vascular volume and surface area in distal villus trees as the defining abnormality in IUGR]

14. Richardson BS. Fetal adaptive responses to asphyxia. Clin Perinat 1989: 595. [Review]

15. Harman CR. Fetal biophysical variables and fetal status. In Maulik D (ed): Asphyxia and Brain Damage. New York, Wiley-Liss, 1998; 279–320. [review]

16. Baschat AA, Gembruch U, Weiner CP, Harman CR. Qualitative venous Doppler waveform analysis improves prediction of critical perinatal outcomes in premature growth-restricted fetuses. Ultrasound Obstet Gynecol 2003; 22(3): 240–5. [II-3 Large cohort (224) of FGR fetuses studied with multivessel Doppler shows best correlation between Doppler changes and outcome prediction]

17. Arduini D, Rizzo G. Fetal behavioral states. In Dawes GS, Burruto F, Zacutti A, et al (eds): Fetal Autonomy and Adaptation. Chichester, Wiley. 1990: 117–124. [review]

18. Morrow RJ, Adamson SL, Bull SB, Ritchie JW. Acute hypoxemia does not affect the umbilical artery flow velocity waveform in fetal sheep. Obstet Gynecol 1990; 75(4): 590–3. [II-2; Controlled fetal sheep experiments demonstrate acute severe hypoxemia does not result in abnormal umbilical artery waveform – affirming the chronic nature of placental vascular resistance]

19. ACOG Practice Bulletin #9, October 1999. Antepartum Fetal Surveillance. [review]

20. Visser GH, Sadovsky G, Nicolaides KH. Antepartum heart rate patterns in small-for- gestational-age third-trimester fetuses: correlations with blood gas values obtained at cordocentesis. Am J Obstet Gynecol 1990; 162(3): 698–702. [II-2 Case control study of fetal heart rate patterns correlated with cordocentesis-derived blood gas values]

21. Lavin JP jr, Miodovnik M, Barden TP. Relationship of nonstress test reactivity and gestational age. Obstet Gynecol 1984; 63: 338–44. [II-3]

22. Manning FA. The Fetal Heart Rate. In Fetal Medicine Principles and Practice. Norwalk, Conn. Appleton & Lange, 1995, 13–111. [review]

23. Nathan EB, Haberman S, Burgess T, Minkoff H. The relationship of maternal position to the results of brief nonstress tests: a randomized trial. Am J Obstet Gynecol 2000; 182: 1070–2. [RCT, $n = 108$]

24. Manning FA, Lange IR, Morrison I, Harman CR. Fetal biophysical profile score and the nonstress test: A comparative trial. Obstet Gynecol 1984: 326–31. [RCT]

25. Keane MW, Horger EO 3rd, Vice L. Comparative study of stressed and nonstressed antepartum fetal heart rate testing. Obstet Gynecol 1981; 57(3): 320–4. [II-1 Sequential testing used each high-risk fetus ($n = 566$) as its own control. Only 24.8% of nonreactive NST had positive CST]

26. Pattison, N. McCowan, L. Cardiotocography for antepartum fetal assessment. Cochrane Database of Systematic Reviews. 4, 2005. [4 RCTs, $n = 1,588$. Demonstrated no significant benefit of cardiotocography on perinatal mortality]

27. Morrison I, Menticoglou S, Manning FA, Harman CR, Cheang M. Comparison of antepartum results to perinatal outcome. J Maternal Fetal Med. 1994; 3: 75–83. [II-2 All FGR fetuses underwent all tests: NST, BPS, umbilical artery Doppler and OCT. The best prediction of poor outcome used all tests. NST alone predicted only 32% of compromised fetuses]

28. Visser GH, Dawes GS, Redman CW. Numerical analysis of the normal human antenatal fetal heart rate. Br J Obstet Gynaecol 1981; 88(8): 792–802. [III-Original development of the System 8000, with 196 fetal heart records]

29. Dawes GW, Moulden M, Redman CW. Improvements in computerized fetal heart rate analysis antepartum. J Perinat Med 1996; 24(1): 25–36. [II-3]

30. Devoe LD, Searle N, Searle J, Phillips M, Castillo RA, Saad S, Sherline DM. Computer-assisted assessment of the fetal biophysical profile. Am J Obstet Gynecol 1985; 153(3): 317–21. [II-3]

31. Bracero LA, Morgan S, Byrne DW. Comparison of visual and computerized interpretation of nonstress test results in a randomized controlled trial. Am J Obstet Gynecol 1999; 181(5 Pt 1): 1254–8 .[RCT, n=410; computerized evaluation of fetal heart rate testing may be superior to standard visual interpretation]

32. Devoe LD, Jones CR. Nonstress test: evidence-based use in high-risk pregnancy. Clin Obstet Gynecol 2002; 45(4): 986–92. [review]

33. Manning FA, Platt LD, Sipos L. Antepartum fetal evaluation: development of a fetal biophysical profile. Am J Obstet Gynecol 1980;

136(6): 787–95. [II-1 Blinded study of first clinical BPS application, $n = 216$]

34. Manning FA, Morrison I, Lange IR, Harman CR, Chamberlain PF. Fetal assessment based on fetal biophysical profile scoring: experience in 12,620 referred high-risk pregnancies. I. Perinatal mortality by frequency and etiology. Am J Obstet Gynecol 1985; 151(3): 343–50. [II-3;-Combined variables provided best indication of perinatal mortality]

35. Manning FA, Morrison I, Harman CR, Menticoglou SM. The abnormal fetal biophysical profile score. V. Predictive accuracy according to score composition. Am J Obstet Gynecol 1990; 162(4): 918–24. [II-3-Different adverse outcomes are predicted better by different combinations of variables. This study included only fetuses with abnormal scores 131 – 6/10, 258 – 4/10, 113 – 2/10]

36. Bocking AD, Harding R. Effects of reduced uterine blood flow in electrocortical activity, breathing and skeletal muscle activity in fetal sheep. Am J Obstet Gynecol 1986; 154(3): 655–62. [II-1 Controlled study of fetal sheep model showed increased sensitivity to hypoxia in abolishing FBM as gestation progresses]

37. Harman CR, Manning FA, Bowman JM, Lange IR. Severe Rh disease - poor outcome is not inevitable. Am J Obstet Gynecol 1983; 145(7): 823–9. [II-3 Application of BPS and other ultrasound methods of fetal transfusion improves outcome]

38. Ribbert LS, Nicolaides KH, Visser GH. Prediction of fetal acidaemia in intrauterine growth retardation: comparison of quantified fetal activity with biophysical profile score. Br J Obstet Gynecol 1993; 100(7): 653–6. [II-2; Comparative trial of multivariable testing methods]

39. Harman CR, Menticoglou S, Manning FA. Assessing Fetal Health. In James DK, Steer PJ, Weiner CP, et al (eds). High Risk Pregnancy Management Options. New York, WB Saunders, 1999: 249–289. [Review]

40. Magann EF, Doherty D, Field K, Chauhan SP, Muffley PE, Morrison JC. Biophysical profile with amniotic fluid volume assessments. Obstet Gynecol 2004; 104(1): 5–10. [RCT. Demonstrates lower false-positive cases, fewer iatrogenic interventions, more accurate depiction of fetal status with single pocket method compared to AFI]

41. Chauhan SP, Doherty D, Magann EF, Cahanding F, Moreno F, Klausen JH. Amniotic fluid index vs. single deepest pocket technique during modified biophysical profile: a randomized clinical trial. Am J Obstet Gynecol 1004; 191(2): 661–7. [RCT. Included 1088 women, showed improved specificity, no change in outcome with single deepest pocket]

42. Vergani P, Ceruti P, Strobelt N, Locatelli A, D'Oria P, Mariani S. Transabdominal amniofusion in oligohydramnios at term before induction of labor with intact membranes: a randomized clinical trial. Am J Obstet Gynecol 1996; 175(2): 465–70. [RCT. Demonstrates safety of transabdominal amnioinfusion in oligohydramnios at term, reducing the Cesarean section rate for fetal distress by 78%, RR 0.22, CI 0.4 to 0.90]

43. Harman CR. Biophysical Profile Scoring. In Rumack C, Wilson S, Charboneau W, Johnson J 9eds). Diagnostic Ultrasound, 3rd Edition. Toronto, Mosby, 2004. [review]

44. Chamberlain PF. Later fetal death – has ultrasound a role to play in its prevention? Irish J Med Science. 1991; 160: 251–4. [II-3. Application of Biophysical Profile Score in an Irish healthcare region dropped PNM by more than 60%. Historical/concurrent non-randomized controls]

45. Baskett TG, Allen AC, Gray JH, Prewett SJ et al. Fetal biophysical profile and perinatal death. Obstet Gynecol 1987; 70: 357–60. [II-2. Concurrent controls had PNM more than double those managed by BPS]

46. Miller DA, Rabello YA, Paul RH. The modified biophysical profile: antepartum testing in the 1990s. Am J Obstet Gynecol 1996; 174: 812–17. [II-2. Large comparative trial of biophysical methodology demonstrated significant difference in outcome of cases managed or not managed by BPS]

47. Vintzileos AM, Campbell WA, Rodis JF, McLean DA, Flemin AD, Scorza WE. The relationship between fetal biophysical assessment, umbilical artery velocimetry and fetal acidosis. Obstet Gynecol 1991; 77: 622–26. [II-3.Clinical study showed BPS was superior and Doppler added nothing, in detection of fetal acidosis, n = 62]

48. Soothill PW, Ajayi RA, Campbell S, Nicolaides LH. Prediction of morbidity in small and normally grown fetuses by fetal heart rate variability, biophysical profile score and umbilical artery Doppler studies. Br J Obstet Gynaecol 1993; 100: 742–45. [II-3. Prospective longitudinal study of 191 women studied with all 3 methods. Doppler discriminated small "sick" fetuses from small normal fetuses, while the other tests did not]

49. Shalev E, Zalel Y, Weiner E. A comparison of the nonstress test, oxytocin challenge test, Doppler velocimetry and biophysical profile in predicting umbilical vein pH in growth-retarded fetuses. In J Gynaecol Obstet 1993; 43: 15–19. [II-3. Clinical series of 23 IUGR fetuses studied by all methods. NST, OCT and BPS all had positive predictive values of 57%, while Doppler was only 14%]

50. Yoon BH, Romero R, Roh CR, Kim SH, Ager JW, Syn HC, Cotton D, Kim SW. Relationship between the fetal biophysical profile score, umbilical artery Doppler velocimetry and fetal blood acid-base status determined by cordocentesis. Am J Obstet Gynecol 1993; 169: 1586–94. [II-2. Interventional cohort study. Doppler and BPS both had statistically significant association with acidemia and hypercarbia at cordocentesis, but Doppler scored higher in logistic regression, n = 24]

51. Alfirevic, Z. Neilson, JP. Biophysical profile for fetal assessment in high risk pregnancies. Cochrane Database of Systematic Reviews. 4, 2005. [meta-analysis; 4 RCTs, n = 2,828]

52. Dayal AK, Manning FA, Berck DJ, Mussalli GM, Avila C, Harman CR, Menticoglou S. Fetal death after normal biophysical profile score: an eighteen-year experience. Am J Obstet Gynecol 1999; 181(5 Pt 1): 1231–6. [II-2, n = 87,000]

53. Manning FA, Snijders R, Harman CR, Nicolaides K, Menticoglou S, Morrison I. Fetal biophysical profile score. VI. Correlation with antepartum umbilical venous fetal pH. Am J Obstet Gynecol 1993; 169(4): 755–63. [II-2 Multicenter clinical trial demonstrates close relationship of multivariable testing to fetal pH determined by antenatal cordocentesis, n = 493]

54. Manning FA, Harman CR, Morrison I, Menticoglou S. Fetal assessment based on fetal biophysical profile scoring. III. Positive predictive accuracy of the very abnormal test (biophysical profile score = 0). Am J Obstet Gynecol 1990; 162(2): 398–402. [II-2. A score of 0/10 is rare (9.2/10,000 tests), but has 100% positive predictive value for death or severe permanent handicap, justifying immediate delivery]

55. Nageotte MP, Towers CV, Asrat T, Freeman RK. Perinatal outcome with the modified biophysical profile. Am J Obstet Gynecol 1994; 170(6): 1672–6. [RCT. Clinical trial evaluating BPS (NST plus AFI) with randomized back-up testing (full BPS or CST) for abnormal values. MBPS discrimination well between adverse outcome (RR 2.0) and IUGR (RR 2.2) and those without these outcomes. CST was without benefit and led to iatrogenic morbidity compared to BPS]

56. Petrovic O, Skunca E, Matejcic N. A simplified fetal biophysical profile. Int J Gynaecol Obstet 1998;61(1): 9–14. [II-2. Sequential testing in large clinical study. 168 fetuses who were quiet on ultrasound examination had VAS to arouse them. The 326 fetuses who moved at once at modified BPS. BPS detected 6/10 adverse outcomes, VAS 2/3. This trial demonstrates the limitations of comparisons between tests when adverse outcomes are so infrequent]

57. Ott WJ, Mora G, Arias F, Sunderji S, Sheldon G. Comparison of the modified biophysical profile to a "new" biophysical profile incorporating the middle cerebral artery to umbilical artery velocity flow systolic/diastolic ratio. Am J Obstet Gynecol 1998; 178(6): 1346–53. [RCT. The addition of Doppler studies enhances Cesarean section rate in IUGR, but makes no other difference in outcome, compared to BPS alone]

58. Arabin B, Snyjders R, Mohnhaupt A, Ragosch V, Nicolaides K. Evaluation of the fetal assessment score in pregnancies at risk for intrauterine hypoxia. Am J Obstet Gynecol 1993; 169(3): 549–54. [II-3. Fetal Apgar score including cerebral and placental Doppler was compared with standard BPS in 213 at-risk fetuses. Both tests correlated well with adverse outcome, but the addition of Doppler was a significant advantage in IUGR cases]

59. Harman CR, Baschat AA. Arterial and venous Dopplers in IUGR. Clin Obstet Gynecol 2003; 46(4): 931–46. [Review]

60. Baschat AA, Gembruch R, Reiss I, et al. Relationship between arterial and venous Doppler and perinatal outcome in fetal growth restriction. Ultrasound Obstet Gynecol 2000; 16:407–13. [II-3. Time sequence of Doppler in IUGR]

61. Bellotti M, Pennati G, De Gasperi C, Bozzo M, Battaglia FC, Ferrazzi E. Simultaneous measurements of umbilical venous, fetal hepatic and ductus venosus blood flow in growth-restricted human fetuses. Am J Obstet Gynecol 2004; 190(5): 1347–58. [II-2. Case-control study depicting the progression of ductal opening and increased flow as condition deteriorated in 56 IUGR fetuses]

62. Kiserud T. The ductus venosus. Semin Perinatol 2001; 25(1): 11–20. [Review]

63. Harman CR, Baschat AA. Comprehensive assessment of fetal wellbeing: which Doppler tests should be performed? Curr Opin Obstet Gynecol 2003; 15(2): 147–57. [Review. Integration of arterial and venous vessel Dopplers]

64. Baschat AA, Gembruch U, Reiss I, Gortner L, Weiner CP, Harman CR. Relationship between arterial and venous Doppler and perinatal outcome in fetal growth restriction. Ultrasound Obstet Gynecol 2000; 16(5): 407–13. [II-2. Multicenter cohort study using multivessel Doppler to evaluate severe IUGR. Abnormal venous patterns denoted the worst outcomes, while prematurity retains a critical role]

65. Soregaroli M, Bonera R, Danti L, et al. Prognostic role of umbilical artery Doppler velocimetry in growth-restricted fetuses. J Matern Fetal Neonatal Med 2002; 11: 199–203. [II-2. Very large IUGR population (n = 578 studied from 1991–1999)]

66. Baschat AA, Weiner CP. Umbilical artery Doppler screening for the small for gestational age fetus in need of antenatal surveillance. Am J Obstet Gynecol 2000; 182: 154–8. [II-2. Umbilical artery Doppler differentiates small fetuses who do not need intensive surveillance, from those with serious IUGR]

67. Alfirevic Z, Neilson JP. Doppler ultrasonography in high-risk pregnancies: systemic review with meta-analysis. Am J Obstet Gynecol 1995; 172(5): 1379–87. [meta-analysis. Umbilical artery Doppler application reduces perinatal mortality and critical neonatal impacts in IUGR and pre-eclampsia]

68. Divon MY. Randomized control trials of umbilical artery Doppler velocimetry: how many are too many? Ultrasound Obstet Gynecol 1995; 6: 377–9. [review]

69. Neilson, JP. Alfirevic, Z. Doppler ultrasound for fetal assessment in high risk pregnancies. Cochrane Database of Systematic Reviews. 4, 2005. [11 RCTs, n = about 7,000]

70. Goffinet F, Paril-Llado J, Nisand I, et al. Umbilical artery Doppler velocimetry in unselected and low risk pregnancies: a review of randomized controlled trials. Br J Obstet Gynaecol 1997; 104: 425–30. [review]

71. Divon MY, Girz BA, Lieblich R, Langer O. Clinical management of the fetus with markedly diminished umbilical artery end-diastolic flow. Am J Obstet Gynecol 1989; 161(6 Pt 1): 1523–7. [II-2. Case-control study of 51 fetuses with severe elevation of umbilical artery resistance. Immediate delivery may not be necessary. Combined surveillance can safely prolong the pregnancy]

72. Baschat AA, Gembruch U, Weiner CP, Harman CR. Qualitative venous Doppler waveform analysis improves prediction of critical perinatal outcomes in premature growth-restricted fetuses. Ultrasound Obstet Gynecol 2003; 22(3): 240–5. [II-2. Cohort study

demonstrates combined arterial and venous Doppler maximized prediction of critical outcomes, $n = 224$]

73. Williams KP, Farwuharson DF, Bebbington M, Dansereau J, Galerneau F, Wilson RD, Shaw D, Kent N. Screening for fetal well-being in a high-risk pregnant population comparing the nonstress test with umbilical artery Doppler velocimetry: a randomized controlled clinical trial. Am J Obstet Gynecol 2003; 188(5): 1366–71. [RCT Randomized "high-risk" patients, beyond 32 weeks, to umbilical artery Doppler or nonstress testing as primary monitoring, amniotic fluid volume as secondary test]

74. Zelop CM, Richardson DK, Heffner LJ. Outcomes of severely abnormal umbilical artery Doppler velocimetry in structurally normal singleton fetuses. Obstet Gynecol 1996; 87: 434–8. [Review]

75. Baschat AA, Gembruch U, Harman CR. The sequence of changes in Doppler and biophysical parameters as severe fetal growth restriction worsens. Ultrasound Obstet Gynecol 2001; 18(6): 571–7. [II-2]

76. Baschat AA, Galan HL, Bhide A, Berg C, Kush ML, Oepkes D, Thilaganathan B, Gembruch U, Harman CR. Doppler and biophysical assessment in growth restricted fetuses: distribution of test results. Ultrasound Obstet Gynecol 2006; 27(1): 41–7. [II-1. Multicenter study of combined Doppler and biophysical profile in IUGR suggests both should be used to maximize gestational age, $n = 328$]

77. Tyrrel SN, Lilford RJ, MacDonald HN, Nelson EJ, Porter J, Gupta JK. Randomized comparison of routine vs. highly selective use of Doppler ultrasound and biophysical profile scoring to investigate high risk pregnancies. Br J Obstet Gynaecol 1990; 97(10): 909–16. [RCT demonstrating combined Doppler and BPS reduced neonatal morbidity by directing intervention, but did not increase iatrogenic prematurity, $n = 500$]

78. Habek D, Hodek B, Herman R, Jugovic D, Cerkez- Habek J, Salihagic A. Fetal biophysical profile and cerebro-umbilical ratio in assessment of perinatal outcome in growth-restricted fetuses. Fetal Diagn Ther 2003; 18(1): 12–6. [II-2. Clinical trial demonstrated the complimentary positive predictive values of biophysical profile and Doppler, $n = 87$ FGR fetuses]

79. Baschat AA. Integrated fetal testing in growth restriction: combining multivessel Doppler and biophysical parameters. Ultrasound Obstet Gynecol 2003; 21(1): 1–8. [Review]

80. Maulik D, Lysikiewicz A, Sicuranaza G. Umbilical arterial Doppler sonography for fetal surveillance in pregnancies complicated by pregestational diabetes mellitus. J Matern Fetal Neonatal Med 2002; 12(6): 417–22. [Review]

81. Harman CR, Menticoglou SM. Fetal surveillance in diabetic pregnancy. Curr Opin Obstet Gynecol 1997; 9(2): 83–90. [Review]

82. Sokol RJ, Chik L, Dombrowski MP, Zador IE. Correctly identifying the macrosomic fetus: improving ultrasonography-based prediction. Am J Obstet Gynecol 2000; 182(6): 1489–95. [Meta-analysis demonstrates the difficulty in identifying fetal macrosomia using standard ultrasound biometry]

83. Hannah ME, Hannah WJ, Hellmann J, Hewson S, Milner R, Willan A. Induction of labor as compared with serial antenatal monitoring in post-term pregnancy. A randomized controlled trial. The Canadian Multicenter Post-term Pregnancy Trial Group. N Engl J Med 1992; 326(24): 1587–92. [RCT showed induction of labor at 41 weeks results in lower Cesarean rate, and non-significant lower stillbirth rate]

84. A clinical trial of induction of labor versus expectant management in post-term pregnancy. The National Institute of Child Health and Human Development Network of Maternal-Fetal Medicine Units. Am J Obstet Gynecol 1994; 179(3): 716–23. [RCT of induction vs. fetal monitoring concluded either approach was satisfactory. This RCT is much smaller than the Canadian trial, but used more reliable testing (modified BPS) and showed no difference in Cesarean section rate or perinatal outcome]

85. Alfirevic Z, Walkinshaw SA. A randomized controlled trial of simple compared with complex antenatal fetal monitoring after 42 weeks gestation. Br J Obstet Gynaecol 1995; 102(8): 638–43. [RCT comparing post-term two modified BPS management schemes. The simpler assessment was superior based on use of single pocket depth]

86. Weiner Z, Farmakides G, Schulman H, Kellner L, Plancher S, Maulik D. Computerized analysis of fetal heart rate variation in post-term pregnancy: prediction of intrapartum fetal distress and fetal alkalosis. Am J Obstet Gynecol 1994; 171(4): 1132–8. [II-2 Cohort study evaluating multiple methods of assessing post-term pregnancy. CTG>BPS , Doppler did not help with management]

87. Arabin B, Becker R, Mohnhaupt A, Vollert W, Weitzel HK. Prediction of fetal distress and poor outcome in prolonged pregnancy using Doppler ultrasound and fetal heart rate monitoring combined with stress tests (II) [II-2. CTG was the only reliable prediction of acidemia in post-term pregnancy. Doppler, CST, and OCT were all irrelevant to predicting acidemia, while none were effective in predicting low Apgar scores].

88. Hershkovitz R, Kingdom JC, Geary M, Rodek CH. Fetal cerebral blood flow redistribution in late pregnancy: identification of compromise in small fetuses with normal umbilical artery Doppler. Ultrasound Obstet Gynecol 2000; 15(3): 209–12. [II-3. MCA abnormality indicated an increased likelihood of perinatal complications in small fetuses with normal umbilical artery Doppler. However, indicators for delivery were multiple and unregulated. Physicians were not blinded to results (although none would know what the abnormal MCA meant), and cases were not controlled]

89. Vintzileos AM, Bors-Koefoed R, Pelegano JF, Campbell WA, Rodis JF, Nochimson DJ, Kontopoulos VG. The use of fetal biophysical profile improves pregnancy outcome in premature rupture of the membranes. Am J Obstet Gynecol 1987; 157(2): 236–40. [II-2]

90. Carroll SG, Papaioannou S. Nicolaides KH. Assessment of fetal activity and amniotic fluid volume in the prediction of intrauterine infection in preterm prelabor amniorrhexis. Am J Obstet Gynecol 1995; 172(5): 1427–35. [II-3]

91. Gauthier DW, Meyer WJ, Bieniarz A. Biophysical profile as a predictor of amniotic fluid culture results. Obstet Gynecol 1992; 80(1): 102–5. [II-2. Cohort study of non-invasive (BPS) vs. invasive (amniocentesis) detection of infection]

92. Del Valle GO, Joffe GM, Izquierdo LA, Smith JF, Gilson GJ, Curet LB. The biophysical profile and the nonstress test: poor predictors of chorioamnionitis and fetal infection in prolonged preterm premature rupture of membranes. Obstet Gynecol 1992; 80(1): 106–10. [II-2]

93. Lewis DF, Adair CD, Weeks JW, Barrilleaux PS, Edwards MS, Garite TJ. A randomized clinical trial of daily nonstress testing versus biophysical profile in the management of preterm premature rupture of membranes. Am J Obstet Gynecol 1999; 181(6): 1495–9. [RCT of two schemes of monitoring patients after PPROM. Both NST and BPS had good specificity, but detected less than half the babies who developed infectious complications]

94. Harman CR. Ultrasound in the management of the alloimmunized pregnancy. In Fleischer AC, Manning FA, Jeanty P, Romero R (eds). Sonography in Obstetrics and Gynecology. 5th edition, Norwalk, Connecticut: Appleton & Lange. 1996: 583–609. [review]

95. Mari G. Middle cerebral artery peak systemic velocity: is it the standard of care for the diagnosis of fetal anemia? J Ultrasound Med 2005; 24(5): 697–702. [Review]

96. Divakaran TG, Waugh J, Clark TJ, Khan KS, Whittle MH, Kilby MD. Noninvasive techniques to detect fetal anemia due to red blood cell alloimmunization: a systemic review. Obstet Gynecol 2001 98(3): 509–17. [Meta-analysis suggests MCA Doppler lacks precision and the studies are incomplete]

97. Deren O, Karaer C, Onderoglu L, Yigit N, Kurukan T, Bahado-Singh RO. The effect of steroids on the biophysical and Doppler indices of umbilical and middle cerebral arteries in healthy preterm fetuses. Eur J Obstet Gynecol Reprod Biol 2001; 99(10): 72–6. [II-2, $n = 35$]

98. Mushkat Y, Asche-Landsberg J, Keidar R, Carmon E, Pauzner D, David MP. The effect of betamethasone vs. dexamethasone on fetal

biophysical parameters. Eur J Obstet Gynecol Reprod Biol 2001; 97(1): 50–2. [RCT, double blinded, comparing effects of betamethasone and dexamethasone]

99. Nageotte MP, Towers CV, Asrat T, Freeman RK, Dorchester W. The value of a negative antepartum test: contraction stress test and modified biophysical profile. Obstet Gynecol 1994; 84(2): 231–4. [II-1 Controlled study, not randomized. New surveillance method, modified BPS was compared in a high risk population to CST. The authors agreed that CST was no longer first-line]

100. Merrill PA, Porto M, Lovett SM, Dorchester W, Nageotte MP, Garite TJ, Freeman RK. Evaluation of the nonreactive positive contraction stress test prior to 32 weeks: the role of the biophysical profile. Am J Perinatol 1995; 12(4): 229–31. [II-3]

101. Newnham JP, Burns SE, Szczygielski C, Roberman B. Nonstress and contraction stress fetal heart rate monitoring. A randomized trial to determine which is the faster primary test. J Reprod Med 1988; 33(4): 354–40. [RCT Despite provoking fetal responses, the CST is not more efficient than NST, requiring back-up testing in one third]

102. Gagnon R, Patrick J, Foreman J, West R. Stimulation of human fetuses with sound and vibration. Am J Obstet Gynecol 1986; 155(4): 484–51. [II-3. Development of VAS]

103. Smith CV, Phelan JP, Platt LD, Broussard P, Paul RH. Fetal acoustic stimulation testing. II. A randomized clinical comparison with the nonstress test. Am J Obstet Gynecol 1986; 155(1): 131–4. [RCT showed shorter testing time, fewer nonreactive results]

104. Kamel HS, Makhlouf AM, Youssef AA. Simplified biophysical profile: an antepartum fetal screening test. Gynecol Obstet Invest. 1999; 47(4): 223–8. [II-2. Although vibroacoustic stimulation shortened the testing time for normal results, 67% of the abnormal results were false-alarms]

105. Serafini P, Lindsay MP, Nagey DA, Pupkin MJ, Tsent P, Crenshaw C Jr. Antepartum fetal heart rate response to sound stimulation: the acoustic stimulation test. Am J Obstet Gynecol 1984; 148(1): 41–4. [II-2. Comparative study showed testing efficiency of VAS, but included 55% false-negative results for prediction of fetal distress]

106. Arabin B, Becker R, Mohnhaupt A, Entezami M, Weitzel HK. Prediction of fetal distress and poor outcome in intrauterine-growth retardation—a comparison of fetal heart rate monitoring combined with stress tests and Doppler ultrasound. Fetal Diagn Ther 1993; 8(4): 234–40. [II-2 IUGR fetuses ($n=103$) were studied with NST/CST, VAS and Doppler. The passive tests – Doppler and NST – were better predictors of adverse outcome. The authors recommended abolishing the stress test]

107. Tan, KH. Smyth, R. Fetal vibroacoustic stimulation for facilitation of tests of fetal wellbeing. Cochrane Database of Systematic Reviews 1, 2007. [meta-analysis; 9 RCTs, $n=4,838$]

108. Caridi BJ, Bolnick JM, Fletcher BG, et al. Effect of halogen light stimulation on nonstress testing. Am J Obstet Gynecol 2004; 190(5): 1470–2. [RCT Fetal light perception shortens NST time]

109. Tan, KH. Sabapathy, A. Maternal glucose administration for facilitating tests of fetal wellbeing. Cochrane Database of Systematic Reviews 4, 2005. [meta-analysis; 2 RCTs, n=708]

110. Tan, KH. Sabapathy, A. Fetal manipulation for facilitating tests of fetal wellbeing. Cochrane Database of Systematic Reviews 4, 2005. [3 RCTs, n=1,100]

111. Grant A, Chalmers I. Randomized trial of fetal movement counting. Lancet 1982; 2(8296): 501. [RCT, n=68,000]

112. Neldam S. Fetal movements as an indicator of fetal well-being. Dan Med Bull 1983; 30: 274–8. [RCT, n=3,111]

113. Olesen AG, Avare JA. Decreased fetal movements: background, assessment, and clinical management. Acta Obstet Gynecol Scand 2004; 83(9): 818–26. [Review]

114. Mohide P, Grant A. Evaluating Diagnosis and Screening in Pregnancy and Childbirth. In Chalmers I, EnkinM, Keierse MJNC (eds). Effective Care in Pregnancy and Childbirth, Vol. 1. Oxford:Oxford University Press 66–80. [review]

115. Vintzileos A, Ananth CV, Smulian JC, Scorza WE, Knuppel RA. The impact of prenatal care on postnatal deaths in the presence and absence of antenatal high-risk conditions. Am J Obstet Gynecol 2002; 187(5): 1258–62. [II-2 Population-based study identified significantly increased risks of post-term, pre-eclamptic, IUGR and infectious complications in women with inadequate prenatal care]

116. Scholl TO, Hediger MO, Belsky DH. Prenatal care and maternal health during adolescent pregnancy: a review and meta-analysis. J Adolesc Health 1994; 15(6): 444–56. [Meta-analysis]

117. Knight M, Plugge E. The outcomes of pregnancy among imprisoned women: a systematic review. BJOG 2005; 112(11): 1467–74. [Meta-analysis, review]

118. Canella BL. Maternal–fetal attachment: an integrative review. J Adv Nurs 2005; 59(1): 60–8. [Meta-analysis]

119. Castles A, Adams EK, Melvin CL, Kelsch C, Boulton ML. Effects of smoking during pregnancy. Five meta-analyses. Am J Prev Med 1999; 16(3): 208–15. [Meta-analysis]

120. Neri M, Ugolini D, Bonassi S, Fucic A, Holland N, Knudsen LE, Sram RJ, Ceppi M, Bocchini V, Merlo DF. Children's exposure to environmental pollutants and biomarkers of genetic damage. II. Results of a comprehensive literature search and meta-analysis. Mutat Res 2006; 612(1): 14–39. [Meta-analysis]

121. Stanley FJ, Blair E. Why have we failed to reduce the frequency of cerebral palsy? Med J Aust 1991; 154(9): 623–6. [Meta-analysis]

52

Fetal lung maturity

Sarah Poggi

KEY POINTS

- Possible indications for assessment of fetal pulmonary maturity include a **high chance for spontaneous preterm birth** from preterm labor, PPROM, **or iatrogenic preterm delivery**, or the **need to plan delivery** in the presence of **unsure dates** or **obstetric complications affecting lung maturity.**
- The American College of Obstetricians and Gynecologists has recommended that **fetal pulmonary maturity should be confirmed before any *elective* delivery at less than 39 weeks of gestation.**
- The probability for RDS should be calculated as **a function of gestational age** and the specific fetal lung maturity test.
- **Lamellar body count** or **surfactant/albumin ratio** can be used as **the initial and only test** given their high negative predictive value, ease and low cost. **L/S ratio can be used** as a confirmatory test, if necessary.
- For diabetic pregnancies, positive PG, surfactant/albumin ratio ≥ 70 mg/g, L/S > 3, or a combination of these tests have a high predictive value for maturity.

HISTORIC NOTES

The lecithin/sphingomyelin (L/S) ratio for assessment of fetal pulmonary maturity was first introduced by Gluck and colleagues in 1971 and over 35 years later this test is still the standard to which others are compared.[1]

DEFINITIONS

Surfactant is a complex substance containing phospholipids and apoproteins produced by the Type II alveolar cells. It reduces surface tension throughout the lung, contributing to its compliance, leading to alveolar stability, and reducing the likelihood of alveolar collapse. Surfactant is 'packaged' in lamellar bodies.

Neonatal respiratory distress syndrome (RDS) occurs when the lungs fail to produce an adequate amount of surfactant. RDS is defined in many different ways, but in general involves mechanical ventilation and oxygen requirement at ≥ 24–48 hours of life, and radiographic chest findings (air bronchograms and reticulogranular appearance), without any other explanation for the respiratory insufficiency. The natural (without steroids) incidence depends on gestational age: about 80–90% at 25–27 weeks, 55–65% at 28–30 weeks, 30–40% at 31–33 weeks, 13% at 34 weeks, 6% at 35 weeks, 3% at 36 weeks, and 1% or less at ≥ 37 weeks. Therefore **the probability for RDS should be calculated as a function of gestational age.** RDS affects approximately 1% of all live births. Complications of its treatment are associated with an increased risk of serious acute and long-term pulmonary and nonpulmonary morbidities. Although the frequency and severity of RDS are worse for delivery remote from term, the pulmonary system is the last organ systems to mature, and RDS can occur even near term.

INDICATIONS FOR ASSESSMENT OF FETAL PULMONARY MATURITY

- High chance for **spontaneous preterm birth** from preterm labor, PPROM, **or iatrogenic preterm delivery.**
- **Need to plan delivery in the presence of unsure dates or obstetric complications affecting lung maturity.**

As the probability for RDS depends on gestational age, **accuracy of gestational age estimation is of outmost importance when assessing fetal maturity.** A first trimester ultrasound is associated with the most accurate estimation of gestational age (see Chapter 3 in *Obstetric Evidence Based Guidelines*). **The American College of Obstetricians and Gynecologists has recommended that fetal pulmonary maturity should be confirmed before any elective delivery** at less than 39 weeks of gestation.[2] For maternal HIV infection, prior uterine surgery with extensive myomectomy or vertical CD, placenta previa, and other selected indications, proof of lung maturity before 39 weeks might not be necessary. Tests for fetal lung maturity are not warranted before 33 weeks, because they are rarely positive this early in gestation.

TECHNIQUES FOR OBTAINING AMNIOTIC FLUID

Amniocentesis

Third trimester amniocentesis performed under ultrasonographic guidance in experienced hands is associated with low rates of failure or of bloody fluid collection, and a < 1% risk of complications, such as emergent delivery.[3]

Vaginal pool collection

The assessment of fetal pulmonary maturity can be obtained from vaginal pool specimens in the presence of premature rupture of membranes. Blood, meconium, and mucus can alter the results. In the absence of these contaminants, vaginally free-flowing collected fluid can be evaluate for determination of L/S ratio, surfactant/albumin ratio, PG, and LBC yielding results similar to those observed with samples obtained with amniocentesis (Table 52.1).

SPECIFIC TESTS FOR LUNG MATURITY (TABLE 52.1)

Lecithin/sphingomyelin ratio

The concentrations of these two substances are approximately equal until the mid-third trimester of gestation, when the concentration of pulmonary lecithin (phosphatidylcholine, most common of surfactant compounds) increases significantly while the nonpulmonary sphingomyelin concentration remains unchanged.

Technique

Following amniocentesis, the sample should be kept on ice or refrigerated if transport to a laboratory is required. Thin-layer chromatography after centrifugation to remove the cellular component and organic solvent extraction is used.

Interpretation of results

An L/S ratio of 2.0 or greater predicts absence of RDS in 98% of neonates. With a ratio of 1.5 to 1.9, approximately 50% of infants will develop RDS. Below 1.5, the risk of subsequent RDS increases to 73%.

Special considerations

Maternal serum has a L/S ratio ranging from 1.3 to 1.9; thus blood-tinged samples could falsely lower a mature result. The presence of meconium can interfere with test interpretation increasing the L/S ratio by 0.1–0.5, thus leading to an increase in falsely mature results.

Phosphatidylglycerol

Phosphatidylglycerol (PG) is a minor constituent of surfactant that becomes evident in amniotic fluid several weeks after the rise in lecithin.[4] Its presence indicates a more advanced state of fetal lung development and function, as PG enhances the spread of phospholipids on the alveoli.

Technique

The original PG testing was performed by thin-layer chromatography and required time and expertise. More recently enzymatic assay or slide agglutinations have been used successfully to determine the presence of PG. Amniostat-FLM (Irvine Scientific) is one such test.

Interpretation

The results are typically reported qualitatively as positive or negative, where positive represents > 3% of total phospholipids, and an exceedingly low risk of RDS.

Special considerations

PG determination is not generally affected by blood, meconium, or vaginal secretion.

Surfactant/albumin ratio

The fluorescence polarization assay uses polarized light to evaluate the competitive binding of a probe to both albumin and surfactant in amniotic fluid.[5]

Table 52.1 *Characteristics of fetal lung maturity tests*

Test	Technique	Threshold	Predictive value mature test (%)	Predictive value immature test (%)	Accurate with blood contamination	Accurate with meconium contamination	Accurate in vaginal pool	Difficulty	Cost
L/S ratio	Thin-layer chromatography	2/1	95–100	33–50	No	No	No	High	High
PG	Thin-layer chromatography	Present (usually means > 3% of total phospholipids)	95–10	23–53	Yes	Yes	Yes	High	High
	Slide agglutination	Positive (> 2%)							
Surfactant/ albumin ratio (TDx–FLM)	Fluorescence polarization	> 55 mg (of surfactant)/g (of albumin)	96–100	47–61	No	No	Yes	Low	Moderate
LB	Cell counter	30 000– 50 000/μL	97–98	29–35	No	Yes	Yes	Low	Low
FSI	Ethanol dilution	> 47	95	51	No	No	No	Moderate	Moderate

See text for abbreviations.

Technique

The TDx-FLM (Abbott) analyzer provides a quantitative and automated measurement of the amniotic fluid surfactant/albumin ratio. The test is simple, rapid, objective, reproducible, and can be performed with equipment commonly available in clinical laboratories.

Interpretation

A TDx FLM value above 55 has similar predictive ability of pulmonic maturity as positive PG test or L/S of 2 or greater.[6] As per other tests, **the probability for RDS should be calculated as a function of gestational age and the fetal lung maturity test results** (Table 52.2). In other words, other pre-test probabilities for maturity should be taken into account when interpreting these tests.[7]

Special considerations

A disadvantage of the TDx-FLM method is the large quantification scale. Values greater than 55 are regarded as mature, however, values of 35 to 55 are considered 'borderline'. As for L/S ratio, red blood cell phospholipids may falsely lower the TDx FLM result, but a mature test can reliably predict pulmonary maturity.

Lamellar body counts

Lamellar bodies (LB) are produced by type II pneumocytes and are a direct measurement of surfactant production because they represent its storage form.

Technique

Lamellar bodies are quantified with a commercial blood cell analyzer, which takes advantage of the similar size between lamellar bodies and platelets. The results can be obtained quickly, with a small fluid volume, and the test is less expensive than traditional phospholipid analysis. Although initial studies employed centrifugation, it is now agreed that the sample should be processed without spinning as centrifugation reduces the number of LB.

Interpretation

Values of 30 000 to 50 000/μL (least false positives) generally indicate pulmonary maturity.[8,9] Values of <15 000/μL are usually associated with immaturity. The test compares favorably with L/S and PG with a negative predictive value of a mature cutoff of 97.7% vs 96.8% and 94.7% respectively.[10] A meta-analysis calculated receiver-operating characteristic curves based upon data from six studies and showed the lamellar body count performed slightly better than the lecithin/sphingomyelin ratio in predicting RDS.[11]

Special considerations

Meconium has a marginal impact on LB counts, increasing the count by 5 000/mcL. Bloody fluid can initially slightly increase the count because the platelets are counted as LB. Afterwards the procoagulant activity of AF produces an entrapment of both, platelets and LB, causing a decrease of LB counts.

Foam stability index

The foam stability index (FSI) is a simple and rapid predictor of fetal lung maturity based upon the ability of surfactant to generate stable foam in the presence of ethanol.

Technique

After centrifugation ethanol is added to a sample of amniotic fluid to eliminate the contributions of protein, bile salts, and salts of free fatty acids. The mixture is shaken for 30 second and will demonstrate generation of a stable ring of foam if surfactant is present in the amniotic fluid. Amniotic fluid samples should not be collected in silicone tubes as the silicone will produce 'false foam'.

Interpretation

The FSI is calculated by utilizing serial dilutions of ethanol to quantitate the amount of surfactant present. RDS is very unlikely with an FSI value of 47 or higher. A positive result virtually excludes the risk of RDS; however a negative test often occurs in the presence of mature lung.

Special considerations

Contamination of the amniotic fluid specimen by blood or meconium interferes with the FSI results.

SINGLE TEST, MULTIPLE TESTS OR CASCADE

Faced with different assays for fetal lung maturity, some laboratories perform multiple tests simultaneously, leaving the clinician with the possibility of results discordant for pulmonary maturity from the same amniotic fluid specimen. In general, any 'mature' test result is indicative of fetal

Table 52.2   Probability of RDS on the basis of gestational age and S/A ratio (TDx–FLM)

	27[a]	28	29	30	31	32	33	34	35	36	37	38	39	40
0[b]	72%	66%	59%	51%	44%	37%	30%	24%	19%	15%	12%	9%	7%	5.1%
10	67%	60%	53%	46%	39%	32%	26%	20%	16%	12%	9.6%	7.3%	5.5%	4.2%
20	62%	55%	48%	40%	33%	27%	22%	17%	13%	10%	7.8%	6%	4.5%	3.4%
30	57%	50%	42%	35%	29%	23%	18%	14%	11%	8.4%	6.4%	4.8%	3.6%	2.7%
40	51%	44%	37%	30%	24%	19%	15%	12%	9%	6.8%	5.2%	4%	3%	2.2%
50	46%	39%	32%	26%	21%	16%	13%	10%	7.4%	5.6%	4.2%	3.2%	2.4%	1.8%
60	40%	34%	27%	22%	17%	13%	10%	8%	6%	4.5%	3.4%	2.5%	1.9%	1.4%
70	35%	29%	23%	18%	14%	11%	8.5%	6.4%	4.9%	3.7%	2.7%	2%	1.5%	1.1%
80	31%	25%	20%	15%	12%	9.1%	7%	5.2%	4%	3%	2.2%	1.7%	1.2%	0.9%
90	26%	21%	16%	13%	10%	7.4%	5.6%	4.2%	3.2%	2.4%	1.8%	1.3%	1%	0.7%
100	22%	17%	14%	10%	8%	6%	4.6%	3.4%	2.6%	2%	1.4%	1%	0.8%	0.6%
110	19%	14%	11%	9%	6.5%	4.9%	3.7%	2.8%	2.1%	1.5%	1.2%	0.9%	0.6%	0.5%
120	15%	12%	9%	7%	5.3%	4%	3%	2.2%	1.7%	1.2%	1%	0.7%	0.5%	0.4%
130	13%	9.8%	7.5%	6%	4.3%	3.2%	2.4%	1.8%	1.3%	1%	0.7%	0.6%	0.4%	0.3%
140	10%	8%	6.1%	4.6%	3.5%	2.6%	2%	1.4%	1.1%	0.8%	0.6%	0.5%	0.3%	0.25%
150	9%	6.6%	5%	3.7%	2.8%	2.1%	1.6%	1.2%	0.9%	0.6%	0.5%	0.4%	0.3%	0.2%
160	7%	5.3%	4%	3%	2.3%	1.7%	1.3%	1%	0.7%	0.5%	0.4%	0.3%	0.2%	0.2%
170	5.7%	4.3%	3.2%	2.4%	1.8%	1.4%	1%	0.8%	0.6%	0.4%	0.3%	0.2%	0.2%	0.1%
180	4.7%	3.5%	2.6%	2%	1.5%	1.1%	0.8%	0.6%	0.4%	0.3%	0.2%	0.2%	0.2%	0.1%
190	3.8%	2.8%	2.1%	1.6%	1.2%	0.9%	0.7%	0.5%	0.4%	0.3%	0.2%	0.1%	0.1%	0.1%
200	3%	2.3%	1.7%	1.3%	0.9%	0.7%	0.5%	0.4%	0.3%	0.2%	0.1%	0.1%	0.1%	0.1%

[a]Gestational age (weeks); [b]S/A (surfactant/albumin) ratio (TDx–FLM); RDS, respiratory distress syndrome.

pulmonic maturity given the high predictive value of any single test (5% or less of false mature rates). Conversely the use of a 'cascade' approach has been proposed to minimize the risk of delivery of an infant with immature lungs, while avoiding unnecessary delay in delivery and costs. According to this approach, a rapid and inexpensive test is performed first, with follow-up tests performed only in the face of immaturity of the initial test (e.g. **lamellar body count or surfactant/albumin ratio as the initial and only test, and L/S ratio as the confirmatory test, as necessary**).

CLINICAL CONDITIONS AFFECTING RISK OF RDS AND PREDICTIVE VALUE OF PULMONARY MATURITY TESTS

Several maternal/fetal clinical or nonclinical circumstances can affect the risk of RDS and modifies the predictive value of pulmonary maturity tests, including:

- African-American race: lung maturity is achieved at lower gestational ages and at lower L/S ratios (1.2 or greater) than in Caucasians.
- Female gender is associated with acceleration of lung maturation.
- Intrauterine growth restriction and preeclampsia are possibly associated with an acceleration of fetal lung maturity.
- **Maternal diabetes** and Rh-isoimmunization are associated with a delay in fetal lung maturation. Some authors have recommended the use of higher thresholds of L/S ratio (e.g. a cut-off ratio of 3) to establish pulmonic maturity in these conditions. Presence of a lamellar body count 50 000/mcL has similarly been recommended to indicate mature fetal lungs in diabetic women.[12] **Presence of PG** is commonly considered as gold standard for documentation of fetal lung maturity with diabetes or Rh-isoimmunization. For diabetes, also a TDx FLM value of ≥ 70 mg/g, or a L/S ≥ 3, or the combination of the two, have been associated with >95% predictive value for a mature test.

- In twin gestations it is commonly recommended that the sac of the male twin or the larger twin be sampled at amniocentesis. The reasoning is that if the sampled twin has mature pulmonic results, the co-twin is even more likely to be mature.

REFERENCES

1. Gluck L, Kulovich MV, Boerer RC Jr, et al. Diagnosis of the respiratory distress syndrome by amniocentesis. Am J Obstet Gynecol 1971; 109: 440. [II-2]
2. American College of Obstetricians and Gynecologists. Assessment of Fetal Lung Maturity. ACOG Educational Bulletin #230. Washington, D.C. ACOG, 1996. [review]
3. Stark CM, Smith RS, Lagrandeur RM, Batton DG, Lorenz RP. Need for urgent delivery after third-trimester amniocentesis. Obstet Gynecol 2000; 95: 48–50. [II-3]
4. Hallman M, Kulovich M, Kirkpatrick E, et al. Phosphatidylinositol and phosphatidylglycerol in amniotic fluid: indices of lung maturity. Am J Obstet Gynecol 1976; 125: 613. [II-2]
5. Russell JC, Cooper CM, Ketchum CH, et al. Multicenter evaluation of TDx test for assessing fetal lung maturity. Clin Chem 1989; 35: 1005. [II-2]
6. Standards of Laboratory Practice: Guidelines for the Evaluation and Management of the Newborn. Nat Acad Clin Biochem, 1998. [II-2]
7. Pinette MG, Blackstone J, Wax JR, Cartin A. Fetal lung maturity indices-a plea for gestational age-specific interpretation: a case report and discussion. Am J Obstet Gynecol 2002; 187: 1721–2. [II-3]
8. Dubin, SB. The laboratory assessment of fetal lung maturity. Am J Clin Pathol 1992; 97: 836. [II-2]
9. Ghidini A, Poggi SH, Spong CY, Goodwin KM, Vink J, Pezzullo JC. Role of lamellar body count for the prediction of neonatal respiratory distress syndrome in non-diabetic pregnant women. Arch Gynecol Obstet 2005; 271: 325–8. [II-2]
10. Neerhof MG, Haney EI, Silver RK, Ashwood ER, Lee I, Piazze JJ. Lamellar body counts compared with traditional phospholipid analysis as an assay for evaluating fetal lung maturity. Obstet Gynecol 2001; 97: 305–9. [II-2]
11. Wijnberger LD, Huisjes AJ, Voorbij HA, Franx A, Bruinse HW, Moll BV. The accuracy of lamellar body count and lecithin/sphingomyelin ratio in the prediction of neonatal respiratory distress syndrome: A meta-analysis. Br J Obstet Gynaecol 2001; 108: 585–8. [II-2]
12. Ghidini A, Spong CY, Goodwin K, Pezzullo JC. Optimal thresholds of lecithin/sphingomyelin ratio and lamellar body count for the prediction of the presence of phosphatidylglycerol in diabetic women. J Maternal Fetal Neonatal Med 2002; 12: 95–8. [II-2]

Index

Note: Diagrams and tables are indicated by *italic* page numbers. There is an *Abbreviations list* on *pages xv to xvii*. The method of indicating *Levels of evidence* is explained on *page xxi*.

abacavir *229*
abdominal decompression 290
abdominal trauma 183–91
    focused abdominal sonography
        for trauma (FAST) 188
abruptio placentae 278
acupressure bands 75
acute chest syndrome, sickle cell disease 93
acute fatty liver, multiple gestations 278
acyclovir, herpes 313
adefovir dipivoxil, hepatitis B 218
adenomas, micro and macroadenomas,
    preconception counseling 70–1
agranulocytosis 65
AIDS *see* HIV infection/AIDS
albuterol, asthma *161*
alloimmune thrombocytopenia
    (NAIT) 337–43
alloimmunization,
    sickle cell disease 93
alpha fetoprotein 288
alternative therapy, smoking 142
amitryptyline 151
amniocentesis
    for fetal lung maturity 384
    non-immune hydrops fetalis 350
    OD$_{450}$ 330–3
    for polyhydramnios 358
amniotic fluid index (AFI) 352–4, *353*
amniotic fluid volume (AFV)
    amnioreduction 281
    antepartum testing 283
    fetal monitoring 283, *365–6, 366*
    measurement 352–4
    multiple gestations 353
    qPCR, CMV infection *299*
    SDP vs AFI estimates 354
    singleton pregnancies 352–3
    ultrasound 352–3
        oligohydramnios in
            singleton pregnancies 353
        pregnancy outcome prediction 354
        single deepest pocket (SDP) 352–4
    vaginal pool collection 384
amoxapine, depression 151

ampicillin, bacterial endocarditis
    prophylaxis 26
anemia, chronic hemolytic,
    sickle cell disease 92
anemia, fetal 375
    bilirubin levels 95
    middle cerebral artery PSV 308, 330
    ultrasound 330
anemia, maternal 86–90
    algorithm, work-up *88*, 89
    complications 87
    etiology/pathophysiology 87
    genetics 86–7
        alpha and beta thalassemia types *86–7*
        hemoglobins *86*, 87
    management 89–90
    prevention 89–90
    risk factors 87
    sickle cell disease 93
    therapy 90
anesthesia
    cardiac disease 25–6
    HELLP 18
    hypertensive disorders 15–16
angiotensin-converting enzyme (ACE)
    inhibitors, contraindications
    in pregnancy 6
antepartum testing *see* fetal monitoring
anthrax (inactivated bacteria), vaccine 266
antibiotics
    chlamydia 242, *243*
    group B streptococcus, intrapartum
        antibiotic prophylaxis
        259, 260–1, *260, 261*
    penicillin allergy 250, *250*
    pneumonia 167–8
antibody testing, antiphospholipid syndrome
    (APS) 175–6
anticardiolipin antibodies 175, 180
anticholinergics, asthma *161*
anticoagulation 197–202, *197*
    acute venous thromboembolism 199
    prevention 199–201
    aspirin 199
    at delivery 201–2

breastfeeding 202
heparin 177, 197–9, *198*
    low molecular weight
        heparin (LMWH) 198
    unfractionated heparin (UFH) 197–8
mechanical heart valves, maternal 27
prophylactic vs therapeutic 209
warfarin 199
anti-D immunoglobulin, prophylaxis 328–9
antidepressants 144, 148–52
    tricyclics 151
    see also specific agents
antiepileptic drugs (AEDs) 114, *115*
    pharmacokinetic profile *115*
antihypertensive drugs 5–7
    prevention of pre-eclampsia 15
    see also specific agents
antinuclear antibodies 179
antioxidants, prevention
    of pre-eclampsia 12
antiphospholipid antibodies 207
antiphospholipid syndrome (APS) 175–8
    anesthesia 178
    antepartum testing 178
    antibodies (APAs) 175–6
    clinical criteria 175
    complications 176
    diagnosis 175–6
    laboratory criteria 175–6
    management 176–8, *198*
        aspirin 177
        prophylactic anticoagulation 177, *198*
        therapeutic anticoagulation 177, *198*
        unfractionated heparin 177, *198*
    postpartum breastfeeding 178
    pregnancy loss 177
    screening 177
    symptoms 176
    venous thromboembolism (VTE) 177
antiplatelet agents, prevention
    of pre-eclampsia 15
antiplatelet IgG 337
antiretroviral therapy 226–7, *227–8*
anti-SSA/Ro, anti-SSB/La 180
antithrombin III deficiency 207, *210*

antiviral drugs 217–18
  herpes 313
aortic graft, post liver transplantation 83
aortic insufficiency, maternal 27
aortic stenosis, maternal 27
L-arginine, post-partum,
      hypertensive disorders 20
aspirin
  antiphospholipid syndrome 177
  prevention of fetal growth
      restriction 288, 290
  prevention of pre-eclampsia 10–11
  safety in pregnancy 10
assisted reproductive
      technologies (ART) 273–4
asthma 155–65
  classification 156
  complications 156
  diagnosis 155–6
  environmental control measures *158*
  management 157–65
    anesthesia 165
    delivery 165
    exacerbations *163–4*
    intubation criteria 165, *165*
    medications *157–8*, 159, *160–4*
    postpartum/breastfeeding 165
    prevention 157, *158*
    specific management and medications
      157–8, 159–65, *160–2*
  National Asthma Education and Prevention
      Program (NAEPP) *157–8*, *160–4*
  peak expiratory flow rate
      (PEFR) 156–8, *157*, 163–5
  pulmonary function work-up 158
autonomic dysreflexia (ADR) 124–5
  differentiating ADR from
      pre-eclampsia *125*
autonomy of patient 101–2
azathioprine
  side effects 84, 108
  systemic lupus erythematosus (SLE) 181

bacterial endocarditis, prophylaxis 26
BCG (bacille Calmette–Guérin)
      vaccine 170–1, *267*
beclomethasone, asthma *160*
bed rest 290
beta-blockers
  antihypertensives 6
  hyperthyroidism 65
  mitral stenosis, maternal 27
beta$_2$ agonists, asthma *160*, *161*, 162
bile acids, intrahepatic cholestasis 78–80
Biophysical Profile Scoring
      (BPS) 365, *365–7*, 368, 372–5, *372–4*
  and cerebral palsy 361–2, *362*
birth, increase of cardiac output 24
bitolterol, asthma *161*
blood groups
  hemolytic disease of fetus/neonate,
      CDE system antigens 335
  MNS system 335
blood pressure
  maternal measurement 3, 5
  pre-eclampsia 8

blood transfusion
  Jehovah's Witness pregnancies 101–2
  maternal anemia in sickle
      cell disease 91, 93
'blueberry muffin baby'
      (CMV infection) 297–301
breast cancer 128–30
  chemotherapy 129–30
  delay in diagnosis 128
  diagnostic tests and safety 128
  sentinel node biopsy 129
  staging 12
  surgery 129
  termination of pregnancy 129
  treatment 129–30
breastfeeding, and
  adenomas 71–2
  anticoagulation 202
  cyclosporine 85, 108
  diabetes mellitus 50, 54
  hepatitis C 220–1
  HIV infection/AIDS 232
  hypertensive disorders 7
  post liver transplantation 85
  smoking 142
bromocriptine, adenoma 69
budesonide, asthma *160*
buproprion 151

cabergoline, adenoma 69
calcium, prevention of pre-eclampsia 11–12
calcium channel blockers 6, 290
cancer *see* chemotherapy; *specific cancers*
carbon monoxide, smoking 138
cardiac disease, maternal 23–30
  anesthesia 25–6
  complications 24–5
  epidemiology/incidence 23
  etiology/basic pathophysiology 23–4
  genetics 23
  labor in lateral decubitus 25
  management 25–9
  management of specific diseases 26–9
  New York Heart Association classification *24*
  preconception counseling 25
  prenatal care/antepartum testing 25
  risk factors 24, *25*
  symptoms/signs 23
cardiac output, at parturition 24
cardiomyopathies 28
cardiotocography (CTG) 291, 363–7, *364*, *365*
  fetal monitoring 291, 363–7, *364*
cardiovascular disorders, non-immune
      hydrops fetalis 346, *349*
CDE system antigens, hemolytic disease of
      fetus/neonate 335
cerclage 280
cerebral palsy, Biophysical Profile Scoring
      (BPS) 361–2, *362*
cervical cancer 133
cervicitis/urethritis 240
cesarean delivery, elective
  fetal macrosomia 295
  severe PUPPP 34
cesarean delivery, prior method, and fetal
      macrosomia 295

chemotherapy
  breast cancer 129–30
  complications during pregnancy 134
  fetal surveillance and
      timing of delivery 134–5
  long-term follow up 128
  maternal surveillance 134
  neonatal evaluation after
      chemotherapy during pregnancy 135
chickenpox (varicella zoster) 231, 315–19
chlamydia 239–44
  cervicitis/urethritis 240
  chlamydial conjunctivitis 240
  classification 240
  complications/risks 241
  diagnosis 241–2, *242*
  epidemiology/incidence 239–40, *240*
  etiology/basic pathophysiology 240
  lymphogranuloma
      venereum (LGV) 240
  management 241–3
  maternal genital infections 240
  prevention 241
  proctitis/proctocolitis 240
  screening 241
  symptoms 240
  transmission 240–1
  treatment 242–3, *243*
cholestasis of pregnancy 78–80
chorio-amnionicity 275, *275–7*
chromosomal abnormalities
  amniocentesis 350
  non-immune hydrops fetalis 346, *349*
chronic hemolytic anemia,
      sickle cell disease 92
chronic hypertension 3–7
  classification 4
  complications, maternal and fetal 4
  diagnosis/definition/history 4
  epidemiology/incidence 4
  etiology/basic pathophysiology 4
  management 4–7
    antihypertensive drugs 5–7
    laboratory and other tests 4–5
    physical examination 4
    prenatal care 5
    screening/diagnosis 5
  preconception counseling 5
  prevention 5
  risk factors/associations 4
citalopram, depression 150
clomipramine 151
clonidine, contraindications,
      smoking cessation 141
coagulation cascade 193, *193*
coarctation of the aorta, maternal 27
congenital heart block (CHB), systemic lupus
      erythematosus (SLE) 181–2
congenital (inherited) thrombophilia 206–7
congestive heart failure, maternal 27
conjunctivitis, chlamydial 240
consent, Jehovah's Witness pregnancies *102*
contraction stress test 375
cordocentesis, and other
      invasive procedures 350
coronary artery disease 28

corticosteroids
  HELLP syndrome 17–18
  pre-eclampsia 14
  systemic lupus erythematosus
    (SLE) 181
  see also steroids
counseling see specific subjects
cranberry juice 109
creatinine clearance 5
  calculation 4
  renal disease 104
cromolyn, asthma 160, 162
cutaneous melanoma 38–40, 39
cyanide, smoking 138
cyclosporine
  contraindications to
    breastfeeding 85, 108
  drug interactions 109
  side effects 84, 108
cytomegalovirus infection 297–301
  after liver transplantation 83
  CMV-specific hyperimmune
    globulin 300
  complications 298–9
  HSV 313
  epidemiology 297
  infant viremia 298
  management 299–301
  qPCR of amniotic fluid 299
  recurrent infection 298
  risk factors 297–8
  screening 299–300
  ultrasound fetal findings 300
  vaccine 299

D-dimer testing 195
deep vein thrombosis (DVT) 193–6, 195
delivery
  mode 292
    see also cesarean delivery; labor; preterm
    birth; timing of delivery
depression 144–54
  complications 146
  diagnosis/definitions 145
  Edinburgh Postnatal Depression Scale
    (EPDS) 146–7
  etiology/basic pathophysiology 145
  historic notes 145
  major depressive disorder
    (MDD) 144–52, 146–7
  management 146–8
  prevention 147
    trials on interventions 148
  resources 152
  risk factors/associations 145
  screening 146, 147
  therapy 148–52
    antidepressants 144, 148–52
    electroconvulsive therapy 152
    hormonal therapy 152
    support/psychotherapy 148, 149
dermatoses 31–42, 31
diabetes mellitus, gestational 50–4
  fetal macrosomia 295
  multiple gestations 278
  one and two step testing 50–1, 51

prenatal care 52–4, 52
  diet and exercise 52–3
  glucose monitoring and
    management 53–4
  insulin 53
  oral hypoglycemic agents 53
  post partum /breastfeeding 54
  risk factors 50, 51, 52
  screening/diagnosis 50–4
diabetes mellitus, pregestational 43–50
  after liver transplantation 83
  antepartum testing 48–9, 49
  complications 44–5
  diabetic ketoacidosis 48, 49
  diet 47, 47
  future therapeutic approaches 50
  glucose monitoring 47, 47
  insulin 47, 48
  intrapartum glucose management 49–50, 50
  management 45–50, 46
  postpartum/breastfeeding 50
  preconception counseling 45–6, 47
diabetic ketoacidosis 48, 49
diabetic vasculopathy 373
dialysis, counseling 106–7
diazepam, vs magnesium, eclampsia 19
didanosine 229
dilated cardiomyopathy 28
diphtheria vaccine 264
diuretics 6
dopamine antagonists, prolactinoma 69, 70
Doppler surveillance 291, 369–72, 369
  abnormal test results 371–2
  abnormal uterine, Doppler prevention
    of pre-eclampsia 10–11
  in FGR 291
  multivessel assessment 368–9, 369–71
  vs BPS 372
Doppler waveform, middle cerebral
  artery PSV 308, 330, 331–3, 368, 369
doxylamine 75
dysplastic nevus syndrome 39

eclampsia 9, 19–20
Edinburgh Postnatal Depression
  Scale (EPDS) 146–7
Eisenmenger's syndrome/pulmonary
  hypertension, maternal 26
electroconvulsive therapy 152
emtricitabine 229
encephalitis, toxoplasmic 231
end-diastolic flow in umbilical artery
  absent (AEDF) 290, 292
  reversed (REDF) 291, 292
enteric nutrition, nasogastric tube 76
epinephrine, asthma 161
estriol levels 291
ethambutol, TB 173
ethical issues, autonomy of patient 101–2

Factor V Leiden (FVL) 206–7, 206, 210
Fallot's tetralogy, maternal 27
famciclovir, herpes 313
fetal blood sampling (FBS)
  cumulative effect 337
  indications 341–2

and platelet transfusion 340–1
risk of hemorrhage 340
fetal breathing movements 365–7
fetal death 320–6
  associations/risk factors/etiologies 320–1, 322
  counseling 321
  definition 320–6, 321
  delivery/anesthesia 323–4
    expectant management 323
    induction 323–4
    postpartum 324–5
  prevention of recurrence and
    future management 324–5
  sickle cell disease 92
  smoking 138
  work-up 321–3, 322
fetal echocardiography 350
fetal growth restriction 286–93
  antepartum testing and follow-up 290–2
    changes in testing
      parameters 291, 291
  classification 288
  counseling
    for future 293
    preconception 289
    prognosis 289
  definitions 286–7
  delivery 292
    mode 292
    preparation, steroids for fetal
      lung maturity 292
    timing 292
  diagnosis 289
  discordant twins 281
  fetal intervention 289–90
  management 288–93, 374
  neonatology management 292
  oxygen therapy 290
  post liver transplantation 84
  prevention 288
    aspirin 288, 290
  risk factors/associations 287, 288
  screening 288–9
  sickle cell disease 93
  smoking 138, 290
  teratology/etiology/basic
    pathophysiology 287–8
  testing interval 291
  ultrasound and Doppler
    ultrasound 290–1
  work-up 289
fetal heart rate 65, 291–2, 363–5, 364
  assessment 65, 363–5
  non-reassuring (NRFHR) 291, 292
fetal lung maturity 383–8
  amniocentesis 384
  amniotic fluid collection 384
  assessment 283
  definitions 383
  fetal pulmonary maturity 383–4
  foam stability index 386
  historic notes 383
  lamellar body counts 386
  lecithin/sphingomyelin ratio 384
  neonatal respiratory distress syndrome
    (RDS) 383–8

phosphatidylglycerol 384
    specific tests 384–6, *385*
    steroids 351
    surfactant/albumin ratio 334, 384–6, *387*
    testing methods 386–8
    vaginal pool collection 384
fetal macrosomia 294–6
    complications 294
    definition 294
    diabetes 295, 373
    management 294–5
    prevention 294–5
    prior cesarean delivery 295
    prior shoulder dystocia 295
    risk factors 294
fetal monitoring 360–82
    abnormal test results 365, 367,
        368, 371–2, 372
    amniotic fluid volume 283, 366, *366*
    ancillary testing methods 375–6
    antenatal steroid administration 375
    antenatal testing 376–7, *377*
    Biophysical Profile Scoring (BPS) 365,
        365–7, 368, 372–5, *372–4*
        and cerebral palsy 361–2, *362*
    cardiotocography (CTG) 291,
        363–7, *364, 365*
    condition-specific testing 373–5
    diabetic fetal macrosomia 373
    diabetic vasculopathy 373
    Doppler surveillance 291, 369–72, *369*
    fetal anemia 375
    fetal body movements 366
    fetal breathing movements 365–7
    fetal heart rate (FHR) testing
        65, 292, 363–5, *364*
    fetal movement counting 376
    fetal tone 366
    Growth Restriction Intervention Trial
        (GRIT) 361, *361*
    hemolytic disease of fetus/neonate 334
    intervals 291
    movement counting 376
    multiple gestations 283
    non-immune hydrops fetalis 351
    non-reassuring fetal heart rate
        (NRFHR) 65, 291, 292
    non-stress tests (NST) 291, 363–5
        see also fetal heart rate
    oxygen 362–3
    perinatal injury 362
    prenatal care 378
    preterm premature ruptured
        membranes (PPROM) 375
    small normal fetus near term 374–5
    suggested surveillance program 377
    testing parameters, progressive
        change in FGR *291*
    timing of delivery 292
        and chemotherapy 134–5
    ultrasound 290
fetal pulmonary maturity 383–8
fetal vibroacoustic stimulation 376
flunisolide, asthma *160*
fluoxetine 150
fluticasone, asthma *160*, 162

fluvoxamine 150
foam stability index 386
focused abdominal sonography
        for trauma (FAST) 188
folate supplements
    maternal seizures 116
    prevention of maternal anemia 89–90
folinic acid, toxoplasmosis 305
formoterol, asthma *160*, 162
furosemide, post-partum, hypertensive
        disorders 20

ganciclovir
    CMV infection 300–1
    cytomegalovirus (CMV) 300–1
gastrointestinal anomalies, non-immune
        hydrops fetalis 346
genetic syndromes, non-immune hydrops
        fetalis 346, *349*
genital infections
    maternal 240
    see also specific subjects
genitourinary anomalies, non-immune
        hydrops fetalis 346
gentamicin, bacterial endocarditis
        prophylaxis 26
gestational diabetes *see* diabetes
        mellitus, gestational
gestational hypertension 7
gestational trophoblastic disease 64
ginger (for N/V) 75
Glanzmann disease 100
glucose monitoring and
        management 49–50, 53–4
    criteria for standard glucose load *51*
    intrapartum 49–50, *50*
goiter 57
gonorrhea 234–8
    complications 235
    concomitant infections 237
    diagnosis 235–6, *236*
    epidemiology/incidence 234
    etiology 234
    management 235–7
    pathophysiology/transmission 234–5
    prevention 235
    screening 235, *236*
    symptoms 235
    treatment 236, *237*
Graves' disease
    antepartum testing 65–6
    defined 63
    diagnosis 64
    management 64–6
    neonatal 66
group B streptococcus *see* streptococcal
        infections, GBS
Growth Restriction Intervention
        Trial (GRIT) 361, *361*

hemodialysis 107
Hashimoto's thyroiditis 57
headache 118–22
    background/epidemiology 118
    diagnosis 119, *119*
    epidemiology/basic pathophysiology 119–20

evaluation in pregnancy 120
    International Headache Society *119*
    primary (benign) causes 119
    prophylaxis in pregnancy 122
    secondary (ominous) causes 119
    therapy 120–1, *121*
        algorithm *121*
heart valves, mechanical, maternal 27–8
helical CT scan 196
HELLP syndrome 9, 17–19
    anesthesia 18
    delivery 18–19
    recurrence 20
    signs and symptoms 17, *17*
    specific therapy 17–18
hematological disorders,
        non-immune hydrops fetalis 347
hemoglobins
    hemoglobin E, sickle cell disease 96
    maternal anemia 86, *87*
    types 86, *87*
Hemolysis, Elevated Liver enzymes and Low
        Platelet count (HELLP) syndrome 9, 17–19
hemolytic disease of fetus/neonate 327–36, 334
    amniocentesis, OD_{450} 330–3
    anti-D immunoglobulin, prophylaxis 328–9
    counseling 329–30
    delivery/anesthesia *331–2*, 334
    epidemiology/incidence 327–8
    etiology/basic pathophysiology 328
    evidence for dosing and timing 329
    fetal intervention 333–4
    fetal monitoring/testing 334
    Kell alloimmunization 334–5
    MNS system 335
    natural history 328
    neonatology management 334
    other atypical antibodies 334–5
    patient with previously affected fetus *332*
    prevention (anti-D immunoglobulin) 328–9
    red blood cell (RBC) alloimmunization 327,
        328, 329–34
    special clinical situations 329
    work-up/investigations
        required 330–3, *331–3*
heparin 177, 197–9, *198*
    low molecular weight heparin (LMWH) 198
    mechanical heart valves, maternal 27
    prophylactic vs therapeutic 209
    unfractionated heparin (UFH) 197–8
heparinoids, danaparoid sodium 198
hepatitis A 213–14
    vaccine 265
hepatitis B 215–18
    classification 216, *216*
    conditions 217
    diagnosis/definition 215, *216*
    drugs 217–18
    epidemiology/incidence 215
    etiology/basic pathophysiology 215
    exposure to HB in pregnancy 217
    HB vaccine 217
    HBIg 217
    maternal chronic hepatitis B 217
    prenatal care 217
    prevention/preconception counseling 217

recombinant vaccine *265*
risk factors/associations 216
hepatitis C 219–22
  diagnosis/definition 219
  epidemiology/incidence 219–20
  management 221–2
  mother-to-infant transmission 220–1
  preconception/pregnancy counseling 221
  risk factors/associations 220, *220*
  screening 221
hepatitis D virus 218
herpes 310–14
  antiviral drugs 313
  classification/pathophysiology 311
  CMV infection 313
  complications 311–12
  delivery mode 314
  first episode HSV 313
  gestationis 34
  history 313
  incidence/epidemiology 310
  maternal–fetal transmission 311
  postpartum/neonate 314
  pregnancy management 312–14
  prevention 312
  reactivation (recurrent) genital herpes 311
  screening 312–13, *312*
  therapy 313
  work-up/diagnosis 313
HIV infection/AIDS 223–33
  antiretroviral therapy 226–7, *227–8*
  breastfeeding 232
  classification 224, *225*
  complications 224
  delivery 230–1
  diagnosis 223
    infants 232
  epidemiology 223–4, *224*
  follow-up of infants 232
  historic notes 223
  immunizations 228–30
  intrapartum care 231–2
  maternal postpartum care 232
  monitor for side effects 227–8
  non-nucleoside reverse transcriptase
    inhibitor–nevirapine 228
  nucleoside analog drugs 227, *229–30*
  nucleoside reverse transcriptase
    inhibitor–AZT 227
  preconception counseling 225
  prenatal care 225–6
  preterm premature rupture
    of membranes 230
  prophylaxis for opportunistic
    infections 228, *231*
  protease inhibitors 227
  risk factors 224
  screening 225
Hodgkin's disease 130–1
  diagnostic tests and safety 130
  effects on pregnancy 130
  staging 130
  surgery 130
  termination of pregnancy 130
  treatment, chemotherapy and
    radiotherapy 130–1

homocysteinemia 207
hormonal therapy, depression 152
human chorionic gonadotropin, suppression
  of TSH 58
human platelet antigens (HPA series) *338*
hydralazine 15
hydramnios
  see polyhydramnios
hydration, maternal 356
hydronephrosis 110
hydrops
  middle cerebral artery PSV 308, 330
  non-immune 344–51
  parvovirus-induced 309
  see also non-immune hydrops fetalis
hydroxychloroquinine sulfate,
  systemic lupus erythematosus (SLE) 181
hydroxyurea 94
hypercoagulability 24
hyperemesis gravidarum 64, 73–7
hyperglycemia, gestational diabetes 50–4
hyperhomocysteinemia 206, 207, *210*, 211
hypertensive disorders 3–22
  after liver transplantation 83
  anesthesia 15–16
  antepartum testing 7
  antihypertensive drugs 5–7
  chronic hypertension 3–7
  complication of renal disease 105, 106
  complications, maternal and fetal 4
  delivery 7
  epidemiology/incidence 4
  etiology/basic pathophysiology 4
  gestational hypertension 7
  post-partum/breastfeeding 7
  pre-eclampsia 7–19
  preconception counseling 5
  prevention of hypertension 5
  risk factors/associations 4
  severe pre-eclampsia 7–8, 13, 16–17
  therapy 5
hyperthyroidism 63–7
  defined 63
  neonatal 66
  subclinical 63
hypertrophic cardiomyopathy 28
hypoglycemic agents 47–8, 53
hypothyroidism 56–62
  complications 57
  congenital hypothyroidism 60
  definitions 56
  fetal 65
  management 57–9
    antepartum and postpartum 60
  pathophysiology 57
  physiology 57–9
    fetal 58
    placental *57*, 58–9
  postpartum thyroiditis 60–1
  pregnancy considerations 57–9
  screening/diagnosis 59
    primary vs secondary
      hypothyroidism *59*
  subclinical hypothyroidism 60
  thyroid nodule 60
  treatment 59

IgG antibody levels
  anticardiolipin antibodies 175
  antiplatelet antibodies 337
  CMV infection 299–300
  IgG thrombocytopenia 197–8
  parvovirus 308
  toxoplasmosis 304
IgG-negative patients,
  CMV infection 297
IgM antibody levels
  anticardiolipin antibodies 175
  CMV infection 299–300
  toxoplasmosis 304
iliac vein thrombosis 194–5
imaging see specific techniques
imipramine 151
immune-mediated IgG
  thrombocytopenia 197–8
immunoglobulin, intravenous 340, 343
immunosuppressive agents
  renal transplantation *108*
  side effects 84, *84*, 108
impetigo herpetiformis 36–8, *37*
indirect Coombs' test 329
induction of labor
  fetal death 323–4
  in fetal macrosomia 295
infections, see also specific infections
infections, intrauterine/congenital
  cytomegalovirus 297–301
  toxoplasmosis 302–5
infections, maternal
  cytomegalovirus 297–300
  toxoplasmosis 302–5
infections, perinatal *298*
inferior vena caval filters 199
infertility 105
influenza (inactivated) vaccine *264*
inherited thrombophilia 205–12
  see also thrombophilia
insulin
  diabetes, prenatal care 53
  pregestational diabetes 47, *48*
    requirements *48*
  types/pharmacokinetics *48*
insulin resistance, gestational diabetes 51–4
interferon alpha-immunomodulator 217
  hepatitis B 217
intracranial hemorrhage, in-utero 340–3 *341*
intrahepatic cholestasis 78–80
intrauterine growth restriction
  management *374*
  post liver transplantation 84
  see also fetal growth restriction
intrauterine transfusion 340–3
intravascular volume increase 24
intravenous immunoglobulin 340, 343
iodine
  deficiency 59
  radioiodine, contraindications 65
  supplements 59
ipratropium bromide, asthma *161–2*
iron supplements, prevention of
  maternal anemia 89–90
isocarboxazid 152
isoniazid, TB 171, *173*

Japanese encephalitis (inactivated virus)
vaccine *266*
Jarisch–Hexheimer reaction 250–1
Jehovah's Witness pregnancies 101–2
complications 101
diagnosis/definition 101
historic notes 101
management 101–2
prenatal care 101–2

Kell alloimmunization 334–5
ketoacidosis 48, *49*
Kleihauer–Betke (KB) test 188–9, 327–329

L-arginine, post-partum,
hypertensive disorders 20
labetalol 6, 15, 65
labor
induction
fetal death 323–4
in fetal macrosomia 295
issues in liver transplantation 85
in lateral decubitus, cardiac disease 25
preparation for
GBS infection 258
spinal cord injury 125
preterm birth 280–1
preterm complications, renal
disease 105, 106
see also delivery
Lactobacillus GG 109
lamellar body counts 386
lamivudine *229*
lamivudine–nucleoside analog 218
hepatitis B 218
large fetus *see* fetal macrosomia
laser therapy, striae gravidarum 31–3
lecithin/sphingomyelin ratio 384
leukemia (acute and chronic) 131–2
leukotriene receptor antagonists,
asthma *160*, 162, 163–5
levalbuterol, asthma *161*
Levels of evidence, using,
explanation *xxi*
levothyroxine 59
ligase chain reaction 241
liver transplantation 81–5
antepartum testing 85
breastfeeding 85
comorbidities/risk factors 82–3
etiology of original disease 82–3
rejection 83
historic notes 81
immunosuppressive agents and their side
effects 84, *84*
labor and delivery issues 85
orthotopic liver transplantation
(OLTx) 81–4
preconception counseling 82
pregnancy complications 83–4
blood chemistry tests and
liver function 84
intrauterine growth restriction 84
preterm birth and low birth weight 84
timing of pregnancy 82
work-up 84–5

low birth weight
complication of renal disease 105
liver transplantation 84
and smoking 138
genetic factors 137
see also fetal growth restriction
lupus, historic notes 175
lupus anticoagulant
antiphospholipid syndrome, algorithm *176*
SLE 180
lupus nephritis 104
lymphogranuloma venereum (LGV) 240
lytic cocktail, vs magnesium, eclampsia 19

macroadenomas 68–72
macrosomia 294–6
complications 294
epidemiology 294
management 49, 294–6
risk factors 294
magnesium
eclampsia
vs diazepam 19
vs lytic cocktail 19
vs phenytoin 19
pre-eclampsia, renal disease 106
prevention of pre-eclampsia, and eclampsia
9, 12, 14–15, *15*, 19
route of administration 14
major depressive disorder
(MDD) 144–52, *146–7*
mammography 128
maprotiline, depression 151
Marfan syndrome, maternal 28
maternal hydration 356
maternal serum alpha fetoprotein
(MSAFP) 288
maternal–fetal transmission of
infection *see* vertical transmission
MDI, asthma *161–2*
measles, MMR vaccine *267*
mechanical heart valves, maternal 27–8
melanoma 132
cutaneous 38–40, *39*
metastasis to placenta 132
meningococcal (polysaccharide) vaccine *265*
metabolic diseases, non-immune
hydrops fetalis 347
metastasis, melanoma, to placenta 132
methimazole 65
methyldopa 5–6
methylxanthines, asthma *160*, 162
metoclopramide 75
metronidazole 254–5
microadenomas 68–72
preconception counseling 70–1
middle cerebral artery PSV
Doppler waveform 308, 330, *331–3*, 368, *369*
fetal anemia/hydrops 308, 330, *331–3*
mifepristone, fetal death 324
mirtazapine 152
misoprostol 324
mitral stenosis, maternal 27
MMR (live viral) vaccine *267*
moclobemide, contraindications,
smoking cessation 141

moles, cutaneous melanoma 38–40, *39*
monoamine oxidase inhiitors,
depression 152
montelukast, asthma *160*, 162
MTHFR/homocysteinemia 207
multiple gestations 273–85, 279–84
acardiac twin 279, 282
actual/natural incidence 273, *274*
amniotic fluid assessment 283, 353
antepartum testing 283
assisted reproductive
technologies (ART) 273–4
complications 276–9
conjoined twins 279, 282
definition 273
delivery 283–4
delayed interval delivery 284
fetal lung maturity assessment 283
route/timing 283–4
determination of chorio-amnionicity
275, *275–7*
diagnosis 275
etiology 274
fetal complications 276–8
higher rates of chromosomal and
congenital anomalies 276–7
immaturity 277
intrapartum complications 277
intrauterine growth restriction and
discordant growth 277
perinatal mortality 278
perinatal neurological damage 277
preterm birth 277, *277*
single fatal demise 277
spontaneous reduction and loss 276
fetal growth restriction/discordant
twins 281, 283
maternal complications 278
monoamniotic twins 282
monochorionic gestation
complications 278–9
monoamniotic twins 279
non-immune hydrops fetalis 347
neonatal 284
nutrition 279
pregnancy reduction 280
prenatal diagnosis 279
preterm birth 279–81
prevention and management of
complications 280–2
selective fetocide 282
anomalous fetus 280
single fetal death 281
twin–twin transfusion syndrome
(TTTS) 278–9, *278*, 281–2
ultrasound 283
zygote division, timing, and
types of twins *274*
mumps, MMR (measles-mumps-rubella)
vaccine *267*
Mycobacterium avium complex,
disseminated 231
Mycobacterium tuberculosis infection 168, 231
mycophenolate mofetil,
side effects 84, 108
myocardial infarction 28

narcotics, sickle cell disease 94
nasogastric tube, enteric nutrition 76
nausea/vomiting and hyperemesis
    gravidarum 64, 73–7, 74–7
    complications 74
    diagnosis/definition 73
    etiology 73
    risk factors/associations 74
nefazodone 152
Neisseria gonorhoeae 234
neonatal alloimmune thrombocytopenia
    (NAIT) 337–43
    classification of HPA series 338, *338*
    diagnosis 339
    early fetal blood sampling (FBS) 343
    etiology/basic pathophysiology 337–8
    fetal monitoring/testing *341–2*, 343
    future pregnancy preconceptional
        counseling 343
    intrauterine transfusion 340–3
        previous sibling with in-utero intracranial
            hemorrhage (ICH) 341–3, *341*
        previous sibling without in-utero
            intracranial hemorrhage
            (ICH) 340–1, *341*
    intravenous immunoglobulin 340, 343
    investigations and consultations 339–40
    management 339–43
    natural history/complications 338
    prevention 339
    testing 339
    therapy, general issues 343
neonatal withdrawal syndrome
    paroxetine 150
    SSRIs 150
neonates
    algorithm
        GBS streptococcal infection *262*
        management, maternal intrapartum
            antibiotic prophylaxis *262*
    alloimmune thrombocytopenia
        (NAIT) 337–43
    complications post maternal trauma 184–5
    complications of trauma 184–5
    evaluation after chemotherapy
        during pregnancy 135
    GBS streptococcal infection 258–9, *262*
    Graves' disease 66
    hemolytic disease 334
    herpes 314
    HSV infection 314
    hyperthyroidism 66
    lupus 182
    management
        fetal growth restriction 292
        FGR 292
    multiple gestations 284
    non-immune hydrops fetalis 351
    parvovirus infection 309
    respiratory distress syndrome (RDS) 383–8
    syphilis 251
    varicella zoster virus infection
        (chickenpox) 318
nephrolithiasis 110–11
neural tube defects 279
nicotine 138

nicotine replacement therapy (NRT) 140, *141*
nifedipine
    hypertensive disorders 6, 15
    post-partum 20
nitroimidazoles 254–5
non-Hodgkin's lymphoma 131
non-immune hydrops fetalis 344–51
    amniocentesis 350
    anatomy ultrasound 348–50
    associated conditions *349–50*
    associations/possible etiologies/differential
        diagnosis 346–7
    cardiovascular disorders 346, *349*
    chromosomal abnormalities 346, *349*
    congenital infections 346–7
    cordocentesis and other
        invasive procedures 350
    counseling/prognosis 347
    diagnosis/definition 344, *345*
    etiology/basic pathophysiology 344, *345*
    extracardiac anomalies 346
    fetal echocardiography 350
    fetal monitoring/testing 351
    gastrointestinal anomalies 346
    genitourinary anomalies 346
    hematological disorders 347, *349*
    maternal complications 347
    metabolic diseases 347
    monochorionic twin pregnancies 347
    neonatology management 351
    postpartum 351
    skeletal dysplasias 346
    thoracic anomalies 346
    treatment 351
    work-up diagnosis 347–51, *348*
non-nucleoside reverse transcriptase
    inhibitor–nevirapine 228
non-stress tests (NST) *see* fetal heart rate
norethisterone enanthate, and postpartum
    depression 147
nortriptyline
    contraindications, smoking cessation 141
    depression 151
NSAIDS (non-steroidal anti-inflammatory
    drugs) 181
nuchal translucency 279
nucleic acid amplification test (NAAT) 241, *242*
nucleoside analog drugs 227, *229–30*
nucleoside reverse transcriptase inhibitor
    (NRTI) 227

odansetron 75
oligohydramnios 278, 354–7
    amnioinfusion 356–7
    management 355–7, *356*
    maternal hydration 356
    singleton pregnancies 353
opioids, contraindications,
    smoking cessation 141
opportunistic infections, prophylaxis 228, *231*
oral hypoglycemic agents 47–8, 53
osteopenia 198
oxygen availability, perinatal injury 362–3
oxygen therapy, fetal growth restriction 290
oxytocin, fetal death 324
oxytocin challenge test 375

palpitations, maternal 26
paroxetine
    in depression 150
    neonatal withdrawal syndrome 150
parvovirus 306–9
    complications 307–8, *307*
    management 308–9, *308*
    maternal–fetal transmission 307, *307*
    neonate 309
    non-immune hydrops fetalis 346, *349*, 351
    pathophysiology 306–7, *307*
    ultrasound fetal findings 308
pelvic muscle training,
    urinary incontinence 111
penicillin 249–50
    allergy 250, *250*
penicillin allergy 250, *250*
peniclovir, herpes 313
perinatal injury, oxygen availability 362–3
peripartum cardiomyopathy 28
phenelzine 152
phenytoin, vs magnesium, eclampsia 19
phosphatidylglycerol, fetal lung maturity 384
pituitary adenomas 68–72
placenta
    metastases, melanoma 132
    thyroid physiology *57*, 58–9
placenta previa, smoking 138
placental abruption, smoking 138
plasma volume expansion
    prevention of FGR 290
    prevention of pre-eclampsia 15
platelet disease 337–8
platelets
    antiplatelet antibodies 337
    human platelet antigens (HPA series) *338*
    normal adhesion at vascular injury site *98*
    transfusion, fetal blood sampling (FBS) 340–1
pneumococcal (polysaccharide) vaccine *265*
Pneumocystis jiroveci pneumonia 231
pneumonia 165–8
    classification 166
    complications 166
    diagnosis 166
    management 166–8
    risk factors 166
    treatment 167–8
polio
    inactivated polio vaccine (IPV) *265*
    oral polio vaccine (OPV) *266*
polyarteritis nodosa 104
polyhydramnios 278, 357–8
    amniocentesis 358
    labor precautions 358
    management 358
    ultrasound 357–8
    work-up and differential diagnosis 357–8
polymerase chain reaction (PCR)
    chlamydia 241
    qPCR of amniotic fluid, CMV infection *299*
post-partum, hypertensive disorders 7, 20
potassium iodide, SSKI 66
pre-eclampsia 7–19
    after liver transplantation 84
    complication of renal disease *104*, 105
    complications 10, 16–20

HELLP 9, 17–19, *17*
  management 17, *18*
  severe pre-eclampsia 13, 16–17
  superimposed pre-eclampsia 16
counseling 14
delivery 15–16
  anesthesia 15–16
diagnoses/definitions 8–9
eclampsia 9, 19–20
epidemiology/incidence 9
etiology/basic pathophysiology 9
management 10–16, *11–13*, 17, *18*
mild 8–9
multiple gestations 278
physical examination 14
prevention 10–16
  antepartum testing 15
  antihypertensive therapy 15
  antioxidant therapy 12
  antiplatelet agents 15
  aspirin 10–11
  calcium 11–12
  corticosteroids 14
  magnesium 12, 14–15, *15*
  plasma volume expansion 15
proteinuria 8–9
renal disease 106
risk factors/associations 10
severe pre-eclampsia 7–8, 9, 13, *13*, 16–17
smoking and 138
superimposed pre-eclampsia 9
symptoms 9
preconception counseling
  see specific subjects
prednisone, side effects 84, 108
pregestational diabetes 43–50
pregnancy
  after liver transplantation 81–5
  general risk factors, contact with children 299
pregnancy loss
  antiphospholipid syndrome 177
  multiple gestations 276
  sickle cell disease 92
  and thrombophilia 211
premature rupture of membranes (PROM) 375
  HIV infection 230
  smoking 138
preterm birth
  complication of renal disease 105
  labor 280–1
  liver transplantation 84
  multiple gestations 280–1
  secondary to early-onset fetal growth
    restriction, other signs of placental
    insufficiency or severe pre-eclampsia 177
  smoking 138
  threatened, GBS streptococcal infection 261
preterm premature rupture of membranes 375
  HIV infection/AIDS 230
prochlorperazine 75
proctitis/proctocolitis 240
prolactinoma 68–72
  complications 68–9
  management 69–72
    dopamine antagonists 69, *70*
    work-up 69, *70*

preconception counseling 69–71
  micro and macroadenomas 70–1
  pregnancy considerations 69
promethazine 75
propranolol 65
  headache prophylaxis in pregnancy 122
propylthiouracil 65
prostaglandins, fetal death 324
protease inhibitors 227
protein C, protein S deficiency 207, *210*
proteinuria
  complication of renal disease 105
  pre-eclampsia 8–9
prothrombin G20210A deficiency 207, *210*
protriptyline, depression 151
prurigo of pregnancy 35–6, *36*
pruritic folliculitis 34–5, *34*
pruritic urticarial papules and plaques
  of pregnancy (PUPPP) 33–4, *33*
pruritus, intrahepatic cholestasis 78–80
Pseudomonas infection 167
ptyalism 74
pulmonary angiography 197
pulmonary artery catheter, indications 26
pulmonary edema 27
pulmonary embolism (PE) 196–7, *196*
pulmonary hypertension, maternal 26
purified protein derivative (PPD) test *169*
pyrazinamide, TB *173*
pyrimethamine, toxoplasmosis 305

rabies vaccine *265*
radiation 189–90, *189–90*
radioiodine, contraindications 65
radiotherapy, Hodgkin's disease 130–1
red blood cell (RBC) alloimmunization,
  hemolytic disease 327, *328*, 329–34
renal disease 103–12
  classification of renal insufficiency *104*
  complications 104–5, *104*
    hypertension 105
    low birth weight 105
    perinatal mortality *104*, 105
    pre-eclampsia *104*, 105
    preterm labor 105
    proteinuria 105
  diagnosis/definitions 103
  dialysis 106–7
  historic notes 103
  management 105–7
    asymptomatic bacteriuria 106
    hypertension 106
    pre-eclampsia 106
    prenatal care 105
    preterm labor 106
    therapy 106
  physiologic renal
    changes in pregnancy 103–4
  postpartum urinary retention 111
  pregnancy, special considerations 106–11
  prenatal care 107–8
    drug interactions with cyclosporin *109*
    immunosuppressive agents *108*
    renal graft rejection 108
    resources, USA National Transplant
      Pregnancy Registry 108

pyelonephritis 109
renal transplantation 107–8
risk factors/preconception counseling 104
urinary nephrolithiasis 110–11
urinary tract infections 108–10
renal insufficiency
  classification *104*
  rate of complications *104*
renal transplantation 107–8
  immunosuppressive agents *108*
  preconception counseling 107–8
respiratory disease 155–74
  physiology in pregnancy 155
respiratory distress syndrome (RDS) 383–8
  probabilities of RDS (GA and S/A ratio) *387*
  risk and predictive value of pulmonary
    maturity tests 388
Rh(D) antibody titers 329–30
rifampin, TB *173*
rubella, MMR (measles-mumps-rubella)
  vaccine *267*

S-adenosyl-L-methionine (SAMe) 79
Sabin–Feldman dye test,
  toxoplasmosis-specific antibodies 304
salmeterol *160*, 162
salt intake, and prevention of pre-eclampsia
  12–13
scleroderma 104
seat belts 185
seizures 113–17
  antiepileptic drugs (AEDs) *114*, *115*
  complications 114
    fetal 114
    maternal 114
  delivery 117
  diagnoses/definitions 113
  effect of pregnancy on disease 115
  history 113–14
  postpartum/breastfeeding 117
  preconception counseling 115–16
  prenatal counseling 116
  therapy 116–17
sentinel node biopsy/mapping,
  Tc-99m sulfur colloid 129, 132
septostomy 282
sertraline, depression 147, 150
sexually transmitted diseases,
  prevention 235, 241
shingles, varicella zoster
  virus infection 318
shock wave lithotripsy 111
shoulder dystocia, prior labor, and
  fetal macrosomia 294
sickle cell disease 91–6, *93–5*
  acute chest syndrome 95
  alloimmunization 95
  anemia 94–5
  complications 92–3
    acute anemia 93
    antepartum admissions 93
    fetal growth restriction 93
    painful crisis 93, 94
    postpartum complications 93
    pre-eclampsia 93
    pregnancy loss 92

preterm birth 93
small for gestational age (SGA) 93
urinary tract infections 93
definition 91
epidemiology/incidence 91
genetics/inheritance 91–2
HbSC disease 96
hemoglobin E 96
maternal mortality 93
pathophysiology 92
sickle beta-thalassemia disease 96
sickle cell trait 95
symptoms 92
sickle cell trait 95
single deepest pocket (SDP), ultrasound of
amniotic fluid 352–4
skeletal dysplasias, non-immune
hydrops fetalis 346
small for gestational age *see* fetal growth
restriction
smallpox (live vaccine virus) vaccine *267*
smoking 137–43, *139–40*
5 'As' and 5 'Rs' *139*
alternative treatments 142
assessment for intervention *139*
basic pathophysiology 137–8
breastfeeding 142
complications 138–9
maternal lifetime complications 139
pregnancy complications 138–9
diagnosis/definition 137
epidemiology/incidence 137
fetal growth restriction 138, 290
genetics 137
management 139
nicotine replacement therapy
(NRT) 140, *141*
other pharmacotherapies 141
postpartum 142
practical counseling/prevention
139–40, *140*, 142
results of cessation in pregnancy 139
risk factors 138
sodium nitroprusside 15
spinal cord injury 123–6
anesthesia 126
autonomic dysreflexia (ADR) 124–5
delivery 125–6, *126*
diagnosis/definition 123
injury during pregnancy 124
National Spinal Cord Injury Association
(NSCIA) 126
postpartum/breastfeeding 126
preconception counseling 123–4
preparation for (preterm or term) labor 125
spiramycin, toxoplasmosis 305
SSRIs
contraindications, smoking cessation 141
neonatal withdrawal syndrome 150
stavudine *229*
steroids
administration 375
asthma 159–62, 165
fetal lung maturity 292
nausea/vomiting 75
see also corticosteroids

streptococcal infections, GBS 256–63
complications 257–8, *257*
diagnosis/definition 256–63
early vs late onset 257
epidemiology/incidence 256, *257*
management 258–62
collection of screening specimen 259–60
delivery *259*, 261
intrapartum antibiotic
prophylaxis *259*, 260–1, *260*
neonatal management algorithm *262*
neonatal screening and
treatment only 258–9
no prenatal maternal screening,
intrapartum treatment 258
prenatal maternal screening, and
intrapartum treatment 258, *259*
screening/diagnosis 259–60, *259*
threatened preterm delivery 261
vaccination, maternal 258
streptomycin, TB *173*
striae gravidarum 31–3
sulfadiazine, toxoplasmosis 305
surfactant 383
surfactant/albumin ratio 334, 384–6, *387*
syphilis 245–52
complications 248
definition 245–52
diagnosis 249
incidence/epidemiology 245
late benign (tertiary) 247
latent syphilis 246–7
management 248–51
neonatal 251
neurosyphilis 247–8
pathophysiology and transmission 245–6
prevention 248
primary/secondary syphilis 246
risk factors 248
screening *248*, 249
symptoms and classification 246–8
treatment 249–51, *250*
follow-up 251
Jarisch–Hexheimer reaction 250–1
penicillin allergy 250, *250*
systemic lupus erythematosus (SLE) 179–82
antepartum testing 181
azathioprine 181
complications 180
congenital heart block (CHB) 181–2
corticosteroids 181
diagnosis 179
American College of Rheumatology
(ARA) criteria 179
differential diagnosis 180
epidemiology/incidence 179–80
historic notes 179
hydroxychloroquinine sulfate 181
management 180–1
neonatal lupus 182
NSAIDS (non-steroidal
anti-inflammatory drugs) 181
prenatal care 181

tacrolimus 107
side effects 84, 108

Tc-99m sulfur colloid
breast cancer 129
sentinel node mapping 129, 132
tenofovir *229*
terbutaline, asthma *161*
tetanus/diphtheria (Td) (toxoids)
vaccine *264*, *267*
tetralogy of Fallot, maternal 27
thalassemia
genetics *86–7*
sickle beta-thalassemia disease 96
theophylline, asthma *160*, 162
thioacetazone, TB *173*
thionamides 65
thoracic anomalies, non-immune
hydrops fetalis 346
thrombocytopenia
gestational 338
multiple gestations 278
see also neonatal alloimmune
thrombocytopenia (NAIT)
thrombolytic agents 199
thrombophilia
acquired 207
antithrombin III 207
complications 207–9
adverse pregnancy outcome 208–9, *208*
venous thromboembolism 208, *208*
definition 206
diagnosis 210–11, *210*
epidemiology/incidence 206, *206*
Factor V Leiden (FVL) 206–7, *206*
fetal thrombophilias 209
genetics/classification 206–7
historic notes 205–6
management *198*, 209–11
MTHFR/homocysteinemia 207
protein C 207
protein S 207
prothrombin G20210A 207
screening 209–10
current VTE 209–10
family with thrombophilia 210
multiple risk factors for VTE 210
prior adverse pregnancy outcome 210
prior VTE and recurring/non-recurring
etiology 209
therapy 211
hyperhomocysteinemia 211
pregnancy loss
10 weeks onwards 211
recurrent pregnancy loss 211
thrombophilia, inherited 205–12
thyroid
physiology
changes in pregnancy *57*
transplacental passage *57*, 58–9
thyroid cancer 134
thyroid nodule 60
thyroid storm 66–7
defined 63
thyroid surgery 60
thyroid-stimulating hormone,
changes in pregnancy *58*
thyroid-stimulating immunoglobulin,
changes in pregnancy *57*

thyrotoxicosis, defined 63
thyrotropin-releasing hormone,
    changes in pregnancy *57*
thyroxine replacement, treatment for
    hypothyroidism 59
thyroxine-binding globulin,
    changes in pregnancy *57*
timing of delivery
    chemotherapy 134–5
    fetal monitoring 292
    and GA 292
    multiple gestations 283
tinidazole 254–5
tocodynamometer monitoring (Toco) 188
tocolytics 280
toxoplasmosis 302–5
    complications 303
    epidemiology 302
    management in pregnancy 303–5
    natural history 303
    pathophysiology 302
    prevention *304*
    screening 304
    toxoplasmic encephalitis 231
trauma 183–91
    blunt abdominal 188, *189*
        focused abdominal
            sonography (FAST) 188
    complications 184–5
        fetal/neonatal complications 184–5
        maternal 184
        special considerations, assault 185
    definition 183
    etiology/basic pathophysiology 184, *184*
    evaluation and diagnostic studies 188–90
    history and physical examination 188
    Kleihauer–Betke (KB) test 188–9
    prevention/preconception counseling 185
    radiation dosage 189–90, *189–90*
    seat belts 185
    stabilization 185–7, *187*
    tocodynamometer monitoring (Toco) 188
    work-up 185–90, *186–7*
trazodone 152
Treponema pallidum, syphilis 245
tretinoin, striae gravidarum 31–3
triamcinolone acetonide *160*
trichomoniasis 253–5
    diagnosis 254, *254*
    etiology/basic pathophysiology 253
    management 254–5
tricyclic antidepressants 151
trimethobenzamide 75
tuberculosis 168–73
    diagnosis 168
    epidemiology/incidence 168–9
    etiology/basic pathophysiology 169
    management 169–73
    purified protein derivative (PPD) test *169*, 170
    risk factors/associations 169
    screening 169–70
        algorithm *171*
    therapy 171–3
        active infection 172, *172–3*
        control issues 171–3
        latent infection 171–2
        WHO recommendations *172*

tuberculin skin testing 169–70, *170*
    work-up 170
T$_{DAP}$ (toxoid/Acellular) vaccine *267*
twin–twin transfusion
    syndrome 278–9, *278*, 281–2
twinning *see* multiple gestations
typhoid vaccines *266*

ultrasound
    compressive 194–5
    fetal anemia 330
    fetal growth restriction 290–1
    multiple gestations 283
    see also Doppler ultrasound
umbilical artery, AEDF, RDEF 290, 291, 292
umbilical artery Doppler 361,
    369–71, *370–1*, 376
urethritis, chlamydia 240
urinary incontinence,
    pelvic muscle training 111
urinary nephrolithiasis 110–11
urinary retention, postpartum 111
urinary tract infections 108–10
    complications 108–9
    diagnosis 109
    prevention 109
    screening 108
    treatment 109
ursodeoxycholic acid (UDCA) 79
urticaria (PUPPP) 33–4, *33*

vaccination 264–9
    contraindications 268
    in HIV infection/AIDS 228
    preconception 264–6
    in pregnancy 266–9
    streptococcal infection
        (GBS) maternal 258
vaccines
    cytomegalovirus (CMV) 299
    hepatitis B 217
    inactivated or killed vaccines, toxoids,
        immune globulins, antisera 268
    live attenuated vaccines 266–8
    not recommended in pregnancy *267*
        BCG (bacille Calmette–Guérin) *267*
        MMR (measles-mumps-rubella) (live
            viral) *267*
        smallpox (live vaccine virus) *267*
        T$_{DAP}$ (toxoid/Acellular) *267*
        varicella (live virus) *267*
    recommended for all pregnant women *264*
        influenza (inactivated) *264*
        tetanus/diphtheria (Td) (toxoids) *264*
    recommended for pregnant women at risk
        for exposure 265–6
        anthrax (inactivated bacteria) *266*
        hepatitis A (inactivated) *265*
        hepatitis B (recombinant) *265*
        Japanese encephalitis
            (inactivated virus) *266*
        meningococcal (polysaccharide) *265*
        pneumococcal (polysaccharide) *265*
        polio: inactivated polio vaccine (IPV) *265*
        polio: oral polio vaccine (OPV) *266*
        rabies *265*
        typhoid *266*

        inactivated whole cell vaccine *266*
        injectable Vi (polysaccharide) *266*
        oral TY2 (live attenuated) *266*
        yellow fever (live virus) *266*
vaginal birth after cesarean
    delivery (VBAC), fetal macrosomia 295
valacyclovir, herpes 313
varicella zoster virus infection
    (chickenpox) 231, 315–19
    clinical neonatal findings of CMV 318
    complications 316
    counseling 317, *317*
    maternal shingles 318
    maternal–fetal transmission 316
    pathophysiology 316, *316*
    prevention 317
    risk factors/associations 315
    therapy 318
    vaccine *267*, 318
    work-up/diagnosis 317–18
vascular injury, platelet adhesion *98*
vasculopathy, diabetic 373
vaso-occlusive episodes, acute,
    in sickle cell disease 92
vasopressin (DDAVP), von
    Willebrand disease 97, 99
venlafaxine 152
venography 195
venous thromboembolism 192–7
    antiphospholipid syndrome (APS) 177
    deep vein thrombosis
        (DVT) 194–6, *195*
    definition 193
    diagnosis 194–7, *194*
    embolectomy 199
    etiology/basic pathophysiology 193
    and inherited thrombophilia 208, *208*
    pulmonary embolism (PE) 196–7, *196*
    risk factors/association 193–4, *194*
ventilation–perfusion scan 196
ventricular septal defects 24
    maternal 26
vertical transmission
    chlamydia 240–1
    CMV infection 298, 300
    gonorrhea 234–5
    hepatitis B 82, 217
    hepatitis C 82, 217, 220–1
    herpes 311
    parvovirus 307, *307*
    toxoplasmosis 303
vibroacoustic stimulation 376
vitamin antioxidants, prevention
    of pre-eclampsia 12
von Willebrand disease 97–100
    diagnosis/definition 97
    etiology/basic pathophysiology 97

warfarin, mechanical heart valves 27

yellow fever (live virus) vaccine *266*

zafirlukast, asthma *160*, 162
zalcitabine *230*
zidovudine (AZT) 227, *229*
zygote division, timing,
    and types of twins *274*

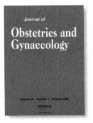
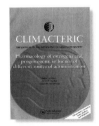
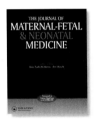
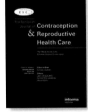
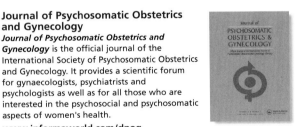
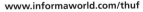
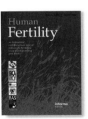
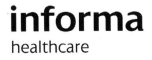